(10)

MD

NUTRIENT ADDITIONS TO FOOD

Nutritional, Technological and Regulatory Aspects

PUBLICATIONS IN FOOD SCIENCE AND NUTRITION

Journals

JOURNAL OF MUSCLE FOODS, N.G. Marriott and G.J. Flick, Jr.
JOURNAL OF SENSORY STUDIES, M.C. Gacula, Jr.
JOURNAL OF FOOD SERVICE SYSTEMS, O.P. Snyder, Jr.
JOURNAL OF FOOD BIOCHEMISTRY, J.R. Whitaker, N.F. Haard and H. Swaisgood
JOURNAL OF FOOD PROCESS ENGINEERING, D.R. Heldman and R.P. Singh
JOURNAL OF FOOD PROCESSING AND PRESERVATION, D.B. Lund
JOURNAL OF FOOD QUALITY, R.L. Shewfelt
JOURNAL OF FOOD SAFETY, T.J. Montville and A.J. Miller
JOURNAL OF TEXTURE STUDIES, M.C. Bourne and P. Sherman

Books

NUTRIENT ADDITIONS TO FOOD, J.C. Bauernfeind and P.A. Lachance
NITRITE-CURED MEAT, R.G. Cassens
THE POTENTIAL FOR NUTRITIONAL MODULATION OF THE AGING PROCESSES, D.K. Ingram et al.
CONTROLLED/MODIFIED ATMOSPHERE/VACUUM PACKAGING OF FOODS, A.L. Brody
NUTRITIONAL STATUS ASSESSMENT OF THE INDIVIDUAL, G.E. Livingston
QUALITY ASSURANCE OF FOODS, J.E. Stauffer
THE SCIENCE OF MEAT AND MEAT PRODUCTS, 3RD ED., J.F. Price and B.S. Schweigert
HANDBOOK OF FOOD COLORANT PATENTS, F.J. Francis
ROLE OF CHEMISTRY IN THE QUALITY OF PROCESSED FOODS, O.R. Fennema, W.H. Chang and C.Y. Lii
NEW DIRECTIONS FOR PRODUCT TESTING AND SENSORY ANALYSIS OF FOODS, H.R. Moskowitz
PRODUCT TESTING AND SENSORY EVALUATION OF FOODS, H.R. Moskowitz
ENVIRONMENTAL ASPECTS OF CANCER: ROLE OF MACRO AND MICRO COMPONENTS OF FOODS, E.L. Wynder et al.
FOOD PRODUCT DEVELOPMENT IN IMPLEMENTING DIETARY GUIDELINES, G.E. Livingston, R.J. Moshy, and C.M. Chang
SHELF-LIFE DATING OF FOODS, T.P. Labuza
RECENT ADVANCES IN OBESITY RESEARCH, VOL. V, E. Berry et al.
RECENT ADVANCES IN OBESITY RESEARCH, VOL. IV, J. Hirsch et al.
RECENT ADVANCES IN OBESITY RESEARCH, VOL. III, P. Bjorntorp et al.
RECENT ADVANCES IN OBESITY RESEARCH, VOL. II, G.A. Bray
RECENT ADVANCES IN OBESITY RESEARCH, VOL. I, A.N. Howard
ANTINUTRIENTS AND NATURAL TOXICANTS IN FOOD, R.L. Ory
UTILIZATION OF PROTEIN RESOURCES, D.W. Stanley et al.
VITAMIN B_6: METABOLISM AND ROLE IN GROWTH, G.P. Tryfiates
FOOD POISONING AND FOOD HYGIENE, 4TH ED., B.C. Hobbs et al.
POSTHARVEST BIOLOGY AND BIOTECHNOLOGY, H.O. Hultin and M. Milner

Newsletters

MICROWAVES AND FOOD, R.V. Decareau
FOOD INDUSTRY REPORT, G.C. Melson
FOOD, NUTRITION AND HEALTH, P.A. Lachance and M.C. Fisher
FOOD PACKAGING AND LABELING, S. Sacharow

NUTRIENT ADDITIONS TO FOOD

Nutritional, Technological and Regulatory Aspects

Edited by

J. Christopher Bauernfeind, Ph.D.
FORMERLY DIRECTOR, FOOD AND AGRICULTURAL PRODUCT
DEVELOPMENT; NUTRITION RESEARCH COORDINATOR
HOFFMANN-LA ROCHE
NUTLEY, NEW JERSEY

and

Paul A. Lachance, Ph.D., FACN
DIRECTOR, GRADUATE PROGRAM
DEPARTMENT OF FOOD SCIENCE, RUTGERS UNIVERSITY
NEW BRUNSWICK, NEW JERSEY

**FOOD & NUTRITION PRESS, INC.
TRUMBULL, CONNECTICUT 06611 USA**

Copyright © 1991 by
FOOD & NUTRITION PRESS, INC.
Trumbull, Connecticut 06611 USA

All rights reserved. No part of this publication may be reproduced, stored in a retrieval system or transmitted in any form or by any means: electronic, electrostatic, magnetic tape, mechanical, photocopying, recording or otherwise, without permission in writing from the publisher.

Every attempt was made by the authors and editors to obtain all necessary permissions for use of previously published material. If there has been any omission of source credits or specific wording of permissions, such omission is sincerely regretted, and all deficiencies will be corrected in future printings.

Library of Congress Catalog Card Number: 91-70657
ISBN: 0-917678-29-X

Printed in the United States of America

CONTRIBUTORS

BAILEY, LYNN B., Ph.D., Food Science and Human Nutrition Dept., University of Florida, Gainesville.

BAUERNFEIND, J. CHRISTOPHER, Ph.D., Formerly Director Food and Agricultural Product Development; Nutrition Research Coordinator, Hoffmann-La Roche, Nutley, New Jersey.

DU BOIS, IRINA, Soms-Directeur, Service Alimentaires, Nestec Ltd., Vevey, Switzerland.

BRIN, MYRON, Ph.D., Research Fellow, The Charles A. Dana Research Institute for Scientists Emeriti, Drew University, Madison, New Jersey; formerly Director, Vitamin and Clinical Nutrition, Hoffmann- La Roche, Nutley, New Jersey.

BUSHNELL, JOHN J., Regulatory Affairs and Data Management, Mead Johnson Nutritional Group, Evansville, Indiana.

CHRISTAKIS, GEORGE J., M.D., M.P.H., Department of Epidemiology and Public Health, University of Miami School of Medicine, Boca Raton, Florida.

CLYDESDALE, FERGUS M., Ph.D., Department of Food Science, University of Massachusetts, Amherst.

DeRITTER, ELMER, Formerly, Analytical Services; Food and Agricultural Product Development, Hoffmann-La Roche, Nutley, New Jersey.

EITENMILLER, RONALD R., Ph.D., Department of Food Science and Technology, University of Georgia, Athens.

GREGORY, III, JESSE F., Ph.D., Department of Food Science and Human Nutrition, University of Florida, Gainesville.

HAGEN, RICHARD E., Ph.D., Environmental Affairs, Mead Johnson Nutritional Group, Evansville, Indiana.

IANNARONE, ANTHONY J., LL.M., Associate Vice President, Associate General Counsel, Hoffmann-La Roche, Nutley, New Jersey.

JOHNSON, LEONARD E., Ph.D., Vitamins and Fine Chemical Division, Hoffmann-La Roche, Nutley, New Jersey.

LACHANCE, PAUL A., Ph.D., FACN, Director, Graduate Program, Department of Food Science, Rutgers University, New Brunswick, New Jersey.

LUND, DARYL B., Ph.D., Department of Food Science; New Jersey Agricultural Experiment Station, Rutgers University, New Brunswick, New Jersey.

MERGENS, WILLIAM J., Ph.D., Vitamins and Fine Chemical Division, Hoffmann-La Roche, Nutley, New Jersey.

MOLINA, MARIO R., Ph.D., Instituto de Nutricion de Centro America y Panama, Guatemala, Centro America.

PHILLIPS, R. DIXON, Ph.D., Department of Food Science and Technology, University of Georgia, Griffin.

RANHOTRA, GUR S., Ph.D., Nutrition Research, American Institute of Baking, Manhattan, Kansas.

ROE, DAPHNE A., M.D., Division of Nutritional Sciences, Cornell University, Ithaca, New York.

SEBRELL, W. HENRY, M.D., FACP, FAPHA, Emeritus Professor of Nutrition, Columbia University, College of Physicians and Surgeons; formerly, Assistant Surgeon General USPHS and Director, National Institutes of Health.

THOMAS, M. RITA, Ph.D., R.D., Research Department, Mead Johnson Nutritional Group, Evansville, Indiana.

VETTER, JAMES L., Ph.D., Vice President, Technical, American Institute of Baking, Manhattan, Kansas.

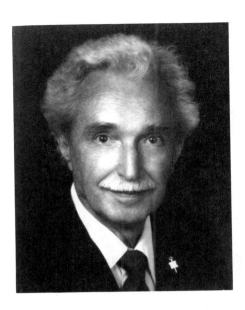

J. CHRISTOPHER BAUERNFEIND, Ph.D.

Born in Rip Van Winkle's Catskill Mountains of New York, 1914, Dr. Bauernfeind attended the North Branch one-room grade school and Callicoon High School. He then entered Cornell University for his B.S. degree in Agriculture and Chemistry and M.S. and Ph.D. degrees in Nutrition, Biochemistry, and Physiology. After a four-year nutrition-teaching assistantship at Cornell he joined Hiram Walker & Sons in Illinois as Research Biochemist and Nutritionist to investigate the nutritive value of fermentation products. In 1943 he moved to the New Jersey Research Center of Hoffmann-La Roche Inc. in the progressive positions of Chief of Applied Nutrition, Director of Food and Agricultural Product Development, Technical Director of Animal Nutrition, Director of Agricultural Research, Director of Agrochemistry and Nutrition Research Coordinator until retirement in 1979. Dr. Bauernfeind has published over 150 scientific papers, patents, reviews and edited 3 books involving nutrient delivery systems, feeding of animals, use of vitamins, antioxidants, carotenoids and drugs in human and agricultural applications, animal health, veterinary medicine, food technology and food preservation projects. He was a recipient of several awards and member of various chemical, food science and nutrition organizations including the American Institute of Nutrition, the American Society for Clinical Nutrition, the Institute of Food Technologists (Fellow) and the American Chemical Society (50-year member).

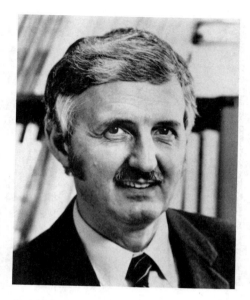

PAUL A. LACHANCE, Ph.D.

Dr. Lachance is a native of Vermont. He earned the BS degree at St. Michael's College and his Ph.D. in Biology and Nutrition from the University of Ottawa, Canada. He joined Rutgers University in 1967. In the Graduate School he is a member of the Food Science, Nutrition and Home Economics graduate programs. He is director of the graduate program in Food Science, considered to be among the five leading programs in the hemisphere.

In addition to his teaching career, Dr. Lachance has played a pivotal role in developing national food and nutrition programs for the United States, and in designing inflight food systems for the Manned Spacecraft Center of NASA. He was the first individual to serve as flight food and nutrition coordinator for NASA (1963–67), where he established the Gemini/Apollo flight food systems. His contributions in this area earned him the John C. Hartnett Award and an honorary D.Sc. degree from his alma mater, St. Michael's College in Vermont. In the late 1960s, Dr. Lachance was a participant in the White House Conference of Food, Nutrition and Health and presented the National Nutrition Objective at the White House. He also served as a liaison member for the USAF and NASA to the Food and Nutrition Board of the National Academy of Sciences/National Research Council.

His professional affiliations include the American Society for Clinical Nutrition, American College of Nutrition (Fellow), Institute of Food Technologists (Fellow), American Public Health Association, American Dietetic Association and American Institute of Nutrition. He has published more than 200 technical papers and scholarly chapters and articles.

"Nutrification" and "Nutrified Foods" were proposed in 1970 by Dr. Lachance and Dr. Bauernfeind, respectively, as more descriptive terminology for adding nutrients to food than previously used terms.

PREFACE

At the 50th anniversary national meeting of the Institute of Food Technologist in 1989, food nutrification, was listed among the top 10 food science innovations of the past 50 years. Nutrification, a term introduced 20 years ago, is used in this volume as an all-inclusive term in place of the older nomenclature (restoration, supplementation, fortification, etc.) and means the addition of one or more nutrients to food. The nutrifying process makes a food more nutritious: it increases the nutrient density of the nutrified food. Nutrification of food is a flexible, economical and socially acceptable method of improving nutritive value without significantly changing the chemical and physical properties of food or the sensory appeal and food consumption practices of the consumer.

Consumer concern about nutritive value of foods and diet-disease relationships has never been higher than it is today, as shown by current surveys. The public wants to know what nutrients and in what quantity they should be consumed daily not only for the maintenance of life but for the optimization of health. Scientific journals, trade publications and advertisements, household magazines, TV talk shows and, yes, the daily press all interact in the search for and/or in discussions about the diet-health connection. Educators are challenged as never before on communicating complex nutritional information to a public which has little basic background knowledge to comprehend and utilize it. Labels of packaged foods are undergoing scrutiny in the hope that their updating and presentation will improve understanding and use of the product. For many decades food guidelines in vogue were devised around daily servings of certain foods; more recently dietary goals or guidelines have been promulgated advising limitations on the consumption of some nutrients and certain ingredients.

In developed countries, changes in living and marketplace patterns have stimulated changes in food industry practices, the result being a diversity of food processing technologies bringing forth an ever changing number and types of foods on market shelves. People are more mobile; family units are smaller; there is less time for home food preparation; sophisticated cooking skills are not required. In addition, the past concept of three meals a day has evolved to include snacking, sometimes referred to as "grazing," leading to increases in the number of daily eating occasions, with significant calorie intakes in addition to the three-meal routine, or as a substitute for one or more meals. This trend increases demand for ready-to-eat or easily prepared food items. The low total calorie intakes of the present sedentary population, complicated by dieting fads, adds to the difficulty of providing and assuring the recommended daily allowances of nutrients in the daily diet.

Developing countries, on the other hand, often face the uncertainty of providing for adequate food supplies when populations are expanding. Currently, people affected by preventable malnutrition are numbered in the millions. Economic, social, and political practices complicate simple nutritional and technological solutions to the problems. Intervention strategies must be developed for specific situations and be ready for insertion into national plans of a given country when opportunity occurs.

This volume has been prepared to pull together a comprehensive compendium of the knowledge on the nutritional, technological and regulatory aspects of the nutrification of foods. Heretofore, the information has existed in fragmented documents. The expectancy is that if this knowledge were located between two covers in a single location, the result will be a greater appreciation of the contributions of added nutrients that have already been made to the food supply of the world. Further, by having a history of the prior use of added nutrients to various foods, a more thorough analysis can be made of present food nutrification practices and the needed improvement in future applications. Lastly, this compilation of information on added nutrients to foods may serve to provide a recognition of their significance and a priority in future national dietary surveys.

It must be recognized that food nutrification practices add to the quality of a given food and much less to quantity. Considering the marginal nutrient insufficiencies, and in some situations definite deficiencies of nutrients, it appears that there is a greater potential for continued food nutrification practices in both developed and developing countries. Food with an improved nutrient distribution pattern relative to calorie content of the food continues to have merit where technical, economic and regulatory considerations permit the adoption of sound nutrification programs. While food nutrification is one of the great accomplishments of humankind in improving nutritional status and preventing disease, it by no means should be regarded as a panacea for all malnutrition ills. It has its limitations. Both technological and economic barriers exist. Some regulatory barriers prevent addition of nutrients to certain foods, such as barriers set up by prior food laws which never were envisaged to limit nutritive improvements when promulgated. Such regulatory practices stifle nutritional advances and need to be changed.

It is hoped that this volume will provide (1) the food technologist with some of the technology involved; (2) the food manufacturer with pilot and/or commercial trial experience on various nutrified food products; (3) the student, educator, physician, public health worker, nutritionist and dietitian with a better understanding of the variation in nutrient content of foods, and the nutritional contribution to foods by the nutrification process; (4) the legal advisors with some understanding of regulatory practices controlling the nutrification of food; and (5) the policy makers with an information source presenting the nutrification concept and practices, the foods which can be nutrified, the need for proper production, safety and distribution controls of the nutrified product, and governmental support for adopted practices.

1991 is the 50th anniversary year of the enrichment of flour and bread with four nutrients: thiamin, riboflavin, niacin and iron. Nutrification of food has been made possible by the availability of pure nutrients in relatively unlimited quantities. Through the utilization of industrially produced nutrients for nutrifying food or food ingredients, as the quantitative needs of more of these nutrients are established and their interrelationships for humans are expanded, the more sophisticated will be our ability to prepare diets intended to optimize health.

J. CHRISTOPHER BAUERNFEIND
PAUL A. LACHANCE

FOREWORD

As a pioneer in the food enrichment program I would like to comment on the public health value of the addition of nutrients to foods, what has been accomplished and the opportunities for the future.

I doubt that many today realize what a great change has occurred in the nature of malnutrition in this country in the last 60 years as a result of the addition of nutrients to foods, nutrition education and food assistance programs. Sixty years ago severe cases of vitamin deficiency disease took thousands of lives every year. Today they are rare and are usually found as a complication of alcoholism or some other disease. Instead, there is much evidence that a large proportion of our population is getting food supply that is less than optimum in nutritive value. However, our greatest nutritional health problem is obesity which is estimated to affect about 25% of our population and is increasing. This is serious because of its complications of diabetes, hypertension, heart disease and other conditions. The obese individual needs to pay particular attention to the nutritive content of food.

The increasing use of convenience foods and calorie-restricted foods which require factory fractionating, refining and processing further decreases available nutrients unless they are added to the ingredients. For example, the milling of white flour from wheat removes most of the germ and the bran. This reduces the thiamin by about 90% and the niacin, riboflavin and iron by about 70–80%. Since white flour products, refined carbohydrates, oils and fats constitute a large part of convenience foods, their "nutrification" is very important.

The proposal to add nutrients to foods has always resulted in controversy between those who support it and those who think that the problems can be solved by nutrition education. As a matter of fact, both are needed. Nutrition education is slow and does not reach everyone. It is likely to be least effective in the less educated and lowest economic groups where the need is greatest. "Nutrification" helps to correct the problem at once and in all groups as food is purchased.

The first program of nutrification in this country was the addition of iodide to table salt for the prevention of endemic goiter. This was a large health problem in the early 1900s, especially in adolescents. Even the dogs in Chicago had goiters. In the military draft of World War I many draftees were rejected because of goiters. David Marine and his associates succeeded in having iodide added to salt in Ohio in 1924 in spite of strong opposition. All efforts to enact laws requiring this health measure have failed because of opposition supported by the canning and salt industries. Today, because of the decreasing use of table salt, lack of knowledge of the health importance of iodized salt, and failure to real labels, it seems likely that we will have an increase in endemic goiter especially in adolescent girls in the Great Lakes area.

A more successful project was the addition of vitamin D to milk to prevent rickets. It had been known for centuries that cod liver oil would prevent and cure rickets. It was also known that exposure of the bare skin to direct sunlight would prevent rickets. However, the disease was widely prevalent in babies, especially those born in the fall in the Northeastern United States. When vitamin D became available in large quantities at an economical price, its addition to whole milk, skim milk, dried milk and evaporated milk became possible. With the cooperation of the dairy industry, practically all milk now contains a specified and controlled amount of vitamin D. The result has been that rickets, with its serious bone deformities, has become so rare that most people no longer recognize the importance of vitamin D in milk. If the use of vitamin D milk for babies declines, we are almost certain to have a return of rickets.

Since a large overdose of vitamin D may have serious toxic effects, there was much controversy over the amount of vitamin D to be added, and the foods to be approved for the addition. It was finally decided that 400 IU per quart of milk was a safe and effective amount if permitted in a limited number of foods.

The addition of vitamin A to margarine in the United States is required by law and is an important factor in preventing blindness. This is of continuous importance because of the increasing use of margarine. Butter is not required to carry a vitamin A content label.

Citrus fruits and juices are major sources of vitamin C, but the amount is unregulated and may be very low unless protected from deterioration. Much of our commercial orange juice is imported from Brazil and mixed with orange juice reconstituted from concentrate. No statement of vitamin C content is required. Many synthetic products or mixtures of juices may contain a measured amount of vitamin C as stated on the label. There is still need for better regulation of the vitamin C content of many foods. Apple juice containing a regulated amount of vitamin C can be a useful product.

The most important addition of nutrients to food with the most far-reaching effect on public health was the "enrichment" program for wheat flour, white bread, cereals and corn meal products. This program was not possible until the required nutrients, thiamin, riboflavin and niacin, became available in large amounts at reasonable prices. The big breakthrough was the synthesis of thiamin by R. R. Williams in the 1930s and the donation of his patent to the Research Corporation. Niacin (nicotinic acid had been synthesized in 1894) only needed Elvehjim's discovery in 1937 that it was the nutrient (nicotinic acid amide) that prevented pellagra. Riboflavin was available and only needed the discovery of human riboflavin deficiency in man by Sebrell and Butler in 1939. Iron was added to the mixture because of the wide prevalence of iron deficiency anemia and the fact that it was removed from wheat in the milling process. A large number of sources of iron were also available.

Beriberi heart disease and Korsakoff's syndrome due to thiamin deficiency were prevalent in many of our large cities, especially in alcoholics. Pellagra due to niacin deficiency had been brought under control by the medical use of niacin. There was evidence of riboflavin deficiency in the south and iron deficiency anemia was everywhere. The time seemed right for the addition of these nutrients to some economical and widely used foods. Bread, flour, cornmeal and cereals seemed obvious choices.

The idea was enthusiastically supported by many nutritionists, and opposed by others. Because of my 10 years of clinical experience with pellagra I knew that this program would save thousands of lives and rehabilitate many additional thousands who were sick or weakened by severe malnutrition. I, therefore, took the leadership in getting the idea officially endorsed by the Public Health Service, the American Medical Association, the American Public Health Association and others. The Food and Nutrition Board of the National Research Council under Dr. Russell Wilder took the leadership for the entire project and played a large role in securing the active support of the baking and milling industry as well as professional nutritionists.

The Food and Drug Administration held extensive hearings at which many of us testified. The term "enriched" was officially defined and approved and the quantity of each nutrient was specified.

The program became official policy on May 27, 1941, with the strong support of both the baking and milling industries.

War Food Administration Order No. 1 in January 1943 made the enrichment of commercial white bread and flour mandatory and settled the controversy for the duration of World War II.

The program was so successful that at the end of the war it was continued by state law and as of 1977 the law covered at least 35 states and Puerto Rico. The baking and milling industries throughout the United States voluntarily continued enriching white bread and flour.

Few nutritional advances have had such a lasting effect on so many people as "enrichment." In 1956 the American Bakers Association presented me a special "Golden Loaf" Award. The citation read "In recognition of and appreciation for his untiring efforts in bringing into being the enrichment of bread, thereby contributing to a healthier, stronger people."

There are still many possible benefits from the further "nutrification" of foods. For example, at least 10 nutrients have been suggested for addition to the enrichment formula. However, nutritionists, physicians and health officials still have to agree on which ones are needed, how much to add and which foods to select for "nutrification." These are all difficult questions to answer. Nutrition education is just as important as food nutrification. We have made great progress in this area, but we need to direct more attention to the food shopper at the point of purchase where the decisions on family nutrition are really made. The buyer must read the labels and understand what they mean as the food is purchased. Preparing a nutritionally adequate meal for the family without excess calories requires a knowledge of nutrition and close attention to labels. The design of such a diet should be about 20% of the calories from protein, about 30% from fats and oil and about 50% from carbohydrates, with adequate vitamins and minerals, without excessive cholesterol and a limited use of foods containing saturated fats. All of this must be held to a total energy intake that does not lead to obesity and takes into account a wide range of consumer preferences, income and seasonal variations in supply. It cannot be accomplished with convenience foods unless they contain added nutrients.

Although the nutritional content of the product is given on the label in accordance with federal regulations, much of the advertising stresses popular subjects such as fiber, cholesterol, cancer and good health. The educated food shopper has to avoid being misled by persuasive advertising and attractive displays.

The nutrition educators (the physician, nutritionist, nurse, dietitian, health officer, school teacher, dentist or other community leaders) should concentrate their efforts not only on guiding the individual to a proper diet, but also on how to obtain a nutritionally adequate food supply for the family, taking into consideration family preferences, availability and cost. If foods are properly selected by a healthy individual, extra nutrient supplements are not necessary.

Nutrient supplements beyond dietary sources are important and may be required by individuals with medical problems or by those who fail to select an adequate, normal diet. If the individual is in ill health, supplements should be used as advised by a physician. If the food supply is restricted or abnormal, supplements should be used only in maintenance doses. The excessive quantities in many mixtures are unnecessary, expensive and may be harmful. Large doses should be used only under the supervision of a physician.

This book, by bringing together the information on nutrition, technology and regulations is a valuable source of food and nutrition information. It should be available to educators, dietitians, nutritionists, physicians and public health personnel.

W. H. SEBRELL, M.D., FACP, FAPHA

CONTENTS

CHAPTER	PAGE
1. MARGINAL MICRONUTRIENT DEFICIENCY, *Myron Brin*	1
2. CONCEPTS AND PRACTICES OF NUTRIFYING FOODS, *Paul A. Lachance and J. Christopher Bauernfeind*	19
3. MINERAL ADDITIVES, *Fergus M. Clydesdale*	87
4. VITAMIN AND AMINO ACID ADDITIVES, *Lynn Bailey*	109
5. FOODS CONSIDERED FOR NUTRIENT ADDITION: CEREAL GRAIN PRODUCTS, *J. Christopher Bauernfeind and Elmer DeRitter*	143
6. FOODS CONSIDERED FOR NUTRIENT ADDITION: FOOD ANALOGS AND EXTRUDED OR BLENDED FOOD MIXTURES, *R. Dixon Phillips and Ronald R. Eitenmiller*	211
7. FOODS CONSIDERED FOR NUTRIENT ADDITION: ROOTS AND TUBERS, *J. Christopher Bauernfeind*	243
8. FOODS CONSIDERED FOR NUTRIENT ADDITION: SUGARS, *Mario R. Molina*	251
9. FOODS CONSIDERED FOR NUTRIENT ADDITION: FATS AND OILS, *J. Christopher Bauernfeind*	265
10. FOODS CONSIDERED FOR NUTRIENT ADDITION: JUICES AND BEVERAGES, *Elmer DeRitter and J. Christopher Bauernfeind*	281
11. FOODS CONSIDERED FOR NUTRIENT ADDITION: SNACKS AND CONFECTIONERIES, *Gur S. Ranhotra and James L. Vetter*	319
12. FOODS CONSIDERED FOR NUTRIENT ADDITION: CONDIMENTS, *J. Christopher Bauernfeind*	347
13. FOODS CONSIDERED FOR NUTRIENT ADDITION: DAIRY PRODUCTS, *Elmer DeRitter*	367

14. FOODS CONSIDERED FOR NUTRIENT ADDITION: FORMULATED SPECIAL PURPOSE FOODS, *Richard E. Hagen, M. Rita Thomas and John J. Bushnell* 395

15. ADDED ASCORBATES AND TOCOPHEROLS AS ANTIOXIDANTS AND FOOD IMPROVERS, *Leonard E. Johnson and William J. Mergens* 433

16. BIOAVAILABILITY OF NUTRIENTS ADDED TO HUMAN FOODS, *Daphne A. Roe* 459

17. ENGINEERING ASPECTS OF NUTRIFYING FOODS, *Daryl B. Lund* 473

18. NUTRIENT INFLUENCE ON OPTIMAL HEALTH, *George Christakis* 495

19. CONSUMER NUTRIENT LABELING ISSUES, *Jesse F. Gregory, III* 519

20. REGULATION OF FOOD FORTIFICATION: UNITED STATES, *Anthony J. Iannarone* 535

21. REGULATION OF FOOD FORTIFICATION: OTHER COUNTRIES, *Irina Du Bois* 589

DIRECTORY: 1990 LIST OF CODEX CONTACT POINTS 601

INDEX 613

CHAPTER 1

MARGINAL MICRONUTRIENT DEFICIENCY

MYRON BRIN, Ph.D.

INTRODUCTION

Nutrition is one of the most popular topics for discussion wherever people gather, whether the group may be lay or scientific. All aspects of nutrition, obesity, cholesterol, vitamins, minerals, fad diets, etc., evoke comment. Whatever the interest in small conversations, nutritional inadequacy is considered of sufficient importance to result in congressional support for the spending of billions of dollars annually on federally funded food programs.

Although the physician in the United States rarely encounters classical clinical deficiency disease syndromes in his daily practice, he constantly contends with problems associated with low-calorie dieting, chronic alcoholism, the taking of vitamin supplements, etc. We hope to put this into perspective by presenting the concept of the "marginal micronutrient deficiency" state. This is based upon experience with controlled studies on the biochemical aspects of human vitamin nutrition, and in the the context of findings in various government and other surveys of nutritional status in various countries.

Following a presentation of methods for the evaluation of nutritional status in human subjects, there will be presented summaries of the major surveys of nutritional status in United States and other populations. Based upon the foregoing, we will define our concept of the marginal deficiency state and refer to the scientific basis for it. Also, following a discussion of the implications of marginal deficiency on experimental animal and human performances, there will be proposals for preventive and corrective measures in man.

METHODS FOR THE EVALUATION OF NUTRITIONAL STATUS

There are four modes for evaluating nutritional status.[1] In the *demographic mode* one depends largely upon the cultural and socioeconomic background of the subject as these may be correlated with the dietary habits of the appropriate population group. This mode is no doubt, at best, the least quantitative for one may be using a grossly generalized background to focus on an individual subject who may not fit the group criteria. The second mode, *dietary history*, is the traditional one by which a trained health professional either interviews the patient to develop a 24 h recall of his or her intake for a time period of no less than one day and usually several days.

When recorded precisely and analyzed accurately for nutrient content the dietary history coupled with tables of food composition, can serve as a reasonable measure of the nutritional status of the individual. The limitations of this mode, however, are those of human frailty; namely, poor record keeping and self-esteem etc., and therefore drawing conclusions may require some judgment on the part of the professional.[2]

The third mode, *physical examination*, has the capability of revealing profound severe vitamin deficiency states which result from a very long nutrient depletion process. In fact, the classical deficiency diseases were identified by this method. An earlier stage of depletion may be over looked, however, because there are no obvious clinical manifestations. The fourth mode, *laboratory assessment*, is the preferred technique.[3] It is the least vulnerable to subjective factors and serves as one of the more quantitative tools for the evaluation of nutrient status.

Examples for laboratory assessment include chemical assay of nutrient or coenzyme levels in blood or urine, as well as more specific functional tests by which the adequacy of a vitamin or mineral for a specific physiological or biochemical function can be demonstrated. For instance, while blood or urine levels of a vitamin (or a nutrient controlled by a vitamin such as calcium in the case of vitamin D) are known to be generally reduced in blood in the deficiency state, such levels often may not be appropriate to define the extent of the deficiency. There are, therefore, some limits to the usefulness of laboratory assays. For instance, in the case of vitamin A, the blood level is not markedly reduced until liver stores are virtually depleted.[4] Also in the case of vitamin B_1, urinary excretion drops to minimum levels quickly, and then levels off making it difficult to estimate the extent of the depletion.

On the other hand, functional assays may contribute more information. For instance, night blindness presents a test of physiological function for vitamin A independent of a chemical analysis for the level of the vitamin. Also, one may use bone density to assess vitamin D or calcium adequacy by specific X-ray techniques, or prothrombin time to reveal the adequacy for vitamin K, etc. In other words, the functional assay presents evidence of adequate utilization and/or need, as well as availability.

For thiamin there has been developed a novel biochemical approach of determining the level of saturation of an enzyme for its vitamin cofactor.[5,6,7] Ideally for human evaluation, this is measured in readily available red blood cells, used as a biopsy tissue. In the case of thiamin, the coenzyme is thiamin pyrophosphate (TTP) which is required for the activity of the erythrocyte enzyme transketolase. In the case of riboflavin, the coenzyme is flavin adenine dinucleotide (FAD) which is an essential cofactor for the activity of the erythrocyte enzyme glutathione reductase.[8] For vitamin B_6, the coenzyme is pyridoxal phosphate which is required for erythrocyte transaminase activity.[9,10] In these enzyme assays, data are expressed as "TPP-effect" (or index), FAD-effect, B_6P-effect, etc. These "effects" (or indices) express the proportion (in percentage) of the enzyme which is unsaturated with coenzyme.[11] Correlation of blood (urine) levels with clinical findings has resulted in criteria by which vitamin and other nutritional status can be estimated.

Evidence for the usefulness of enzyme/coenzyme functional tests were obtained from thiamin studies done under controlled laboratory conditions with volunteer subjects.[5] These showed that urinary thiamin reaches minimal values after only 10 days of depletion while the TPP-effect shows a gradual increase over a depletion period of 6 to 7 weeks. Accordingly, the level of TPP-effect is much more useful than other techniques in determining the actual adequacy of a person for thiamin during the time interval between the onset of depletion and the appearance of classical clinical deficiency. These phemomena are similar for the evaluation of riboflavin and the effect on FAD. This is also the case with vitamin B_6 and several other nutrients.

Criteria for adequacy have been established for the separation of individuals into vitamin nutritional status categories such as "acutely deficient," "marginally deficient," and "adequate" for a large variety of biochemical tests in the evaluation of vitamin status. For vitamin B_1 the criteria are greater than 25%, 15-24%, and less than 15%, respectively, for the aforementioned three categories. [11,12] The methodology and the criteria are available in a number of publications for various assay techniques.[3,13] Current laboratory tests for nutrient adequacy and their relative degrees of sensitivity as tabulated by McLaren and McQuid are found in Table 1.1.[14] Not all agree on the appropriate interpretation of survey data. But, the presence of a biochemical marker along with dietary survey data in the same population group are strongly suggestive of a dietary intake problem.[15]

The tools by which to assess the quality of social performance at work and at home are not as objective or quantitative as chemical/enzyme tests, although all are subject to interpretation. The wide variability in the emergence of clinical signs and symptoms when deficiency levels of thiamin, for instance, are present, was demonstrated with the determination of blood thiamin levels over 35 years age.[16] Functional enzyme tests on the other hand which measure the percentage of enzyme which is unsaturated with coenzyme are particularly useful, therefore. Despite early predictions to the contrary,[17] the usefulness of these tests is becoming more widely recognized[18]

NUTRITIONAL STATUS IN THE UNITED STATES

The U.S. Department of Agriculture (USDA) performs a national food consumption survey (NFCS) approximately every 10 years. This market basket food survey also includes a subpopulation who completed a dietary survey. The questionnaire is given to the homemaker for the members of the family and describes the type of foods purchased, as well as uses, the cost, family socioeconomic, and demographic

TABLE 1.1.
RELATIVE SENSITIVITIES OF LABORATORY TESTS FOR NUTRIENTS AND METABOLITES

Nutrient	Most Sensitive	Less Sensitive	Least Sensitive
Protein	plasma, amino acids, transferrin, prealbumin urine 3-methyl histidine	serum albumin, urine hydroxyproline, urea/creatinine	total serum protein
Lipids	serum high density lipoproteins	serum cholesterol triglycerides	
Vitamin A		serum vitamin A, retinol-binding protein	
Vitamin D	serum $25(OH)D_3, 1,25(OH)_2D_3$	serum alkaline phosphatase	serum calcium and phosphorus
Vitamin E	serum tocopherol	H_2O_2 erythrocyte fragility	
Vitamin K	prothrombin time (PT)	bleeding and coagulation times	
Vitamin C	whole blood ascorbic acid	serum ascorbic acid	
Thiamin	erythrocyte transketolase	urine thiamin	blood pyruvate
Riboflavin	erythrocyte glutathione reductase	urine riboflavin	
Nicotinic Acid		urine N_1methyl nicotinamide and its pyridone	
Folic Acid	erythrocyte folate	serum folate	bone marrow film, thin blood film
Vitamin B_6		tryptophan load test and urine xanthurenic acid, plasma and urine pyridoxine	erythrocyte glutamic pyruvate and oxalo-acetic transaminase
Vitamin B_{12}	serum vitamin B_{12}, thymidylate synthetase	urine methylmalonic acid	bone marrow film, thin blood film
Iron	serum ferritin, iron in bone marrow	serum iron saturation transferrin	blood film
Iodine	T_3, T_4	serum protein-bound iodine	urine iodine
Zinc	serum zinc	hair zinc	
Selenium	erythrocyte glutathione peroxidase	serum selenium	

Source: McLaren and McQuid.[14]

data. In comparing the relative nutritional status for nutrients between the surveys of 1955 and 1965, it was noted that 5 to 9% of diets in 1955 provided less than ⅔ of the RDA for calcium, vitamin A, and vitamin C, and that in 1965 the gap ranged from 8 to 13% of the level recommended. These data revealed that not everyone in the United States was consuming certain vitamins and minerals at recommended levels. The diets in 1965 were somewhat poorer than a decade earlier, despite several federally funded food programs.[19] Additional summaries for the 1965 survey noted that 18 to 21% of meals were rated poor (less than ⅓ of an RDA for 1 or more nutrients) for calcium, iron, and vitamins A and C. In the case of the vitamins, the problems were more severe in rural than urban areas at all seasons of the year.[20] Although vitamins B_6, B_{12} and magnesium were not studied in as complete detail, it was suggested that they also were problem nutrients.

A review of studies of vitamin and mineral nutrition in the United States for the years 1950 to 1968[21] was made in anticipation of the White House Conference on Food Nutrition and Health convened in 1969. It was concluded that a significant proportion of the examined population had intakes below 1/2 RDA and biochemical indices in the deficient range for calcium, iron, vitamins A, B_1, B_2, and C and niacin. It was also concluded that dietary habits of the American public had become worse since 1960. This compilation[21] of the findings by various investigators over almost two decades was an independent confirmation of the findings of the earlier 1955 and 1965 NFCS results.

In the 1970s the U.S. Department of Health, Education, and Welfare (USHEW) launched the Ten State Nutrition Survey.[22] The results[23] confirmed the findings of the prior USDA NFCS and also the conclusions drawn by others.[21] This was followed by a more comprehensive Health and Nutrition Examination Survey (HANES 1974) which included physical examinations as well as biochemical evaluation between the years 1973 and 1975.[24] Those results revealed that between the ages of 19 and 59, approximately 10% of those examined had bleeding and swollen gums suggesting inadequacy for vitamin C, and bowed legs suggesting inadequacy for vitamin D. Also, above the age of 60 there were loss of ankle jerks often correlated to vitamin B_1 inadequacy and fissured tongue often associated with niacin deficiency. The associated dietary and biochemical studies essentially confirmed and extended the findings of the Ten State Nutrition Survey[23] and the USDA NFCS previously described.[20,25] Another reevaluation of the NFCS's of 1955, 1965, and 1977 revealed that the percentage of diets delivering less than 100% RDA for vitamins A, B_1, B_2 and C, of iron, more than doubled during the intervening 22 years.[26] Although there were downward adjustments for vitamins B_6, B_2, folate, magnesium and iron in the 1989 RDA, most of the conclusions drawn on the bases of the previous RDAs are still valid.

As a reflection of the public concern over the nutritional status of school children, Congress enacted the National School Lunch Act in 1946 which required by regulation the "type A" meal distribution of food from the four major food groups. This assumed that a single meal representing a proportion of the four food groups would result in the provision of approximately ⅓ of an RDA of the major nutrients (being proportional to ⅓ of the daily food intake). A report to Congress by the Comptroller General in 1977 questioned whether these goals were being met.[27] A school site study by the USDA Agricultural Research Service suggested that nutrient levels were low.[28] A more extensive study involved the collection and analysis of entire meals from 29 schools in North Carolina (on the assumption that the entire meal was eaten)[29] and confirmed 3 prior pilot studies.[30] It was noted that for all of the 8 nutrients listed, over 28% of meals contained less than ⅓ of an RDA and that the "adequate" nutrient levels for protein and riboflavin would be inadequate if the milk was not consumed. Considering that there is about a 30% waste of food in lunch programs and the equivalent amount of wasted milk if only white milk is served, the gap reported by Head et al.[29] could be even greater.

The elderly have been observed, in a diverse group of studies, to be less than adequate for vitamins A, C, D, E, B_1, B_2, B_6, B_{12} and niacin and folacin in various combinations[9,12,31,32,34] with differences apparent between fall and spring.[33] Rural elderly were less well-nourished that those in urban areas.[35] Of interest is a study of 473 elderly observed to have below adequate intakes of vitamin B_6, B_{12} and niacin. Thirty-nine percent showed deficits despite oral supplementation. It was noted that the natural folylpolyglutamate was a poor supplement compared to the synthetic monoglutamate form of folic acid.[36,37]

In 1985, an analysis of the NFCS data revealed that diets of women in particular failed to contain recommended levels of calcium, iron, magnesium, zinc, vitamin B_6 and folacin, and there was an increase in carbohydrate intake.[26] A further study of this data base revealed that women smokers, compared to never smokers, had significantly lower intakes per 1,000 kcal of protein, dietary fiber, vitamin C and thiamin.[38] An analysis of the popular weight-reducing diets revealed the marginal nature of these regimens[39] for micronutrients.

In a subgroup of sports participants, gymnasts[40], ballerinas[41], and volley ball players,[42] there were inadequate intakes of calcium, iron, zinc, magnesium, and vitamin B_6. A study of female cyclists revealed more than ⅓ of the group having a below optimal calorie intake, as well as a below ⅔ RDA for magnesium, iron, zinc, folacin and vitamins B_6, B_{12} and E.[43]

Micronutrient deficiencies are particularly noted in chronic alcoholics and include vitamins A, B_1, B_6 and folate.[44] In adequately nourished nonalcoholic elderly subjects, the influence of alcohol is smaller and variable depending upon the specific nutrient examined. The significance of the biochemical indices must be judged with knowledge of the adequacy of the subjects diet.[45]

One, therefore, is faced with a dilemma.[46] On the one hand, there are but few instances of overt clinical micronutrient deficiency in the U.S. population, but there is evidence for the presence of pervasive biochemical inadequacy for many micronutrients. Also, while we assume that nutrient intake would be adequate when eating "balanced" meals, however, a balanced regimen such as the Type A school lunch *as served* does not meet the criteria of ⅓ of the RDA as expected.[28,29,30] Further, national food consumption survey data indicate that the intake of several nutrients are below 70% of the RDA.[25] Accordingly, the true functional nutritional status of the U.S. population with regard to human health performance remains to be clarified.

NUTRITIONAL STATUS IN OTHER COUNTRIES

During the decade 1956-1967, nutrition problems were shown to be widespread in 33 countries of the world, including countries in Latin America, Africa, the Near East, and the Far East, as examined and reported by the Interdepartmental Committee for National Defense.[47,48] A summary for thiamin status[49] indicated 54% of the Army personnel (Uruguay) and 49% of civilian groups (Thailand) were inadequate. As of 1985, approximately 400 million people were considered undernourished according to the Fifth World Food Survey of the United Nations Food and Agricultural Organization.[50] Nutrient deficiencies in European populations[50a] were reviewed in 1989.

Australia

Thiamin is one of the marginally adequate nutrients in some Australian diets.[51] The incidence and prevalence of Wernicke-Korsakoff syndrome in this country is maybe one of the highest in the world. Blood levels of thiamin, folate, ascorbate, pyridoxine and zinc were found to be low in attendees of clinics.[51a] In a randomly selected group of 2195 people, 65 years and older, a proportion with dietary intakes below two-thirds of the recommended daily allowances was greatest for folate, calcium, magnesium, copper and zinc and varied from about 10 to 35% of the total group. The mean intakes of the total group, however, were adequate.[51b]

England

A recent study indicates that adolescents have been found to have nutrient intakes below recommended levels for calcium, iron and vitamins A, B_1, B_2 and C even though mean intake values may be greater than the RDA and no overt clinical signs of malnutrition are apparent.[52]

France

The study on Vitamin Status in Three Groups of French Adults (ESVITAF) which was published in 1986 has shown that of the vitamins studied, the average dietary consumption of thiamin, riboflavin, and folic acid was below the French RDA.[53]

At the same time, the determination of biochemical parameters of vitamin nutrition status has shown that up to 30% of the subjects had borderline deficiencies of thiamin, folic acid and vitamin A.

In the region of Burgundy, a report indicates that up to 86% of the adult population consumed only 50-80% of the French Recommended Dietary Allowances for thiamin, riboflavin, nicotinic acid and vitamins C, A, D, and E.[54]

Germany

A comprehensive report on food and nutrition in the former Federal Republic of Germany[55] provides evidence that qualitative nutritional deficiencies, which include vitamin nutrition status, also occur in certain population groups. The problem of inadequate intake was more prevalent among teenagers and young adults; in these groups other risk factors affecting vitamin nutrition status such as smoking, alcohol consumption and use of oral contraceptives were also present. On the basis of biochemical assessment of vitamin nutrition status, these age groups show inadequate levels of vitamin A, thiamin, riboflavin, pyridoxine and especially folic acid. In adults aged 20-50 years, the frequent inadequacies were found for vitamin A and pyridoxine, followed by thiamin and folic acid.[56]

Switzerland

Studies in the Swiss populations[57] have shown that despite the adequate average supplies of most of the vitamins, the intake of vitamins A and C, thiamin and riboflavin may still represent a problem in some population age groups. More specifically, as much as 30% of young children do not reach a daily intake of even 70% of the RDA for thiamin, vitamin C and pyridoxine. Among older school children, biochemical measurements of vitamin blood levels have shown that up to 25% do not have the expected levels for thiamin, vitamin C, pyridoxine and riboflavin. Even in adults, inadequate levels can be found for thiamin, vitamin C, pyridoxine, riboflavin and vitamin A.

Canada

In the "Nutrition Canada" study, a marginal deficiency of certain vitamins was also found.[58] Between 6.5 and 20% of the investigated adult population showed inadequate blood levels for vitamin C, folic acid and thiamin.

The prevalence of vitamin A deficiency was very low, perhaps due to the addition of vitamin A to foods, particularly margarine, of which consumption has increased constantly in the last 20 years and has contributed to a better vitamin A nutrition status in Canada.

THE CONCEPT OF MARGINAL VITAMIN DEFICIENCY

Clinical deficiency findings for specific nutrients include one or more of anemia, exfoliative dermatitis, xerophthalmia, cheilosis, stomatitis, purpura, coiled hairs, hyperkeratosis, some cases of congestive failure, dementia, diarrhea, poor bone calcification, facial erythema, convulsions, rickets, etc.[59] To the trained physician, these findings suggest specific deficiency states when they appear in proper combinations. On the other hand, findings in marginal deficiency include reduced growth and appetite, feeling of lack of well-being, anxiety, somnolence or insomnia, loss of attention span, lethargy, headache, infection susceptibility, drug potentiation, etc. Clearly, the findings in marginal deficiency states are nonspecific, highly subjective and could be identical to those resulting from many stresses of daily living, as well as nutritional in origin. The specific relationship to marginal nutrient deficiency, however, is the appearance of both the nonspecific findings along with specific biochemical defects before clinical signs appear when single nutrient depletion is studied under controlled laboratory conditions.[5]

From studies on thiamin depletion in human subjects during which thiamin supplemented and unsupplemented persons were studied biochemically, physically, and behaviorally throughout their depletion period, it was possible to segregate the sequence of events in the development of thiamin vitamin deficiency, into five stages as shown in the Table 1.2 entitled "Sequence of Events in Development of Vitamin Deficiency".[6] In the first or "preliminary stage," there is the reduction of tissue stores of the vitamin and marked drop in its urinary excretion. As the studies progressed through the second or biochemical state, the depletion became more severe. There is then a reduction in coenzyme formation consistent with a reduction in biochemical function of the observed enzyme activity which requires that specific vitamin coenzyme. These are preclinical "biochemical" findings which would not be evident by physical examination. With continued depletion into stage 3, however, there are "physiological" changes as a consequence of vitamin depletion but which still are nonspecific and, therefore, nonobjective. These include behavioral effects such as insomnia, sommolence, changes in the Minnesota Multiphasic Personability Index (MMPI) scores, irritability accompanied by loss of appetite and reduced body weight. There are also animal and human studies in which modified drug metabolism and reduced immunocompetence can be observed.[60] Physical activity may be impaired. This list of physiological, physical, and behavioral changes are directly related to specific nutrient deficiencies when developed under controlled laboratory conditions, but which otherwise would be explained by daily living stresses. With further depletion, the fourth stage of classical "clinical" deficiency, disease syndromes would appear. If continued to stage 5, severe tissue pathology would be encountered, resulting in death unless the subject is repleted with the missing vitamin.

In summary, vitamin deficiency, therefore, is the result of a gradual depletion process during which there are subliminal but progressive biochemical changes. As

TABLE 1.2
SEQUENCE OF EVENTS IN DEVELOPMENT OF VITAMIN DEFICIENCY

Sequence	Stage	Findings and Comments
1	Preliminary	Reduction of tissue stores, depression of urinary vitamin excretion
2	Biochemical	Reduction in certain enzyme activity due to insufficient coenzyme, urinary excretion at minimum levels
3	Physiological	Behavioral effects such as insomnia or somnolence, adverse behavioral MMPI scores, irritability, accompanied by loss of appetite and reduced body weight. Modified drug metabolism and reduced immunocompetence. Biochemical findings more severe than stage 2
4	Clinical	Classical deficiency disease syndromes
5	Terminal	Severe tissue pathology resulting in death unless repleted promptly

the depletion becomes more severe, there emerge measurable physiological changes in behavior, physical performance, drug metabolism, and immunocompetence. All of these occur before there is any identifiable clinical deficiency syndrome, and at least at early stages they are totally reversible by administering the missing vitamin.

This table has stimulated others to describe the depletion process in a similar fashion.[61] Stages 1 through 3 are called the condition of "marginal deficiency," because in fact, there is a marked impairment in human physiological, physical, behavioral, and immunologic function, without any clear definition of a vitamin deficiency state. It is proposed that this multiple effect of marginal micronutrient deficiency results in an impairment to the individual's health, as well as to his/her function in society.

IMPLICATIONS OF MARGINAL VITAMIN DEFICIENCY ON HUMAN PERFORMANCE

A description of behavioral effects of vitamin depletion is appropriate. Depletion studies by the U.S. Army Medical Nutrition laboratory on marginal deficiencies for thiamin and riboflavin were carried out on human volunteers under carefully controlled conditions.[62,63] Similar studies on ascorbic acid deficiency (vitamin C) were done at the University of Iowa with similar collaboration.[64] In each case the adverse effects on the MMPI scores were clearly evident long before any specific signs of clinical disease appeared. In marginal thiamin and ascorbic acid depletion, there were adverse scores for hypochondriases, depression, and hysteria, and additionally in the case of riboflavin for psychopathic deviation and hypomania. Subsequent and less detailed studies also showed behavioral changes in rats and man when depleted of vitamin B_1.[65]

In the case of riboflavin, there were reductions in grip strength as measured by a hand dynamometer, and it took more than 2 weeks of high level repletion for the MMPI scores and other observations to return to normal values. This suggested that behavioral changes resulting from vitamin depletion may not always be immediately reversible upon administering the particular vitamin. This again reinforces the recommendation that a balanced diet should be consumed daily or that daily proper nutrient intakes should be maintained, in order to prevent the onset of slowly reversible effects.

Young men fed diets under controlled conditions but containing a maximum of 35% of the Dutch RDA developed borderline indices of vitamin adequacy in 4 weeks. This resulted in impaired performance on a bicycle ergometer, as measured by oxygen intake and lactate production. All values reverted to normal with a 2 week repletion period. The control group remained normal throughout.[66]

Non-institutionalized elderly scored worse on the Halstead-Reitan Categories Test (a nonverbal test of abstract thinking ability) when low dietary levels of vitamins C, B_{12}, B_2 or folacin[67] were in evidence. These findings appear to be important in the light of major efforts to reduce morbidity in this rapidly increasing segment of the population. Also in adolescents, an association between folacin status and school performance[68] has been reported.

Another area of interest in marginal vitamin deficiency is the metabolism of drugs and environmental chemicals. A number of studies have shown that marginal deficiencies of vitamins A, E, and C result in markedly reduced rates of drug metabolism.[69,70] Exposure to drugs and/or environmental chemicals, such as antibiotics, anticonvulsants, oral contraceptives, etc. can result in reduced vitamin levels in blood or tissues in experimental animals and man.[69] For instance, vitamin A blood levels are reduced by exposure to the environmental chemicals: PCB, benzopyrine, and DDT, and the drug spironolactone. Also, it is generally recognized now that anticonvulsants given to children can result in folacin deficiency or in rickets, both of which are reversible with appropriate vitamin administration.[70] Similarly, oxygen, ozone, and nitrosamines may increase the need for vitamin E.[71] One of the vitamins which has a broad spectrum of drug interactions is vitamin B_6 for which blood levels are reduced by isonicotinic hydrazide, oral contraceptive analogs, alcohol, penicillamine, thiosemicarbazide and hydralazine,etc.[72] Vitamin/vitamin interaction may also result in marginal deficiency.[73] Supplementation is often recommended in these cases. One of the correlaries of drug-vitamin interactions is that if the metabolism of the drug is reduced by vitamin inadequacy, then the action of the drug might be potentiated.

Immunocompetence is very sensitive to vitamin status in man[74] and experimental animals.[75] These effects are seen on humoral and cell mediated immunity. Serum thymic factor activity is reduced in deficiencies of calories, zinc, vitamin A, and pyridoxine,[76] and vitamin A influences the immune response in children with Down's syndrome,[77] childhood morbidity in general,[78] and nonspecific resistance to infection.[79]

Accordingly, the adverse effects consequent to marginal vitamin deficiency relate to impaired immune response, adverse effects on behavior and the altered metabolism of drugs and environmental chemicals, and thus impaired human function in society and adverse health consequences.

PREVENTIVE/CORRECTIVE PROPOSALS FOR MARGINAL MICRONUTRIENT DEFICIENCY

Top priority should be given to both food and nutrition education programs for age groups and for the general population. Objective programs should be incorporated with priority at the elementary school and high school levels, and certainly in all medical and paramedical training programs, which provide captive groups. Curriculae should include information of the function of nutrients and the nutrient content of foods as these may directly influence proper food choices whether in the marketplace, or restaurant, and in the home. They should also be related to good health and should include cost/benefit information. For instance the provitamin A carotenes can be obtained more cheaply from vegetables than vitamin A from dairy products, and furthermore, carotenes are nontoxic. The concept of eating a large variety of foods should prevail with proper proportion of the four good groups at every meal, where possible. These include the vegetable/fruit group, the milk group, the meat group, and the bread-cereal group. The proportions should be ⅔ plant foods to ⅓ or less animal foods. Physicians in particular should be knowledgeable about good dietary practices for nutrient intake. Also, the public should be educated on a continuing basis with emphasis on nutrition labeling by which they can assess calories, as well as a nutrient profile per serving portion.[80] Realistically, however, the consumption of a highly varied and balanced diet may not necessarily guarantee the proper intake of all nutrients, whether micro or macro.[25,26,39] Nevertheless, judicious food choices would accomplish a great deal toward gaining this goal, and the ultimate purpose is to consume a balanced diet resulting in proper consumption of the entire array of nutrients.[80,81]

As mentioned previously, food as well as nutrition education programs should be undertaken for both parents and children. When 2250 grade school children were studied following an extensive educational program in school, versus a parent education program, a significant contribution by the home environment was observed.[82]

Another suggestion which has been forthcoming since 1974 is the proposal from the Food and Nutrition Board of the National Academy of Sciences/National Research Council to broaden the enrichment of cereal grain food.[83] The current fortification of wheat flour comprises 3 vitamins and 1 mineral, namely, vitamins B_1, B_2, niacin and iron. A report from an expert committee of the Food and Nutrition Board which reviewed all of the data available on the nutrition status of U.S. populations recommended that it would be a public health benefit to broaden the enrichment of cereal grain products to include 6 vitamins and 4 minerals, essentially restoring these nutrients to levels found in whole grain cereals.[83,84] The additional vitamins proposed to be added to the original formula are vitamins A, B_6 and folacin, and the additional minerals are calcium, magnesium and zinc. It is noteworthy that the human requirements for magnesium and zinc have been highlighted only within the last few decades, and the metabolism and function of vitamins B_6 and folacin have been studied largely within the last 3-4 decades. In this regard it should be noted that the original fortification program now in use was devised in 1942 when these four nutrients just mentioned were not widely recognized to be essential in human nutrition. Therefore, this proposal should be considered as desirable not only for the United States but internationally as well.[85,86]

Technological studies on the baking of bread, cookies, cakes, etc. have shown that the enrichment mixture suggested is a feasible one and appropriate for the purposes intended.[84] The advantage of delivering micronutrients through food in this manner is that is is delivered to the consumer irrespective of income or ethnicity, without any change in the hedonistic qualities of appearance or flavor of the food product and without the fear of toxicity. Another consideration is that wherever applied, the probability of enhanced nutritional status increases and is accomplished at the least possible cost per person.

The last mode of nutrient delivery would be the nutrient supplementation of the subject consuming an inappropriate diet with a vitamin and/or mineral supplement or a specially designed food supplement. Although this should be a last resort solution, it is quite obvious that significant portions of our population are not consuming properly balanced diets. An expert committee has described a large number of health stresses under which conditions vitamin and mineral needs may be increases beyond those of an otherwise healthy person.[81] One could include situations such as the finicky eater, the persistent dieter, the drinker, the smoker, and some women who are pregnant, nursing or on oral contraceptive steroids, etc. The committee recommended avoiding excessive intakes suggesting that the RDA provides safe and adequate levels. The recognition of the need for nutrients, but the need for caution at levels exceeding the RDA was restated in the Surgeon General's Report[87] and NAS report on Diet and Health.[88]

In addition, the USDA concluded that at an average calorie intake in women of 1,500 calories per day, it is difficult for the individual to consume adequate micronutrient levels in all cases.[89] This level of calorie consumption is only slightly in excess of that generally followed for weight-loss dieting,[39] and below that recognized by the NAS/NRC RDA as needed to assure the adequate intake of all nutrients.[90]

SUMMARY

Four modes available for the evaluation of nutritional status have been described. Surprisingly, significant portions of the U.S. population and other populations are below optimal in a variety of vitamins and minerals, despite the belief that the consumption of balanced diets could theoretically deliver the necessary levels of these nutrients. Yet, these below-adequate populations do not show clinical signs of nutritional deficiency. However, there is the potential of markedly impaired physical activity, behavior change, impaired immunocompetence, and altered drug and environmental chemical metabolism thereby resulting in below-optimal health and performance in society, for these subjects. This condition is what we define as marginal deficiency.

In discussing preventive or corrective proposals for marginal deficiency, it was pointed out that educational programs for disseminating information on the function of nutrients, the nutrient composition of foods, food labeling and judicious food choices toward eating a balanced diet, comprise the highest priority and should be directed at parents, as well as children and medical professionals. Coordinating these educational programs in concert with a broadened enrichment of cereal grain foods to 6 vitamins and 4 minerals as proposed by the Food and Nutrition Board of the NAS/NRC would be an important intervention in the United States and internationally. Lastly, for those who have difficulty eating balanced meals, such as the finicky eater, the dieter, etc., or those who are exposed to various stresses, such as smoking, oral contraceptive steroids, pregnancy, and various drugs or intercurrent diseases, etc., there is the optional avenue of micronutrient supplementation, sometimes with special formulations, although this should be done at least at present, on an individual basis with professionally trained supervision.

REFERENCES

1. ANON. 1973. Nutritional Assessment in Health Programs. Am. J. Pub. Health *63*, Suppl.
2. GUTHRIE, H. D. 1989. Interpretation of data on dietary intake. Nutr. Rev. *47*, 33–38.
3. ANON. 1973. Laboratory assessment. *In* Nutritional Assessment in Health Programs, G. Christakis, (ed.). Am. J. Pub. Health *63* (Suppl.), 33–37.
4. RAICA, N., SCOTT, JR., LOWRY, L. and SAUBERLICH, J. E. 1972. Vitamin A concentration in human tissues collected from 5 areas in the United States. Am. J. Clin. Nutr. *25*, 291–296.
5. BRIN, M. 1962. Erythrocyte transketolase in early thiamine deficiency. Ann. N.Y. Acad. Sci. *98*, 528–551.
6. BRIN, M. 1964. Erythrocyte as a biopsy issue in the functional evaluation of thiamin status. JAMA *187*, 762–766.
7. BRIN, M., TAI, M. and KALINSKY, H. 1960. The effect of thiamin deficiency on the activity of erythrocyte hemolysate transketolase. J. Nutr. *71*, 273–281.
8. BAMJI, M. S. 1969. Gluthathione reductase activity in red blood cells and riboflavin nutritional status in humans. Clin. Chem. Acta *26*, 263–269.
9. ROSE, C. S. *et al.* 1976. Age differences in vitamin B_6 status of 617 men. Am. J. Clin. Nutr. *29*, 847–853.
10. BRIN, M. 1964. Use of the erythrocyte in functional evaluation of vitamin adequacy. *In* The Red cell, D. Surgenor and C. F. Bishop (eds.). Academic Press, New York.

11. BRIN, M., CHODOS, R. B., VINCENT, W. A. and WATSON, J. M. 1964. Erythrocyte transketolase activity and the TPP-effect in Wernicke's Encephalopathy (Color, Sound, 19 min.). U. S. Veterans Admin. Hosp., Audio Visual Dept., Washington, DC.
12. BRIN, M., DIBBLE, M. V., PEEL, A., MCMULLEN, E., BOURQUIN, A. and CHEN, N. 1955. Some preliminary findings on the nutritional status of the aged in Onondaga County, NY. A. J. Clin. Nutr. *17*, 240–258.
13. SAUBERLICH, H. E., DOWDY, R. P. and SKALA, J. H. 1974. Laboratory tests for the assessment of nutritional status. CRC Press, Boca Raton, Fla.
14. MCLAREN, D. S. and MCQUID, M. M. 1988. Nutrition and its Disorders, 4th Ed. Churchill Livingstone, London.
15. WOTECKI, C., JOHNSON, and MURPHY, R. 1986. Nutritional status of the US population for iron, vitamin C and zinc. *In* What Is America Eating? NAS/NRC, Washington, DC.
16. BURCH, H. B., BESSEY, O. A., LOVE, R. H. and LOWRY, O. H. 1952. The determination of thiamin and thiamin phosphates in small quantities of blood and blood cells. J. Biol. Chem. *198*, 477–490.
17. WILLIAMS, R. H. 1960. Toward the Conquest of Beriberi, Williams-Waterman Fund, NY. Harvard Univ. Press, Cambridge, Mass.
18. TANPHAICHITR, V. 1984. Thiamine. *In* Present Knowledge of Nutrition. Nutrition Foundation Washington, DC.
19. U.S.Department of Agriculture. 1965. Household Food Consumption Survey. USDA/ARS, Washington, DC.
20. U.S. Department of Agriculture. 1968. Dietary levels of households in the U.S. Agricultural Research Service ARS 62-17.
21. DAVIS, T. R. A., GERSHOFF, S. N. and GAMBLE, D. F. 1969. Review of Studies of vitamin and mineral nutrition in the U.S. (1950-1968). J. Nutr. Education *1* (Suppl. 1).
22. U.S. DHEW 1972. Ten State Nutrition Survey. Publ. 72-8130 to 72-8134. Washington, DC.
23. SCHAEFER, A. E. 1977. Nutritional needs of special populations at risk. Ann. N.Y. Acad. Sci. *300*, 419–427.
24. US DHEW. 1974. HANES. Health and Nutrition Examination Survey. Publ. (HRA) 74-12191-1, Rockville, MD.
25. PAO, E. M. and MICKLE, S. J. 1981. Problem Nutrients in the United States. Food Technol. (35(9), 58–69.
26. PETERKIN, B. M. 1986. Women's diets, 1977 and 1985. J. Nutr. Ed. *18*, 251–257.
27. U.S. Comptroller General. 1977. The National School Lunch Program—Is it working? Report to Congress. U.S. Government Printing Office, Washington, DC.
28. MURPHY, E. W., KOONS, P. C. and PAGE, L. 1968. Vitamin content of Type A school lunches. J. Am. Dietet. Assoc. *55*, 372–378.
29. HEAD, M. K., WEAKS, R. J. and GIBBS, E. 1973. Major nutrients in the Type A lunch. J. Am. Dietet. Assoc. *63*, 620–625.
30. LACHANCE, P. A. 1977. The U.S. School Food Service Program—Successes, Failure and Prospects. Ann. N.Y. Acad. Sci. *300*, 411–418.
31. BRIN, M., SCHWARZBERG, S. H. and ARTHUR-DAVIES, D. 1964. A vitamin evaluation program as applied to 10 elderly residents in a community home for the aged. J. Am. Geriat. Soc. *12*, 493–499.
32. BRIN, M. and BAUERNFEIND, J. C. 1978. Vitamin needs of the elderly. Post. Grad. Med. *63*, 155–163.

33. DIBBLE, M. V., BRIN, M., THIELE, V. F., PEEL, A., CHEN, N. and MCMULLEN, E. 1967. Evaluation of nutritional status of elderly subjects with comparison between fall and spring, J. Am. Geriat. Soc. *15*, 1031–1060.
34. THIELE, V. F., BRIN, M. and DIBBLE, MV. 1968. Preliminary biochemical findings in Negro migrant workers at Kings Ferry, NY. Am. J. Clin. Nutr. *21*, 1229–1238.
35. NORTON, L. and WOZNY, M. C. 1984. Residential location and nutritional adequacy among elderly adults. J. Gerontol. *39*, 592–595.
36. BAKER, H. and FRANK O. 1985. Clinical vitamin deficits in various age groups. Intern. J. Vit. Nutr. Res. (Suppl. 27).
37. GUPTA, K., DWORKIN, B. and GRAMBERT, S. R. 1988. Common nutritional disorders in the elderly: atypical manifestations. Geriatrics *43*, 87–97.
38. LARKIN, F. A., BASIOTIS, P. P., RIDDICK, H. A., SYKES, K. E. and PAO, E. M. 1990. Dietary patterns of women smokers and non-smokers. J. Am. Dietet. Assoc. *90*, 230–237.
39. FISHER, M. C. and LACHANCE, P. A. 1985. Nutrition evaluation of published weight-reducing diets. J. Am. Dietet. Assoc. *85*, 450–454.
40. MOFFAT, R. 1984. Dietary status of elite female high school gymnasts: inadequacy of vitamin and mineral intake. J. Am. Dietet. Assoc. *84*, 361–363.
41. BENSON, J. D. M., GILLIEN, D. M., BOURDET, K. and LOOSLI, A. R. 1985. Inadequate nutrition and chronic calorie restriction in adolescent ballerinas. Phys. Sports Med. *13*, 79–80, 83–87, 90.
42. PERRON, M. and ENDRES, E. 1985. Knowledge, attitude and dietary practices of female athletes. J. Am. Dietet. Assoc. *85*, 573–576.
43. KEITH, R. E., O'KEEFE, K. A., ALT, L. A. and YOUNG, R. L. 1989. Dietary Status of trained female cyclists. J. Am. Dietet. Assoc. *89*, 1620–1623.
44. HOYUMPA, A. M. 1986. Mechanisms of vitamin deficiency in alcoholism. Clin. Exp. Rsch. *10*(6), 573–581.
45. JACQUES, B. F., SALCKY, S., HARTZ, S. G. and RUSSEL, R. M. 1989. Moderate alcohol intake and nutritional status in nonalcoholic elderly subjects. Am. J. Clin. Nutr. *50*, 875–883.
46. BRIN, M. 1972. Dilemma of vitamin deficiency. *In* Proc. 9th Intern. Congr. Nutr. *4*, 103–115. Karger, Basel.
47. Interdepartmental Committee on Nutrition for National Defense. 1963. Manual for Nutrition Surveys. U.S. Agency for International Development, Washington, DC.
48. MCKIGNEY, J. I. 1974. Malnutrition in world populations. Office of Nutrition, U.S. Agency for International Development, Washington, DC.
49. BRIN, M. 1976. Recent information on thiamin nutritional status in selected countries. *In* Thiamin, C. Gubler, M. Fujiwara, and P. Dreyfus (eds.). John Wiley & Sons, New York.
50. DICHTER, C. R. 1987. The Fifth World food survey: an estimate of food supplies and malnutrition. J. Am. Dietet. Assoc. *87*, 1668–1672.
50a. SOMOGYI, J. C. and HEJDA, S. (eds.). 1989. Nutrition in the prevention of disease (Symp. of European Nutritionists). Bibl. Nutr. Dieta *44*, 51–84.
51. YELLOWLEES, P. M. 1986. Thiamin deficiency and the prevention of the Wernicke-Korsakoff syndrome: a major public health problem. Med. J. Austr. *145*, 216–219.
51a. DARNTON-HILL, I. and TRUSWELL, A. S. 1990. Thiamin status of a sample of homeless clinic attenders in Sydney. Med. J. Austr. *152*(1), 5–9.

51b. HORWATH, C. C. 1989. Dietary survey of a large random sample of elderly people: energy and nutrient intakes. Nutr. Res. 9(5), 479–492.
52. BULL, N. L. 1988. Studies of the dietary habits, food consumption, and nutrient intake of adolescents and young adults. World Rev. Nutr. Diet. 57, 24–78.
53. LEMOINE, A., LE DEVEHAT, C. and HERBETH, B. 1986. ESVITAF. Enguête sur le statut vitaminique de trois groupes l'adultes fraçais: Temoins, obêses, buveurs excessifs. Ann. Nutr. Metab. 30, (Suppl. 1), 1–94.
54. GUILLAND, J. C., BOGGIO, V., MOREAU, D. and KLEPPING, J. 1986. Evaluation de l'apport alimentaire vitaminique en Bourgogne (France). Ann. Nutr. Metabl. 30, 21–24.
55. ERNÄHRUNGSBERICHT. 1988. Deutsche Gesellschaft fur Ernährung. E. V., Frankfurt.
56. KÜBLER, W. 1987. Vitaminversorgung: Risikogruppen. Fortbildungskongress fur Apotheker "Die Empfehlung in der Selbstmedikation," Frankfurt.
57. AEBI, H. et al. (eds.). 1984. Zweiter Schweizerischer Ernährungsbericht. Hans Huber, Bern.
58. MONGEAU, E. 1983. Carences et subcarences en vitamines et mineraux au Canada. Can. Nutr. Diet. 3, 145.
59. ANON. Present Knowledge in Nutrition. 1984. Nutrition Foundation, Washington DC.
60. ROE, D. 1985. Drug Induced Nutritional Deficiencies, 2nd Ed. Van Nostrand Reinhold/AVI Publishing Co., New York.
61. SAUBERLICH, H. 1984. Implications of nutritional status on human biochemistry, physiology and health. Clin. Biochem. 17, 132–142.
62. BROZEK, J. 1951. Physiological effects of thiamin restriction and deprivation in young men. Am. J. Clin. Nutr. 5, 109–120.
63. STERNER, R. T. and PRICE, W. R. 1973. Restricted riboflavin: Within subject behavioral effects in humans. Am. J. Clin. Nutr. 26, 150–160.
64. HODGES, R. E., BAKER, E. M., HOOD, J., SAUBERLICH, H. E. and MARCH, S. C. 1969. Experimental scurvy in man. Am. J. Clin. Nutr. 22, 535–548.
65. BRIN, M. 1979. Example of behavioral changes in marginal vitamin deficiency in rat and man. In Behavioral Effects of Energy and Protein Deficits, J. Brozek (ed.). Nat. Inst. Health Publ. 79-1906.
66. VAN DER BEEK, E. J., VAN DOKKEN, W., SCHRYVER, J. and HERMUS, R. J. J. 1984. Impact of marginal vitamin intake on physical performance in healthy young men. Proc. Nutr. Soc. Mtg., Sept. 11/12.
67. GOODWIN, J. S., GOODWIN, J. M. and GARRY, P. 1983. Association between nutritional status and cognitive functioning in a healthy elderly population. JAMA 249, 2917–2921.
68. TSUI, J. C., NORDSTROM, J. W. and KOHRS, M. B. 1985. Association between folacin status and school performance in adolescents. Fed. Proc. 44, 1283.
69. BRIN, M. 1978. Drugs and environmental chemicals in relation to vitamin needs. In Drug Interrelations. Academic Press, New York.
70. BRIN, M. and ROE, D. 1979. Drug-diet interactions. J. Fla. Med. Assoc. 66, 4221–4228.
71. LUBIN, B. and MACHLIN, L. J. (eds.). 1982. Vitamin E: Biochemical, Hematological and Clinical Aspects. Ann. New York Acad. Sci. 393.
72. BHAGAVAN, H. N., and BRIN, M. 1983. Drug-vitamin B_6 interaction. In Nutrition and Drugs, M. Winick (ed.). John Wiley & Sons, New York.

73. MACHLIN, L. J. and LANGSETH, L. 1988. Vitamin-vitamin interactions. *In* Nutrient Interactions. C. E. Bodwell and J. W. Erdman (eds.). Marcel Dekker, New York.
74. ANON. 1985. Nutrition and the immune response. Dairy Council Dig. 56, 10–12.
75. KUMAR, M. and AXELROD, A. E. 1978. Cellular antibody synthesis in thiamin, riboflavin, biotin and folic acid deficient rats. Proc. Soc. Exp. Bio. Med. *157*(3), 421–423.
76. CHANDRA, R. K., HERESI, G. and AN, B. 1980. Serum, thymic factor activity in deficiencies of calories, zinc, vitamin A and pyridoxine. Clin. Exp. Immunol. *42*, 333–335.
77. PALMER, S. 1977. Influence of vitamin A nutriture on the immune response: Findings in children with Down's Syndrome. Intern. J. Vit. Nutr. Res. *48*, 188–216.
78. MILTON, R. C., REDDY, V. and NAIDU, A. N. 1987. Mild vitamin A deficiency childhood morbidity. Am. J. Clin. Nutr. *46*, 827–829.
79. COHEN, B. E. and ELIN, R. J. 1974. Vitamin A induced nonspecific resistance to infection. J. Infect. Dis. *129*, 597–600.
80. LACHANCE, P. A. and FISHER, M. C. 1986. Educational and technological innovations required to enhance the selection of desirable nutrients. Clin. Nutr. *5*, 257–264.
81. CALLAWAY, C. W., MCNUTT, K. W., RIVLIN, R. S., ROSS, A. C., SANDSTEAD, H. H. and SIMOPOULIS, A. P. 1987. Statement on vitamin and mineral supplements (Joint Public Information Committee of the AIN/ASCN). J. Nutr. *117*, 1649.
82. PERRY, C. L., LENPKER, R. V., MURRAY, D. M. and KURTH, C. 1988. Parent involvement with children's health promotion. Am. J. Pub. Health *78*, 1156–1160.
83. Food and Nutrition Board. 1974. Proposed fortification policy for cereal-grain products. NAS/NRC, Washington, DC.
84. LACHANCE, P. A. 1986. The cereal grain fortification gap. Public Issue Report. Hoffmann-LaRoche Inc., Nutley, NJ.
85. HORNSTEIN, I. 1982. Nutritional assessment and food fortification. *In* Adding Nutrients to Food—Where Do We Go From Here? J. L. Vetter (ed.). Am. Assoc. Cereal Chemists, St. Paul, MN.
86. COUNSELL, J. N. 1988. Vitamin fortification of foods. *In* Food Technology International Europe, A. Turner (ed.). Sterling Publications, London.
87. Surgeon General of the United States. 1988. Report on Nutrition and Health. DHHS (PHS) Publ. 88-50211. Washington, DC.
88. Food and Nutrition Board. 1989. Diet and Health: Implication for Reducing Chronic Disease Risk. NAS/NRC, Washington, DC.
89. ANON. 1981. II: Menus to get you going. *In* Ideas for Better Eating, Science and Education Admin./Human Nutrition. U.S. Dept. Agr., U.S. Government Printing Office, Washington, DC.
90. Food and Nutrition Board. 1989. Recommended Dietary Allowances, 10th Ed. NAS/NRC, Washington, DC.

CHAPTER 2

CONCEPTS AND PRACTICES OF NUTRIFYING FOODS

PAUL A. LACHANCE, Ph.D.

and

J. CHRISTOPHER BAUERNFEIND, Ph.D.

INTRODUCTION

What distinguishes humans from other animals are the advanced development of the brain and the hands. Humans have devised tools and developed a technology which enables them to cause the earth to yield more food.[1] There was no single type of food used by primitive people everywhere. The supply of food was related to climate, geographical and environmental conditions.

A continuous food supply has always been the critical factor in the survival of humankind and in the rate of population growth.[2] Whereas humanity has existed for about 2 million years, it took until 1850 for the world's population to grow to one billion persons.[3] For each succeeding billion, a decreasing time interval has elapsed, namely 80, 30, 16 and 10 years respectively, bringing the world's population to over 5 billion, and approaching 6 billion today (Fig. 2.1). Predictions from the United Nations are that the world's population will stabilize around 10 billion by approximately the year 2100.

Feeding this increasing population is a major concern with an agricultural economy highly dependent upon climate and pest control challenges. To date, remarkable success has been achieved in producing an ample food supply to feed the expanding population. Distribution inequalities—a result of faulty economic political systems due to ignorance, indifference or even deliberate actions—have resulted in famine in some countries.[3] But what about the future? While attempts have and are being made to stem the upward spiral of population growth, there is little evidence of success in drastically changing this pattern. Will the limitation of food supplies from agriculture and aquaculture in the future be the dominant determinant? When food supplies fail, famine follows. This has been evidenced regionally in the past, is happening today and undoubtedly will happen in the future. Not only food production problems are involved, but food distribution problems as well.[4]

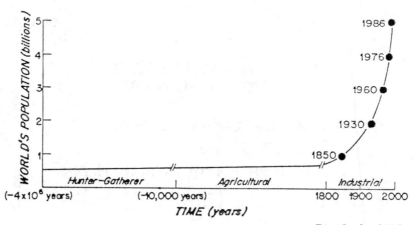

From Leaf and Weber[3]

FIG. 2.1. THE WORLD'S POPULATION GROWTH

Humankind has managed to survive due to flexibility[5] to utilize and modify a wide range of substances for nutritional needs. Only through timely adaptations will food production continue to meet human needs. Development of alternative food resources provides some assurance against the future challenge. Future world needs demand the fullest application of technological knowledge and resources both in agriculture and the food processing industry for the efficient production and distribution of food.[6]

Various attempts have been made to describe food. An individual food such as honey can be described[7] as being made by a six-legged creature, the bee, wandering in fields and forests, partaking of pollen and nectar. The bee ingests the nectar into its stomach, which mixes it with a natural secretion, an additive called invertase, converts the nectar to sugar as the bee flies back to the hive, and then regurgitates this mixture all over the floor of the wax cell, with other bees vibrating their wings in unison to evaporate the contents to about an 80% sugar concentrate called honey. Food is any substance that is eaten or otherwise taken into the body to provide physiological and psychological life, provide energy and promote nutrition. The substance of food is an array of chemicals that impart color, flavor, texture and nutritive values. The risk benefit of food[8] can be described as follows:

> Food = an array of known chemicals and unknown chemicals which *may be modified* by maturation, storage, processing, preparation, *which may be modified* by digestion, absorption, metabolism, the end product of which have a good, bad, or no effect on body cells and tissues.

So, individual foods, themselves, are groups of chemicals. In plant foods these chemicals are present in the soil and water, with carbon dioxide of the air. Many more chemicals are synthesized by the action of sunlight on the chlorophyll-containing plants and by further interchemical reactions.[9] Animals eat the plant chemicals, and by catabolism, and synthesis, form other chemicals to make up the chemical distribution in animal products. In all there are probably thousands of chemicals making up our plant and animal food supply. Whether they are good or bad depends on the amount consumed. There are chemical toxins occurring naturally in our food supply, such as methyl alcohol, benzene, alkaloids, cyanides, solanine and others. In addition there are microbiological byproducts such as the carcinogenic aflatoxins which can contaminate the food. Some foodborne toxicants (Table 2.1) influence nutrient availability or utilization.[10]

In the past 50 years much has been learned about the nutritional requirements of humankind in terms of specific nutrients such as the essential amino acids, fatty acids, minerals and vitamins and their interrelationships, however, there are many unknowns, particularly the precise metabolic functions of each nutrient, yet to be discovered. Today, laboratory animals can be grown, maintained and be reproduced while fed on purified diets of known composition. The current state of knowledge of human nutritional needs is illustrated by the success[11] that has been achieved in providing nutritional support intravenously. Many seriously ill patients can now be maintained for months with parenterally administered fluids containing only known purified or crystalline substances. Persons with substantial loss of gastrointestinal function have been able to live reasonably active lives for over 10 years with such solutions administered from portable infusion units as their sole source of food. Young ambulatory phenylketonuric patients[12] have been kept on a chemically defined diet as a sole nutrition for a three or four year period in a "good health" condition. Thus, we are approaching a better understanding of the chemistry of the essential nutritional needs of the human.

With increasing population growth, it would seem prudent to search for new food sources for future use, if and when needed.[13] One possibility is single-cell-protein, produced by microbial fermentation. One organism can grow rapidly on an inorganic medium supplied by a mixture of hydrogen, oxygen and carbon dioxide; others can convert oils to protein.[14] In another technology, protein structures can be modified in the form of covalent attachment of suitable amino acid esters with the aid of protease action. Some examples can be mentioned. One meat substitute (Provesteen) is made in the United States from high-protein yeast and other ingredients. A fungal fermentation product is used in frozen meat pies in England.[15] Amino acids have been blended physically with inferior proteins to upgrade foods and diets.[16] Improved amino acid production[17] by means of fermentation, enzymatic synthesis, chemical synthesis and extraction is proceeding with new production technologies, cost reduction and utilization of unused resources resulting. Raw materials can be macromolecules of plant sources or fossil petroleum, and the goal is to use the nitrogen and carbon dioxide of the air. More control of nitrogen fixation, photosynthesis and genetic manipulations offer promise. The chemical and food industries need to be partners[18] of government and consumers, for only through such cooperation can safe and wholesome conditions for the production of the required foods (as well as their convenient storage and processing, leading to the manufacture of final products of high nutritive value with acceptable characteristics) be realized.

TABLE 2.1
EFFECT OF TOXICANTS ON NUTRIENT AVAILABILITY AND UTILIZATION

Foodborne Toxicants That Decrease Nutrient Availability

Toxicant	Nutrients Affected	Sources in the Diet
Dietary fiber	Minerals, vitamins, protein	Plants
Phytates	Zinc, other minerals	Oilseeds, grains
Oxalates	Calcium	Spinach, rhubarb, tea, cocoa
Plant phenolics		
Gossypol	Iron, other minerals, protein	Cottonseed
Tannins	Protein, vitamin B_{12}, glucose	Many plants
Other phenolics	Protein, vitamins	Many plants
Heavy metals		
Iron	Vitamin A, vitamin E, polyunsaturated fatty acids	Animal tissues
Vitamin antagonists		
Avidin	Biotin	Eggs
Phenolics	Thiamin	Many plants
Linatine	Pyridoxal	Linseed meal
Unknown	Vitamin B_{12}	Raw soybeans
Thiaminase	Thiamin	Shellfish, carp
Enzymes		
Thiaminase	Thiamin	Shellfish, carp
Lipoxygenase	Vitamin A	Raw soybeans, other plants
Tocopherol oxidase	Vitamin E	Raw soybeans and kidney beans
Insect toxins		
p-Benzoquinones	Protein, thiamin	Foods infested with flour beetles
Nitrite	Protein	Additive, certain plants

Foodborne Toxicants That Decrease Nutrient Utilization

Toxicant	Nutrients Affected	Mechanism	Sources
Enzyme inhibitors			
Trypsin inhibitors	Protein	Inhibit protein digestion	Legumes
Ovomucoid	Protein	Inhibits protein digestion	Eggs
Ovoinhibitor	Protein	Inhibits protein digestion	Eggs
Amylase inhibitors	Carbohydrate	Inhibit carbohydrate digestion	Legumes
Vitamin antagonists			
Linatin	Pyridoxal	Complex formation	Linseed meal
Dicumerol	Vitamin K	Interferes with thrombin production	Sweet clover
Goitrogens	Iodine	Inhibit iodine uptake by thyroid	*Cruciferae* plants
Phenolics			
Tannins	Glucose, methionine	Inhibit intestinal absorption	Many plants
Phlorizin	Glucose	Inhibits intestinal absorption	Apples
Saponins	Cholesterol	Inhibit cholesterol absorption	Alfalfa, soybeans
Heavy metals			
Lead	Calcium	Inhibits calcium absorption and deposition into bone; interferes with other Ca-dependent processes	Contaminant
Cadmium	Calcium, zinc	Induces metallothionein formation	Contaminant
Mercury	Selenium	Complex formation	Fish, contaminant
Canavanine	Arginine	Interferes with arginine-dependent processes	*Papilionoidae* plants
Nitrite	Iron	Decreases incorporation	Additive, certain plants

Source: Taylor.[10]

FOOD INDUSTRY TRENDS

The consumer remains uncertain as to whether natural foods should receive industrial processing treatments which would alter substantially their physical and chemical characteristics, believing that foods closer to their native state are preordained to better serve humankind. This view is challenged by changes in career/family and recreational lifestyles under which there is less time for meal preparation and a demand for convenience.

Food processors take animal, marine, vegetable and inorganic materials and transform them into more useful edible products with extended shelf-life through the application of scientific knowledge, labor, machinery, and energy, while simultaneously having to consider consumer preferences, distributor practices, ingredient availability and technological feasibility.[19] Household (at home or away from home) expenditures account for 89% of the retail value of processed foods sold in the United States. Business, government and exports account for 11% of the value of processed foods sold in the United States. The average food supermarket may offer 7,000–17,000 items; about 1,000 new processed food products are introduced annually, a considerable number (90%) of which are not continued because of insufficient consumer interest.

Another indicator of an increased availability of a greater variety of U.S. foods is the number of items shown in the USDA Handbook on Composition of Food.[20] In 1950 there were over 700 items, in the 1963 version over 2,400, and in the current edition over 4,000. The problem of food composition data is compounded markedly by the enormous diversity of food processing technology and the equally diverse and ever-changing number and types of foods on supermarket shelves.

Foods are being formulated and fabricated with the philosophy of making foods fit taste and health preferences and still be nourishing but low calorie.[15,21] Attempts are being made to lower the cholesterol and fat of animal products and to increase the fiber content of foods in general. New food ingredients are proliferating, as the following trends indicate.

Protein emulsions which emulate fat (Simplesse®) and nonassimilated fats (Olestra®) are developments to reduce the fat content of food and still retain the texture and mouthfeel that fat previously provided, but now without the associated lipid calories. Fat microemulsions are prepared by high shear homogenization with fat spheres less than one micron in diameter. Reduction of the fat microspheres and protein stabilization of the emulsion are the two key elements needed to duplicate smooth, fat-like textures.[22]

Sucrose polyesters, produced by reacting sucrose molecules with any of several food grade fatty acids, act as a very efficient class of fat substitutes that are not absorbed through the intestine and hence do not contribute to calories.[22] They are used in Japan, but not yet in the United States. Their proposed uses are as a partial fat substitute in shortenings, cooking oils, frying oils, and ice cream. They can "pull" bile cholesterol (also some fat-soluble pesticides) from blood plasma by binding the recycling of these compounds in the gut. However, sucrose polysters reduce the absorption of fat soluble vitamins.

Noncaloric sweeteners are a familiar additive[23] in low-calorie beverages and other foods. Saccharin, aspartame and acesulfame-K are approved for use in the United States. Sucralose (600 times sweeter than sucrose) is pending approval in the United States, and other sweeteners, e.g., L-sugars, PS-99 and PS-100, are at various stages in test programs for possible future approval for food use.

Interest in fiber is stimulated by observations that populations with higher fiber intakes show a lower incidence of cancer of the colon, diverticulitis, appendicitis, etc. In populations consuming less fiber, there is a higher incidence of these diseases. Sales of high fiber breakfast cereals have increased. Bakers have added fiber to bread. Soft drinks with added soluble fiber are marketed in Japan. For example, fluffy cellulose, is a noncalorie supplement made from straw, citrus pulp or sugar beets.[15] Research on fiber continues.

LOSS OF NUTRIENTS IN FOOD PROCESSING

With the population growth of the past decades, processing of food has been essential to convert the foods of the land and the waters (usually perishable, at times bulky, parts of which may be inedible) into relatively stable, convenient, packaged products subject to wide distribution and storage environments for year-round availability in the feeding of humankind. To reach this objective, there occurs an inevitable loss of some nutrients, depending on the processing methodology.[24]

Evaluation of the nature and extent of losses of nutrient content from food processing methods and storage is a difficult task because of the diverse nature of the various nutrients, their chemical heterogeneity within each class of compounds and the fact that most foods are complex systems.[25-27] Because of these variables and their interactions, generalization about losses to be expected are not always trustworthy guides in specific cases.

Generally, the water soluble vitamins, especially thiamin, riboflavin, and ascorbic acid, are more susceptible to losses due to leaching during washing and blanching.[27] Water soluble vitamins are generally more heat sensitive than fat soluble vitamins. Ascorbic acid, thiamin and folate are the most heat sensitive. Riboflavin is sensitive to light. The fat soluble vitamins, particularly A, D, and E, are more sensitive to oxidation during processing and storage. Minerals which are water soluble are also susceptible to leaching. Minerals are not heat sensitive, but their bioavailability may be altered as a result of chemical interactions within the food. Additionally, some small losses in soluble protein and changes in protein bioavailability may occur, as a result of nonenzymatic browning (Maillard reaction) occurring between certain amino acids, in particular lysine and reducing sugars. However, the resultant flavor and color changes which are characteristic of the browning reaction are very desirable in many foods.

TABLE 2.2
SUMMARY OF VITAMIN LOSSES FROM VARIOUS CLASSES OF FOODS DURING FREEZING-PROCESSING AND COOKING

Processing Step	Vegetables	Fruits	Animal Tissues
Prefreezing treatments	10–44% loss of vitamin C during blanching; substantial losses can occur during storage if time-temperature conditions are abusive	Slight if properly handled prior to freezing	Slight if properly handled prior to freezing
Freezing	Slight	Slight (two studies)	Insignificant, except perhaps for B vitamins in pork
Frozen storage	Substantial losses of vitamin C and pantothenic acid; moderate losses of vitamins B_1 and B_2; losses of vitamin C are highly temperature dependent (Q_{10} = 6–20)	Substantial losses of vitamin C except in citrus juice concentrate; losses of vitamin C are highly temperature dependent (Q_{10} = 30–70)	Data limited; substantial losses of pyridoxine from beef, pork, oysters; moderate losses of vitamins B_1 and B_2 in pork; substantial losses of B vitamins in oysters

Thawing	Slight	Little data; probably slight, except perhaps for loss of vitamins in the syrup and thaw-exudate	Moderate losses of B vitamins and amino acids in thaw-exudate
Total freezing process	Many common vegetables lose ~50% of their original vitamin C contents	Losses of vitamin C are usually less than 30%, except in citrus juice concentrate, where losses of vitamin C are less than 5%	Losses of B vitamins are highly variable; losses of B_1 usually 25%, B_2 often 15%, niacin often 10%, pyridoxine about 25-50% (few data)
Cooking of frozen food	Mean values (variability large): vitamin C, 30%; β-carotene, 5%; folic acid, 15%; niacin, 12%; B_1, 12%; B_6, 25%; B_2, 10%; pantothenic acid, 17%; leaching is an important factor	Not applicable for most fruits	B_1, 15-40%; B_2, 0-40%; niacin, 0-15%; pantothenic acid, 0-15%; pyridoxine, 0-1%; B_{12}, 0-25%; substantial losses in cooling exudate

Source: Fennema.[28]

As an example of a mild food preservation method, one can examine what happens to nutrients during freezing, thawing, and the subsequent heat preparatory step prior to consumption where applicable (Table 2.2). Even in a processing method where the food in question remains intact and does not usually undergo physical partitioning, there are significant losses in vitamin content. During the freezing process vitamin losses are caused in vegetables primarily by blanching and prolonged frozen storage, in fruits by prolonged frozen storage and thawing, and in animal tissues by prolonged frozen storage and by thawing.[28] Losses[29] of nutrients in vegetables occurring with freezing as compared to canning are shown in Fig. 2.2.

In the situation where a food is partitioned and parts removed during the initial processing operation, a prime example being the milling of wheat grain into white flour, nutrient losses[30] can be more substantial (Fig. 2.3), as is evident when one compares the extraction rate (the percentage of the wheat grain remaining in the

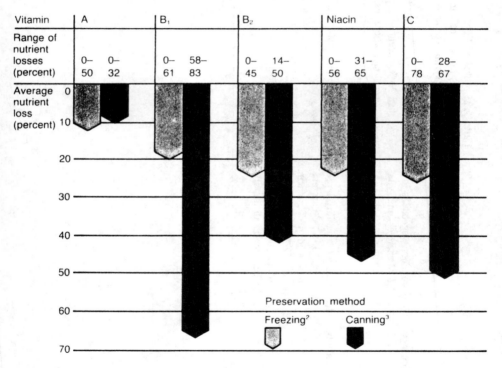

[1]Boiled and drained.
[2]Frozen, boiled and drained. The vegetables analyzed were asparagus, lima beans, green beans, broccoli, brussel sprouts, cauliflower, corn, peas, potatoes and spinach.
[3]Canned, drained and heated. Same vegetables except broccoli, brussel sprouts and cauliflower excluded.

From Roberts[29]

FIG. 2.2. VITAMIN LOSSES IN FROZEN AND CANNED VEGETABLES COMPARED TO FRESH-COOKED[1] PRODUCTS

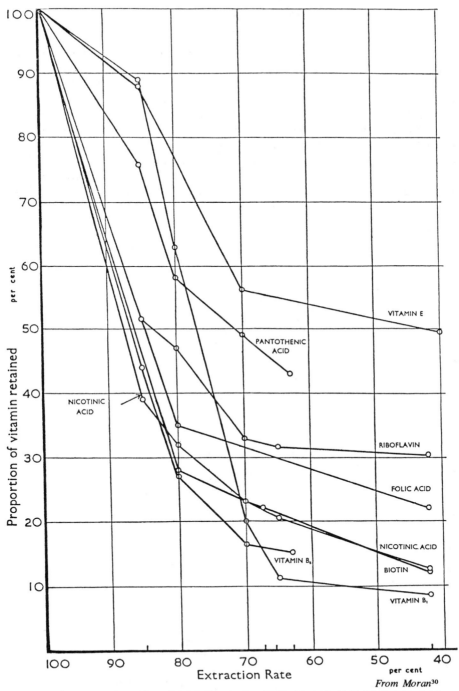

FIG. 2.3. THE RELATION BETWEEN EXTRACTION RATE AND PROPORTION OF THE TOTAL VITAMINS OF THE GRAIN RETAINED IN FLOUR

flour) against the proportion of vitamin retained and similar losses of minerals (Fig. 2.4).[31-33]

When specific vitamins[26] are investigated in food processing, their peculiar nature must be considered. For example, the term, vitamin B_6, in foods refers to a group of 2-methyl-3-hydroxy-5-hydroxymethylpyridine compounds and the active vitamin B_6 compound can be either an alcohol (pyridoxine), an aldehyde (pyridoxal) or an amine (pyridoxamine) or a phosphate ester of either of the above 3 forms, all 6 compounds differing in thermal and storage ability properties. Likewise folate in food tissue exists in the methyl, formyl and other forms of folylpolyglutamates of at least five glytamyl residues. These different forms again have different stability char-

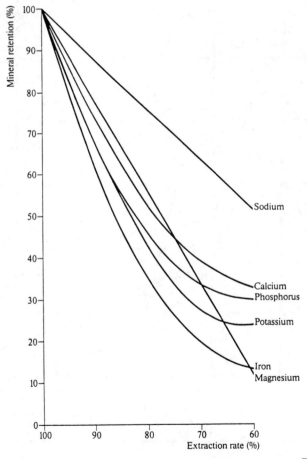

From Thomas[31]

FIG. 2.4. CHANGES IN MINERAL CONTENT OF WHEAT GRAIN WITH MILLING

acteristics influencing their behavior in food processing and storage operations. The pyridoxine form of vitamin B_6, and the folic acid form of folate are the more stable ones and are the ones produced chemically for additions to food. For a more extensive and detailed discussion of the influence of food processing on the nutrient content of food the reference book of Karmas and Harris[34] should be consulted as well as current reviews.[24,27,35]

CHANGING LIVING AND MARKET PLACE PATTERNS

There is a new style of living,[36,37] with more mobility, job changing, divorces and one parent homes. Food consumption in the United States has shifted from traditional to varying patterns. Eating habits no longer follow a routine of three meals a day at home. A majority of women are in the workforce, more two-income households, more male and female single homemakers, all with less time for meal preparation. Skipped meals are more commonplace. Peterson and Stone[38] raised the issue more than 20 years ago, namely, will fabricated foods revolutionize mealtime? They proclaimed that new manufactured foods would first imitate, then evolve from the natural, then become increasingly novel. They also foretold of kitchen changes, the eventual disappearance of the conventional oven and less time in food preparation.

There are fewer occasions where household members eat together. From National Food Consumption Survey (NFCS) data, Evans and Cronin[39] report that 29–50% of eating occasions of individuals age 6–18 and 35–50 years of age were shared with nonhousehold members or were eaten alone. Snacking is a common practice regardless of age, providing about 20% of calories in this form of eating. The share of the food dollar spent to eat away from home[40] was 25% in 1954 and was approximately 45% in 1985 at food costs 2½ times greater than that prepared at home. Much of this money[40] goes to the fast food restaurants (Fig. 2.5). An impact study of eating away from home indicated that persons 22 years old and younger favored fast food establishments; those over 22 years old favored restaurants.[41] Although the nutrient density of food eaten away from home is slightly lower than at home, individuals (1977–79 NFCS and 1985 CSFII) did not eat out frequently enough to shift the adequacy of their diets significantly. However, if the practice continues, individuals will be putting themselves at greater risk of certain nutrient inadequacies (calcium, magnesium, vitamin A, vitamin B_6 and ascorbic acid) and of caloric excess with evidence for predisposition to obesity which already exists.[41]

There are present concerns about eating right in order to remain healthy. Decades ago, when daily life was less sedentary, the volume of food consumed would contain 3,000–4,500 calories. Because of the amount of energy needed to perform physical work extended over long periods, it was more likely that daily nutrient needs were met. With present day food consumption supplying only 1,500–2,400 calories daily, the choices of individual foods must be very carefully made to meet micronutrient needs.[42] In a 1986 consumer attitude and supermarket survey (1,004

Shares of Away-from-Home Food Market Sales

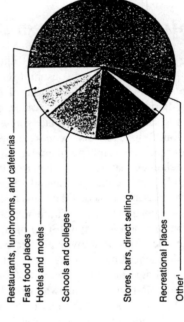

- Restaurants, lunchrooms, and cafeterias
- Fast food places
- Hotels and motels
- Schools and colleges
- Stores, bars, direct selling
- Recreational places
- Other[1]

Food Away from Home...
At a Glance

This country has more than 700,000 places to eat out, ranging from hot dog vendors at the ball park to school cafeterias. In 1985, these establishments sold $168 billion worth of meals and snacks (excluding alcoholic beverages). Fast food establishments have been big winners in the market share battle. These restaurants accounted for 32 percent of away-from-home sales in 1985, compared with 5 percent in 1958. At the same time, however, conventional restaurants, lunchrooms, cafeterias, and other commercial food-service establishments have seen their share of away-from-home sales decline from 54 percent to 42 percent.

CONCEPTS AND PRACTICES 33

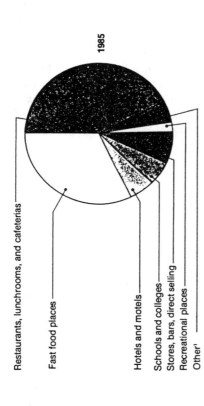

FIG. 2.5. FOOD AWAY FROM HOME: CONSUMPTION PATTERNS

From Anon.[40]

¹ Includes military clubs and exchanges, civic clubs and organizations, manufacturing plants, offices, child day care, and dining cars.

telephone interviews), 93% indicated they were very or somewhat concerned about the nutritive content of the foods they eat.[43] They were interested in "healthy foods" and their specific concerns were tabulated (Table 2.3). Yet, in choosing main course items, the most common reason given was taste, followed by ease of preparation, then nutrition and health value and economy.

American households[44] are getting smaller, from 3.7 persons in 1940 to 2.7 in 1982, with ¼ of all households having only one member. The cooking skills of younger people are minimal, hence they prefer "ready-to-eat" food. The future indicates an increased demand for convenience food at home, an increased demand for quick service when eating out and an increased use of food take-out services.[45] The emphasis is on foods that are fully prepared, tasty, healthy and nutrient-dense. There is an increased demand for diet-health information. Shoppers show interest in low or limited calorie, low cholesterol and low sodium foods.[46] With the new more convenient foods, more than half of all adults eat breakfast and another 19% try to. Menus are simpler, but more dinners are eaten in family shifts. Sales of dried fruit snacks and granola-based bars are up. There is a "grazing" trend[47] leading to an increase in the sale of finger foods, snacks for microwave preparation, single serve portion, and takeout from convenience stores. A current study comparing a grazing pattern of 17 hourly snacks during the day to the regular pattern of 3 daily meals revealed lower serum cholesterol and serum insulin levels in the subjects when nibbling.[48] Almost 75% of U.S. homes have one microwave oven and 15% have two. The microwaveable ready-to-eat food industry in the United States, Japan, and United Kingdom is booming.[49]

FOOD GUIDES

There is a fairly universal human desire to eat a so-called "balanced diet," meaning that it should provide proper nutrition. When discussing the balanced diet,[50] is it to be judged in terms of foods or nutrients or dietary goals? Food is the input to nutrition, but it is not nutrition itself. Food is any substance taken into the body to sustain physiological and psychological life, to provide energy and to promote nutrition. Most foods will have some nutritive value depending on a number of variables. There is a difference between a food delivery system and a nutrient delivery system. Nutrition is the sum of all the biochemical and physiological processes that are concerned with growth, maintenance and repair of the living organism. Within the food delivery systems there exist degrees of possible food combination choices spanning a continuum from voluntary to involuntary choices (Table 2.4). In everyday life, consumer experience varies on a continuum between voluntary (free choice) food and meal selection and involuntary (restricted) or no choice (prescribed) food and meal selection. The priorities which shift are sensory appeal, cost and perceived health benefits.

TABLE 2.3
NATURE OF SHOPPERS' CONCERN ABOUT THE
NUTRITIONAL CONCEPT OF FOOD (VOLUNTEERED)[1]

Base: The shopping public

Q: What is it about the nutritional content of what you eat that concerns you and your family the most? What else?

Response	1983 Total (%)	1984 Total (%)	1985 Total (%)	1986 Total (%
Vitamin/mineral content	24	19	17	22
Salt content, less salt	18	17	19	20
Sugar content, less sugar	21	22	20	18
Fat content, low fat	9	8	13	17
Chemical additives (e.g., flavoring, MSG, steroids)	27	25	18	16
No preservatives	22	17	13	15
Making sure we get a balanced diet	10	9	11	14
Cholesterol levels	5	8	10	13
Food/nutritional value	10	19	14	11
Calories, low calories	6	9	9	11
Freshness, purity, no spoilage	14	12	8	8
Desire to be healthy/eat what's good for us	0	0	3	6
No harmful ingredients, nothing that causes illness/cancer	10	6	5	5
Protein value	5	6	4	5
As natural as possible, not overly processed	12	6	5	3
Fiber content	2	1	2	3
Empty calories, junk food	4	4	5	2
Excess food coloring/dyes	6	4	3	2
Carbohydrate content	1	2	2	2
Less red meat	0	0	2	2
Artifical sweetener	0	0	2	1
Quality of food	3	5	1	1
Starch content	1	1	1	1
Other	2	4	1	5
Don't know/refused	5	5	6	5

Source: Farr.[43]
From *Trends— Consumer Attitudes and the Supermarket*. Reprinted with permission of the Food Marketing Institute.

About 100 years ago menu or meal planning was started,[51] applying the early knowledge of nutrition. Later, food guidelines by the USDA were devised for the consumer around daily selections of the number of servings of 7 groups of foods. This was revised in 1956 for greater ease of understanding and use into 4 food groups (milk and dairy products; meat, poultry and fish; vegetables and fruit; bread and

TABLE 2.4
FOOD DELIVERY SYSTEM ON A VOLUNTARY/INVOLUNTARY CONTINUUM

	Category I Voluntary	Category II Voluntary	Category III Involuntary	Category IV Involuntary
Menu	Full	Limited	Offer vs. serve	Prescribed
Choice	Free	Free	Limited or preplanned	Little or none
Place	Home or restaurant	Home or restaurant; fast food restaurant	Educational or penal institution	Health care institution
Example of federal program	Food stamps	WIC; supplemental feeding	Title III & nutrition programs	Meals on Wheels
Balanced diet?	Maybe	Maybe if planned	Likely because it is program goal	Yes, with additional health aspects also
Uses dietitian?	No	In some cases	Likely	Required
Priorities of food selection	1. Appeal 2. Cost 3. Balance	1. Appeal 2. Cost 3. Balance	1. Cost 2. Balance 3. Appeal	1. Balance 2. Cost (variable) 3. Appeal

Source: Lachance.[50]

cereal products) (Fig. 2.6). A study of the underlying assumptions for U.S. food guides from 1917 through the basic four food groups guide is available.[52] Present food guides have been in usage for over 30 years but have limitations. Serving numbers and the amount recommended for each food group are indicated but have not been followed;[37] see Fig. 2.7. Dietary guidelines simply state, eat a variety of foods. What does this mean? Do food guides translate into diet patterns providing an adequate intake of micronutrients conducive to good health? With thousands of items in large food stores, ponder the problem of dividing them into 4 or 5 food groups. The food group concept sounds good and is a widely used teaching tool but some wonder if the food group concept hasn't been simplified to the point where it is useless[53] in the present day food markets.

The use of the basic food group guide is questioned periodically. Analyzing data from the 1977–78 Nationwide Food Consumption Survey (NFCS), it appears that only about 3% of the U.S. population actually follows the recommendation to the letter and the majority of those who do so consume excessive amounts of fat.[54] A Secretary of Agriculture in 1977 commented that it is no longer enough to recommend a regular diet from the four basic food groups and that this kind of advice has produced a nation malnourished in a new way, leading to overindulgence and obesity.[55] The nutrient content of 20 daily menus published as examples of well-balanced diets based on the four food groups as determined by computer analyses[56] revealed that they provided 60% or less of the adult RDA for vitamin E, vitamin B_6, magnesium, zinc and iron. Modifications of the basic four food groups were suggested for diet improvement but extensive nutrition education will be needed at all levels, if the food choices of the population are to be improved. A similar study of frozen meals approved for school lunches revealed analogous results.[57]

A major problem is not with the thousands of consumer food items but with the consumer's ability to deal effectively with the food choices presented.[58] The consumer either does not know how to put these foods together to make a suitable diet or does not desire to do so. The marketing component of the food industry may also confuse the consumer and create a credibility gap. The consumer must have the education to choose a balanced diet among the types of foods, food substitutes and fabricated products offered today because foods of the future will continue to be less traditional.[59] Food nutrification is needed particularly for the low calorie diet consumers and to assure against nutrient dilution by formulated and fabricated foods that are not nutrified.

The nutritional labeling laws, approved in 1975, provided the U.S. consumer, on a voluntary basis, with additional information on food content and nutritive value

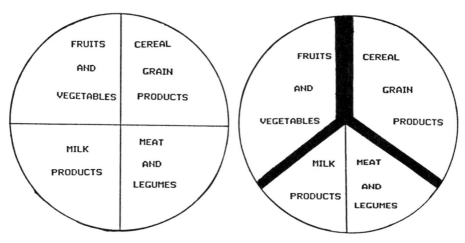

FIG. 2.6. THE BASIC FOUR FOOD GUIDE

Left: The Basic Four food guide, as shown in a four-leaf-clover array, is the most established food combination education scheme in the United States (USDA/AS-62-4, 1956). The number of servings of food to be consumed from each food group (4-4-2-2) was taught separately.

Right: The proportion of the food groups recommended can be represented graphically in a manner representing the plate at each meal, wherein two thirds of the food is of plant origin and only one third is of animal origin. (Reprinted with permission from Lachance, PA. Food Technology. 1981:35:58. Copyright © by Institute of Food Technologists.)

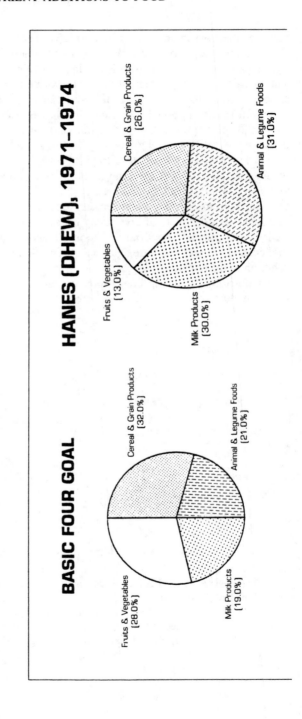

CONCEPTS AND PRACTICES 39

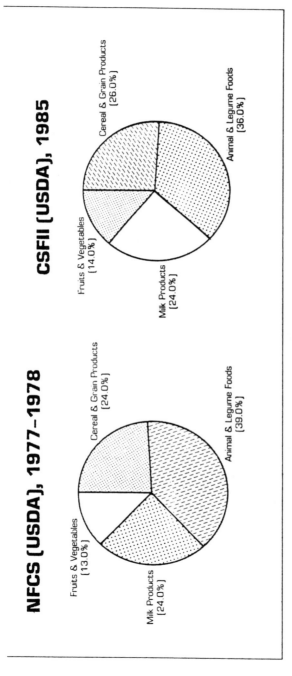

FIG. 2.7. BASIC FOUR COMPARISONS

A comparison of the Basic Four recommendation to actual eating patterns. The Basic Four recommendation approximates the recommended 4:4:2:2: servings per day of key food groups. What Americans have been eating is reflected in the 1971-74 HANES data, the 1977-78 NFCS data, and the 1985 CSFII data. Rather than consuming 2 servings of plant derived food for each serving of animal derived food, as recommended by the Basic Four food guide concept, the consumer is doing the opposite. Copyright © Institute of Food Technologists.

of food purchases with specific items being required on the food label.[60] Label information includes serving size, and calorie, carbohydrates, fat and protein content. Protein content and the content of five vitamins (vitamins A, C, thiamin, riboflavin and niacin) and two minerals (calcium and iron) are required as the percentage of the USRDA in one serving. Optionally, the content of other vitamins (vitamin B_6, B_{12}, D, E, biotin, folate and pantothenate) and other minerals (iodine, copper, magnesium, phosphorus and zinc) may also be listed in the same manner. Sodium content is optional and can be reported without triggering full nutritional labeling. Nutrient contents of less than 2% of the USRDA per serving are designated by an asterisk. The latter also means that a product with zero nutrients content is labeled as having 2% or less!

After more than a decade of use, how helpful has the food labeling program been in enabling the consumer to prepare a balanced diet? By 1985 it was estimated that nutritional labeling had expanded to include more than 50% of the foods regulated by FDA in supermarkets.[61] Surveys have indicated that consumers have used the food label to avoid or to control purchase based on the calorie, fat, salt and sugar content of foods. Consumers also reported that the presently used label format is difficult to use. Pressure is being applied on the FDA to improve the format, and labeling changes are now underway. However, little information is available to indicate that the food labeling program greatly helps the consumer to formulate and put into practice nutrient-balanced meals. As predicted,[60] the initial regulation has increased our knowledge of the nutrient content of foods by requiring the industry to collect such data for labeling and/or consumer inquiries.

Legislation has been passed by Congress (Public Law 1) requiring food labeling on all food and to alter the current labeling to provide more information on ingredients relative to meeting dietary goals, e.g., *percent* saturated fat. The FDA has held[62] a series of regional hearings to answer a number of questions concerning a new nutrition labeling format. A likely outcome is the label format given in Fig. 2.8. Also at issue[63] is the use of the food label to provide specific health claim information, which the FDA must regulate.

The consumer, not being able to readily use the initial format, has voted for a label change. Consumer activists are promoting a new format which provides information relative to health risks, rather than nutrients and nutrition needs. It is predicted that the new format will not provide nutrient density information nor food combination information, both of which are needed to improve food combinations for nutrient balance. As a result, nutrification will continue to be an essential deterrent to marginal and outright malnutrition.

DIETARY AND HEALTH SURVEYS

Concern was expressed[64] more than 10 years ago about elevated blood cholesterol levels in the U.S. population and the prevalence of obesity in the population. In

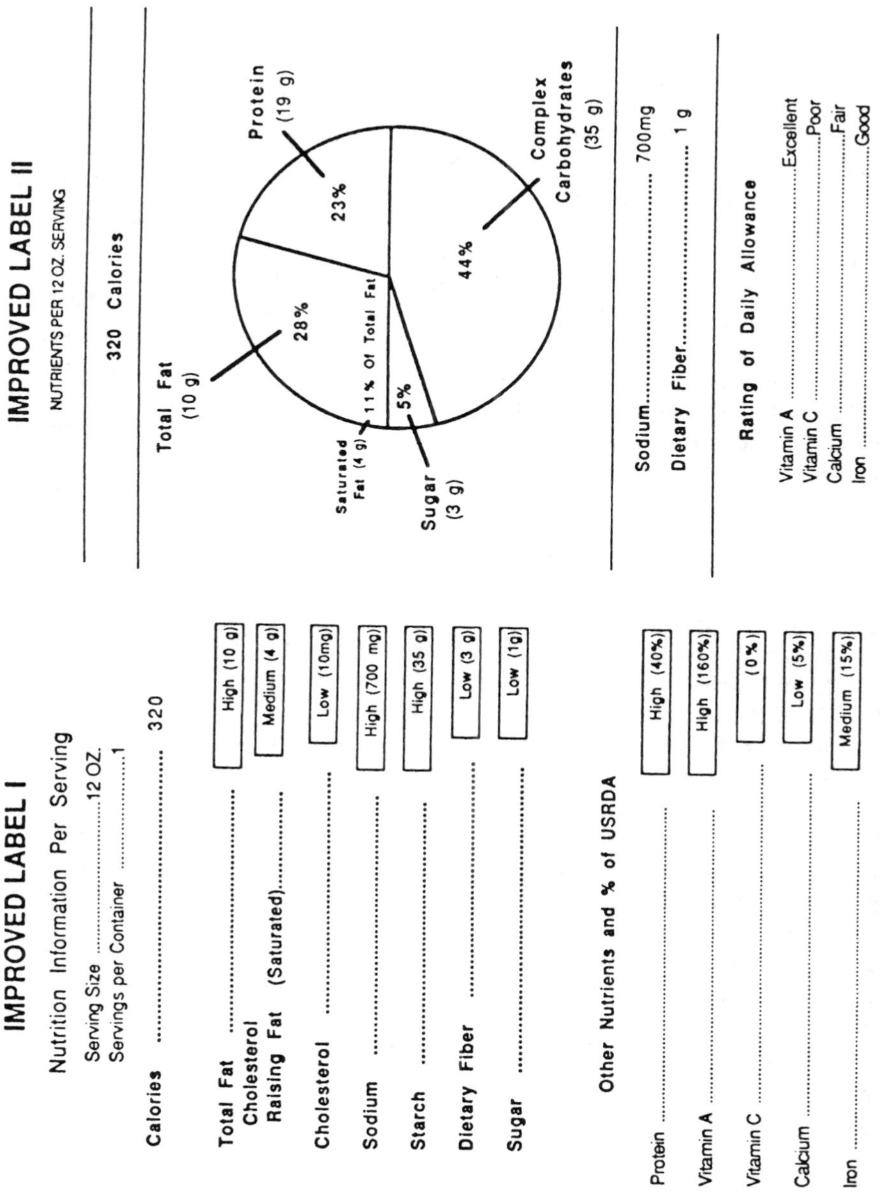

CONCEPTS AND PRACTICES 41

IMPROVED LABEL I

Nutrition Information Per Serving

Serving Size .... 12 OZ.
Servings per Container 1

Calories 320

Total Fat .... [High (10 g)]
Cholesterol
Raising Fat (Saturated)........ [Medium (4 g)]

Cholesterol .... [Low (10mg)]

Sodium .... [High (700 mg)]

Starch .... [High (35 g)]

Dietary Fiber .... [Low (3 g)]

Sugar .... [Low (1g)]

Other Nutrients and % of USRDA

Protein .... [High (40%)]

Vitamin A .... [High (160%)]

Vitamin C .... [(0%)]

Calcium .... [Low (5%)]

Iron .... [Medium (15%)]

IMPROVED LABEL II

NUTRIENTS PER 12 OZ. SERVING

320 Calories

Total Fat (10 g) — 28%
Saturated Fat (4 g) 11% Of Total Fat
Sugar (3 g) — 5%
Protein (19 g) — 23%
Complex Carbohydrates (35 g) — 44%

Sodium 700mg
Dietary Fiber............................ 1 g

Rating of Daily Allowance

Vitamin A .... Excellent
Vitamin C .... Poor
Calcium .... Fair
Iron .... Good

FIG. 2.8. LABEL PROJECTIONS

1977 the Senate Select Committee on Nutrition and Human Needs published dietary goals linking 6 major causes of death (heart attack, stroke, arterioscelorsis, cancer, cirrhosis of the liver and diabetes) to diet and recommended quantitative decreases in fat (to 30% of calories) refined sugars (to 10% of calories) and salt consumption (to less than 4 g) and an increase in complex carbohydrate consumption.

A Nationwide Food Consumption Survey (NFCS) was carried out in 1977-78. Over the following years a number of reports were published based on data collected during the survey. In the 1977-78 NFCS survey, the average intakes for teenage girls and adult women (over 50%) were substantially below 70% of the RDA for both calcium and iron.[39] Alcohol consumption and the nutrient density of diets in the 1977-78 NFCS survey was examined by Windham et al.[65] The food consumption data available indicated that for those individuals who reported consuming alcohol, an average of 388 calories, or approximately 19% of total dietary calories, were contributed by alcoholic beverages and that the nutrient density of diets of drinkers was significantly lower than that of nondrinkers with respect to protein, fat, carbohydrate, calcium, iron, phosphorus, vitamin A and thiamin. Soft drink and milk intake were negatively correlated,[66] indicating that soft drink consumption may contribute to lower intakes of calcium, magnesium, riboflavin, vitamin A and vitamin C.

Based on diets[67,68] of 1,503 women (19-50 years of age) reported in the Spring of 1985 in the USDA's Continuing Survey of Food Intakes by individuals compared with diets of women of the same ages reported in the NFCS survey of spring 1977, the 1985 diets failed to provide recommended levels of several nutrients, calcium, iron, magnesium, zinc, vitamin B_6, and folate (Fig. 2.9). Fat supplied less energy in 1985 and carbohydrates more energy. Food eaten away from home supplied 25-30% of the nutrients examined; snacks provided 9-16%.

During 1976-80 the National Health and Nutrition Examination Survey (NHANES II) was conducted which indicated a mean energy intake of approximately 2,400 calories for males and 1,600 calories for females. These data for calories match CSFII findings in 1985. Processed foods were an important contributing source of many vital nutrients in the U.S. diet. Iron, zinc, folate, vitamin A, vitamin C and protein nutritional status are of concern.[69] Low iron status is apparent, but the degree of it varies according to which of the five measures of iron status is used for comparison. Poor zinc nutrition is also evident. Prevalence of low serum and red blood cell folacin values are compared with low hemoglobin levels. Poor persons had higher prevalences of low serum vitamin A value for all ages except adults. Low vitamin C plasma values were associated with low dietary intakes, smoking and low economic status.[69]

In a May 1986 Joint Nutrition Monitoring Evaluation Committee report,[70] 28% of Americans were reported as overweight. Intakes of iron and vitamin C were low in certain subgroups, also there were low intakes of calcium. From the NHANES survey, data are most complete for energy, protein, vitamins A and C, and iron; less complete for vitamins B_1, B_2, B_6, B_{12}, niacin, calcium and phosphorus; and least complete for fatty acids, fat, cholesterol, carbohydrates, added caloric sweeteners, fiber, folate, magnesium, sodium and zinc values. In a 1988 workshop on nutrition monitoring activities[71] there was general agreement that good nutrition is essential for good health and if earlier indicators could be established at various life cycle stages for encouraging health, health care costs could be significantly lowered through a preventative approach to the pathogenesis of metabolic and chronic diseases. Toward that goal an effort is being made to improve the current methodologies and systems of gathering, recording, interpreting and retrieving data taken in dietary surveys, biochemical studies and clinical surveys to arrive at nutritional status as it relates to health in the population.

The dietary goals set forth by the Select Senate Committee on Nutrition and Human Needs are directional indicators intended for better health, but with only average consumer understanding and ability for making the dietary adaptations required, more nutrition knowledge is needed.[53] The USDA/DHHS Dietary Guidelines provide a broader (qualitative) set of general directions. A summary of U.S. guidelines is available.[72] In the last 10 years, national dietary guidelines have emerged in several countries. These guidelines (Table 2.5) go beyond nutritional goals and can be re-

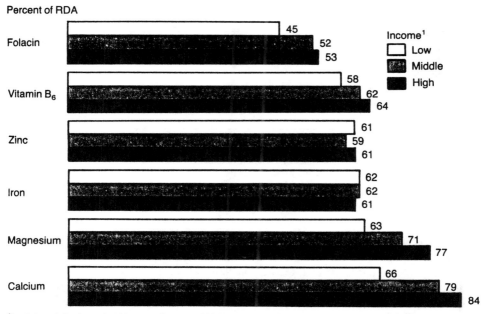

[1]Low income defined as under 131 percent of poverty; middle income, 131 to 300 percent; high income, over 300 percent.
Source: CSFII-85, HNIS, USDA.

From Peterkin and Rizek[68]

FIG. 2.9. DIETS OF HIGH- AND LOW-INCOME WOMEN ARE SHORT OF RDA GOALS FOR SOME NUTRIENTS

TABLE 2.5
THEMES OF VARIOUS NATIONAL DIETARY GUIDELINES

Recommendation	1968 Sweden	1980, 1985 USA	1985 Japan	Most Common in 17 Sets[3]	1987 Korean Proposal	1987 Brazilian Proposal
Eat						
A variety of foods		+	+	+	+	+[6]
Selected foods	+[1]			+[4]	+[5]	
Starch and fiber		+		+[4]		
Enjoy						
Meals with family			+		+	+
Maintain						
Desirable weight	+	+		+	+	
A balance between calories and physical activity	+		+			
Good traditional food habits						+
Limit						
Fat, mainly saturated fat	+	+	+[2]	+		
Sugar	+	+		+		
Salt (sodium)		+	+	+	+	
Alcohol		+		+		
Provide						
Inexpensive local foods						+

Source: Olson.[73]
[1]Vegetables, fruits, potatoes, skim milk, fish, lean meats, and cereal products.
[2]Be aware that the quality and quantity of fat are important.
[3]Analysis of guidelines from 13 industrialized countries.
[4]Includes fiber, starch, fruits, vegetables, and cereals.
[5]Two guidelines: 1) legumes and fish and 2) milk.
[6]Ensure enough nutritious food.

garded as general health guidelines and are especially applicable to persons at higher risk.[73]

The 1988 Surgeon General's Report[74] on Nutrition and Health contains 5 generally applicable recommendations, namely, reduce dietary saturated fats and *blood* cholesterol, maintain desirable weight, increase complex carbohydrates and fiber, reduce sodium and reduce alcohol; for some people, use sources of fluorides, limit sugars, increase calcium and consume more iron.

In the 1989 National Academy Press publication, "Diet & Health" dietary recommendations[75] include daily consumption of 5 or more servings of a combination of vegetables and fruits, increasing intake of starches and complex carbohydrates by eating 6 or more daily servings of a combination of breads, cereals and legumes, maintaining adequate calcium intake, maintaining protein intake at moderate levels, maintaining adequate intake of fluoride, reducing total fat intake, reducing saturated fatty acid intake, reducing cholesterol intake, limiting salt intake, limiting dietary supplement consumption, limiting alcohol intake by drinkers and balancing food intake against physical activity for maintenance of body weight.

In the opinion of many, optimal health is closely aligned with proper nutrition and dietary habits practiced over a lifetime. Dietary practices and nutrition are believed to have a major influence on the etiology of chronic diseases, such as hypertension, diabetes, heart disease and some types of cancer for some population segments. There is, however, some disagreement[11] both among and between public health officials over the use of scientific knowledge in associations between diet and the incidence of chronic and degenerative disease in establishing public health policy. Such a situation, in the opinion of one nutritionist[11] brings about conflicts which could undermine the confidence of the public in both the science of nutrition and in public health policy. Communicating current nutrition information to the public deserves a high priority.[76]

The growing complexity of nutrition monitoring is illustrated by the number of activities under way or in planning in federal agencies and departments involved (Table 2.6) on the Washington scene. Nutrients included in past U.S. surveys[75] have been tabulated (Table 2.7). Nutrition monitoring, not only of the general population but for U.S. population segments at risk (such as the 10 million alcoholics, the 25 million aged and about 40 million on some kind of a weight reduction program), ought to be included in future studies.

NUTRIFICATION OF FOOD

With the general public consuming fewer calories than in decades past, according to recent dietary surveys,[68,69] women are taken in 1500–1600 calories and men, 2300–2400 calories. There is also a dieting population of millions of people with daily intakes of 900–1200 calories to reduce weight, and the elderly are curtailing food consumption in the range of 1250–1650 calories compared to earlier stages in a more active lifestyle. As a result, there is concern about the need to increase the nutrient density of foods to assure that diets of lower calorie intake supply the required daily allowance of known micronutrients. In one study an examination of 11 weight reducing diets, thiamin, vitamins B_6, B_{12}, calcium, iron, zinc and magnesium levels were below recommendations.[77] The trend[78] toward the modification of traditional food and the fabrication of new foods will likely accelerate in the future as the consumer will demand: (1) better nutrient balance and delivery in food products to ensure healthy fitness and longevity; (2) more convenience in terms of portion size, packaging, preparation, cooking or microwaving; (3) safety and wholesomeness; and (4) most importantly, quality characteristics such as good flavor, tex-

TABLE 2.6
NUTRITION MONITORING AND RELATED ACTIVITIES OF THE FEDERAL GOVERNMENT

Category	Activity	Department[1]	Agency[1]	Population	Timing
Health and nutritional status measurements	National Health and Nutrition Examination Surveys	DHHS	NCHS	U.S. population, special groups	
	NHANES I			1–75 yr	1971–1974
	NHANES II			6 mo–74 yr	1976–1980
	Hispanic HANES			6 mo–74 yr	1982–1984
	NHANES III			2 mo+	1988–1994
	National Health Interview Survey	DHHS	NCHS	U.S.	Annual
	NHIS Special Topics	DHHS	NCHS	U.S.	Selected topics
	NHANES I Epidemiologic Followup	DHHS	NCHS	NHANES I elderly	1982–1984, 1987, 1986
	National Survey of Family Growth	DHHS	NCHS	Women 15–44	1976, 1983, 1987
	National Maternal and Infant Health Survey	DHHS	NCHS		Planned 1988
	National Mortality Survey	DHHS	DCHS		Annual 1961–1968, 1986
	Vital Statistics	DHHS	NCHS	U.S., states, counties, local areas	Annual
	Coordinated State Surveillance System	DHHS	CDC	Pregnant women, children	Continuous
	Behavioral Risk Factor Surveillance System	DHHS	CDC	Adults	Continuous
	Nutrition Research in Support of Nutrition Monitoring[2]	DHHS USDA	NIH, ARS CDC, FDA	Varies	Ongoing

CONCEPTS AND PRACTICES

Category	Survey/Study	Agency	Subagency	Population	Frequency
Food consumption measurements	Nationwide Food Consumption Survey	USDA	HNIS		Every 10 years Current 1987–88
	Continuing Survey of Food Intakes by Individuals (CSFII) 1985 and 1986	USDA	HNIS	U.S. low-income sample Women 19–50, their children, low-income men, low-income sample	Annual
	1989 and beyond			U.S. population, low-income sample, Other	Annual (planned)
	NHANES	DHHS	NCHS	U.S. population	See above
	Total Diet Study	DHHS	FDA	Specific age-sex groups	Annual
	Vitamin/Mineral Supplement Adverse Reactions	DHHS	FDA	U.S.	Continuous
Food composition measurements	Nutrient Data Bank	USDA	HNIS		Continuous
	Nutrient Composition Laboratory	USDA	ARS		Continuous
	Food Labeling and Package Survey	DHHS	FDA		Annual and biennial parts
	Total Diet Study	DHHS	FDA		Annual
	Fiber, Carotenoid and Vitamin A Comparison	DHHS	NIH/NCI NIH/NIDDK		Ongoing
	Studies: Taurine and Biotin Comparison Studies			Ongoing	
Dietary knowledge and attitude assessment	Health and Diet Survey	DHHS	FDA	U.S. adults	18–22 month intervals
	Survey of Infant Feeding Practices	DHHS	FDA	Pregnant women	1988 or 1989
	Survey of Weight-Loss Practices		FDA, NIH/NHLBI		
	Cholesterol Awareness Survey	DHHS	FDA, NIH/NHLBI	U.S. adults	1987 or 1988
	Nursing and Dietitian Survey	DHHS	NIH/	Physicians	1986

TABLE 2.6 (Continued)

Category	Activity	Department[1]	Agency[1]	Population	Timing
	NHIS Special Topics	DHHS	NHLBI	Nurses, dieticians	1986, 1987
	Health Promotion/Disease Prevention	DHHS	NCHS	U.S. adults	1985
	Vitamin/Mineral Supplement/Cancer Control		+NIH/NCI		1986
	CSFII Followup (Consumer Perceptions Survey)	USDA/DHHS	HNIS FSIS, FDA NIH/	U.S. population	1987
	Physician Knowledge Survey on Hypertension	DHHS	NHLBI	Physicians	Planned 1989–1996
	Cancer Prevention Awareness Program	DHHS	NIH/NCI	U.S. adults	1978–1988
Food supply determinations	Supply Data	USDA	ERS/HNIS	U.S. population	1984–Ongoing
	Demand Studies	USDA	ERS	U.S. population	Annual
					Continuous

[1]Abbreviations used are: ARS, Agricultural Research Service; CDC, Centers for Disease Control; DHHS, Department of Health and Human Services; ERS, Economic Research Service, FDA, Food and Drug Administration; FSIS, Food Safety and Inspection Service; HNIS, Human Nutrition Information Service; NCHS, National Center for Health Services; NCI, National Cancer Institute; NHIS, National Health Interview Survey; NHLBI, National Heart, Lung, and Blood Institutes; NIDDK, National Institute of Diabetes and Digestive and Kidney Diseases; NIH, National Institutes of Health; USDA, U.S. Department of Agriculture.

[2]Includes research on nutritional status assessment and requirements throughout the life cycle. The nutritional status research focuses on (1) indices of nutritional status, (2) micromethods to measure nutrient concentrations in various tissues and plasma and (3) methods that improve accuracy of dietary intake data.

ture and mouthfeel. This signals that the market will need to provide more food products that have been totally engineered and fabricated from functional components (protein, fat, carbohydrates, vitamins and minerals).

Among the interventions to be considered in national or international food programs, nutrification,[79-81] the addition of one or more nutrients to one or more commonly consumed foods or food mixtures can, if properly introduced and controlled, improve the dietary intake of a group, community or population. The term, to nutrify, or the process of nutrification, merely means to make a food more nutritious. Nutrification increases the nutrient density of food products. Nutrification is used here as a replacement term for fortification, enrichment, restoration, supplementation, etc., terms which originally had different meanings and were borrowed from disciplines or applications other than food use. Nutrification is the most rapidly applied, the most flexible, and the most socially acceptable intervention method of changing the intake of nutrients without a vast educational effort and without changing the current food patterns of a given population. The principle of nutrification challenges a long-standing belief that the consumer must consciously desire and be involved in nutritional change.[82] Food nutrification usually has a favorable cost-benefit ratio compared to other intervention methods. Once a nutrification program involving the addition of a single nutrient has been initiated, adding a second or subsequent nutrients is an easier task and per nutrient costs are lower. An educational effort along with any nutrification plan may be used to explain the goal of the program and to introduce, if warranted, other interventions, such as improved agricultural and health practices.

One can envision at various periods in past history that on more than one occasion some individual did make an addition to a food item which was based on the state of knowledge at the time. Such an early nutrification attempt[83] occurred in 4000 B.C. when the Persian physician, Melampus, medical advisor to Jason and the Argonauts, prescribed sweet wine laced with iron filings to strengthen the sailors resistance to spears and arrows and to enhance their sexual potency. Boussingault, a French physician recommended in 1831 the addition of iodine to table salt to prevent the development of goiter. Realistic large-scale nutrient additions to food, however, could not take place until the 20th century when both biochemical and physiological knowledge and the availability of economical pure forms of the nutrients and technology were on hand so the additions could be carried out in a meaningful and controlled manner. Between the end of World War I and the end of World War II, iodine was added to salt, vitamins A and D to margarine, vitamin D to milk, and thiamin, riboflavin, niacin and iron to flour and bread.

PROS AND CONS OF NUTRIFICATION

Some phases of nutrification of food have been in effect for over 80 years, yet its merits and demerits continue to be expressed in the literature.

TABLE 2.7
NUTRIENTS AND OTHER FOOD CONSTITUENTS REPORTED BY NATIONAL STUDIES[1]

Nutrient or Food Constituent	Historical Food Supply[2]	1977-1978 NFCS[3] House-hold	1977-1978 NFCS[3] Individual	1985 CSFII[4]	NHANES[5] I	NHANES[5] II	Total Diet Study[6]	Food Composition[7]
Water	−	−	−	−	−	−	−	+
Energy (kcal)	+	+	+	+	+	+	−	+
Protein, total	+	+	+	+	+	+	−	+
Amino acids	−	−	−	−	−	−	−	*/**
Carbohydrates, total	+	+	+	+	−	+	−	+
Sugars	+	−	**	−	−	−	−	−
Lipids								
Total fat	+	+	+	+	−	+	−	+
Saturated fat	+	−	−	+	−	+	−	*
Oleic acid	+	−	−	−	−	+	−	*
Total mono unsaturated fat	−	−	−	+	−	−	−	*
Linoleic acid	+	−	−	−	−	+	−	*
Total polyun-saturated fat	−	−	−	+	−	−	−	*
Cholesterol	+	−	**	+	−	+	−	*
Vitamins								
A, IU	+	+	+	+	+	+	−	+
A, RE	−	−	−	−	−	−	−	*
Carotene	−	−	−	+	−	−	−	−
E	−	−	−	+	−	−	−	*/**
Thiamin (B$_1$)	+	+	+	+	+	+	−	+
Riboflavin (B$_2$)	+	+	+	+	+	+	−	+
Niacin (preformed)	+	+	+	+	+	+	−	+
Pantothenic acid	**	−	−	−	−	−	−	*/**
B$_6$	+	+	+	+	−	−	−	+
Folate	**	−	−	−	−	−	−	*/**
B$_{12}$	+	+	+	+	−	−	−	+
C	+	+	+	+	+	+	−	+
Minerals								
Calcium	+	+	+	+	+	+	+	+
Phosphorus	+	+	+	+	−	+	+	+
Magnesium	+	+	+	+	−	−	+	+
Iron	+	+	+	+	+	+	+	+
Iodine	−	−	−	−	−	−	+	−
Sodium	+	−	**	+	−	+	+	+
Potassium	+	−	−	+	−	+	+	+

TABLE 2.7 (*Continued*)

Nutrient or Food Constituent	Historical Food Supply[2]	1977-1978 NFCS[3] House-hold	1977-1978 NFCS[3] Individual	1985 CSFII[4]	NHANES[5] I	NHANES[5] II	Total Diet Study[6]	Food Composition[7]
Copper	−	−	−	+	−	−	+	*/**
Zinc	+	−	−	+	−	−	+	*
Manganese	−	−	−	−	−	−	+	*/**
Selenium	−	−	−	−	−	−	+	−
Chromium	−	−	−	−	−	−	+	−
Fiber, crude	+	−	−	−	−	−	+	+
Dietary	−	−	−	+	−	−	−	**
Alcoholic beverages	−	+	+	+	−	+	+	+

Source: Anon.[75]
NOTE: +, Data reported; −, data not reported; *, nutrient data will be available in revised USDA Agriculture Handbook No. 8 (USDA, in press); **, data incomplete or questionable.
[1]Table based on information from USDA (1987a) and Woteki (1986).
[2]USDA's food supply data indicating disappearance of food into consumer channels.
[3]Nationwide Food Consumption Survey (USDA, 1984).
[4]Continuing Survey of Food Intakes of Individuals (USDA, 1985, 1986b).
[5]National Health and Nutrition Examination Survey I (1971-1974) and II (1976-1980).
[6]Total Diet Study of Food and Drug Administration (unpublished data).
[7]Woteki (1986).

Kline (1974)

Food fortification recommendations were highly visible in the 1969 White House Conference Final Report. The panel on new food proposed an immediate food fortification program to provide to the public nutritionally complete food to relieve under- and malnutrition. The food quality panel recommended mandatory fortification to the original nutrient content or above, where appropriate, be established for certain basic foods. The panel on food manufacturing and processing specifically favored enrichment efforts and proposed that the food industry accelerate its efforts to make available nutritious snack foods. Kline[84] favored improvement of snack foods (as well as other between-meal foods used by teenagers) by application of enrichment and protein supplementation proportionate to caloric contribution.

Beaton (1976)

Food fortification[85] can be an extremely important intervention procedure for improving or maintaining the nutritional qualities of the food supply, depending on local situations, nutrient needs, food consumption patterns, including processed foods.

Berg (1973)

Fortification[82], one of the most attractive alternatives available to the government office responsible for nutritional betterment, has a small expense and can quickly be introduced to reach large numbers of people without the need of a massive organizational or administrative apparatus.

Tannenbaum (1979)

Food fortification[86] is a social policy, adopted on the basis of sound scientific information to correct a public health problem.

Stare (1979)

Human nutrition in a progressive environment with far more people will depend more and more on fortified foods, particularly fortified cereal products.[87] One might add fortified potatoes and fortified sugars, cheap and efficient sources of energy. We will be fortifying these basic foods, possibly even tea, coffee and soft drinks.

Hegsted (1976)

Fortification of food with nutrients is a logical tool[88] for the control of malnutrition, and undoubtedly fortification will increase in the future. The major and unresolved problems of the immediate future, considering our fragmentary knowledge of the nutritional need of humans, is to develop a rational policy that prevents overreliance on fortification.

Darby and Hambraeus (1978)

A major contribution to an increased food supply can be made through developing nutritionally designed processed products based in large measure on cereal, tuber or other primarily carbohydrate crops and utilizing nutrients that can be produced through chemical and microbiological procedures, either directly for mankind or indirectly by first feeding them to animals producing edible products.[6] The great potential offered by wise utilization of industrially produced nutrients (edible byproducts, isolates, manufactured vitamins, minerals, amino acids, other enzymatically or microbiologically produced nutrients) is rarely fully realized.

Russo (1977)

"Let people eat what they want, but make sure the foods provide good nutrition" is a concept which emerged at the White House Conference. If a segment of the population is not receiving adequate vitamins, minerals and/or protein, then the foods that are being consumed should be fortified to provide appropriate nutrient values.[89]

Tepley (1974)

It seems reasonable to expect that the science and technology of food formulation and fortification will gradually be applied in all countries of the world; hopefully, this will promote a just distribution of the world's resources to provide a good diet for all.[90]

Quick and Murphy (1982)

When individuals decrease the quantity of food they consume, the requirements for most essential nutrients do not decrease in the same manner. As less foods are consumed it becomes important to increase the nutrient density of the energy foods consumed. Fortification of foods is one means of increasing nutrient density.[91]

Mertz (1977)

Fortification of foods with essential micronutrients is one of the great accomplishments of nutritional science. Fortification is only one solution to nutritional problems, and any effective program must be dynamic, utilizing new advances in nutritional knowledge as they become available.[92]

Latham (1984)

It can be agreed that because adequate nutrients are available, knowledge of requirements are inadequate, and greater potential with nutrition education, fortification should be limited. Supplementation is not the answer; it is nutrition education. Those favoring fortification say education is not the all-problem solver, that education assumes nutritional value of key foods, and there are built-in technological controls for overfortification. It can also be argued that nutrition education and nutrification are complementary. Food habits are difficult to change, and the rise of convenience foods also tends to support the need for food fortification.[93]

Lachance (1980)

Because of the changes in lifestyles and the nature of the food supply itself, and because of the loss of nutrients in food handling and preparation, fortification and restoration are logical and progressive steps toward the insurance of adequate nutrition on a national basis.[94]

Guthrie (1980)

Fortification should be limited to cases of adequately tested, clearly defined health problems. Left unregulated or unchecked it could become a costly promotional vehicle which will create a false sense of nutritional adequacy and ultimately undermine the quality of the food supply.[95]

Caliendo (1979)

Fortification limitations[96] are that (1) it can be used only with foods centrally processed; (2) it does not reach those who grow their own food or do not participate in a market economy; (3) it may reach those who do not need fortification; (4) it is a recurring cost; (5) the consumption of the carrier used may be a function of income, and (6) it does not add to calorie density needs of individuals.

Reidy (1981)

Obstacles and risks cited for fortification are: (1) identifying natural nutrient needs; (2) technological concerns of adding nutrients; (3) risk of toxic doses; (4) risks of exclusion of nutrients; and (5) consumers inability to discriminate between fortified and nonfortified foods.[97]

Christopher (1978)

Because we are a culture enchanted with technology, fortification has an immediate, popular appeal. Unfortunately, technology has a way of instituting change for the sake of change, without necessarily offering any new direction. Can we really accept that superfortification will eliminate our need to select widely from conventional foods to balance nutrient intake?[98]

Dymsza (1974)

The fortification case has not been adequately supported on the basis of need or social or scientific merit. There is an inadequate base of knowledge to support increased fortification programs, especially with fabricated or engineered foods. Other problems may include hidden costs, more regulations and increased chance of excessive nutrient intake. The education approach offers more potential at less cost and risk.[99]

Richardson (1990)

Many nutrition surveys in developed and developing countries continue to indicate that an appreciable fraction of the population, particularly young children, adolescents, the elderly and women of child-bearing age can suffer from nutrient deficiencies at a borderline or pathological level. In the developed nations, nutrient needs and food choices of these specific population groups, the increasing use of dietetic and low-energy products, the overall trend towards consuming fewer calories and the greater reliance on commercially prepared foods are just some of the reasons why it is essential to reexamine policies and guidelines for the addition of nutrients to foods.[99a]

ALTERNATIVES TO NUTRIFICATION

Alternatives to nutrification for improved nutritional status have been considered at various times in the past and will continue to be considered. This should be the case whenever a policy is extended or a new one is about to be adopted. As alternatives[82] to early cereal enrichment, scientists and public health officials considered the vitamin pill, but recognized the difficulty of getting them to those who needed them most. Next were considered public programs designed to increase the consumption of nonprocessed (i.e., whole) grains but discarded because of lack of success of earlier efforts and slowness of nutrition education. Large-scale distribution of special foods to the needy was also considered, but was not regarded as economically feasible. Nutrification won out with four nutrients added to key cereal flours and bread in 1941. Alternative interventions[100] have inherent advantages and disadvantages with respect to certain criteria. These criteria include costs, skill, number of personnel, delivery system infrastructure, technical feasibility, role of the beneficiary, and impact. Attempts have been made (Table 2.8) to rank different interventions, however, it should be kept in mind that the individual situation, and the nutrients involved, may influence the ranking and the appropriateness of interventions and hence have a major influence on the intervention selected for the particular population segment in a given country.

POLICY ASPECTS OF NUTRIFICATION

The Food and Nutrition Board of the National Academy of Sciences and the Council on Foods and Nutrition of the American Medical Association issued their last policy

TABLE 2.8
COMPARISON OF ALTERNATIVE INTERVENTIONS

Criteria	Fortification	Tablets	Injections	Nutrition Education	Home Gardens	Plant Breeding
Costs						
Initial capital investments	Moderate	Low	Low	Low	Low	High
Continuing personnel	Low	High	High	High	Low	High
Continuing materials	Low[1]	Low	Moderate	Low	Moderate	High
Personnel Requirements						
Skill level	Moderate	Moderate	High	Low	Moderate	High
Numbers	Low	High	High	Moderate	High	Low
Administrative Requirements						
Supervision	Moderate	High	High	Moderate	Moderate	High
Health system organization	Low	High	High	Moderate	Low	Low
Technical Feasibility						
Technology dependability	High[2]	High	Moderate	Moderate	High	Moderate
Side effects risk	Low	Moderate	High	Low	Low	Moderate
Beneficiary Rule						
Acceptability	High	Moderate	Moderate	Moderate	Moderate	Moderate
Community involvement	Low[3]	Moderate	Moderate	High	High	Low
Impact						
Population coverage	High	Moderate[4]	Moderate[4]	Moderate	Moderate	Moderate
Time needed to show benefit	Moderate	Low	Low	Moderate	Low	High
Permanency of benefit	High	Low	Low	Moderate	High	High

Source: Austin and Hitt.[100] Adapted from World Food Council 1977.

[1]An exception is protein fortification, which is expensive relative to micronutrient fortification.
[2]Iron fortification has encountered technical difficulties, but recent improvements appear to have resolved these.
[3]In contrast to a central processing plan, village-level fortification could have high community participation.
[4]Direct-dosage coverage is a function of the outreach capacity of the delivery system, but coverage is constrained by the one-to-one system.

statement[101] on food fortification in 1982. The statement confirmed the previous conditions and again endorsed the traditional enrichment and fortification programs, such as iodine to salt,, vitamin D to milk, thiamin, riboflavin, niacin and iron to cereal grain products, vitamin A to margarine, low fat and nonfat milks, and fluoride to water. Important guidelines for both food restoration and fortification were included. It recognized the concept of nutrient density related to caloric food value, urged improvement of processing techniques rather than only dependence on addition of nutrients, and endorsed the continued development of improved foods that will assure an overall diet of superior nutritional quality and economic advantage to the total population. Snack foods are recognized as contributors to the total food intake and may be carriers of nutrients in some circumstances.

The Food and Drug Administration's basic mission in nutrition[102] is to improve and maintain the quality of the national food supply, and its role is limited to situations which involve health and safety or which involve a need to respond to consumer request for information. There is concern about the food supply, one current problem being meeting nutrient needs in the presence of the declining calorie energy intake of the U.S. population. FDA's present policy supports nutrient addition[103] under the following principles:

(1) to conform with current food standards,
(2) to replace nutrients to a level representative of those in the food prior to storage, handling and processing,
(3) to avoid nutritional inferiority in a food that replaces a traditional food in the diet,
(4) and to balance the vitamin, mineral and protein content of a food in proportion to its total caloric content.

FDA has identified 22 nutrients as candidates for addition to foods namely, protein, vitamins A, B_1, B_2, B_6, B_{12}, C, D, E, biotin, folic acid, niacin, pantothenate, calcium, phosphorus, magnesium, potassium, manganese, iron, copper, zinc and iodine. The levels of nutrients can be related to each 100 calories of a food (Table 2.9) when a nutrient to caloric balance concept is considered.

FDA has concluded[103] from the evidence obtained in the 1977–78 NFCS and NHANES surveys that further additions to the food supply of nutrients are unnecessary at the present time, although both national and international needs demand continued surveillance. Will FDA concern themselves only with the issues of deficiency disease or will they devise a reasonable fortification program to deal with the issue of the role of low-calorie diets and chronic degenerative diseases? Goals for fortification today are to further improve public health and to thereby enhance the quality of life. In terms of fortification, the shift from deficiency disease prevention to health promotion opens a complex realm in which earlier scientific data were deficient.[103] There is a need to better understand the dynamics of nutrient requirements, better understand nutrient toxicities not only in the traditional sense

TABLE 2.9
FDA-RECOMMENDED FORTIFICATION LEVELS
BASED ON A CALORIC STANDARD

Nutrient	USRDA	Level of nutrients per 100 kcal
Protein (PER < casein), g	65	3.25[1]
Protein (PEr < casein), g	45	2.25[1]
Vitamin A, IU	5000	250
Vitamin C, mg	60	3
Thiamin, mg	1.5	0.075
Riboflavin, mg	1.7	0.085
Niacin, mg	20	1.0
Calcium, g	1	0.05
Iron, mg	18	0.9
Vitamin D, IU	400	20[1]
Vitamin E, IU	30	1.5
Vitamin B_6, mg	2	0.1
Folic acid, mg	0.4	0.02
Viamin B_{12}, mcg	6	0.3
Phosphorus, g	1	0.05
Iodine, mcg	150	7.5[1]
Magnesium, mg	400	20
Zinc, mg	15	0.75
Copper, mg	2	0.1
Biotin, mg	0.3	0.015
Pantothenic acid, mg	10	0.5
Potassium, g	[2]	0.125
Manganese, mg	[2]	0.2

[1]Optional.
[2]No USRDA has been established for these nutrients.

of individual nutrients, but even more so when considering the impact of several nutrients. There has been approximately a century's accumulation of knowledge on the macronutrients, protein, fat and carbohydrate, about 30–50 years of knowledge for most of the vitamins and some of the minerals such as calcium and iron, and little on newer trace elements such as molybdenum, manganese, chromium, selenium and silicon.[104]

In the context of the modern consumer-oriented food industry, traditional production technologies and regulations concerning labeling and standards of identity may be occasionally incompatible with modern scientific knowledge particularly in the area of nutritional needs. In many instances, these may represent constraints to the development of products with the most desirable nutrient balance and may need to be reevaluated.[78]

The four principles upon which USDA's fortification position is based are:

(1) There is a demonstrated need for the nutrient in a specified population.
(2) The use of the product is not likely to create a dietary imbalance.
(3) The vehicle to which nutrients are added is an appropriate one.
(4) The use of the product will not be confusing or misleading to the consumers.

In USDA food assistance programs,[105] nutrient levels in foods are specified for populations with demonstrated needs. In the WIC (Women, Infant and Children) food program, recommended foods have high levels of vitamin A, C, calcium, iron and protein. Cereals are fortified with iron (45% of U.S. RDA per one ounce dry serving). There are 20 adult dry cereals which meet the iron and other requirements for WIC cereals. In the child nutrition and needy family programs, only fortified foods having an FDA standard are used. One exception is a vitamin A and C dehydrated mashed potato product. There are also some exceptions in the child nutrition (school food service) program with cheese alternative products, vegetable protein products and enriched macaroni products.

One wonders if the nutrification efforts had kept pace better with the increased production of processed and fabricated foods over the past decades, whether the consumer would have initiated their "do it oneself" program of daily vitamin and mineral supplements to the extent that it is practiced today, namely about 30–40% of the population. While such supplements have their place, they are not a substitute for nutrified foods which would reach all economic levels of consumers, with greater safety and with inherently greater balance.

NUTRIFICATION OF MILITARY RATIONS

Prior to the administration of the Department of Defense by Secretary Donald S. McNamara, each branch of the U.S. military services (Army, Navy, Air Force) had its own specifications and research progarms for food to be used in food service and during military operations. Today, the Surgeon General of the Army acts as the Department of Defense (DOD) executive agent for nutrition matters. The Surgeon Generals of the Army, Navy and Air Force evaluate, recommend and review all aspects of the DOD nutrition policies. This includes (1) establishing dietary allowances for military feeding; (2) prescribing nutrient standards for packaged rations and (3) providing basic guidelines for nutrition education.[106]

The joint regulation provides a military recommended dietary allowance (MRDA) adopted from the NAS/NRC Recommended Dietary Allowances. The MRDA is defined as the daily essential nutrient intake levels presently considered to meet the known nutritional needs of practically all 17–50 year old, moderately active military personnel (Table 2.10).

TABLE 2.10
MILITARY RECOMMENDED DIETARY ALLOWANCES (MRDA) FOR SELECTED NUTRIENTS[1]

Nutrient	Unit	Male	Female
Energy[2,3]	kcal	3200 (2800-3600)	2400 (2000-2800)
	MJ	13.4 (11.7-15.1)	10.0 (8.4-11.7)
Protein[4]	gm	100	80
Vitamin A[5]	mcg RE	1000	800
Vitamin D[6,7]	mcg	5-10	5-10
Vitamin E[8]	mg TE	10	8
Ascorbic Acid	mg	60	60
Thiamin (B_1)	mg	1.6	1.2
Riboflavin (B_2)	mg	1.9	1.4
Niacin[9]	mg NE	21	16
Vitamin B_6	mg	2.2	2.0
Folacin	mcg	400	400
Vitamin B_{12}	mcg	3.0	3.0
Calcium[7]	mg	800-1200	800-1200
Phosphorus[7]	mg	800-1200	800-1200
Magnesium[7]	mg	350-400	300
Iron[7]	mg	10-18	18
Zinc	mg	15	15
Iodine	mcg	150	150
Sodium	mg	See note[10]	See note[10]

[1]MRDA for moderately active military personnel, ages 17-50 years, are based on the *Recommended Dietary Allowances*, 9th Rev. Ed., 1980.

[2]Energy allowance ranges are estimated to reflect the requirements of 70% of the moderately active military population. One megajoule (MJ) equals 239 kcals.

[3]Dietary fat calories should not contribute more than 35% of total energy intake.

[4]Protein allowance is based on an estimated protein requirement of 0.8 gm/kg desirable body weight. Using the reference body weight ranges for males of 60-79 kg and for females of 46-63 kg, the protein requirement is approximately 48-64 g for males and 37-51 g for females. These amounts have been approximately doubled to reflect the usual protein consumption levels of Americans and to enhance diet acceptability.

[5]One microgram of retinol equivalent (mcg RE) equals 1 mcg of retinol, or 6 mcg betacarotene, or 5 mcg IU.

[6]As cholecalciferol, 10 mcg of cholecalciferol equals 400 IU of vitamin D.

[7]High values reflect greater vitamin D, calcium, phosphorus, magnesium, and iron requirements for 17-18-year olds than for older ages.

[8]One milligram of alpha-tocopherol equivalent (mg TE) equals 1 mg d-alpha-tocopherol.

[9]One milligram of niacin equivalent (mg NE) equals 1 mg niacin or 60 mg dietary tryptophan.

[10]The safe and adequate levels for daily sodium of 1100-3300 mg published in the RDA are currently impractical and unattainable within military food service systems. However, an average of 1700 mg of sodium per 1000 kc of food served is the target for military food service systems. This level equates to a daily sodium intake of approximately 5500 mg for males and 4100 mg for females.

The regulation sets nutrient standards for packaged rations (Table 2.11). Operational rations include the individual combat ration (MCI), the meal ready-to-eat (MRE)

TABLE 2.11
NUTRIENT DENSITY INDEX PER 1000 CALORIES FOR MENU PLANNING

Nutrient	Unit	Military Diet Amount	Reduced Calorie Menu Amount
Protein	gm	33	53
Vitamin A	mcg RE	333	533
Ascorbic Acid	mg	25	40
Thiamin (B_1)	mg	0.5	0.7[1]
Riboflavin (B_2)	mg	0.6	0.8[2]
Niacin	mg	6.7	8.7[3]
Calcium	mg	333	533
Phosphorus	mg	333	533
Magnesium	mg	125	200
Iron	mg	6.0[4]	6.0[4]
Sodium	mg	1700	1700

[1]NDI for thiamin is based on a minimum recommended allowance of 1.0 mg/day.
[2]NDI for riboflavin is based on a minimum recommended allowance of 1.2 mg/day.
[3]NDI for niacin is based on a minimum recommended allowance of 13.0 mg/day.
[4]Iron supplementation is recommended for female personnel subsisting on a 1500 kcal diet. Levels higher than 6 mg/1000 calories are difficult to attain in a conventional U.S. diet.

and other rations identified as A, B, or T. The regulation states that "it is essential that ration planners compensate for losses of nutrients, such as ascorbic acid, thiamin, riboflavin, niacin and pyridoxine which may occur during storage of operational and restricted rations." It is desirable that each combat meal (MCI, MRE) provides one-third of the nutrient standard. A restricted ration is intended for subsistence up to 10 days under certain operation scenarios. The nutrient standard does not apply to the survival food packet (food bar) designed to be consumed for periods of less than four days.

The regulation provides a nutrient density index (NDI) for normal and reduced calorie planning. Personnel subsistence on a 1,500 calories meal plan requires a diet that is nutritionally more dense. The NDI serves as a basic tool for nutrition education within the military in promoting a healthful diet.

In addition to foods commercially fortified, the military practices the nutrification of selected foods to assure key nutrients in operational rations. Investigators, particularly at the U.S. Army Quartermaster Food and Container Institute, were leaders in the study of the effects of processing such as canning,[107] electronic cooking,[108] sulphite use in dehydrated foods,[109] irradiation,[110] and food dehydration.[111] These and many other scientists at the U.S. Army Natick Laboratories provided development and specifications for food and nutritional analysis support to: the Navy for nuclear submarine needs; the USAF high altitude balloon flights and the U-2 and high performance aircraft needs, and NASA for manned spaceflight.[112]

Fortified components in packaged operational rations include the nutrification with ascorbic acid of coffee, cocoa and orange beverage powders. Additional nutrients are added to survival-type cereal bars and to several components of the meal-ready-to-eat.

The meal-ready-to-eat is aseptically processed and the package configured to meet the dimensions of military "fatigue" pockets. In the absence of vegetables and fruits, or microbiologically safe-to-eat fresh vegetables and fruit, peanut butter, cheese spread, cocoa, sweet chocolate candy and coatings for cookies and brownies are fortified with A, C, B_1 and B_6. Aseptic pouch bread will replace crackers and will be fortified, but values are not available.

NUTRIFICATION IN DEVELOPING COUNTRIES

Malnutrition[113] has many roots: inadequate food supply, limited purchasing power, poor health conditions, incomplete knowledge about nutrition, often aggravated by uncertain political commitment. Adding to the complexity is the lack of an organizational focus for carrying out programs. Nutrition is not a sector; it is a universal need. Solutions must cut across disciplines and organization charts. Malnutrition is everybody's business, but a focus of responsibility is lacking. Recognition of the consequences of malnutrition for national development is growing and is being seen as both a cause and an effect of underdevelopment. Improved food production and consumption is the main need in countries where decreasing proportions of the poor have access to land. But, for the vast majority of the world's malnourished, increased production is not the only need, as evidenced by countries which have become self-sufficient and yet malnutrition continues. Health delivery system approaches have been used but where nutrition deficiencies are so vast these limited efforts are costly and inadequate to alleviate health problems and productivity remains low.

Transfer in the past three decades of modern agricultural technology[114] to developing countries has led to a steady improvement of global food production, but with a high energy cost. Since the early 1970s, economic growth has slowed and cost of input on which improved performance of green revolution crops was based, rose dramatically. Since 1979 worldwide average economic growth rate is closely matched or even exceeded by population growth. In countries where population growth is under control, conditions are better than where it is not. Other environmental changes (excess cutting of forests causing permanent loss of fragile soils, expanding deserts, deteriorating air quality, acid rain and soil erosion caused by poor agricultural practices on better farm lands) all attest to poor stewardship over natural resources and add to uncertainty in keeping food supplies ahead of population expansion.

The best foods to subsidize are those that are consumed predominantly by the poor and have little appeal to others, grains such as sorghum and millet, processed cassava flour, legumes, etc. Political commitment is the first requisite to solving the problem of malnutrition, and as experience is gained with the nutritional intervention, progress will follow. Nutritional considerations must be integrated into agricultural economies, extension, medicine and public health. Coordination is necessary among the efforts of government, private and foreign-assistance organizations and generally requires some kind of organizational focal point. Support can most profitably be concentrated on projects to combat energy-protein malnutrition and the diseases and handicaps caused by deficiencies of vitamin A, iodine and iron. These types of malnutrition are widespread and their consequences severe.[113]

World-wide estimates[93] are made from time to time on the extent of total malnutrition. Currently, people affected by preventable malnutrition are estimated in the millions. Protein-energy malnutrition (PEM) affects about 500 million people. More severe forms are characterized by retarded growth, apathy, loss of appetite, and fluid accumulation (kwashiorkor) due to severe protein deficiency, or retarded growth, and extreme thinness (marasmus) caused by deficiency of both calories and protein, or a mixture of the two states. PEM exists in many developing countries, parasitic infections and diarrhea are complicating factors. Approaches to control or prevent PEM include increase in cereal-legume foods, more oil and fat in the diet, protein or amino acid supplemental additions to the low protein foods, a greater effort on immunization, parasitic disease control and oral rehydration treatment for diarrhea.

Vitamin A deficiency (VAD) is a leading cause of childhood blindness (xerophthalmia). Most nutritionists now agree that if an appropriate food carrier exists, to which Vitamin A can be added, fortification is the cheapest and most effective means of controlling xerophthalmia in most countries. Since this intervention can be quickly initiated, it provides time for other approaches, such as an improved horticulture, to be introduced. VAD also results in an increased incidence of childhood infections and mortality.[93]

Endemic goiter and cretinism (dwarfness), a result of iodine deficiency disease (IDD), is influenced primarily by a lack of sufficient iodine in the inland soils in which food crops are grown. In industrialized countries, control of IDD has generally come about by means of mandatory or voluntary iodization of salt, a cheap and simple delivery system. In some countries there remain implementation problems. Delivery of an iodized product to remote population segments continues.[115]

Nutritional anemias, more prevalent in poor communities, are not uncommon in industrialized countries. Iron deficiency anemia (IDA) is the most prevalent form, but folate deficiency is also quite widespread. IDA is a complex subject. The form of iron in the diet, the form added, the valence of the iron in food products after processing and storage influencing bioavailability, iron metabolism, the role of enhancing substances, like vitamin C on iron metabolism, and the role of iron nutritional status to infections are some factors under study. Nutrification of appropriate foods with iron in food compounds is one approach.[93]

Rather than approach nutrition problems in developing countries today with purely a technical solution as a simple intervention approach, it is believed that nutrition planning integrated as part of primary health care and preventive medical programs or part of an agricultural or social program may result in a more acceptable and sustained effort and provide a better compatibility with administrative and political goals of the country under study.[116] As developing countries struggle with debt, budgetary and refugee crises, there can be a lessened interest in country-wide food distribution and consumption issues, including nutritional deficiencies. Educational efforts in schools about malnutrition and the training of more nutritionists need to be encouraged. Furthermore, plans for the incorporation of specific intervention strategies must be kept ready and adaptable to fit into appropriate national plans when opportunity and economic or political situations appear and will allow their incorporation. Greater recognition needs to be given to nutrition goals as inseparable from broader goals related to how societies function and their provision of benefits. Planners must join in the political process and stay with it until the desired action takes place.[116]

Nutrition interventions are planned actions undertaken for the explicit purpose of improving the nutritional well-being of a specified population group.[117] There are nine types of interventions: (1) enhancing agricultural production, (2) fortification, (3) formulated weaning foods, (4) improved marketing infrastructure, (5) food price subsidies, (6) mass dosage of specific nutrients, (7) supplementary feeding strategy, (8) nutrition education, and (9) an integrated program of the above eight interventions. To be effective, any intervention strategy must be related to national development linked to a national food policy. When resources are scarce, achieving broad coverage may reduce the efforts to nutritional insignificance. Nutrition intervention can generate positive biological improvements at affordable costs. Table 2.12 (note costs are relative to each other and not in today's dollars) presents summary results for various types of interventions.[117]

Interim solutions for the millions of people suffering from undernutrition are applications of direct nutrition and health measures until poverty and economic ills are overcome. Among the major categories of nutrition programs suggested are food nutrification and distribution of nutrient supplements. While greater movement of food to where countries need it is evident, the long-range solution calls for developing countries doing things themselves toward which a greater educational and "hands-on" effort must be directed.[118,119]

FOOD NUTRIFICATION INTERVENTION CONSIDERATIONS

Whether a nutrification program is undertaken with a food will depend on the goal, logic or rationale, technology, nutrient bioavailability, as well as governmental regulations, cost/benefits, and safety. If the food product considered is a regularly consumed food item in a developed country and vitamin and/or mineral content is not in balance with the RDA or the calorie content, the addition of those missing nutrients to the food is warranted, thus providing a balanced food product. Another

TABLE 2.12
SUMMARY ESTIMATES OF INTERVENTION COSTS AND IMPACT

	Costs	Impact
Supplementary feeding	$10–$15 per recipient per year	Positive growth impact over 4- to 24-month period
Nutrition education	$0.05–$3 per recipient	Changes in feeding practices documented; positive biological effects suspected
Formulated foods	$0.001–$.003 per g of protein; $0.007–$.014 per 100 calories	Positive growth impact, particularly when used with severely malnourished
Fortification	$0.002–$0.11 per recipient per year for micronutrients; $2.50 per recipient per year for lysine fortification	Goiter largely eradicated in some areas; vitamin A blood serum levels increased; iron fortification led to increased hemoglobin and hematocrit levels. Lysine fortification did not yield growth improvements where calories were inadequate
Consumer price subsidies	1%–25% of total government expenditures	Has provided up to 30% of calorie requirements of low-income groups
Agricultural production	Depends on nature of project	High potential but depends on income, employment and price effects on target groups
Integrated programs	$15–$50 per beneficiary per year, 5%–20% cost savings over nonintegrated	Infant mortality rates decreased 30%–75%

Source: Autin.[117]

situation may be choosing a food ingredient to serve as the carrier of one or more nutrients to a population in a developing country currently consuming suboptimal nutrient levels in their regular diet. In this latter example, the important considerations which can be adapted to specific projects, depending on local circumstances, involved in a nutrification program are as follows:[120]

Food Carrier or Vehicle for the Added Nutrient

The food ingredient serving as a carrier should be a universally consumed item by the target population, preferably consumed at relatively constant intakes over the seasons of the year. More than one carrier may be chosen if such a selection adds greater assurance that the goal will be achieved. In early nutrification practices the food carrier was often regarded as having to be a staple food such as a cereal-grain product. While this is a commendable concept, realistic and practical considerations dictate that only foods that pass through central, communal or regional processing centers where the nutrification process can take place are useful. From a carrier viewpoint, a food ingredient such as sugar, salt, beverages (tea), seasoning agents, etc., may be the only choice for the project. There may be instances where village nutrification may be better focused on the needs and practices of the target population,[121] rather than that provided by central processing at a remote source.

Nutrient or Nutrients

The nutrient to be added should possess acceptable chemical, physical, and noninterfering organoleptic properties. Likewise the nutrient(s) should demonstrate acceptable bioavailability and stability performances in the food carrier. The physical form of the nutrient in many instances may be critical to the success of the project. The nutrient may need prior chemical and/or physical processing for greater stability in the food product. Also, nutrients may not be added directly in pure form but in a premix, either custom formulated or carried out as a prior stage in the nutrification center. Where a nutrient premix is to be added to the food carrier by automatic or mechanical feeders, it should be free flowing, consistent in bulk density, and nonsettling in transportation and storage.[121] Before large-scale operations are initiated, prior experience and/or pilot feasibility time should determine whether foreign odors or flavors, likewise texture changes, occur during storage and simulated in-use procedures. The quantity to be added to the food carrier can be determined from the knowledge combining the difference between the nutrient daily allowance or requirement and the lowest nutient intake of the chosen food carrier by individuals in the target group.[2] The amount of added nutrient must also reflect consideration for imbalance and safety.

Location of the Nutrification Process

The addition of the nutrient(s) to the food carrier must be carried out in a uniform fashion and produce an adequate volume of nutrified premix and/or food necessary to serve the intended purpose. With well-chosen commercial equipment supervised by trained personnel, the nutrifying operations may be performed by the batch system but more likely from volume considerations, it will be carried out by continuous processing. A premix may be manufactured on a continuous basis and the addition to a food carrier or staple performed on a batch basis at the target site.

Production Controls for the Nutrified Food

Qualitative daily control procedures at the site of the nutrification process and quantitative procedures in a qualified laboratory, periodically applied, will provide assurance of operations at the nutrification center. The laboratory can be located at a remote site serving several centers.

Distribution of the Nutrified Food

Periodic marketplace and home use and check points are desirable to observe continued food use patterns. The home use check will signal any unfavorable unforeseen changes from the use of the food as the nutrient carrier.

Voluntary or Mandated Program

Early determination must be made as to how the program is to be undertaken. Upon setting up a nutrification program, it must be decided whether to make the program compulsory or optional, and whether to encourage the program by incentives as a component of the program or to set up standards in food usage outlets, such as in schools, and whether to institute other support actions for the program.[2]

Overall Program Monitoring

If the nutrification program is to remedy an existing health problem, suitable monitoring of the target population at timely intervals will confirm whether the program is correcting the problem. Ideally, baseline data should be available and concurrent control data as to effectiveness of the intervention collected concomitantly.

Cost of Program

Prior decisions are necessary to determine whether the consumer or government pays for the program. If the food industry is to absorb the cost initially, an understanding with government is desirable on prevailing policy under inflationary situations. Costs need to be weighed against expected benefits.[2] Costs of the program include cost of the added nutrient and premix preparation including the mixing equipment involved, cost of equipment involved, cost of equipment to control the uniform introduction of the additive to the food, analytical tests, monitoring needs and overall personnel.

SITUATIONS FOR NUTRIFICATION

Nutrification of food can be considered as an intervention measure where a substantial segment of a population would benefit from the incorporation of a nutrient or nutrients in its diet, but preferably where the total quantity of food available is reasonably adequate. Nutrification with micronutrients adds to the nutritional quality of the diet, less so to the quantity of the diet. Whether a selected nutrification plan is adopted depends upon many factors, including governmental policies, time period to achieve the goal, economies, and safeguards to ensure that the efficacy and safety of the program are maintained. Situations which might call for nutrification with industrially produced nutrients are described[120] below:

Restoration Concept

Under the restoration concept, some micronutrients originally present in the whole natural food but lost in processing are returned to a processed food. For example, peanuts are roasted prior to the usual manufacture of peanut butter, a process that destroys the thiamin naturally present. It is technically feasible to add thiamin back to the butter during the peanut grinding operation.

Because of the volume consumed, freshly cooked white potatoes have made a substantial contribution of vitamin C and other nutrients to some populations. Currently, more potatoes are consumed in manufactured convenience foods such as fries, powders, buds, flakes, chips or crisps. Processing and storage on supermarket shelves degrade much of the natural vitamin C present in the original potato. Restoring vitamin C to these processed potato products is nutritionally justifiable. Different technologies have been developed for the nutrification process. See Chapter 7 for potato product nutrification information.

Food Class Standardization Concept

If a natural food for a given class of foods is serving as a substantial source of a micronutrient and another food containing little or none of that nutrient is promoted or recommended for the same purpose, some justification exists for adding the missing nutrient(s). One case in point is consumption of juices naturally low in vitamin C in place of citrus juice as a breakfast beverage. Since a good portion of daily vitamin C needs is consumed at breakfast meal, there is merit in having juices such as prune, apricot, pineapple, pear, peach, grape and apple contain standardized vitamin C levels. The consumer can then have variety of juice selections without forfeiting vitamin C nutritional value. Chapter 10 deals with nutrification of juices and beverages. Another case is the vegetable protein food analogues adapted to serve as replacements for animal protein products wherein the vegetable product should be nutrified with nutrients to simulate the composition of the product imitated. A third example is the meal replacers. When a product is developed and promoted to replace a regular meal, a suitable approach is to have the new product provide one third of the daily allowance of micronutrients. Instant breakfast products follow this concept.

Cereal Grain Products as Nutrient Carriers Concept

Cereal grains and tuber foods provide the basic energy sustenance to most of humankind. About 26% of the daily caloric intake in the United States comes from products based on cereal grains. In some developing countries cereal grain products provide up to 70% of the caloric intake. As a class of foods, cereal grains have considerable merit as carriers for added nutrients because (1) they are universally consumed, (2) they are prime suppliers of calories and protein, (3) they provide diet variety by use of industrial and home processing for consumption, (4) they contain complex carbohydrates and (5) they store well if moisture content and insect infestation are controlled. They are logical carriers of nutrients lost in the milling process or nutrients not identified with cereal grain products, such as vitamin A. Chapter 5 may be consulted for a more detailed presentation.

Nutrient Balanced Calorie Concept

Presently, a greater percentage of the population has become involved in more sedentary occupations and hence has lowered daily caloric needs. Advances in food science and technology have led to the development of high-energy food products as well as low-calorie food products, many of which have a refined or highly processed character, or have been fabricated from refined and/or nonabsorbed food ingredients. Although many of these foods provide calories, they do not contain an appropriate level of essential micronutrients. Examples of these high-caloric items are beverages and sweet goods made from sucrose, fructose, glucose, corn sugar syrups and table syrups, as well as high-calorie items made with fats, shortenings and vegetable oils, some of which also have added sugar and/or starch. If all foods contained the required micronutrients at levels comparable to their caloric contribution to the diet, there would be less difficulty with nutritional insufficiencies. Certain high-calorie foods fit less well into a meal pattern. They are frequently consumed between meals. How then should they be considered in nutritional programs, since foods consumed between meals may influence the consumption pattern of foods eaten at meal time? Where no recognized serving size exists, a nutrification program could best be guided by an adjusted caloric density or available protein approach. Chapter 11 deals with nutrification of snack foods.

Special Purpose Food Concept

A number of unique dietary foods are designed to meet specific physiologic states or life cycle stages. They may also be sole sources of nutrient supplies for the time period. Others may be supplemental to the diet. Examples are diets for pregnancy and lactation, for diabetics for allergy control, for control of hypertension, for weight control, for pre- or postoperative periods, and for infants. Those influencing most adult individuals are diets for weight control. Diets containing 900–1,200 calories need close scrutiny regarding adequacy in essential amino acids, vitamins, and minerals. Nutrients in total parenteral or oral nutrition are prepared from carbohydrates, amino acids, vitamins and minerals and from synthetic or purified sources. Chapter 14 deals with some of these special purpose foods.

Improved Bioavailability Concept

When one is dealing with an insufficiency of a mineral element in the diet, two approaches are usually considered: (1) to increase the mineral content by the addition of proper mineral sources, and (2) to attempt to improve the bioavailability of the mineral already in the diet. An approach gaining momentum is to improve the biological availability of existing dietary iron supplies or that of added iron by incorporating in the diet some facilitating substance (Chapter 3) such as L-ascorbic acid[122] or its sodium salt. Enhancement by ascorbic acid is somewhat dose-dependent. An intake of as little as 25 mg at a meal may be significant in enhancing the bioavailability of iron.

Lack of Protective Foods Concept

Some populations in the world do not have access to a sufficient quantity of protective foods or do not consume valuable or protective foods because of beliefs and taboos. Both practices can lead to dietary deficiencies. Although long-range approaches need to be introduced under these circumstances, in many instances a nutrification program can quickly introduce the missing nutrient or nutrients. An example is the insufficient consumption of vitamin A, iron and iodine in some countries. The consumption of protector compounds such as beta carotene, tocopherols and ascorbic acid are believed to be important in disease prevention. Along these lines the National Cancer Institute has evoked a concept of designer foods to thwart certain cancers. Addition of these nutrients to foods could also be considered a public health concept. Chapters 8, 12 and 13 supply additional information.

Gastro-limitations Concept

In young children consideration is not always given to the physical limitation of the size of the stomach or the entire GI tract. If, for example, rice is the only dietary source of certain essential amino acids for the young child, it is not possible for the stomach to hold the amount of rice to meet the daily need.[123]

Allaying Chronic Disease Concept

Since consumers have become more concerned about how foods and nutrients relate to health and disease prevention, a new concept arises for interpreting the need for nutrification of food or food ingredients. Traditionally recommended dietary allowances have been regarded as judgmental levels or estimates of nutrient intakes which would meet the needs of most healthy individuals in the population. Now a controversy has emerged concerning whether these approved allowances based on past criteria are adequate for beneficial influences on the prevention of certain specific degenerative or chronic diseases. Not all nutrients are currently considered in the dispute, but eventually most may need to be reexamined.[75]

Multi-role nutrients,[124] vitamin A and/or β-carotene, ascorbic acid, vitamin E and selenium are in the forefront of a steady stream of literature reports querying optimal daily intake levels for maximum application against diseases, such as cancer, cardiovascular pathology, neurological disorders, cataracts, etc. Nutrients[125-127] which inhibit oxidation reactions from free radicals thereby provide a protective role in maintaining body fluids, cells and tissues. Calcium is being reviewed relative to chronic disease prevention.[128] The outcome of this general controversy should have an influence on food product labeling, which already is engaged in diet-health interrelationships.[63,129] Chapter 18 deals with the diet-health issue. Should intakes be increased and, if so, should it be in the form of nutrified food or as a separate dietary supplement?

Geochemical Environment Deficiency Concept

Soils in wide areas of the world are deficient in certain minerals. This situation can result in low concentrations of major or trace minerals in drinking water, plant crops, and even tissues of farm animals, thus contributing to marginal or deficient dietary intakes in humans. Some minerals in this category are fluorine, iodine, molybdenum, and selenium; in some countries, the first two are added back to the diet in the form of fluoride-treated water and iodized salt. See Chapter 12. Trace mineral elements are gaining increased attention as dietary essentials. Certain areas of the United States, New Zealand and the Peoples Republic of China are known to be selenium-deficient.[81] Estimated safe intakes of selenium have been determined. Nutrification of food with selenium in selected areas may be a consideration in the future. Manganese, copper, chromium, and zinc likewise could become future candidates, depending upon continuing research.[130-133] See Chapter 3.

Changing Economics Concept

Industrially produced nutrients, appropriately utilized in combination with agricultural products, offer protective safeguards or alternative choice products in changing economic conditions.[6] More vegetable protein extenders are utilized in foods in Japan and the United States as more economical and some believe as healthier food sources than animal sources. The initial impetus for the increased use of vegetable protein concentrates in human foods came from the earlier concern of meeting a suspected protein crisis in the developing countries through the supplementation of cereal grain products. See Chapter 6 for an expanded discussion.

Nonnutritional Concept

Several nutrients have dual properties. In addition to serving as dietary essential they contribute some technologic advantage to the food product to which they are added. L-ascorbic acid (vitamin C) may act as: (1) an oxygen scavenging agent in bottled and canned food products; (2) an inhibitor of oxdative rancidity in frozen fish; (3) a stabilizer in cured meats; (4) a flour-maturing agent and dough conditioner; (5) an oxygen acceptor in beer production, and (6) a reducing agent in wine. Alpha-tocopheral (vitamin E) serves as a fat-soluble antioxidant in fats and oils and a retardant to nitrosamine formation. Beta-carotene and beta-apo-8'-carotenal, carotenoid vitamin A precursors, also serve as food colors.[134] Ferrous gluconate improves color in processed ripe olives. See Chapter 15 for a further discussion of food product improvers.

SUCCESSFUL NUTRIFICATION PROGRAMS

Iodine addition in the form of an iodide or iodate compound to salt is one of the earliest successful nutrification programs initiated around the 1920s in the United States. Presently, iodate addition to salt or other carriers has spread around the world as a prophylaxis against goiter, cretinism and other symptoms of iodine deficiency disease (IDD). Apart from salt, many food items[115] such as condiments, sauces, oil, sweets, chocolates, cereal, flour, bread, baby foods, and dry skimmed milk have been used in iodization. Water iodization has been tried successfully in Thailand, Sicily and Malaysia (also sterilizes the water). Iodine nutrification was originally proposed in South America and in France in the early part of the 19th century. Currently, there are three global initiatives:[135] (1) one by the International Council for Control of Iodine Deficiency Disorders (ICCIDD), (2) another as a result of a World Health Organization (WHO) Assembly Resolution to give priority to IDD, and (3) a support program adopted by a Subcommittee on Nutrition of the United Nations Food and Agriculture Organization (FAO). There is a coordinating group for the three agencies. ICCIDD has a global network of over 300 members with expertise to implement programs. Currently, more attention needs to be given to controlled programs in Italy, the German Federal Republic, including the former German Democratic Republic and Spain, where IDD still persists. Accelerated programs are being carried out in Bolivia and Ecuador. Production of iodated salt in India has increased from 100,000 metric tons in 1983 towards a goal of 700,000. Activities are under way in a number of African countries. Chapters 12 and 17 contain more details of salt nutrification with iodine.

Vitamin D deficiency results in rickets, a condition recognized for centuries but not prevented until the early part of this century. If the skin of children is not exposed to direct sunlight by which 7-dehydrocholesterol is converted to active vitamin D in the body, a dietary source of vitamin D is necessary for freedom from this deficiency disease. There is an interesting observation made by a historian visiting a Persian-Egyptian battlefield in 526 B.C. He noted the skulls of the slain Persians were fragile, those of the Egyptians strong and heavier. The observation was attributed to difference in exposure to sunlight: The Persians wore turbans and clothing to shield the sun; the Egyptians went bareheaded since childhood.

Cow's milk contains calcium and phosphorus but little or no vitamin D for absorption of the minerals into the body of the milk-consuming, young child. Vitamin D nutrification of cow's milk and infant formulas has been responsible for the rarity of infantile rickets as a public health problem where vitamin D nutrification is practiced. In the early 1930s vitamin D was first added to milk at the rate of 135 IU which by the early 1940s was increased to 400 IU of vitamin D per quart of reconstituted evaporated milk or per quart of fresh fluid vitamin D milk. The favorable effects of fortification of foods with vitamin D on the health of populations of 19 countries has been recorded by Milot.[136] Chapters 13 and 14 provide further information on vitamin D nutrified milks and nutrified infant formula.

During World War I, Denmark shipped its butter to England and, as a consequence, greatly reduced its availability in the Danish diet. Without an alternative vitamin A source in the diet, vitamin A deficiency symptoms, xerophothalmia, impaired growth and a high incidence of respiratory infections appeared in many Danish children. By adding fish liver oil as a source of vitamin A concentrate to margarine, the symptoms disappeared and Denmark became practically free of vitamin A deficiency. Other countries, Sweden and England, followed the Danish nutrification program, as did the United States. Today, the major portion of the world's margarine production is nutrified with vitamin A. Vitamin A nutrification of margarine and wheat flour enrichment have been credited with significant health improvement in the people of Newfoundland. The local Newfoundland government was so impressed with the benefits of the nutrification program that mandatory continuation of the program was a condition of their annexation to Canada in 1949. Chapter 9 deals further with nutrient addition to fats. Currently, vitamin A is also added to low and nonfat fluid milk and also to nonfat dry milk in the United States. In 1955, WHO and FAO recommended that both vitamins A and D be added to all milks shipped to underdeveloped countries for prevention of nutritional disease. This subject is further discussed in Chapter 13.

The addition of three vitamins (thiamin, riboflavin and niacin) and one mineral (iron) to processed white flour and other processed cereal-grain products has been credited with substantial dietary increases of these nutrients in the United States, with the virtual disappearance of pellagra[137] in the South (Fig. 2.10) and beriberi and pellagra in urban centers. At a large general hospital in Chicago, in which beriberi previously could always be observed, a 3-year search failed to reveal a single case of beriberi, nor did a 1948 and 1949 survey of the Chicago House of Correction.[138] In 1989 it was estimated that nutrification provided 24% of thiamin, 24% of iron, 18% of niacin, and 20% riboflavin in the 1985 United States nutrient supplies.[37] Earlier estimates were made in 1972.[139]

Bakers in the United States voluntarily began to enrich bread with high vitamin yeast and subsequently with added synthetic vitamins three years before the widely published legal acceptance of cereal enrichment in 1941 and establishment of minimum requirements. In 1938 there was an estimate of 100,000 cases of active pellagra in the United States.[147] U.S. Public Health reports show that during the two war years of 1943–1944 there were still over 9,000 pellagrins in the 13 southeastern states. Enactment of state laws in several of the southeastern states requiring enrichment of corn meal and corn grits was followed by a rapid decline in

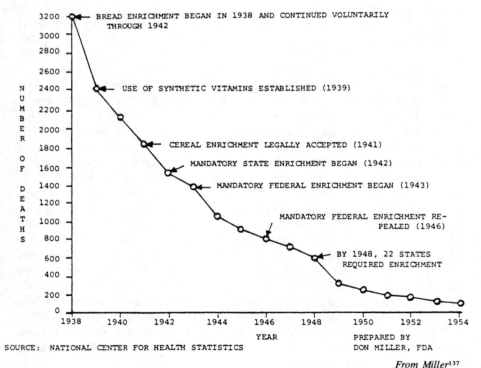

FIG. 2.10. DEATHS FROM PELLAGRA IN THE UNITED STATES (1938–1954)
Reprinted with permission of Am. Assoc. Cereal Chemists.

cases of pellagra.[138] Morbidity data from Mississippi, the state hit hardest by pellagra, indicate that this state solved its grave problem by requiring enrichment. Chapter 5 deals with the nutrification of cereal grain products.

Dietary studies in the 1950s among the Jewish population in Israel indicated the diet, especially of the lower income group, to be low in riboflavin. Furthermore, a survey including clinical observations of pregnant women showed signs of ariboflavinosis. Israel, upon the advice of nutrition experts, enriched all flour with 2.5 mg of riboflavin, 2.5 g of calcium carbonate and 30 g of heat-processed soymeal per killogram. Subsequent clinical and biochemical survey of pregnant women under the same conditions of the early survey demonstrated a marked improvement. Enrichment of flour was credited with the deficiency correction.[140] Enrichment of wheat flour with thiamin, riboflavin and niacin has alleviated riboflavin deficiency in Chile.[141]

Enriched rice by the Furter process was used in the extensive feeding trials made during 1948–1950 in the Bataan province of the Philippines. Two areas were set up, the experimental to consume nutrified rice, the control to consume rice without nutrification. Comparing the incidence of beriberi in the two areas, the data showed conclusively that nutrified rice reduced mortality from beriberi by a marked degree in one year's time.[142]

A new type[143] of enriched rice, "Shingen" containing Ca, Fe, and vitamins B_1, B_2, B_6, E, niacin and pantothenic acid was included in the diet of female students (aged 20 years). Data included calculated thiamin intake, and thiamin, alpha-tocopherol, and triglyceride levels in blood serum, erythrocyte transketolase activity, and thiamin pyrophosphate effects, for students with or without enriched rice in the study. Results suggest that consumption of the new rice improved the nutritional status of the students compared with control groups, some of whom exhibited marginal vitamin B_1 deficiency. An inverse relationship between the number of deaths from beriberi and the annual output of nutrified rice has been reported.[144]

It has been established that pellagra occurs frequently among the Bantu population in South Africa. Confirmatory biochemical data showed a high incidence of subclinical deficiency of both niacin and riboflavin. A two village project was designed in 1969 wherein the school children in the nutrification village would receive 1 mg of riboflavin and 10 mg of niacinamide added to 400 g of maize meal as a daily intake; school children in the control village would continue eating maize (corn) meal without the added nutrients. Clinical and biochemical observations during the study demonstrated the efficiency of the nutrient additions in reducing the incidence of subclinical deficiency. The nutrient addition was judged technologically and economically feasible. A second 9 month study was conducted several years later with children and young adults which confirmed the earlier study. Furthermore, this study showed that the nutrification plan did not aggravate an existing marginal protein calorie malnutrition state. As a result of these studies it was recommended that the nutrification plan be introduced on a national basis.[145]

Folate deficiency is a frequent cause of megaloblastic anemia among pregnant and lactating women in rural areas of South Africa.[146] One solution proposed has been the possibility of nutrifying food with folate. The vehicle chosen for folate nutrification was maize meal. Pregnant (less than 37 weeks) women in a hospital lodging facility who had not received folate or antibiotics, but had received iron supplementation and had a hemoglobin concentration of 11 g/dL or less, were randomly assigned to an experimental or control group. The experimental group received cooked maize meal containing 1 g of pure folic acid with milk and sugar, the control group the same without the added nutrient. At the time of delivery women consuming the nutrified meal showed a marked and statistically significant rise in serum and red cell folates, whereas the control group showed a fall in red cell folates, thus indicating that food nutrification could be used to correct folate deficiency. Folate stability added to maize meal was studied over 6–18 months. Cooking and baking trials revealed high retention values. Bioavailability tests were also satisfactory. Maize nutrification with folate appears to be a practical intervention.[146,147]

The nutritional status of Aborigines was studied in 1974, with particular reference to blood levels of hemoglobin and vitamins, after white bread fortified with iron and thiamin, riboflavin, and niacin had been available for 6½ months in New South Wales, Australia. There were significant increases of the nutrients in blood, less iron deficiency anemia and decreased angular stomatitis and skin xerosis.[148]

One form of blindness, xerophthalmia, occurs in infants and young children in areas of the world such as Asia, the Middle East, Africa, and Latin and South America where the intakes of vitamin A are inadequate.[149] As many as 500,000 children around the world may go blind annually as a result of this nutritional deficiency. In addition to eye symptoms, other signs of vitamin A deficiency are growth depression, greater susceptibility to other disease and, in many instances, eventual death. Through the cooperative efforts of the Agency for International Development, the World Health Organization, UNICEF, the International Vitamin A Consultative Group, the international blindness societies, and national groups, a concerted effort has been made to eradicate vitamin A deficiency.[149,150]

A facet of these intervention program deals with distribution of foods nutrified with vitamin A. Among the vitamin A nutrified foods[150] are dried milk, wheat flour, sugar (sucrose), tea dust and tea leaves and seasonings such as monosodium glutamate (MSG) and salt. The nutrification of sugar with vitamin A, developed by INCAP and practiced in Guatemala, is an outstanding example of the nutrification concept converted to successful practice.[151]

Trials conducted with vitamin A nutrified MSG in the Philippines[152] and in Indonesia[153] have demonstrated by decreased deficiency indicators and higher retinol serum values that MSG will prove to be another practical carrier for vitamin A. Chapters 5, 8, 9, 12 and 13 may be consulted for further information on vitamin A nutrified foods.

It is estimated that about 40% of the iron intake in Sweden[154] is supplied by nutrification compared to an estimated 25% in the United States. The nutrification of foods with iron is commonly accepted as one of the factors responsible for the significant decrease in the incidence of iron deficiency. The prevalence of anemia in women in childbearing age in Sweden dropped between 1965 and 1975 from 30 to 7%. Hallberg estimates that iron nutrification of flour can account for about a third of the reduction.[155]

Iron deficiency anemia in weaned infants can be prevented with iron-fortified powdered milk. Chilean researchers[156] have developed a powdered, full-fat, acidified milk product fortified with 15 mg of elemental iron and 100 mg of ascorbic acid/100 g of powder. When this product was supplied to infants ages three to 15 months, the prevalence of anemia dropped to 2.5%, compared with the nearly 26% rate seen in unsupplemented infants. Acidification of the milk made the product distasteful for adults, preventing other family members from drinking it. The fortified milk proved to be palatable to infants.

Keshan disease, a result of selenium deficiency is found in about 15 provinces in China. It frequently leads to death through heart failure among children and women of childbearing age. Selenium nutrification of food in the affected area has reduced the incidence of Keshan disease.[157]

Successful nutrification projects are also underway with amino acids, largely centered in Japan, in the nutrification of cereal-grain products. In the 1960s, in an investigation in Japanese rural areas with children depending on rice and barley as staple foods, children consuming lysine-fortified bread served in a school lunch program showed increased growth over a control group. A similar urban study revealed no change.[158] Amino acid addition trials in Guatemala, Tunisia and Thailand were less successful.[159] During the past 10 years, oilseed protein mixtures have been prepared with wheat, corn sorghum, oats, and bulgur. In these products, the oilseed or vegetable proteins supplement the proteins from cereal grains, which are inferior. Various baked goods have been developed with oilseed mixtures. One of these is a leavened bread made from wheat flour and soy flour developed by Kansas State University. For some years a nutrified bun (Nutribun) made from soy-wheat flour and added micronutrients has been successfully used in the school nutrition program in the Philippines. In India and Ecuador, a soy-wheat flour has been used with success in production of bread. High-protein pasta and high-protein cookies have elicited some interest. Blends of cereal products that have achieved some success in retail sales are Incaparina and Pronutro. Chapter 6 demonstrates the extensive use of combination foods made from agricultural food ingredients and industrially produced nutrients to meet human needs.

The success of the use of industrially prepared nutrients in special purpose food products used in pregnancy and lactation, for diabetics, for allergy control, for control of hypertension, for weight control, as pre- or postoperative diets and as infant formulas, can be taken as advance support of what technology and nutritional knowledge can formulate, field test, and put in commercial operation. Nutrification of refugee foods has been strongly recommended.[160] These experiences are encouragement for further production of well-fabricated food products to meet the needs for all population groups. Chapter 14 deals with formulated special purpose foods.

NUTRIFICATION IN THE FUTURE

This book provides the first comprehensive overview of the science and technology of nutrient additions to food and the delivery of nutrients through formulated and fabricated food systems. Although the science of nutrition has many gaps in its knowledge, as does food science, the technology of nutrition and food technology have evolved because of the need for practical solutions in spite of the gaps. With small steps in science, technology is able to take giant leaps because educated ideas become plausible inventions and advances. Most advances in medicine and technology, including the landing of man on the moon, did not require that all aspects of the technology be scientifically and completely understood. A major argument opposing nutrification has been the insufficient science is available to justify the practices. Imagine where the world would be if we applied such an argument in all fields of technical endeavor.

Food delivery systems of various types were established and evolved long before food as a nutrient delivery system was discovered. Currently, fabricated food systems have evolved both, with nutrient delivery (infant formula) and without nutrient delivery (spun vegetable protein meat replacers) being a consideration.

The most sophisticated practice of nutrification has occurred with the advances in infant formulas and "medical" foods. The demand for infant formulas was triggered by medical needs (allergy, phenylketonuria and other diseases) and by social needs (death of mother, working mother, etc.). Chemically defined diets in animal research led to similar enteral and parenteral diets for humans to meet specific metabolic diseases and situations of impaired gastrointestinal physiology and are now vital to rehabilitating nutritionally debilitated patients.

The most random practice of nutrification has occurred with public health enrichment, restoration and fortification practices. These practices were initially motivated by the presence of deficiency diseases and the need for intervention on a broad scale. This practice for improving the nutritional and health status of the population is one of the great accomplishments in nutrition and preventive medicine and ranks among the milestones in the history of public health. Some form of public health nutrification is found in practically all countries, either as a matter of policy or as a component of military feeding and child nutrition programs. In these applications, nutrification is not tied to deficiency diseases and medical pathologies but to public health and performance considerations.

Nutrification is an emerging technology in the issues of the nutrition needs of the elderly, the role of food in quality of life styles, the role of designer foods in cancer and other chronic disease prevention, and possibly the role of nutrients and other food ingredients in psychosocial and behavioral phenomena.

Nutrification has its limitations and is certainly not a panacea for all malnutrition situations.

The future state-of-the-art nutrification is dependent on:

(1) the continued ingenuity of chemists and food technologists in food fabrication;
(2) the improved understanding of interactions in nutrition among nutrients, other food ingredients and drugs which alter human performance;
(3) the continued open debate on the role and benefits of nutrification vis a vis education, safety and alternative interventions;
(4) continued dietary, biochemical and clinical survey research; and
(5) new advances in basic nutrition, particularly at the molecular level.

Nutrification is here to stay because there is a demand and a responsibility to apply knowledge, resources and technology in agriculture and food science to the efficient production and distribution of food for the responsible benefit of humankind.

REFERENCES

1. LOWENBERG, M. E., TODHUNTER, E. N., WILSON, E. D., SAVAGE, J. R. and LUBAWSKI, J. L. 1974. Food and Man, 2nd Ed. John Wiley & Sons, New York.
2. ANON. 1972. Food fortification. WHO Chron. 26(7), 307-312.
3. LEAF, A. and WEBER, P. D. 1987. A new era for science in nutrition. Am. J. Clin. Nutr. 45, 1048-1053.
4. CHRISTENSEN, R. P. 1966. Man's historic struggle for food. USDA Yearbook of Agr., NO. 349, Washington, DC.
5. MILLER, S. A. 1986. Synthetic foods:technical, cultural and legal issues. Food Technol. 38(4), 160-164.
6. DARBY, W. H. and HAMBRAEUS, L. 1978. Proposed nutritional guidelines for utilization of industrially produced nutrients. Nutr. Rev. 38(3), 65-71.
7. CLYDESDALE, F. M. 1979. Nutrition realities—where does technology fit? J. Am. Dietet. Assoc. 74(1), 17-22.
8. LACHANCE, P. A. 1973. Basic human nutrition and the RDA. Food Prod. Dev. 6(8), 64-68.
9. ROGERS, R. W. 1987. Foods are chemicals. Sci. Food Agr. 5(3), 16-19.
10. TAYLOR, S. L. 1982. An overview of interactions between food-borne toxicants and nutrients. Food Technol. 36(10), 91-95.
11. HARPER, A. E. 1988. Nutrition; from myth and magic to science. Nutr. Today 23(1). 8-17.
12. BEIGLER, M. A. 1976. Complete synthetic foods. In New Protein Foods, Vol. 2, Part B. A. M. Altschul (ed.). Academic Press, New York.
13. THEMILT, L. W. 1983. Chemistry and World Food Supplies: The New Frontiers. Pergamon Press, New York.
14. LACHANCE, P. A. 1968. Single cell protein in space systems. In Single Cell Protein, R. Mateles and S. Tannenbaum (eds.). MIT Press Cambridge, MA.
15. SUGERMAN, C. 1988. Healthier eating through chemistry. Food Technol. 42(7), 23-24.
16. BRESSANI, R. 1988. Protein complementation of foods. In Nutritional Evaluation of Food Processing, E. Karmas and R. S. Harris (eds.). AVI/Van Nostrand Reinhold, New York.

17. AIDA, K. 1979. Production of amino acids and nucleotides by fermentation. *In* Food Science & Technology, H. Chiba, M. Fujimaki, K. Iwai, H. Mitsuda, Y. Mitsuda and U. Morita (eds.). Kodansha, Tokyo.
18. KUEBLER, W. 1973. Enrichment and fortification of food for infants and children. Bibl. Nutr. Dieta. *18*, 224–285.
19. ANON. 1988. Growth and economic impact of the food processing industry: a summary report. Food Technol. *42*(5). 95–100, 105–110.
20. SHANK, F. R. and WILKENING, V. L. 1986. Considerations for fortification policy. Cereal Foods World *31*(10), 728–740.
21. IFT. 1989. IFT Status Summary—Low Calorie Foods. Food Technol. *43*(4).
22. McCORMICK, R. 1988. The lowdown on low-cal. Dairy Foods *89*(5), 48–49.
23. ANON. 1988. Sweeteners. Food Eng. Int. *13*(3), 35.
24. DIETZ, J. M. and ERDMAN, J. W. 1989. Effects of thermal processing upon vitamins and protein in foods. Nutr. Today *24*(4), 6–15.
25. LEVEILLE, G. A. 1984. Food fortification: opportunities and pitfalls. Food Technol. *38*(1), 58–63.
26. GREGORY, J. F. 1985. Chemical changes of vitamins during food processing. *In* Chemical Changes if Food During Processing, T. Richardson and J. Finley, (eds.). AVI/Van Nostrand Reinhold, New York.
27. ANON. 1986. Effects of food processing on nutritive value. A scientific status summary. IFT Expert Panel on Food Safety & Nutrition, Institute of Food Technologists, Chicago.
28. FENNEMA, O. 1987. Effects of freeze preservation on nutrients. *In* Nutritional Evaluation of Food Processing, 3rd Ed. E. Karmas and R. S. Harris (eds). AVI/Van Nostrand Reinhold, New York.
29. ROBERTS, R. 1983. Food preservation and nutrition. Natl. Food Rev. NFR-*20*, 2–6.
30. MORAN, R. 1959. Nutritional significance of recent work on wheat flour and bread. Nutr. Abstr. Rev. *29*, 1–10.
31. THOMAS, B. 1968. Nutritional-physiological views in processing cereal products. Vegetables *15*, 360–371. (German)
32. LACHANCE, P. A. 1986. The Cereal-Grain Fortification Gap. Public Issue Report, Hoffmann-LaRoche, Nutley, NJ.
33. PEDERSON, B., KNUDSEN, K. C. B. and EGGUM, B. O. 1989. Nutrition value of cereal products with emphasis on the effect of milling. *In* Nutritional Value of Cereal Products, Beans and Starches, G. H. Bourne (ed.). Karger, Basel.
34. KARMAS, E. and HARRIS, R. S. 1987. Nutritional Evaluation of Food Processing, 3rd Ed. AVI/Van Nostrand Reinhold, New York.
35. BORENSTEIN, B. and LACHANCE, P. A. 1988. Effects of Processing Preparation on the Nutritive Value of Food. *In* Modern Nutrition in Health and Diseases, 7th Ed, M. Shils and V. Young (eds.) Lea & Febiger, Philadelphia.
36. LACHANCE, P. A. 1973. The vanishing American meal. Food Prod. Dev. *7*(9), 36–40.
37. LACHANCE, P. A. 1989. Nutritional responsibilities of food companies in the next century.. Food Technol. *43*(4), 144.
38. PETERSON, H. C. and STONE, F. M. 1967. Will fabricated foods revolutionize mealtime? Food Prod. Dev. *1*(4), 26–28, 54.
39. EVANS, M. D. and CRONIN, F. J. 1986. Diets of school-age children and teenagers. Fam. Economics Rev. *3*, 14–20.
40. ANON. 1987. Food service trends. Natl. Food Rev. NFR-*37*, 10–15.

41. RIES, C. P., KLINE, K. and WEAVER, S. O. 1987. Impact of commercial eating on nutrient adequacy. J. Am. Dietet. Assoc. *4*, 463–468.
42. STEPHENSON, M. 1986. A how-to-guide to a balanced diet. FDA Consumer *20*(8), 23–27.
43. FARR, D. T. 1987. Consumer attitude and the supermarket. Cereal Foods World *32*(6), 413–415.
44. KINSEY, J. 1987. Changing food market demographics: implications for food processors. Cereal Foods World *32*(6), 425–428.
45. CHOU, M. 1989. Is cooking becoming a spectator sport? Cereal Foods World *34*(4), 350–351.
46. JACKSON, C. 1987. Today's food consumers: What they are looking for in a supermarket. Cereal Foods World *32*(6), 417–418.
47. SLOAN, A. E. 1987. Change in breakfast patterns may be among current consumer trends. Cereal Foods World *32*(3), 246–247.
48. JENKINS, D. J. A. *et al.* 1989. Nibbling versus gorging: Metabolic advantages of increased meal frequency. N. Engl. J. Med. *321*, 929–934.
49. ANON. 1988. Ready-to-eat foods usage tied to microwave ovens. Food Eng. Int. *13*(4), 23; 1989. *14*(8), 23.
50. LACHANCE, P. A. 1981. The balanced diet as a delivery system. Presentation: VNIS Balanced Diet Conference, St. Lucie, Fla.
51. HERTZLER, A. A. and ANDERSON, H. L. 1974. Food guides in the United States. J. Am. Dietet. Assoc. *64*, 19–28.
52. HAUGHTON, B., GUSSOW, J. D. and DODDS, J. M. 1987. A historical study of the underlying assumptions for U.S. guides from 1917 through the basic four food group guide. J. Nutr. Educ. *19*(4), 169–174.
53. SCHAEFER, A. 1981. The balanced diet: What is it? Presentation: VNIS Balanced Diet Conference, St. Lucie, Fla.
54. CLAPP, S. 1983. Chuck the basic 4, Community Nutritionist *II*(Jan–Feb.), 1.
55. WELLBORN, S. N. 1977. Are you eating right? U.S. News & World Rep. 11/28, 39–43.
56. KING, S. C., COHENOUR, S. H., CORRUCCINI, C. G. and SCHNEEMAN, P. 1978. Evaluation and modification of the basic four food guide. J. Nutr. Educ. *10*(1), 27–29.
57. MISKIMIN, D., BOWERS, J. and LACHANCE, P. 1974. Nutrification of frozen preplated school lunches is needed. Food Technol. *28*(2), 52–56.
58. KIRK, J. R. 1981. They just don't make a balanced diet the way they used to. Presentation: VNIS Balanced Diet conference, St. Lucie, FL.
59. LACHANCE, P. A. and FISHER, M. C. 1986. Educational and technological innovations required to enhance the selection of desirable nutrients. Clin. Nutr. *5*(6), 257–267.
60. LACHANCE, P. A. 1973. A Commentary on the New FDA Nutritional Labeling Regulations. Nutr. Today *8*(1), 18–23.
61. SCHUCKER, R. E. 1985. Does nutrition labeling really affect food choices? Nutr. Today *20*(6), 24–28.
62. FDA. 1989. Nutrition labeling. Fed. Reg. *54*(151), 32610–15.
63. MILLER, S. A. 1989. The sage of health claims labeling: A modern fable, Cereal Foods World *34*(4), 343–346.
64. LEVEILLE, G. A. 1978. Today's American diet—a cause for concern. Food Prod. Dev. *12*(12). 53–54.
65. WINDHAM, C. T., WYSE, B. W. and HANSEN, R. G. 1982. Alcohol consumption

and nutrient density of diets in the Nation-wide Food Consumption Survey. J. Am. Dietet. Assoc. 82(4), 364–372.
66. GUENTHER, P. M. 1986. Beverages in the diets of American teenagers. J. Am. Dietet. Assoc. 86, 493–499.
67. PETERKIN, B. B. 1986. Women's diets: 1977 and 1985. J. Nutr. Educ. 18(6), 251–257.
68. PETERKIN, B. B. and RIZEK, R. L. 1986. Diets of American women: Looking back nearly a decade. Natl. Food Rev. NFR-34, 12–15.
69. YETLEY, E. 1987. Nutritional applications of the health and nutrition surveys (NHANES). Ann. Rev. Nutr. 7, 441–463.
70. ANON. 1986. Joint Nutrition applications of the health and nutrition surveys (NHANES). Nutr. Today 21(3), 23–29.
71. ANON. 1988. Report of the National Food/Nutrition Science Policy Workshop: Research Required to Improve the Validity and Utility of Nutrition Monitoring Activities. Office of Scientific Public Affairs, IFT, Chicago.
72. CRONIN, F. J. and SHAW, A. M. 1988. Summary of dietary recommendations for healthy Americans. Nutr. Today 28(6), 26–34.
73. OLSON, J. A. 1988. Dietary guidelines: International and national perspectives. Nutr. Rev. 46(6), 236–240.
74. ANON. 1988. Surgeon General's report on nutrition and health (summary & recommendations). Nutr. Today 23(5), 22–30.
75. ANON. 1989. Diet and Health: Implications for Reducing Chronic Disease. National Academy Press, Washington, DC.
76. SLAVIN, J. L. 1990. Communicating nutrition information: Whose job is it? Food Technol. 44(10), 70, 72, 74.
77. FISHER, M. C. and LACHANCE. P. A 1985. Nutrition evaluation of published weight-reducing diets. J. Am. Dietet. Assoc. 85, 450–454.
78. KINSELLA, J. E. 1987. Trends in the new product development modifying the nutrient composition of animal products. Food Technol. 41(1), 62–65.
79. LACHANCE, P. A. 1970. Nutrification, a new nutritional concept. Food Technol. 24, 724.
80. BAUERNFEIND, J. C. 1970. Vitamin fortification and nutrified foods. Proc. 3rd Int. Congress, Food Science & Technol. Washington, DC.
81. LACHANCE, P. A. 1972. Nutrification: A concept for assuring quality by bringing intervention in feeding systems. J. Agr. Food Chem. 20, 522–525.
82. BERG, A. 1976. The nutrition factor: Its role in national development. Report of the Brookings Institution, Washington, DC.
83. RICHARDSON, D. 1983. Iron fortification of foods and drinks. Chem. Ind. 13(4), 498–501.
84. KLINE, O. L. 1974. What foods should be fortified? In Nutrients in Processed Foods: Vitamins, Minerals. American Med. Assoc., Publishing Sciences Group, Chicago, IL.
85. BEATON, G. H. 1976. Food fortification In Nutrition in Preventative Medicine: Major Deficiency Syndromes, Epidemiology, and Approaches to Control, G. H. Beaton and J. M. Bengoa (eds.). World Health Organization, Geneva.
86. TANNENBAUM, S. R. 1979. The issue of fortification: The case for broadening. Presentation: VNIS Vitamin Nutrition Issues Conference. Boca Raton, Fla.
87. STARE, F. J. 1979. Fortification of foods in industrial and developing countries. Bibl. Nutr. Dieta. 28, 201–205.

88. HEGSTED, D. M. 1976. Food fortification. *In* in the Community, D. S. McLaren (ed.). John Wiley & Sons, New York.
89. RUSSO, J. R. 1977. Why not fortify doughnuts, potatoes, hot dogs, pizza and similar foods? Food Eng. *49*(10), 81–82.
90. TEPLY, L. J. 1974. Food fortification. *In* Man, Food and Nutrition, M. Recheigl, Jr. (ed.). CRC Press, Boca Raton.
91. QUICK, J. A. and MURPHY, C. W. 1982. The Fortification of Foods: A Review. Agr. Handbook No. 598. USDA, Washington, DC.
92. MERTZ, W. 1977. Fortification of foods with vitamins and minerals. Ann. N.Y. Acad. Sci. *300*, 151–160.
93. LATHAM, M. C. 1984. Strategies for the control of malnutrition and the influence of nutritional sciences. Food Nutr. *11*(1), 5–31.
94. LACHANCE, P. A. 1980. Fortification: Broader. VNIS Vitam. Issues *1*(1), 1.
95. GUTHRIE, H. A. 1980. Fortification: Narrower. VNIS Vitam. Issues *1*(1), 3.
96. CALIENDO, M. A. 1979. Food fortification. *In* Nutrition and the World Food Crisis, M. A. Caliendo (ed.). MacMillan Publishing Co., New York.
97. REIDY, K. 1981. Adding nutrients to foods: The plus and minuses. Natl. Food Rev. NFR-*13*, 29–30.
98. CHRISTOPHER, C. 1978. Is fortification unnecessary technology? Food Prod. Dev. *12*(4), 24–25.
99. DYMSZA, H. A. 1974. Supplementation of food vs. nutrition education: In favor of nutrition education. Food Technol. *28*(7), 55–63.
99a. RICHARDSON, D. P. 1990. Food fortification. Proc. Nutr. Soc. *49*, 39–50.
100. AUSTIN, J. E. and HITT, C. 1979. Nutrition Intervention in the United States. Ballinger Publishing Co., Cambridge.
101. ANON. 1982. The nutritive quality of processed foods; General policies for nutrient addition. Nutr. Rev. *40*(3), 93–96.
102. FORBES, A. 1981. Government regulations and nutrition alternates. Presentation: VNIS Balanced Diet Conference, St. Lucie, FL.
103. MILLER, S. A. and STEPHENSON, M. F. 1987. Food fortification: The need for scientific contribution. Bibl. Nutr. Dieta. *40*, 82–95.
104. FORBES, A. L. 1978. Determining the composition of the U.S. food supply. Food Prod. Dev. *12*(1), 26–28.
105. JARRATT, M. C. 1982. USDA's position on food fortification. Food Eng. *54*(3), 123–124.
106. ANON. 1985. Nutrition Allowances Standards and Education. Army Regulation 40-25/Naval Command Medical Instr. 10110.1 and Air Force Reg. 160-95 (May 15).
107. HINMAN, W. F., HIGGINS, M. M. and HALLIDAY, E. G. 1947. Nutritive value of canned foods 18. Further study of ascorbic acid and thiamine. J. Am. Dietet. Assoc. *23*, 226–231.
108. THOMAS, M. H., BREMER, S., EATON, A. and CRAIG, V. 1949. Effect of electronic cooking on nutritive values of foods. J. Am. Dietet. Assoc. *25*, 39–45.
109. THOMAS, M. and BERRYMAN, G. H. 1949. Effect of sulphite in dehydrated foods on thiamine content of a diet. J. Am. Dietet. Assoc. *25*, 941–942.
110. THOMAS, M. H. and CALLOWAY, D. H. 1957. Nutritive value of irradiated turkey. II. Vitamin losses after irradiation and cooking. J. Am. Dietet. Assoc. *33*, 1030–1033.
111. THOMAS, M. H. and CALLOWAY, D. H. 1961. Nutritional value of dehydrated foods. J. Am. Dietet. Assoc. *39*, 105–116.

112. KLICKA, M. V., HOLLENDER, H. A. and LACHANCE, P. A. 1967. Food for Astronauts. J. A. Dietet. Assoc. *51*, 238–245.
113. BERG, A. 1987. Malnutrition: What can be done? Johns Hopkins University Press, Baltimore.
114. GOODMAN, R. M. 1986. New technology and its role in enhancing global food production. Fed. Proc. *45*(10), 2432–2436.
115. HETZEL, B. S. 1988. The Prevention & Control of Iodine Deficiency Disorders. United Nations Admin. Comm. Coordinator, Subcommittee on Nutrition ACC/SCN, Policy Discussion Paper No. 3. Rome, Italy.
116. BERG, A. and AUSTIN, J. 1987. Nutrition policies and programs: A decade of redirection. *In* Food Policy: Integrating Supply, Distribution and Consumption, J. P. Gittinger, J. Leslie and C. Horsington (eds.). Johns Hopkins University Press, Baltimore.
117. AUSTIN, J. E. 1981. Nutrition Intervention: Scope and Limits. Symp. on Nutrition on Health and Disease and International Development. Proc. XII Int. Congress of Nutrition. Alan R. Liss, New York.
118. DICHTER, C. R. 1987. The fifth world food survey: An assessment of food supplies and malnutrition. J. Am. Dietet. Assoc. *87*(12), 1668–1672.
119. TROSTLE, R. G. 1989. Food aid needs during 1990's. Natl. Food Rev. *12*(1), 31–33.
120. BAUERNFEIND, J. C. 1988. Nutrification of food. *In* Modern Nutrition in Health & Disease. M. E. Shils and V. R. Young (eds.). Lea & Febiger, Philadelphia.
121. AUSTIN, J. E. and ZEITLIN, M. 1981. Nutrition Intervention in Developing Countries: Vol. III. Fortification. Oelgeschlager, Gunn & Hain Publishers, Cambridge.
122. HALLBERG, L. 1982. Effect of vitamin C on the availability of iron. *In* Vitamin C, J. Counsell and D. Hornig (eds.). Applied Science. London.
123. HUANG, P. C. and TUNG, T. C. 1971. Feeding of infants with rice-milk mixtures. J. Formosan Med. Assoc. *70*, 135.
124. MOON, T. E. and MICOZZI, M. S. 1989. Nutrition and Cancer Prevention: Investigating the Role of Micronutrients. Marcel Dekker, New York.
125. International Conference. 1989. Antioxidant Vitamins and β-Carotene in Disease Prevention. Queen Elizabeth II Conference Centre, London, U.K. Oct. 2–4 (in press).
126. SOKOL, R. J. 1989. Vitamin E and neurological function in man. Free Radical Biol. Med. *6*, 189–207.
127. PRYOR, W. A. 1987. Views on the wisdom of using antioxidant vitamin supplements. Free Radical Biol. Med. *3*, 189–191.
128. BERNER, L. A., McBEAN, L. D. and LOFGREN, P. A. 1989. Calcium and chronic disease prevention challenges to the food industry. Food Technol. *44*(3), 50–70.
129. ANON. 1989. Nutrition information on food labels J. Am. Dietet. Assoc. *89*(3), 266–267.
130. MILNER, J. A. 1989. Minerals as modifiers of the cancer process. Abstr. 75, 197th ACS Natl. Meeting, Dallas, April 9–14.
131. GIBSON, R. S. 1989. Assessment of trace element status in humans, Prog. Food Nutr. Sci. *13*, 67–11.
132. MERTZ, W. 1982. Trace minerals and atherosclerosis. Fed. Proc. *41*, 2807–2812.
133. NIELSEN, F. H. 1988. Nutritional significance of the ultratrace elements. Nutr. Rev. *46*(10), 337–339.
134. BAUERNFEIND, J. C. 1981. Carotenoids as Colorants and Vitamin A Precursors: Technological and Nutritional Applications. Academic Press, New York.

135. HETZEL, B. S. 1988. Progress in the prevention & control of iodine deficiency disease 1986-87: A global review. ICCIDD Newsletter 4(1), 1-12.
136. MILOT, R. 1986. Effect of the fortification of foods with vitamin D on the health of populations of 19 countries. Cah. Nutr. Diet. 21(4), 295-299.
137. MILLER, D. F. 1977. Cereal Enrichment/Pellagra-USA in perspective. Presentation: Annual Meeting of Am. Assoc. Cereal Chem. AACC, St. Paul; 1978. Food Prod. Dev. 12(4), 30.
138. WILDER, R. M. 1956. A brief history of the enrichment of flour & bread. J. Am. Med. Assoc. 162(17), 1537-1541.
139. FRIEND, B. 1972. Enrichment and fortification of foods 1966-70. Natl. Food Situation 142, 29-34.
140. GUGGENHEIM, K., BRZEZINSKI, A., ILAN, J. and KALLNER, B. 1959. Nutritional evaluation of flour enrichment with riboflavin in Israel. Am. J. Clin. Nutr. 7, 526-631.
141. PAK, D. N. 1986. The vitamin situation in Chile. Rev. Chilena Nutr. 14(2), 71-84.
142. SALCEDO, J. et al. 1950. Artificial enrichment of white rice as a solution to endemic beriberi. J. Nutr. 42, 501-523.
143. IGARASHI, O., OHZEKI, S., NIHO, Y., ANDO, K., MOHRI, K. and ITOKAWA, Y. 1984. Effect of intake of a new enriched rice, "Shingen," on the levels of vitamin B_1, E and some characteristics of blood of female students. J. Jap. Soc. Nutr. Food Sci. 37(2), 145-150.
144. MITSUDA, H. and YAMAMOTO, A. 1983. Vitamin fortification. In Handbook of Nutritional Supplements: Human Use, Vol. 1, M. Recheigl (ed.). CRC Press, Boca Raton.
145. DuPLESSIS, J. P. et al. 1974. Effect of the enrichment of maize meal with nicotinic acid and riboflavin upon the vitamin and protein nutritional status of young school-going and pre-school children. S.A. Med. J. 48(14), 1641-1648.
146. COLEMAN, N. 1983. The use of food fortification to prevent folate deficiency. In Nutrition Intervention Strategies in National Development, B. A. Underwood (ed.). Academic Press, New York.
147. HAWKES, J. G. and VILLOTA, R. 1989. Folates in foods; reactivity, stability during processing and nutritional implications. Crit. Rev. Food Sci. Nutr. 28(6), 439-538.
148. KAMIEN, M., WOODHILL, J. M., NOBILE, S., CAMERON, P. and ROSEVEAR, P. 1975. Nutrition in the Australian Aborigines—Efforts of the fortification of white flour. Aust. N.Z.J. Med. 5, 123-133.
149. BAUERNFEIND, J. C. 1986. Vitamin A Deficiency and Its Control. Academic Press, Orlando.
150. BAUERNFEIND, J. C. 1983. Vitamin A: Technology and applications. World Rev. Nutr. Dietet. 41, 110-199.
151. ARROYAVE, G. et al. 1979. Evaluation of sugar fortification with vitamin A at the national level. Pan Am. Health Organ. Publ. 384. Washington, DC.
152. SOLON, F. S., LATHAM, . C., GUIRRIEC, R., FLORENTINO, R., WILLIAMSON, D. F. and AGUILAR, J. 1985. Fortification fo MSG with vitamin A: The Philippine experience. Food Technol. 38(11), 71-77.
153. MUHILAL et al. 1988. Vitamin A-fortified monosodium glutamate and vitamin A status: A controlled field trial. Am. J. Clin. Nutr. 48, 1265-1283.
154. BEARD, J. L. 1988. Iron fortification: Rationale & effects. Nutr. Today 23(4), 17-20.

155. HALLBERG, L. *et al.* 1979. An analysis of factors leading to a reduction in iron deficiency in Swedish Women, WHO Bull. *57*, 947–970.
156. STEKEL, A., OLIVARES, M., PIZARRO, F., CHADUD, P., LOPEZ, I. and AMAR, M. 1986. Absorption of fortification iron from milk formulas in infants. Am. J. Clin. Nutr. *43*, 917–922.
157. JAMISON, E. T. and PIAZZA, A. 1987. China's food and nutrition planning. *In* Food Policy: Integrating Supply, Distribution and Consumption, J. P. Gittinger, J. Leslie and C. Horsington (eds.). John Hopkins University Press, Baltimore.
158. ORSO, T. 1971. Clinical studies of amino acid fortification in Japan. *In* Amino Acid Fortification of Protein Foods. M. S. Scrimshaw and A. M. Altschul (eds.). MIT press, Cambridge.
159. GERSHOFF, S. N. 1978. Evaluation of cereal grain enrichment programs. Proc. Western Hemisphere Nutr. Congr. *5*, 41–45.
160. HARRELL-BOND, B. E., HENRY, C. J. K. and WILSON, K. 1989. Fortification of foods for refugees. Lancet, June 17, 1392; 1989. SCN News *4*, 29–30.

CHAPTER 3

MINERAL ADDITIVES

FERGUS M. CLYDESDALE, Ph.D.

INTRODUCTION

The use of mineral additives in food, like other nutrient additives, was used historically as a public health measure to prevent the occurrence of deficiency diseases in large segments of the population. In fact, the first and perhaps most successful use of fortification in the United States involved the element iodine with the development of iodized salt in 1924 to prevent goiter.

Other standards which included minerals were promulgated under the Federal Food and Drug Act of 1938 when in 1940 a hearing was held under this act which resulted in a standard for enriched flour which specified the addition of iron along with thiamine, riboflavin, and niacin and made calcium and vitamin D optional.[1] Over the years, many groups such as the American Public Health Association, the Council on Food and Nutrition of the American Medical Association (AMA), and the Food and Nutrition Board of the National Research Council and the National Academy of Sciences (FNB) have been involved in attempting to establish principles and policies for the fortification of foods culminating in a final policy statement by the FDA in 1980.[2] This policy provides a reasonable umbrella for mineral fortification. Table 3.1 shows some of the mineral additives available for fortification including some listed by the Food Chemicals Codex[3] as a nutrient, dietary supplement or as miscellaneous general purpose. Since there are many suitable forms of most minerals which may be added to food, this list is not complete but it provides some insight into the number of minerals involved.

If current dietary recommendations are reviewed one might speculate that the recommended shift from animal to plant protein and a dramatic decrease in calories from what was consumed at the beginning of the century could lead to a realistic concern about potential mineral deficiency. In fact, such a scenario could easily lead to recommendations for more judicious mineral fortification. Many arguments can be made as to the efficacy or even wisdom of certain types of mineral fortification, but there is evidence that well-focused mineral fortification can indeed be beneficial. A study by Yip et al.[4] involving children aged 6–60 months enrolled in public health programs in 6 states that were monitored by the Centers for Disease Control Pediatric

TABLE 3.1
VARIOUS FORMS OF MINERALS WHICH MAY BE CONSIDERED
FOR ADDITION TO FOOD

Calcium	*Phosphorus*
Calcium Carbonate	Calcium Phosphate, Dibasic
Calcium Chloride	Calcium Phosphate, Monobasic
Calcium Chloride Anhydrous	Calcium Phosphate, Tribasic
Calcium Chloride Solution	Calcium Pyrophosphate
Calcium Gluconate	Phosphoric Acid
Calcium Glycerophosphate	Potassium Phosphate,
Calcium Oxide	mono, di, tri and pyro
Calcium Phosphate, Dibasic	*Zinc*
Calcium Citrate	Zinc Gluconate
Calcium lactate	Zinc Oxide
Calcium lactobionate	Zinc Sulfate
Calcium Phosphate, Monobasic	*Iodine*
Calcium Phosphate, Tribasic	Calcium Iodate
Calcium Pyrophosphate	Potassium Iodate
Calcium Sulfate	Potassium Iodide
Sodium	*Iron*
Sodium Ascorbate	Ferric Ammonium Citrate, Brown
Sodium Chloride	Ferric Ammonium Citrate, Green
Sodium Ferric Pyrophosphate	Ferric Phosphate
Sodium Gluconate	Ferric Pyrophosphate
Sodium Phosphate,	Ferrous Gluconate
mono, di+tribasic	Ferrous Sulfate
Sodium Pyrophosphate	Ferrous Sulfate, dried
Potassium	Iron, Carbonyl
Potassium Chloride	Iron, electrolytic
Potassium Gluconate	Iron, reduced
Potassium Glycerophosphate	Sodium Ferric Pyrophosphate
Magnesium	*Manganese*
Magnesium Phosphate dibasic	Manganese Chloride
Magnesium Phosphate tribasic	Manganese Gluconate
Magnesium Sulfate (Epsom Salt)	Manganese Glycerophosphate
Copper	Manganese Hypophosphate
Copper Gluconate	Manganese Sulfate

Nutrition Surveillance System found that the prevalence of anemia declined steadily from 7.87% in 1975 to 2.9% in 1985. To ensure that the results were not a function of changing socioeconomic status, correlations were conducted that indicated that anemia declined within each socioeconomic group. This means that there was a true decline likely due to improvements in childhood iron nutrition. In the same issue of JAMA in which this paper appeared, an editorial by Stockman[5] names the Special

Supplemental Food Program for Women, Infants and Children (WIC program, Public Law 92-433) begun in the 1970's and the recommendations proposed in 1976 by the Committee on Nutrition of the American Academy of Pediatrics as significant events in the decline of anemia. The recommendations encouraged breast-feeding, the use of iron-supplemented formulas when breast-feeding was not employed, the introduction of iron-fortified cereals, and the avoidance of iron-poor food sources. Additionally it was recommended that universal screening for anemia be undertaken as early as 9 months of age for term infants and at 6 months for preterm infants. Undoubtedly all of these factors played an important role in aiding the decline in anemia, but certainly fortification was an important contributor to the overall effect.

Obviously there are, and will be, other target populations and/or situations which demand fortification of foods with minerals other than iron. The remainder of this chapter will discuss some of the factors which should be considered from a technical point of view if mineral fortification is to succeed.

MINERAL REACTIVITY AND FOOD QUALITY

Successful fortification of a food is dependent upon the fortificant acting in a relatively benign manner in the food. Unfortunately this level of chemical inertness is often associated with insolubility and relatively poor bioavailability. This leads to a situation where some compromises must be made and/or new stable, yet bioavailable, mineral complexes developed. However, prior to making such decisions it is necessary to consider the kinds of reactions which might occur and which we may wish to avoid.

The essential minerals, trace elements and electrolytes are shown in Table 3.2. There are 17 known to be essential and 4 (V, Si, Ni, Sn) suspected of essentiality with boron gathering increasing interest as another mineral of nutritional importance.[6] However, for purposes of fortification this list can be further narrowed to approximately 10: Na, K, Ca, P, Mg, Fe, I, Zn, Cu and Mn. Of these, it is unlikely that Na or K would be added as nutrients, iodine would be mostly in salt, and phosphorus would probably be added only in a calcium complex, thus reducing the list to six, namely, Ca, Mg, Fe, Zn, Cu, and Mn.

Calcium and Mg are in Group 2A of the Periodic Table and as such are divalent, electropositive and form salts with nonmetals and bases in water. The other four, Fe, Zn, Cu and Mn are members of the transition metal series and perhaps their most notable property is their ability to form stable complexes, often as chelates.

The key to proper mineral fortification is to remember that you are dealing with chemically reactive species, not inert compounds as the minerals are often thought of. This reactivity becomes particularly apparent in a food in the presence of moisture and/or adequate water activity when reactions may occur with free radicals, other food components, oxygen or diffused packaging materials. Ionization, dehydration, rehydration or a change in valence, where possible, might also occur. Any, or all

TABLE 3.2
THE ESSENTIAL MINERALS IN NUTRITION

Mineral	Maximum Adult RDA or Estimated Safe and Adequate Intake	Physiological Functions
Calcium (Ca)	1200 mg/day	Structural function, bones, teeth; cofactor; clotting; nerve and muscle action; membrane permeability
Phosphorus (P)	1200 mg/day	Structural function, bones, teeth, acid-base balance; glucose catabolism; component of genetic material and phospholipids
Magnesium (Mg)	350 mg/day	Cofactor in many reactions; energy metabolism, protein synthesis, nerve and muscle action; bone structure
Sulfur (S)	None	Component of several vitamins, amino acids and other compounds
Iron (Fe)	Males 10 mg/day; Females, premenopausal 15 mg/day, postmenopausal 10 mg/day	Hemoglobin formation and oxygen transport; cellular oxidation; cofactor as the nonheme form
Iodine (I)	150 μg/day	Component of the thyroid hormone which regulate cell oxidation
Zinc (Zn)	15 mg/day	Cofactor in many reactions; growth reproduction, wound healing; taste acuity; insulin function
Copper (Cu)	Estimated safe and adequate intake 1.5–3.0 mg/day	Cofactor; facilities iron metabolism
Fluoride (F)	Estimated safe and adequate intake 1.5–4.0 mg/day	Dental health; integrity of teeth and bones
Manganese (Mn)	Estimated safe and adequate intake 2.0–5.0 mg/day	Cofactor for many reactions; urea formation; protein metabolism; glucose oxidation; lipid metabolism; blood clotting
Selenium (Se)	70 mg/day	Associated with fat metabolism, cofactor for an enzyme that neutralizes peroxides
Chromium (Cr)	Estimated safe and adequate intake 50–200 μg/day	Component of glucose tolerance factor for the metabolism of carbohydrates
Molybdenum (Mo)	Estimated safe and adequate intake 75–250 μg/day	Enzyme cofactor
Cobalt (Co)	None	Component of vitamin B_{12}

TABLE 3.2 (*Continued*)

Mineral	Maximum Adult RDA or Estimated Safe and Adequate Intake	Physiological Functions
Sodium (Na)[1,2]	Estimated *minimum* requirement of healthy adults 500 mg/day	Fluid and acid-base balance, nerve and muscle action; involved in glucose and amino acid absorption
Potassium (K)[3]	Estimated *minimum* requirement of healthy adults 2000 mg/day	Fluid and acid-base balance, nerve and muscle action
Chloride (Cl)[1,2]	Estimated *minimum* requirement of healthy adults 750 mg/day	Fluid and acid-base balance; anion of stomach acid
Vanadium (V)	Suspected human essentiality	
Silicon (Si)	Suspected human essentiality	
Nickel (Ni)	Suspected human essentiality	
Tin (Sn)	Suspected human essentiality	

[1]No allowance has been included for large, prolonged losses from the skin through sweat.
[2]There is no evidence that higher intakes confer any health benefits.
[3]Desirable intakes of potassium may considerably exceed these values.
NOTE: The U.S. Recommended Daily Allowance (U.S. RDA) for adults and children (4 or more years of age) are as follows: calcium, 1000 mg; iron, 18 mg; phosphorus, 1000 mg; iodine (optional) 150 µg; magnesium, 400 mg; zinc, 15 mg; copper, 2 mg/day. No U.S. RDA has been established for either potassium or manganese; daily intakes of 2500 mg and 4 mg respectively are based on the 1979 Recommended Daily Allowances of the Food and Nutrition Board, National Academy of Sciences, National Research Council.

of these reactions could result in undesirable quality changes and consideration must be given to such an occurrence. It must be remembered that, ideally, mineral fortification should cause no change in color, flavor, methods of preparation, appearance, or catalyze any other undesirable changes in the food if it is to be used successfully in a general fortification program. This is a difficult ideal to achieve and the following sections will summarize some of the potential problems.

Color

Color is one of the most obvious undesirable changes that minerals can cause in food. Some color changes are due to the reactivity of the mineral used while others may be due to the amount of mineral used. The minerals with a high nutritional requirement such as Ca, P, and Mg present problems somewhat different than those in the lower ranges (Table 3.2). For instance in sterile strawberry and chocolate liquid dietary products, the use of insoluble Ca or Mg salts causes a lighter color than desirable,[7] probably due to a diluent-like effect at high concentrations. The opposite occurs with soluble salts in chocolate dietary products, probably due to reactions with phenolic compounds such as tannins in the chocolate. As well even small amounts of minerals such as iron, if added in a reactive form such as ferrous sulfate, can react with phenolics to form blue-black colors and darken food products containing large amounts of tannin, such as chocolate and barley flour.[8] Iron may also cause color problems in milk[9] and soy isolate infant formulas[10] by giving a gray cast to these products.

Problems may also occur in powdered products and dry blends when liquified. This has been reported[7] in a vanilla-flavored product fortified with ferrous citrate. In the powdered form this product had a normal white appearance but when added to milk it became dark gray. The color was attributed to a reaction between iron, sodium ascorbate and vanilla. Interestingly, vanillin, the most important characterizing agent in vanilla extracts, can be obtained as a lignin byproduct.[11] Perhaps traces of lignin or other polyphenolics in vanilla could explain the darkening with iron.

The use of minerals in products containing either naturally occurring or added-anthocyanin pigments must be also done with care. Several multivalent metal ions can interact with anthocyanins possessing vicinal phenolic hydroxyls and shift the color of the pigment from red to blue. Aluminum, tin, iron, calcium, and potassium have all be reported to affect the color of anthocyanins in some manner.[12] Again the reactivity and/or solubility of the mineral is critical. It should be noted that many fruit-based beverages are of low pH and as a result will tend to solubilize most mineral salts thus increasing their reactivity and potential to cause color problems. Unfortunately this same solubilization increases the potential for bioavailability, thus establishing the inverse relationship between functionality and bioavailability mentioned previously.

Some of these color problems may be eliminated by changing the fortificant source or adding it to the product at a different stage in the process. If iron is dry-blended into the finished powdered product, the color may be better than if added during the liquid stage of processing due to minimization of reactivity in the dry state.

Flavor

The addition or presence of minerals in food can also cause undesirable flavor changes, as well as color changes. As was the case with color, the amount of mineral necessary to achieve nutritional significance has a direct bearing on flavor. For instance large amounts of calcium and magnesium salts are necessary to achieve nutritional significance and at these levels, tribasic calcium phosphate, calcium sulfate, and magnesium oxide can produce chalky flavors. In some cases this chalkiness can be reduced by adding the mineral salt early in the process, particularly prior to homogenization. As well, if a more soluble calcium salt like calcium gluconate is used at high levels, problems can arise due to the undesirable flavor of calcium ions,[13] or problems might arise from high levels of the anion of a salt such as citrate or some amino acids. High levels of calcium and magnesium can also produce astringency while the electrolytes can cause bitterness and off-flavors.

The major flavor problem, however, may arise in foods which contain lipids. Many minerals, particularly the transition metals possessing two or more valence states with a suitable oxidation-reduction potential between them such as cobalt, copper, iron, manganese, and nickel are major pro-oxidants. Even at levels as low as 0.1 ppm they can increase the rate of oxidation under certain circumstances,[14] and cause unacceptable off-flavors. Heavy metals may also cause oxidative problems, but they are usually due to uptake from soil and not from intentional fortification.

Of all the minerals, iron is the one most involved with the formation of off-flavors in lipid-containing foods. It forms complexes and free radicals with oxygen that are energized sufficiently to remove hydrogen from the fatty acid chains and form free-radical derivatives of fatty acids.[15] This process may be simplistically displayed as follows:[16]

$$Fe^2 + O_2 \rightarrow Fe^{3+} + O_2^{\cdot -} \quad \text{(superoxide)}$$

Haber-Weiss mechanism:

$$2O_2^{\cdot -} + 2H^+ \rightarrow H_2O_2 + O_2$$

$$Fe^{2+} + H_2O_2 \rightarrow HO \text{ (hydroxyl radical)} + OH^- + Fe^{3+}$$

It has been shown with model physiological systems in vivo, as well as with non-physiological model systems, that oxidation of lipids is greatly facilitated by the presence of iron whether the lipid peroxidation is dependent on the superoxide radical[17] or the hydroxyl radical.[18] It is also apparent that different forms of iron may act as lipid peroxidation initiators. Ferrous, ferric and EDTA chelated forms in some systems may initiate the peroxidation reactions[18] or the ADP-Fe^2-O_2 (perferryl) complex may be the initiator.[19] Interestingly, it has been reported that ferrous sulfate can be used in pasta without adversely affecting its color, shelf-life or flavor. However, it may require further testing in unusual types of pasta products.[20]

Both ready-to-eat (RTE) breakfast cereals and flours from wheat or corn are shelf-stable for the storage time required. However, reactive forms of iron will accelerate lipid oxidation to the point that rancidity will create flavor problems that prohibit an adequate shelf-life. Elemental iron, ferric orthophosphate and sodium ferric pyrophosphate can be used without causing rancidity. However, due to the poor bioavailability of the latter two iron compounds, elemental iron was chosen as the fortificant of choice in RTE cereals during the 1970's and that practice continues today.[15]

Other Quality Changes

Although color and flavor changes often supersede other quality factors, such changes may still be very important. For instance, in the case of iron fortification, rancidity and off-color generally provide the benchmark for use. However, such factors as particle size are important as a quality factor, since elemental iron if added to granular materials, such as farina or semolina, might be removed along with the dust when run through a purifier or any similar device that uses air separation. This problem can be prevented by addition of reduced iron at the end of the milling process.[20] Elemental iron in ready-to-eat cereals can also cause physical problems, since it can gather on magnets that are in the cereal processing lines to remove tramp metal. Rearrangement of the magnets, however, can minimize this problem.[15]

High concentrations of soluble Mg salts may promote gelation of sterilized liquid dietary products, whereas the insoluble salts precipitate. Destabilization of protein may occur with Ca and Mg interactions causing sedimentation or gelation. If the food system does not provide a buffering effect, the addition of basic or acidic salts could cause problems in sterilization. For instance a change in pH in a liquid product due to MgO could cause changes in viscosity, depending on the components of the liquid, and affect heat transfer and sterilization.

In protein-containing liquid products, care must be taken in the amount and rate at which minerals are added, since an overload might cause protein precipitation and a grainy defect. Some of these functional problems may be addressed by using a combination of insoluble and soluble forms,[7] but care should be taken in the way in which such a choice might affect bioavailability.

The oxidative properties of certain minerals such as Fe and Cu may catalyze the destruction of vitamins A and C,[13] as well as promoting flavor changes through oxidative rancidity. Such an occurrence must be considered. Mineral fortification of breads and, I suspect, other baked products may promote quality problems depending upon the mineral, its form, and the product. Lee and Clydesdale[21] evaluated various iron forms in chemically-leavened bread and found that the baking generated insoluble iron independent of the iron source. This may have been due in part to the alkalinity provided by the baking soda used to leaven the bread, but regardless of the cause it would render the iron non-reactive and therefore not likely to cause quality problems on storage. Unfortunately it would also likely reduce bioavailability. Ranhotra et al.[22] evaluated the effect of eight Ca sources (sulfate, carbonate, chloride, phosphate, acetate, lactate, oxide and hydroxide) on the quality of bread made with flour fortified according to the 1974 recommendations of the NAS/NRC.[23] Six of the eight Ca sources produced quite acceptable breads while two others, the oxide and hydroxide, could be usable if the dough pH was adjusted.

In the fortification of bread with Mg, Ranhotra[24] has suggested that Mg powder, because it is theoretically all magnesium is the fortificant of choice in bread making. However, he warns that the powder, like MgO, Mg(OH)$_2$ and MgCO-, tends to raise bread pH above acceptable limits unless the concentration of Mg added is corrected for Mg in the flour to obtain the final proposed level of 44.05 mg of

Mg/100g flour. Such a concentration adjustment also improves loaf volume and overall bread quality, as does a pH adjustment with acetic acid or the addition of magnesium salt to the dough instead of the sponge in the sponge dough process.[25]

Several forms of zinc including both organic (acetate and stearate) and inorganic (carbonate, chloride, oxide, sulfate and elemental) were evaluated in breads made by the sponge dough process.[26] It was found that none of the zinc sources exerted any adverse effects on loaf volume, flavor or overall quality indicating that zinc has few functional problems in this application.

Cost

Although I do not believe that a chapter such as this is an appropriate vehicle for listing prices which are always changing, I still think that some mention of this important parameter should be made.

Costs are from two major sources: (1) the cost of the mineral to be added, and (2) cost of controlling the levels added to ensure consistency with the label declaration.

The cost of raw ingredients varies considerably with the source, and such factors as functionality, bioavailability, and the percentage mineral in the compound added must be considered. To illustrate this cost differential one can note in Table 3.3 the cost of various forms of iron as reported by Barrett and Ranum.[20] These costs may certainly have changed, but the widespread differences probably still hold and are illustrative of the need to consider all factors.

The second major cost factor, that of control, is one that is less troublesome if analytical equipment, personnel and expertise are available. However, even then costs can be high and for that reason manufacturers often utilize vitamin-mineral premixes which do reduce control costs and add some uniformity. The minerals used must not be hygroscopic because of caking problems, and care should be taken with storage of the premix if it contains vitamins and minerals. Recall that Fe and Cu can cause oxidative damage to Vitamin A and C. Thus some assurance of physical and chemical stability of the premixes must be obtained.[7]

Toxicity

The use of supplements and fortification procedures have raised some concern about the possibility of toxic effects from minerals. Increased iron fortification, in particular, generated much debate when it was proposed in the seventies that the standards for the iron content of flour bread and bakery products be tripled. Concerns about hemochromatosis were raised by Drs. Crosby, Krikker and Stohlman and the ensuing debate resulted in a rejection of this proposal although many scientists believed that an increase would have responded to a public health need.[27]

For those minerals with a large RDA (Table 3.2) such as calcium, phosphorous and magnesium there is little concern about toxicity from individual foods which

TABLE 3.3
RELATIVE COSTS OF COMMONLY USED IRON SOURCES

Iron Source	Cost[1] (U.S. Kg)	Contained Iron (%)	Cost of Iron (U.S. $/kg of Fe)
Ferrous sulfate, dried	1.43	32.1	4.45
Hydrogen-reduced	1.06	97.0	1.09
Electrolytically reduced	3.20	98.0	3.26
Carbonyl-reduced	3.20	98.0	6.50
Ferric orthophosphate	1.70	28.6	5.94
Sodium iron pyrophosphate	1.94	15.7	12.36
Ferrous fumarate	3.28	33.0	9.95

Source: Barrett and Ranum.[20]
[1] 1980, Large volume undelivered.

have been fortified since excessively high levels would cause quality problems such as sandiness or chalkiness. However, concerns could be raised if we were to see indiscriminate fortification of these minerals in a broad spectrum of foods. Of the minerals required at lower levels, aside from iron, it would appear that selenium and iodine might pose toxic hazards because of their high toxicities and increasing intakes.[28]

It is difficult to arrive at a measure of "safe intake" for any compound including the nutrients. However, Hathcock[28] has proposed an interesting technique which he employed to arrive at a "mineral safety index" (MSI). This technique involved the use of a "recommended intake" (RI) which is the highest RDA value for an adult, except those for pregnancy and lactation, or the U.S. RDA, whichever is higher and a "minimum toxic dose" (MTD) estimated from the literature. From these values the mineral safety index is calculated as:

$$MSI = MDT/RI$$

The MSI is thus defined in easily understood terms, and the result is a ratio that is independent of units as long as they are the same for the RI and the MTD. The MSI for several minerals are shown in Table 3.4. It should be noted that the MSI for copper is quite high[28] for most people but much less for those with Wilson's disease, a genetic inability to excrete copper. Safety is an emotional issue with conflicting scientific data and undoubtedly these numbers may be questioned. However, the approach seems rational and provides some measure of assessment.

MINERAL REACTIVITY AND BIOAVAILABILITY

Since minerals are added to food for the purpose of providing nutritive value, it is obvious that the major factor which must be considered in choosing a mineral

TABLE 3.4
MINERAL SAFETY INDEXES

Mineral	Recommended Adult Intake[1]	Estimated Adult Oral MTD	MSI
Calcium	1,200 mg	12,000 mg	10
Phosphorus[2]	1,200 mg	12,000 mg	10
Magnesium	400 mg	6,000 mg	15
Iron	18 mg	100 mg	5.5
Zinc	15 mg	500 mg	33
Copper	3 mg	100 mg	33
		<3 mg[3]	<1
Fluoride[4]	4 mg	20 mg	5
		4 mg[5]	1
Iodine	0.15 mcg	2 mg	13
Selenium	0.2 mcg	1 mg	5

[1]The highest of the individual RDA (except those for pregnancy and lactation) or the U.S. RDA, whichever is higher.
[2]As the orthophosphate ion
[3]For people with Wilson's disease
[4]As fluoride ion
[5]Level producing slight fluorisis of dental enamel.
Source: Hathcock.[28]

additive for a particular food is that it be bioavailable and fulfill its intended purpose. After all it doesn't make sense to use a low cost mineral additive that doesn't degrade food quality if it isn't absorbed and utilized by the body. However, the converse is also true in that it doesn't make sense to use an exceedingly bioavailable form of a mineral if the food is rendered unpalatable due to quality losses.

Unfortunately, bioavailability of a mineral in food is not strictly a function of the bioavailability of the mineral salt or additive chosen. If this were the case then one could simply go to the literature, find the bioavailability of a mineral additive when fed alone and then make a decision. However, minerals are often chemically reactive and their bioavailability will often be greatly affected by interactions with food components when added, or during processing and storage. Such reactivity will of course vary with the mineral additive used, the food, the process, and storage times and conditions. This means that the bioavailability of a mineral in food is ultimately dependent upon its electronic configuration, since this governs its physical and chemical properties which in turn govern its behavior in food. Interestingly, the electronic configuration of the elements is also important, since it has been shown that those elements whose physical and chemical properties (electronic structure) are similar will act antagonistically to each other biologically. This thesis was first presented by Hill and Matrone[29] and explained many of the competitive interactions that had been noted up to that time, and since. Thus, excessively high intakes of zinc can cause copper-deficiency anemia and affect calcium absorption as may phosphorus. Conversely excessive intakes of certain forms of calcium can decrease iron absorption. Such interactions are thought to be due to competition at the intestinal absorption site or during absorption rather than to food interactions.

Therefore, in order to make judgements about both bioavailability and functionality so that an appropriate mineral additive may be chosen, it is essential to understand the major physicochemical properties which affect potential bioavailability and how these may be influenced by their food environment and/or processing and storage.[29a]

Solubility

It is a maxim that in order to be absorbed, minerals must be soluble in the intestinal tract but not all soluble minerals are absorbed. Further, it must be noted that when we speak of solubility we are not only referring to the solubility of an ion, salt, hydrate or complex, but also to the type and strength of chemical bonds involved within and without these species. Therefore, we must understand the totality of the chemical reactions occcurring in the food environment to understand mineral solubility and therefore bioavailability. Such basic properties as the charge density of the mineral, the reduction potential, and pH of the medium and the type and strength of bonding, complex formation or chelation which the mineral undergoes must be considered.

Charge Density

In food, mineral solubility can often only be obtained and sustained by the formation of complexes, and the ability of minerals to form such complexes is often related to their charge density, with those with a relatively higher charge in relation to size forming the more numerous and stable complexes. This is illustrated in the transition metals with the trivalent forms producing more stable complexes than the divalent species. Charge density is also of importance to cell permeability since the rate at which a molecule diffuses across the lipid bilayer of the cell membrane is dependent upon its size and degree of polarity. Small nonpolar molecules readily dissolve in lipid bilayers and therefore diffuse across them. Emery[30] has noted that the neutralization of the change on ferric iron by ferrichrome allows the ferrichrome-iron complex to pass through the bacterial cell membrane thus providing iron to the cell.

Reduction Potential and pH

The effect of pH on the solubility of iron and calcium in particular and minerals in general has been reviewed in some detail.[31-34] The solubility product (Ksp) for a mineral (M) in the presence of hydroxyl ions (OH) may be represented by the following equation:

$$M^2 + 2OH^- \rightleftarrows M^2(OH)_2$$

$$Ksp = [M^{+2}][OH^{-1}]^2$$

Since Ksp is a constant, an increase in pH, [OH^{-1}], causes a decrease in the free metal ion [M^{+2}] which follows first, second, and third powers of hydroxyl ion concentration with the mono, di and trivalent form of the metal respectively. It is therefore evident that metal ions will decrease in solubility as the pH is increased. A dramatic example of this was given by Wien and Schwartz[32] who reported that a pH increase of 0.9 units, from pH 6.2 to 7.1, caused a 40% drop in calcium solubility in three muffin formulations.

Another equally important reaction occurs with transition metal solubility as pH increases. The transition metals, including those nutritionally important, Fe, Ca, Ni, Cu and Zn, exist in solution as hydrates rather than ions. As the pH is raised the hydrates lose protons and form the less soluble or insoluble hydroxides. Iron is the best known example of this phenomenon, existing in solution at low pH as Fe(H$_2$O)$_6^{+3}$ and Fe(H$_2$O)$_6^{+2}$. As the pH is raised, the hydroxides, Fe(OH)$_3$ and Fe(OH)$_2$ form the solubilities of 10^{-16} M and 10^{-1} M, respectively. Although neither of these is very soluble, it is clear that Fe^{+2} is much more soluble than Fe^{+3} and explains the greater bioavailability of Fe^{+2}.

The difference in solubility between ions of different valence states is why the reduction potential of the medium is important. In the above case an environment which promotes reduction will keep the Fe^{+2} form predominating and increase bioavailability. This is one of the reasons why vitamin C, which is a reducing agent, greatly enhances the bioavailability of iron. This means that acidic foods and those that contain vitamin C may be a logical place to consider fortification with iron or other minerals.

Complexation and Chelation

The binding of metals in a complex is an extremely important consideration in both the inhibition and enhancement of mineral bioavailability. Due to its importance it will be discussed in some detail in the next section.

ENHANCEMENT AND INHIBITION OF MINERAL BIOAVAILABILITY

The potential bioavailability of minerals is dependent upon solubility as explained previously. Solubility may be due to the inherent chemical nature of the mineral, its immediate environment and the presence of food components which will bond with the mineral forming a complex or chelate. Both enhancers and inhibitors in food act as mineral binding agents, and it is merely the nature of the bond which they form and the solubility of their complex which determines there role as either an enhancer or an inhibitor. On this basis each may be defined as follows:

Enhancers are molecular species in food which form a compound with the mineral which is soluble and can be absorbed by the mucosal cells as such, and/or may undergo cleavage to release the mineral in a soluble form, and/or has constants which allow the mineral to be transferred to a mucosal or serosal acceptor.

On the other hand, inhibitors are molecular species in food which form an insoluble compound, and/or cannot be absorbed as such, and/or cannot be cleaved, and/or releases the mineral in an insoluble form, and/or has thermodynamic constants which do not allow transfer to a mucosal or serosal acceptor.[34]

Implicit in these definitions is the fact an enhancer must form a complex with a mineral that is soluble and that has a stability constant greater than that formed with the mineral by an inhibitor. Thus the mineral would preferentially bind the enhancer due to its greater binding strength. Further, the strength of the bond must be less than the strength of the bond the mineral has with a mucosal acceptor, so that the mineral will pass from the soluble mineral-enhancer complex to the mucosal acceptor. If this was not the case, the mineral would remain in the soluble complex and the ligand involved would be considered an inhibitor. This is why it was stated previously that a mineral must be in a soluble form to be absorbed, but not all soluble minerals are necessarily absorbed.

There are several recent reviews dealing with the inhibition of mineral bioavailability[33-37] and the ability of various enhancers to counteract these effects.

Berner and Miller[37] have summarized the effects of protein on iron bioavailability and concluded that meat protein enhances, while plant, milk and egg protein inhibit, iron absorption. A recent in-vitro study[38] has found that the compounds responsible for the iron-absorption-enhancing properties of meat may be specific peptides formed during digestion. Another study[39] has indicated that this solubilizing effect is not related to sulfhydryl groups which had previously been suggested as a possible reason for the effect. If indeed this factor is responsible for enhancement of iron bioavailability, its identity and use as a food additive or as a peptide genetically engineered into a plant would increase the absorption of added iron.

Perhaps most important as inhibitors are the dietary fibers and phytates whose effects on mineral absorption are well documented.[36,37] Of the plant foods which all contain dietary fibers, the cereals and legumes are the most important in this respect due to their consumption worldwide. in fact INACG devoted an entire monograph to the effects of cereals and legumes on iron availability.[40]

Many of these inhibitory effects, however, are overcome by the presence of naturally occurring or added enhancers. Perhaps the best studied enhancer mineral relationship is that of ascorbic acid and nonheme iron. Ascorbic acid is extremely effective in increasing nonheme iron absorption, with some studies showing an increase in geometric mean absorption from 1% to 15% as the molar ratio of ascorbic acid: iron increases from 0 to 2.0.[40] Obviously the presence of ascorbic acid in the nutrient package added to cereals is very important to ensure absorption of added iron. Interestingly, the literature has reported little or no effect of ascorbic acid on the enhancement of absorption of other minerals.

Other carboxylic acids have also been shown to increase mineral absorption. Hurley and Lonnerdal[41] have identified citric acid as the low-molecular weight Zn-binding ligand in human milk while Nicar and Pak[42] have shown calcium citrate to be more bioavailable than calcium carbonate in humans. However, Sheikh et al.[43] found that calcium lactate, acetate, gluconate, citrate, carbonate and milk are all absorbed to the same extent when fed alone. This apparent conflict could be due to the precision of the methods or preparation of the samples. However, in either case, care must be taken in the interpretation of studies which are done without food. In our laboratory we found that milk prevented the precipitation of calcium in the presence of phytate with or without the presence of Fe or Zn, whereas precipitation occurred in all cases in an aqueous system.[44] The same effect was noted in a study on the solubility of iron in cereals with and without milk.[45] This indicates that milk may increase bioavailability in the presence of inhibitors of mineral absorption, an effect which would not be noted in an aqueous system or in studies with calcium salts. Further credence is lent to this effect by Sandstrom et al.[46] who found that addition of milk and cheese increased the Zn absorption of wholemeal bread in humans to the level of white bread. However, they did not speculate on the reason for this effect.

Malate and lactate have been evaluated in various studies, as well, and have shown inconsistent results in improving bioavailability. But a recent patent[47] has utilized a combination of citrate and malate with calcium to form a calcium-citrate-malate complex which has been shown to provide calcium bioavailability similar to milk when fed with food and not interfere with iron absorption.

Effects of Processing

The effects of processing on mineral bioavailability involve the form of mineral or mineral salt added to the food followed by the maximization or minimization of the factors discussed previously by processing.

The choice of the form of mineral added will be a compromise between its effect on quality, as discussed previously, and its bioavailability. As a general rule it is wise to choose a mineral additive that will become, at least, partially soluble in the food when eaten or in the acidic medium of the stomach.

When fortifying with iron it is often wise to utilize some form of elemental iron when the food is in the dry form and undergoes storage. It has been shown that the bioavailability of elemental iron powders increases with decreasing particle size and surface volume, within limits.[48] As well it has been shown that in a dry fruit-flavored beverage mix fortified with elemental iron that 30% of the iron was converted to the ferrous form upon rehydration and 90% after standing overnight.[49] Clydesdale and Nadeau[50] found that the addition of whole milk to three different experimental batches of cereal solubilized the elemental iron, and concluded that with our present state of knowledge, elemental iron is probably the best iron additive in dry cereals because it is nonreactive. The solubility of both elemental iron and other sources can be affected by food processes such as drying,[49] thermal processing,[51] and baking.[52] One study[53] found that extrusion had no effect on the apparent absorption of iron and calcium, but significantly decreased the apparent absorption of Zn, Mg, and P. This may be due to the decreased digestion of phytate found in extruded bran products.[54]

In the case of iron it must be remembered that its absorption is inversely related to the amount of storage iron in the body, and therefore, the absorption of fortificant iron of any kind will be influenced by the individual's iron status. Further, it should also be remembered that variability in absorption of minerals does occur. Heaney et al.[55] in studies with calcium estimated that when the standard double-isotope method is used to measure Ca absorption, there is approximately 10% variability around any given absorption value within an individual human subject, and that roughly two-thirds of this represents real biological variability in absorption.

Control of pH at appropriate points during processing may be a simple yet effective role in increasing the final bioavailability of the mineral in question. In our laboratory we have noted some positive effects of an acidic incubation of iron with a ligand, and then a subsequent increase in pH prior to addition to cereals.[56] Other studies have shown that the neutralization of soy products after acid precipitation influenced the bioavailability of Zn but not Mg.[57]

In a recent study[58] it was shown that the acidification of a full-fat milk fortified with 15 mg of iron as $FeSO_4$ and 100 mg of ascorbic acid increased availability of iron in infants. Since the acidification discouraged use by other family members as well as increasing bioavailability, it was recommended for consideration in supplementary food programs in the developing world.

Although the role of ionic calcium versus soluble complexed calcium in bioavailability is not clear, it is interesting to note that a decrease in ionized calcium resulted from heating milk,[59,60] and that the decrease was directly proportional to the temperature of heating. This could have potential effects on bioavailability.

Ranhotra[24] has reviewed many of the studies involving the effects of processing cereal-based foods on the bioavailability of magnesium. Most of the processes discussed had little effect. Clearly there may be losses of minerals during processing aside from effects on bioavailability. Washing, blanching, milling, peeling, etc., all remove endogenous minerals[61] and fortificant mineral if these were added prior to such operations. Therefore, steps should be taken to avoid losses as well as maximizing bioavailability.

There are many other interactions which have been reviewed in some detail,[33-37,62,63] but there is no need to discuss all of these. We should always take care to follow ethical, scientific and legal guidelines so that problems of undersupply nor oversupply are created. Having said that it might be helpful to those researching for a mineral additive to consult Table 3.5 which is a generalized modification of a table originally proposed by Coccodrilli and Shah[9] for the development of iron-

TABLE 3.5
SELECTED CRITERIA FOR DEVELOPMENT OF MINERAL FORTIFIED FOODS

Identification of food-approved mineral compounds
  Bioavailability
  Cost
  Color
  Solubility
  Particle size
  Commercial availability
  Encapsulated
Manufacturing practices and product form
  Heat processing
    Pasteurization, sterilization, spray-drying, evaporation-condensation
  Freeze-dried powders
  Instant powdered beverage mixes
  Method of addition and nutrient dispersibility
    Dry blending-premixes, spray coatings
Product stability
  Packaging
    Foil pouch, can, paperboard, plastic, glass, paper envelope
  Environmental conditions
    Climate, temperature, humidity
  Expected shelf-life
  Interactions with flavor and color systems
Target consumer group
  Serving size
  Frequency of anticipated consumption
  Fortification level (mg/serving)
  Labeling regulations (marketing claims of "fortified with mineral in question")

Source: Modified from Coccodrilli and Shah.[9]

fortified beverages. Such a list will allow the development of a sound, practical and valuable addition to our food supply.

FUTURE EXPECTATIONS

In the future there is no doubt that we shall see the use of nutrient packages designed for specific foods. This will involve minerals in a bound or perhaps encapsulated form to ensure both food functionality and bioavailability during processing and/or storage. Minerals, along with other nutrients, were originally added to food to answer public health needs. The technological advances and increased understanding gained since that time have brought us to a point where we will be able to answer that public health need in an even more meaningful manner. Such a goal will provide more and better nutrition for a public who will require greater nutrient density in food which can be met, in part, by judicious and rational fortification.

REFERENCES

1. SHANK, F. R. and WILKENING, V. L. 1986. Considerations for food fortification policy. Cereal Foods World *31*, 728–740.
2. U.S. Code of Federal Regulations, Title 21, Part 100. 1980. Nutritional quality of goods: addition of nutrients. Fed. Reg. *45* (18), 6314–6324, Jan. 25.
3. Committee on Codex Specifications, Food and Nutrition Board. 1981. Food Chemicals Codex, 3d Ed. National Academy Press, Washington, DC.
4. YIP, R., BINKIN, N. J., FLESHOOD, L. and TROWBRIDGE, F. L. 1987. Declining prevalence of anemia among low income children in the United States. JAMA *258*, 1619–1623.
5. STOCKMAN, J. A., III. 1987. Iron deficiency anemia: have we come far enough? JAMA *258*, 1645–1647.
6. NIELSEN, F. H. 1988. Boron—an overlooked element of potential nutritional importance. Nutr. Today *23*, 4–7.
7. Committee on Food Protection, Food and Nutrition Board. 1975. Technology of Fortification of Foods. Proc. of a Workshop of the Subcommittee on Food Technology. National Academy of Sciences. Washington, DC.
8. WADDEL, J. 1973. The Bioavailability of Iron Sources and Their Utilization in Food Enrichment. FASEB report for FDA. Bethesda, Maryland.
9. COCCODRILLI, G., JR. and SHAH, N. 1985. Beverages. *In* Iron Fortification of Foods, F. M. Clydesdale and K. L. Wiemer (eds.). Academic Press, New York.
10. PURVIS, G. A. 1985. Supplementation of infant products. *In* Iron Fortification of Foods, F. M. Clydesdale and K. L. Wiemer (eds.). Academic Press, New York.
11. LINDSAY, R. C. 1985. Flavors. *In* Food Chemistry, 2nd Ed., O. R. Fennema (ed.). Marcel Dekker, New York.
12. MARKAKIS, P. 1982. Anthocyanins as Food Colors. Academic Press, New York.
13. BORENSTEIN, B. and GORDON, H. T. 1988. Addition of vitamins, minerals, and amino acids to foods. *In* Nutritional Evaluation of Food Processing, 3rd Ed., E. Karmas and R. S. Harris (eds.). AVI, Van Nostrand Reinhold Co., New York.
14. NAWAR, W. W. 1985. Lipids. *In* Food Chemistry, 2nd Ed., O. R. Fennema (ed.). Marcel Dekker, New York.
15. ANDERSON, R. 1985. Breakfast cereals and dry milled corn products. *In* Iron Fortification of Foods, F. M. Clydesdale and K. L. Wiemer (eds.). Academic Press, New York.
16. CHU, N. 1961. Physio-chemical aspects of autoxidation. *In* Autoxidation and Antioxidants, Vol. I, W. O. Lundberg (ed.). John Wiley & Sons, New York.
17. TIEN, M., SVINGEN, B. A. and AUST, S. D. 1981. Superoxide dependent lipid peroxidation. Fed. Proc., Fed. Am. Soc. Exp. Biol. *40* (20), 179–182.
18. TIEN, M., SVINGEN, B. A. and AUST, S. D. 1982. An investigation into the role of hydroxyl radical in xanthine oxidase-dependent lipid peroxidation. Arch. Biochem. Biophys. *216*, 142–151.

19. TIEN, M., SVINGEN, B. A. and AUST, S. D. 1981. Initiation of lipid peroxidation by preferred complex. *In* Oxygen and Oxy-Radicals in Chemistry and Biology, M. A. J. Rodgers and E. L. Powers (eds.). Academic Press, New York.
20. BARRETT, F. and RANUM, P. 1985. Wheat flour and other cereal based products. *In* Iron Fortification of Foods, F. M. Clydesdale and K. L. Wiemer (eds.). Academic Press, New York.
21. LEE, K. and CLYDESDALE, F. M. 1980. Effect of baking on the forms of iron in iron-enriched flour. J. Food Sci. *45*, 1500–1504.
22. RANHOTRA, G. S., LEE, C. and GELROTH, J. A. 1980. Expanded cereal fortification: bioavailability and functionality (breadmaking) of various calcium sources. Nutr. Rep. Intern. *22*, 469–475.
23. Food and Nutrition Board. 1974. Proposed fortification policy for cereal grain products. National Academy of Sciences/National Research Council. Washington, DC.
24. RANHOTRA, G. S. 1983. Bioavailability of magnesium in cereal based foods. Cereal Foods World *28* (6), 349–351.
25. RANHOTRA, G. S., LOEWE, R. J., LEHMAN, T. A. and HEPBURN, F. N. 1976. Effect of various magnesium sources on bread making characteristics of wheat flour. J. Food Sci. *41*, 952–954.
26. RANHOTRA, G. S., LOEWE, R. J. and PUYAT, L. V. 1977. Bioavailability and functionality (breadmaking) of zinc in various organic and inorganic sources. Cereal. Chem. *54*, 496–502.
27. ANON. 1978. Anatomy of a decision. Nutrition Today *13* (1), 6–7.
28. HATHCOCK, J. N. 1985. Quantitative evaluation of vitamin safety. Pharmacy Times, *51* (5), 104–113.
29. HILL, C. H. and MATRONE, G. 1970. Chemical parameters in the study of in vivo and in vitro interactions of transition elements. Fed. Proc. *29*, 1474–1481.
29a. CLYDESDALE, F. M. 1989. The relevance of mineral chemistry to bioavailability. Nutr. Today *24* (2), 23–30.
30. EMERY, T. 1982. Iron metabolism in humans and plants. Am. Scientist *70*, 626–632.
31. CLYDESDALE, F. M. 1982. The effects of physicochemical properties of food on the chemical status of iron. *In* Nutritional Bioavailability of Iron, C. Kies (ed.). ACS Symposium Series. American Chemical Society, Washington, DC.
32. WIEN, E. M. and SCHWARTZ, R. 1985. Dietary calcium exchangeability and bioavailability. *In* Nutritional Bioavailability of Calcium, C. Kies (ed.). ACS Symposium series 275. American Chemical Society, Washington, DC.
33. CLYDESDALE, F. M. 1988. Minerals: Their chemistry and fate in food. *In* Handbook of Trace Minerals in Foods: Their Relationship to Health and Nutrition, K. T. Smith (ed.). Marcel Dekker, New York.
34. CLYDESDALE, F. M. 1988. Minerals interactions in foods. *In* Nutrient Interactions, C. E. Bodwell and J. W. Erdman (eds.). Marcel Dekker, New York.
35. MILLS, C. F. 1985. Dietary interactions involving the trace elements. *In* Annual Review of Nutrition, R. E. Olson, (ed.). Annual Rev., Palo Alto, CA.
36. JAMES, W. P. T. 1980. Dietary fiber and mineral absorption. *In* Medical Aspects of Dietary Fiber, G. A. Spillar and R. McPherson Kay (eds.). Plenum Med. Book Co., New York.
37. BERNER, L. A. and MILLER, D. D. 1985. Effects of dietary proteins on iron bioavailability—a review. Food Chem. *18*, 47–69.

38. SLATKAVITZ, C. A. and CLYDESDALE, F. M. 1988. Solubility of inorganic iron as affected by proteolytic digestion. Am. J. Clin. Nutr. 47, 487–495.
39. GHIA, M. L. and CLYDESDALE, F. M. 1991. Effect of enzymatic digestion, pH and molecular weight on the iron solubilizing properties of chicken muscle. J. Food Sci. (In press).
40. INACG (International Nutritional Consultative Group). 1982. The Effects of Cereals and Legumes on Iron Availability. Nutr. Foundation, Washington, DC.
41. HURLEY, L. S. and LONNERDAL, B. 1982. Zinc binding in human milk: citrate versus picolinate. Nutr. Rev. 40, 65–71.
42. NICAR, M. J. and PAK, C. Y. C. 1985. Calcium bioavailability from calcium carbonate and calcium citrate. J. Clin. End. Met. 61, 391–393.
43. SHEIKH, M. S., SANTA ANNA, C. A., NICAR, M. J., SCHILLER, L. R. and FORDTRAN, J. S. 1987. Gastrointestinal absorption of calcium from milk and calcium salts. NEJM 317 (9), 532–536.
44. PLATT, S. R., NADEAU, D. B., GIFFORD, S. R. and CLYDESDALE, F. M. 1987. Protective effect on milk on mineral precipitation by Na phytate. J. Food. Sci. 52, 240–241.
45. CLYDESDALE, F. M. and NADEAU, D. B. 1984. Solubilization of iron in cereals by milk and milk fractions. Cereal Chem. 61, 330–335.
46. SANDSTROM, B., ARVIDSSON, B., BJORN-RASMUSSEN, E. and CEDERBLAD, A. 1978. Zinc absorption from bread meals. In Trace Elements Metabolism in Man and Animals III. Proc. 3rd Intern. Sym., M. Kirchgessner (ed.). Arpeitskeirs Fuhr Tierernahrungs Forschung: Weihenstephan.
47. HECKERT, D. C. 1988. Fruit juice beverages and juice concentrates nutritionally supplemented with calcium. U.S. Patent No. 4, 722, 847, Feb. 2.
48. PATRICK, J., JR. 1985. Elemental sources. In Iron Fortification of Foods, F. M. Clydesdale and K. L. Wiemer (eds.). Academic Press, New York.
49. LEE, K. and CLYDESDALE, F. M. 1980. Chemical changes of iron in food and drying processes. J. Food Sci. 45, 711–715.
50. CLYDESDALE, F. M. and Nadeau, D. B. 1984. Solubilization of iron in cereals by milk and milk fractions. Cereal Chem. 61, 330–335.
51. LEE, K. and CLYDESDALE, F. M. 1981. The effect of thermal processing on the endogenous and added iron in canned spinach. J. Food Sci. 46, 1064–1068.
52. LEE, K. and CLYDESDALE, F. M. 1980. Effect of baking on the forms of iron in iron-enriched flour. J. Food Sci. 45, 1500–1504.
53. KIVISTO, B., ANDERSSON, H., CEDERBLAD, G., SANDBERG, A. S. and SANDSTROM, B. 1986. Extrusion cooking of a high-fibre cereal product. Br. J. Nutr. 55, 255–260.
54. SANDBERG, A. S., ANDERSSON, H., CARLSSON, N. G. and SANDSTROM, B. 1987. Degradation products of iron phytate formed during digestion in the human small intestine: Effect of extrusion cooking on digestion. J. Nutr. 117, 2061–2065.
55. HEANEY, R. P., RECKER, R. R. and HINDERS, M. S. 1988. Variability of calcium absorption. Am. J. Clin. Nutr. 47, 262–264.
56. CLYDESDALE, F. M. and NADEAU, D. B. 1985. Effect of acid pretreatment on the stability of ascorbic acid iron complexes with various iron sources in a wheat flake cereal. J. Food Sci. 50, 1342–1347.
57. ERDMAN, J. W., JR., WEINGARTNER, K. E., MUSTAKAS, G. C., SCHMUTZ, R. D., PARKER, H. M. and FORBES, R. M. 1980. Zinc and magnesium bioavailabil-

ity from acid precipitated and neutralized soy products. J. Food Sci. *45*, 1193–1199.
58. STEKEL, A., OLIVARES, M., CAYAZZO, M., CHADUD, P., LLAGUNO, S. and PIZARRO, F. 1988. Prevention of iron deficiency by milk fortification. A field trial with a full-fat acidified milk. Am. J. Clin. Nutr. *47*, 265–269.
59. MULDOON, P. J. and LISKA, B. J. 1971. Effects of heat treatment and subsequent storage on the concentration of ionized calcium in skimmilk. J. Dairy Sci. *55*, 35–38.
60. KOCAK, H. R. and ZADOW, J. G. 1984. Short term changes in the ionic calcium content of heat-treated skim milk. Aust. J. Dairy Tech. Mar., 40–43.
61. ROTRUCK, J. T. 1982. Effect of processing on nutritive value of food: trace elements. *In* Handbook of Nutritive Value of Processed Food, Vol. I. Food for Human Use, M. Rechcigl, Jr. (ed.). CRC Press, Boca Raton, FL.
62. GREGER, J. L. 1987. Mineral bioavailability/new concepts. Nutr. Today, *22* (4), 4–9.
63. KOHLS, K. J. 1989. Calcium bioavailability of calcium-fortified food products. FASEB J. *3* (3), A771.

CHAPTER 4

VITAMIN AND AMINO ACID ADDITIVES

LYNN BAILEY, Ph.D.

INTRODUCTION

The vitamins (Table 4.1) are a heterogenous group of organic chemical compounds each of which have essential functions in the maintenance of metabolism and thereby are necessary for life and well-being of humans. Vitamins are differentiated from the essential organic macronutrients, carbohydrates, fats and proteins by the relatively small quantities required, since individual vitamins are only needed in the range of several micrograms to approximately 100 mg daily. The concept of these accessory factors in food was developed in the early part of the 20th century and the word "vitamin" was accepted to designate such factors. Deficiencies of such factors were once widespread and caused the diseases recognized as beriberi, pellagra, rickets, scurvy, xerophthalmia. The actual isolation, identification, and synthesis of the vitamins (Table 4.2) took place between 1910 and 1950, after which time the deficiency conditions could be treated with the pure vitamins and/or foods identified as sources of the specific vitamins.[1-3] The structure of the vitamins is illustrated in Fig. 4.1 and 4.2.

Dietary allowances of vitamins are of importance internationally for planning diets to ensure adequacy of intake. Tabulations of recommended dietary allowances (RDAs) are periodically published by such organizations as the World Health Organization, the U.S. Food and Nutrition Board of the National Research Council, National Academy of Sciences (Tables 4.3), the U.S. Food and Drug Administration and by organizations in many other countries. The USRDAs of the Food & Drug Administration (Table 4.4) apply to labeling claims for food and pharmaceutical products marketed in the United States. A proposal to review these values is under study by the FDA.

Application Forms

In most cases, vitamins produced commercially are chemically identical to those naturally occurring in foods. Most vitamins are produced commercially by chemical synthesis. Riboflavin is produced both by fermentation and chemical synthesis. Vitamin B_{12} is derived commercially by microbial fermentation.

TABLE 4.1
VITAMINS AND PROVITAMINS AND THEIR MOST IMPORTANT FORMS

Vitamin group	Most important representative	Important active compounds	Most important commercial forms
Vitamin A	Retinol	Retinol, retinal, retinoic acid, 3-dehydroretinol (A_2)	Vitamin A acetate, vitamin A palmitate,
Provitamin A	β-Carotene	α-, β- and γ-carotene, β-apocarotenoids, cryptoxanthine, echinenone	β-Carotene β-apo-8'-carotenal, β-apo-8'-carotinic esters
Vitamin D	Cholecalciferol	Ergocalciferol cholecalciferol	Vitamin D_2, vitamin D_3
Vitamin E	α-Tocopherol	α-, β-, γ- and δ-tocopherol α-, β-, γ- and δ-tocotrienol	[d]- and [dl]-α-Tocopherol* [d]- and [dl]-α-tocopherol acetate**
Vitamin K	Phylloquinone	Phylloquinone (K_1) Menaquinone (K_2) Menadione (Menaquinone O)	Vitamin K_1 Menadione Menadiol esters
Vitamin B_1	Thiamin	Thiamin and its salts; thiamin diphosphate (cocarboxylase)	Thiamin chloride hydrochloride, thiamin mononitrate thiamin diphosphate (carboxylase)
Vitamin B_2	Riboflavin	Riboflavin, riboflavin phosphoric acid	Riboflavin, riboflavin sodium phosphate
Niacin	Nicotinamide	Nicotinamide, nicotinic acid	Nicotinamide, nicotinic acid
Vitamin B_6	Pyridoxine	Pyridoxine, pyridoxal, pyridoxamine, pyridoxal 5'-phosphate (codecarboxylase)	Pyridoxine hydrochloride, pyridoxal 5'-phosphate (codecarboxylase)
Vitamin B_{12}	Cyanocobalamin,	Cyanocobalamin, hydroxocobalamin	Cyanocobalamin, hydroxocobalamin
Folic acid	Folic acid	Folic acid, folic acid conjugates	Folic acid
Pantothenic acid	Pantothenic acid	Pantothenic acid Pantetheine Panthenol	Calcium pantothenate Sodium pantothenate
Biotin	d-Biotin	d-Biotin	d-Biotin
Vitamin C	Ascorbic acid	Ascorbic acid Dehydroascorbic acid	Ascorbic acid Sodium ascorbate Calcium ascorbate

Source: Isler and Brubacher.[69]
*More correctly, RRR- and *all-rac*-α-Tocopherol.
** More correctly, RRR— and *all-rac*-α-Tocopheryl acetate.

TABLE 4.2
HISTORY OF THE VITAMINS

Vitamin	First isolated	Discovery	Isolation	Structure elucidated	Synthesis
Vitamin A	Fish liver oil	1909	1931	1931	1947
Provitamin A	Carrot, palm oil		1831	1930	1950
Vitamin D	Fish liver oil, yeast	1918	1932	1936	1959
Vitamin E	Wheat germ oil	1922	1936	1938	1938
Vitamin K	Alfalfa	1929	1939	1939	1939
Vitamin B_1	Rice bran	1897	1926	1936	1936
Vitamin B_2	Egg albumin	1920	1933	1935	1935
Niacin	Liver	1936 (1894)	1935 (1911)	1937	1894
Vitamin B_6	Rice bran	1934	1938	1938	1939
Vitamin B_{12}	Liver, fermentation	1926	1948	1956	1972
Folic acid	Liver	1941	1941	1946	1946
Pantothenic acid	Liver	1931	1938	1940	1940
Biotin	Liver	1931	1935	1942	1943
Vitamin C	Adrenal cortex Lemon	1912	1928	1933	1933

Source: Isler and Brubacher.[69]

The water-soluble vitamins [thiamin, riboflavin, niacin, pyridoxine, folate (as the monoglutamate), biotin, vitamin B_{12}, calcium pantothenate, and ascorbic acid] are produced in pure crystalline form for direct addition to foods or in the form of premixes.[4,5] Biotin and vitamin B_{12}, which are added to foods in very small amounts (micrograms per serving) are supplied as dry concentrates at 0.1% or 1% potencies to facilitate mixing. The mononitrate salt of thiamin is preferred over the hydrochloride for use in dry premixes and in direct food additions due to its lower hygroscopicity. For food nutrification, niacin is normally employed; niacinamide is usually used in pharmaceutical dosage forms, but also may be used as a food additive. Where stability of the water-soluble vitamins is a problem in heat-processed foods such as toasted breakfast cereals, soluble or emulsified formulation of the labile vitamin(s) can be sprayed onto the product after heat treatment.[6] Coated niacinamide, pyridoxine, riboflavin, thiamin, etc., may be useful where taste, flavor, or special protective problems arise. Some vitamins have a dual role such as L-ascorbic acid which acts as a nutrient and as a food product improver.[7]

Retinyl esters, vitamin A palmitate or acetate, of the all-trans type, are employed most frequently in food applications. Either vitamin D_2, calciferol, or vitamin D_3,

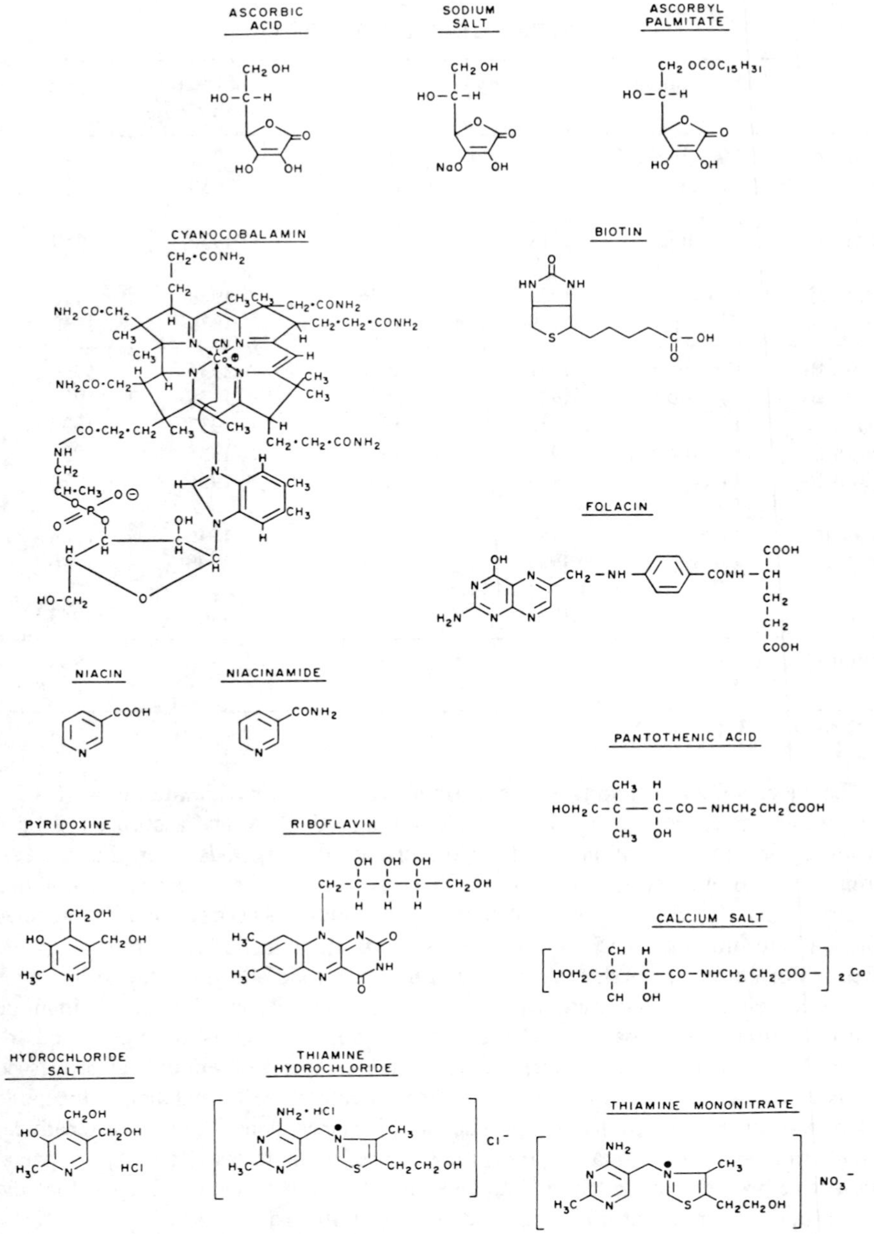

FIG. 4.1. STRUCTURES OF WATER-SOLUBLE VITAMINS

cholecalciferol, serve as added food nutrients. Vitamin E in the form of either dl, α-tocopherol (synthetic) or d,α-tocopherol (natural) provide antioxidant value while the more stable tocopheryl acetates are preferred in applications as added nutrients. The fat-soluble vitamins (A, D, and E) are usually prepared in the form of oil solutions, emulsions or dry, stabilized preparations. The dry forms may be adsorbates, drum-dried, spray-dried, or spray-chilled powders, microcapsules, or beadlets.[8] They can be incorporated into multivitamin-mineral premixes or added directly to food. Typical dry concentrates may contain 250,000–500,000 IU of vitamin A per gram (with or without added vitamin D) stabilized with antioxidants in an oxygen-free protective matrix. Vitamin E emulsions may contain 100 or more IU/g, and dry preparations are available with as much as 50% alpha-tocopheryl acetate content per gram. Dry stabilized, free-flowing vitamin K_1 is produced commercially for the nutrification of food.

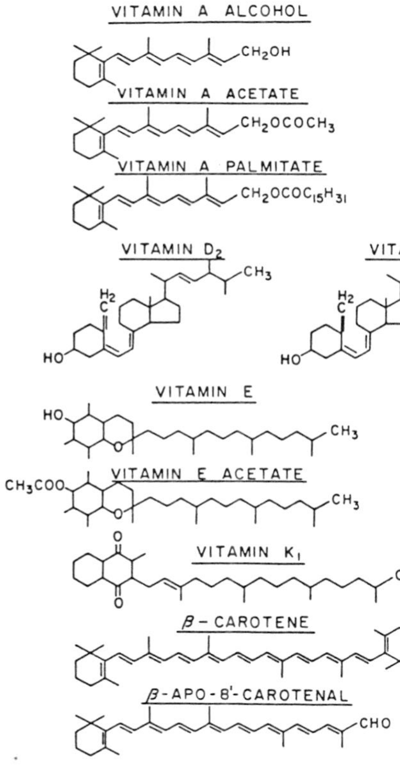

FIG. 4.2. STRUCTURES OF FAT-SOLUBLE VITAMINS

TABLE 4.3
RECOMMENDED DIETARY ALLOWANCES, 10TH EDITION, 1989

Food and Nutrition Board, National Academy of Sciences—National Research Council
Recommended Dietary Allowances,[a] Revised 1989
Designed for the maintenance of good nutrition of practically all healthy people in the United States

Category	Age (yr) or Condition	Weight[b] (kg)	Weight[b] (lb)	Height[b] (cm)	Height[b] (in)	Protein (g)	Vitamin-A (μg RE)[c]	Vitamin D (μg)[d]	Vitamin E (mg α-TE)[e]	Vitamin K (μg)
Infants	0.0–0.5	6	13	60	24	13	375	7.5	3	5
	0.5–1.0	9	20	71	28	14	375	10	4	10
Children	1–3	13	29	90	35	16	400	10	6	15
	4–6	20	44	112	44	24	500	10	7	20
	7–10	28	62	132	52	28	700	10	7	30
Males	11–14	45	99	157	62	45	1,000	10	10	45
	15–18	66	145	176	69	59	1,000	10	10	65
	19–24	72	160	177	70	58	1,000	10	10	70
	25–50	79	174	176	70	63	1,000	5	10	80
	51+	77	170	173	68	63	1,000	5	10	80
Females	11–14	46	101	157	62	46	800	10	8	45
	15–18	55	120	163	64	44	800	10	8	55
	19–24	58	128	164	65	46	800	10	8	60
	25–50	63	138	163	64	50	800	5	8	65
	51+	65	143	160	63	50	800	5	8	65
Pregnant						60	800	10	10	65
Lactating	1st 6 months					65	1,300	10	12	65
	2nd 6 months					62	1,200	10	11	65

[a] The allowances, expressed as average daily intakes over time, are intended to provide for individual variations among most normal persons as they live in the United States under usual environmental stresses. Diets should be based on a variety of common foods in order to provide other nutrients for which human requirements have been less well defined. See text for detailed discussion of allowances and of nutrients not tabulated.
[b] Weights and heights of Reference Adults are actual medians for the U.S. population of the designated age, as reported by NHANES II. The median weights and heights of those under 19 years of age were taken from Hamill et al. (1979) (see pages 16–17). The use of these figures does not imply that the height-to-weight ratios are ideal.
[c] Retinol equivalents, 1 retinol equivalent = 1 μg of retinol or 6 μg of β-carotene. See text for calculation of vitamin A activity of diets as retinol equivalents.
[d] As cholecalciferol, 10 μg of cholecalciferol = 400 IU of vitamin D.
[e] d-Tocopherol equivalents, 1 mg of α-2 tocopherol = 1-α-TE. See text for variation in allowances and calculation of vitamin E activity of the diet as α-tocopherol equivalents.
[f] 1 NE (niacin equivalent) is equal to 1 mg of niacin or 60 mg of dietary tryptophan.
Editor's Notes: Boxed values—new to 10th edition; underlined values—changed from 9th edition.

Estimated Safe and Adequate Daily Dietary Intakes of Selected Vitamins and Minerals[a]

Category	Age (yr)	Vitamins		Trace Elements[b]				
		Biotin (μg)	Pantothenic Acid (mg)	Copper (mg)	Manganese (mg)	Fluoride (mg)	Chromium (μg)	Molybdenum (μg)
Infants	0–0.5	10	2	0.4–0.6	0.3–0.6	0.1–0.5	10–40	15–30
	0.5–1	15	3	0.6–0.7	0.6–1.0	0.2–1.0	20–60	20–40
Children and	1–3	20	3	0.7–1.0	1.0–1.5	0.5–1.5	20–80	25–50
adolescents	4–6	25	3–4	1.0–1.5	1.5–2.0	1.0–2.5	30–120	30–75
	7–10	30	4–5	1.0–2.0	2.0–3.0	1.5–2.5	50–200	50–150
	11+	30–100	4–7	1.5–2.5	2.0–5.0	1.5–2.5	50–200	75–250
Adults		30–100	4–7	1.5–3.0	2.0–5.0	1.5–4.0	50–200	75–250

[a] Because there is less information on which to base allowances, these figures are not given in the main table of RDA and are provided here in the form of ranges of recommended intakes.
[b] Since the toxic levels for many trace elements may be only several times usual intakes, the upper levels for the trace elements given in this table should not be habitually exceeded.

Source: Nutrition Today.[66]

Recommended Dietary Allowances—continued

	Water-Soluble Vitamins						Minerals						
Vita-min C (mg)	Thia-min (mg)	Ribo-flavin (mg)	Niacin (mg NE)[f]	Vita-min B_6 (mg)	Fo-late (μg)	Vita-min B_{12} (μg)	Cal-cium (mg)	Phos-phorus (mg)	Mag-nesium (mg)	Iron (mg)	Zinc (mg)	Iodine (μg)	Sele-nium (μg)
30	0.3	0.4	5	0.3	25	0.3	400	300	40	6	5	40	10
35	0.4	0.5	6	0.6	35	0.5	600	500	60	10	5	50	15
40	0.7	0.8	9	1.0	50	0.7	800	800	80	10	10	70	20
45	0.9	1.1	12	1.1	75	1.0	800	800	120	10	10	90	20
45	1.0	1.2	13	1.4	100	1.4	800	800	170	10	10	120	30
50	1.3	1.5	17	1.7	150	2.0	1,200	1,200	270	12	15	150	40
60	1.5	1.8	20	2.0	200	2.0	1,200	1,200	400	12	15	150	50
60	1.5	1.7	19	2.0	200	2.0	1,200	1,200	350	10	15	150	70
60	1.5	1.7	19	2.0	200	2.0	800	800	350	10	15	150	70
60	1.2	1.4	15	2.0	200	2.0	800	800	350	10	15	150	70
50	1.1	1.3	15	1.4	150	2.0	1,200	1,200	280	15	12	150	45
60	1.1	1.3	15	1.5	180	2.0	1,200	1,200	300	15	12	150	50
60	1.1	1.3	15	1.6	180	2.0	1,200	1,200	280	15	12	150	55
60	1.1	1.3	15	1.6	180	2.0	800	800	280	15	12	150	55
60	1.0	1.2	13	1.6	180	2.0	800	800	280	10	12	150	55
70	1.5	1.6	17	2.2	400	2.2	1,200	1,200	320	30	15	175	65
95	1.6	1.8	20	2.1	280	2.6	1,200	1,200	355	15	19	200	75
90	1.6	1.7	20	2.1	260	2.6	1,200	1,200	340	15	16	200	75

Median Heights and Weights and Recommended Energy Intake

Category	Age (yr) or Condition	Weight (kg)	Weight (lb)	Height (cm)	Height (in)	REE[c] (kcal/day)	Multi-ples of REE	Average Energy Allowance (kcal)[b] Per kg	Average Energy Allowance (kcal)[b] Per day[c]
Infants	0.0–0.5	6	13	60	24	320		108	650
	0.5–1.0	9	20	71	28	500		98	850
Children	1–3	13	29	90	35	740		102	1,300
	4–6	20	44	112	44	950		90	1,800
	7–10	28	62	132	52	1,130		70	2,000
Males	11–14	45	99	157	62	1,440	1.70	55	2,500
	15–18	66	145	176	69	1,760	1.67	45	3,000
	19–24	72	160	177	70	1,780	1.67	40	2,900
	25–50	79	174	176	70	1,800	1.60	37	2,900
	51+	77	170	173	68	1,530	1.50	30	2,300
Females	11–14	46	101	157	62	1,310	1.67	47	2,200
	15–18	55	120	163	64	1,370	1.60	40	2,200
	19–24	58	128	164	65	1,350	1.60	38	2,200
	25–50	63	138	163	64	1,380	1.55	36	2,200
	51+	65	143	160	63	1,280	1.50	30	1,900
Pregnant	1st trimester								+0
	2nd trimester								+300
	3rd trimester								+300
Lactating	1st 6 months								+500
	2nd 6 months								+500

[a] Calculation based on FAO equations, then rounded.
[b] In the range of light to moderate activity, the coefficient of variation is ± 20%.
[c] Figure is rounded.

Equations for Predicting Resting Energy Expenditure from Body Weight[a]

Sex and Age Range (yr)	Equation to Derive REE in kcal/day	R^a	SD^b
Males			
0–3	$(60.9 \times wt^c) - 54$	0.97	53
3–10	$(22.7 \times wt) + 495$	0.86	62
10–18	$(17.5 \times wt) + 651$	0.90	100
18–30	$(15.3 \times wt) + 679$	0.65	151
30–60	$(11.6 \times wt) + 879$	0.60	164
>60	$(13.5 \times wt) + 487$	0.79	148
Females			
0–3	$(61.0 \times wt) - 51$	0.97	61
3–10	$(22.5 \times wt) + 499$	0.85	63
10–18	$(12.2 \times wt) + 746$	0.75	117
18–30	$(14.7 \times wt) + 496$	0.72	121
30–60	$(8.7 \times wt) + 829$	0.70	108
>60	$(10.5 \times wt) + 596$	0.74	108

[a] From WHO (1985). These equations were derived from BMR data.
[b] Correlation coefficient (R) of reported BMRs and predicted values, and standard deviation (SD) of the differences between actual and computed values.
[c] Weight of person in kilograms.

TABLE 4.4
FDA U.S. RECOMMENDED DAILY ALLOWANCES FOR VITAMINS (USRDA)

Vitamins and Minerals	Unit of Measurement	Infants	Children Under 4 Years of Age	Adults and Children 4 or More Years of Age	Pregnant or Lactating Women
Vitamin A	International units	1,500	2,500	5,000	8,000
Vitamin D	do	400	400	400	400
Vitamin E	do	5	10	30	30
Vitamin C	Milligrams	35	40	60	60
Folic acid	do	0.1	0.2	0.4	0.8
Thiamin	do	0.5	0.7	1.5	1.7
Riboflavin	do	0.6	0.8	1.7	2.0
Niacin	do	8	9	20	20
Vitamin B_6	do	0.4	0.7	2.0	2.5
Vitamin B_{12}	Micrograms	2	2	6	8
Biotin	Milligrams	0.05	0.15	0.30	0.30
Pantothenic acid	do	3	3	10	10

Source: Fed. Reg.[67]

BIOAVAILABILITY

Bioavailability may be defined as the relative amount of a nutrient utilized after ingestion. Information on bioavailability of the nutrients is steadily increasing; individual variability, malabsorption conditions, and nutrient interactions are some influencing factors, as well as the form of the nutrient in the diet. In the nutrification of food, the added vitamins and amino acids resulting from chemical syntheses are in a free or unbound form, and hence are likely to be quite bioavailable.

In the natural state of food some vitamin B_1 and B_2 are covalently bound and some vitamin B_6 is in the form of the less stable pyridoxal and pyridoxamine forms. Some vitamin B_6 compounds such as pyridoxine-β-glucoside in plant foods have lower bioavailability.[9] Some niacin exists in the cereal grains in bound form such as niacytin and is not easily available as reviewed in 1988 by Wall and Carpenter.[10] Much of the folate exists in a conjugated form and many factors may influence folate bioavailability.[11] Vitamin B_{12}, in part, is linked to polypeptides; the majority of pantothenic acid is in coenzyme form; and much of the biotin is in complexed form, which influences bioavailability, depending on circumstances. Food processing and dietary effects as they influence bioavailability of vitamin A, carotenoids and vitamin E has been detailed by Erdman et al. in 1988.[12]

Information relating to interactions of vitamins with other nutrients and elements which can influence bioavailability has been reported by Levander and Cheng,[13] and by Machlin and Langseth.[14] The state of knowledge in 1985 on the bioavailability of vitamins was reviewed by Sauberlich.[15] Borenstein *et al.* in 1988 examined the literature and concluded that the bioavailability of vitamins added to foods is at least equivalent to that of vitamins indigenous to foods.[16]

TOXICITY

Citations of toxicity from nutrients such as the vitamins usually originate from two sources. The first is the case study in which a subject voluntarily consumes a high dose level of a dietary supplement well beyond label directions over a period of time, then develops toxic symptoms and seeks out medical treatment, resulting in the case being published in a journal with the recorded vitamin intake of the subject based on memory recall or willingness to admit. The second instance involves supervised programs of megadose vitamin administration to subjects, hence actual intake values are more trustworthy, but the subjects remain on the daily dosage for too long a period or the chosen megadose level was too high at the beginning of the program. Thus, toxic manifestations result from abuse of vitamin supplement usage or inadequate surveillance of adopted programs.

Vitamins added to foods by the process of nutrification are intended to correct insufficient intakes of a population by bringing the total intake at or slightly above values set for recommended daily allowances such as have been provided by the U.S. Food and Drug Administration, the National Research Council or in other recognized standards or goals. In the past there has been no major problem of vitamin toxicity resulting from the nutrification of food. With proper planning and diligent practice in future endeavors on vitamin additions to food, vitamin toxicity should not be a deterrent.

In the matter of avoidance of potential vitamin toxicity for humans, literature surveys reveal that more past data comes as a byproduct of research studies set up for another purpose rather than direct toxicological trials with humans. Hence, data often are fragmentary, sometimes incomplete or even contradictory, but with time quite a mass of overall information has been assembled which serves as a basis for safety judgments. One tends to look for guidelines when undertaking new endeavors. In setting forth a guideline values which would be safe, general minimums are favored. One such guideline on estimated daily oral minimum toxic vitamin dose levels has appeared in the 1989 National Research Council publication entitled "Diet & Health" (Table 4.5).

FOLATE

Nomenclature

Folic acid, pteroylglutamic acid ($C_{19}H_{19}N_7O_6$) is currently referred to by the generic term folate which encompasses the many different forms of the vitamin. In the past

TABLE 4.5
VITAMIN SAFETY INDEXES[a]

Nutrient	Highest Recommended Adult Intake[b]	Source of Recommended Intake	Estimated Daily Adult Oral Minimum Toxic Dose	References
Vitamin A	5,000 IU	USRDA	25,000 to 50,000 IU	Miller and Hayes, 1982
Vitamin D	400 IU	USRDA	50,000 IU	Miller and Hayes, 1982
Vitamin E	30 IU	USRDA	1,200 IU	Miller and Hayes, 1982
Vitamin C	60 mg	RDA	1,000 to 5,000 mg	Miller and Hayes, 1982
Thiamin	1.5 mg	USRDA	300 mg	Itokawa, 1978; Miller and Hayes, 1982
Riboflavin	1.7 mg	USRDA	1,000 mg[c]	Miller and Hayes, 1982; Rivlin, 1978
Niacin (nicotinamide)	20 mg	USRDA	1,000 mg	Miller and Hayes, 1982; Waterman, 1978
Pyridoxine	2.2 mg	RDA	2,000 mg[d]	Schaumburg et al., 1983
Folacin	0.4 mg	USRDA	400 mg	Miller and Hayes, 1982
Biotin	0.3 mg	USRDA	50 mg	Miller and Hayes, 1982
Pantothenic acid	10 mg	USRDA	1,000 mg	Miller and Hayes, 1982

[a]Source: Anon.[69] Adapted from Hathcock, 1985.
[b]Figures represent the highest published value for each nutrient, either the Recommended Dietary Allowances (RDA) (except those for pregnancy and lactation) or Estimated Safe and Adequate Daily Dietary Intakes (ESAADDI) (NRC, 1980), or the U.S. Recommended Daily Allowances (USRDA).
[c]However, only ~25 mg of riboflavin can be absorbed in a single oral dose given to an adult.
[d]More recent data suggest that the toxic dose of pyridoxine for some individuals is much lower.

Addendum. For further discussion on potential toxicological aspects of the vitamins the following general sources are listed:

Buist, R. A. 1984. Vitamin toxicities, side effects and contraindications. Int. Clin.Nutr. Rev. 4(4), 159–171.
Dickinson, A. 1986. Safety of Vitamins and Minerals: A Summary of the Findings of Key Reviews. Council for Responsible Nutrition, Washington, DC.
Friedrich, W. 1988. Vitamins. Walter de Gruyter, New York.
Greger, J. I. 1987. Food supplements and fortified foods; scientific evaluations in regard to toxicology and nutrient bioavailability. J. Am. Dietet. Assoc. 87(10), 1369–1373.
Machlin, L. J. 1991. Handbook of Vitamins. Marcel Dekker, New York.
Marks, J. 1985. The Vitamins: Their Role in Medical Practice. MTP Press Limited, Boston.
Miller, D. R. and Hayes, K. C. 1982. Vitamin Excess and Toxicity. In Nutritional Toxicology, Vol. 1, J. Hathcock (ed.). Academic Press, New York.
NAS/NRC. 1989. NRC Report: Recommended Dietary Allowances, 10th Ed. National Research Council, Washington, DC.
Walter, P., Brubacher, G. and Steahelin, H. B. 1989. Elevated Dosages of Vitamins. Hogrefe & Huber Publ., Lewiston, New York.

it was referred to as folacin, factor U, *L. casei* factor, and vitamin B_c or M. It consists of a pteridine linked to p-aminobenzoic acid and glutamic acid, namely N-[p{[2-amino-4-hydroxy-6-pteridinyl) methyl] amino} benzoyl] glutamic acid. Folate exists in plants, and some animal tissue largely in the form of conjugates of more than one molecule of glutamic acid, linked at the γ carbon positions. Commercially synthesized folic acid has only one glutamic acid group.

Chemical Properties and Stability

Folic acid is a yellow-orange, odorless and tasteless crystalline powder. It is readily soluble in dilute alkali, soluble in dilute acid, sparingly soluble in water (0.16 mg/100 mL at 25°C; 1 g/100 mL at 100°C), and insoluble in acetone, ether and chloroform. The disodium salt is much more water soluble. Crystalline folic acid is degraded by light and ultraviolet radiation but is fairly stable to air and heat. Acids, alkalines, oxidizing and reducing agents have a destructive effect; however, neutral solutions are relatively stable. Folic acid in solution is unstable below pH 5, but its solubility in this acid pH range is very limited.[17]

Function, Deficiency Symptoms, and Safety

Folate functions metabolically in a large number of coenzyme forms required as acceptors and donors of one-carbon units. Folate in the form of 5,6,7,8-tetrahydrofolic acid (THFA) is indispensable for the transformations of the one-carbon compounds in metabolism. The C_1 units can be formed by degradation of purines and histidine, by oxidative cleavage of glycine, by activation of free formate, by elimination of the β-carbon atom of serine with the formation of glycine, or by activation of free formaldehyde. THFA also participates in the reduction of active formaldehyde to the methyl group and the transfer of the latter. The one carbon units then can enter a series of biosynthetic reactions: incorporation into purine bases and histidine; transfer of active formaldehyde to glycine with formation of serine; formation of methionine, choline, thymine, and methylnicotinamide by methylation of the corresponding precursors. The major physiological functions of the folate coenzymes relate to requirements for cell division, amino acid metabolism and nucleotide synthesis.[1,24]

A deficiency of folate is expressed by the development of megaloblastic anemia resulting from blockage of cell division. Other characteristic changes include the development of polymorphonuclear leukocytes, granulocytopenia, and thrombocytopenia. Malabsorption of nutrients may result from abnormal cell division in the intestinal mucosa.[24]

Folate is safe and nontoxic in moderate therapeutic doses with no side effects in the range of 5–10 mg. Folate has a low acute and chronic toxicity for humans. In adults no adverse effects were noted after doses of 400 mg/day for 5 months and after 10 mg/day for 5 years.[2] Therapeutic doses of folate should not be taken indiscriminately as they may obscure the diagnosis of pernicious anemia. The USRDA for folate is 0.4 mg/day.

VITAMIN B_{12}

Nomenclature

Vitamin B_{12} is also known as cyanocobalamin, extrinsic factor, and chemically is 5,6-dimethyl-benzimidazolylcyanocobamide ($C_{63}H_{88}N_{14}O_{14}PCo$). Cyanocobalamin is a permissive name for vitamin B_{12} under the rules of the International Union of

Pure and Applied Chemistry (IUPAC) Commission on Biochemical Nomenclature (CBN). Vitamin B_{12} is used as a generic term for all the active cobalamins. Cobalamin describes the vitamin B_{12} molecule minus a cyano group which cyanocobalamin contains. Other active cobalamins contain such anions as the bromo, chloro, hydroxy, nitro, or nitrito and sulfito groups in place of the cyano group.

Chemical Properties and Stability

Cyanocobalamin is a red, crystalline, hygroscopic compound, soluble in water (1 g/80 mL) and alcohol, but insoluble in acetone, chloroform, or ether. It is unstable in light, strong acid or alkali. Solutions in the pH range of 4–7 are most stable at room temperature. Oxidizing and certain reducing agents and exposure to sunlight have deleterious effects. Iron salts in solution tend to stabilize vitamin B_{12}. The B_{12} molecule is fairly stable to heat and is stable to autoclaving for short periods. Destruction occurs during heating in alkaline solution at temperatures in excess of 100°C.[17]

Functions, Deficiency Symptoms, Safety

Vitamin B_{12} functions in one of two coenzyme forms: adenosylcobalamin or methylcobalamin. Adenosylcobalamin functions in the conversion of methylmalonyl coenzyme A to succinyl coenzyme A in the pathway for the catabolism of propionic coenzyme A, which is derived from the breakdown of valine and isoleucine and odd chain fatty acids. Because coenzymes vitamin B_{12} is required for hydrogen transfer and isomerization whereby methylmalonate is converted to succinate, B_{12} is involved in both fat and carbohydrate metabolism. Vitamin B_{12} is also involved in protein synthesis through its role in the synthesis of methionine and other ways. The one reaction requiring methylcobalamin is the conversion of homocysteine to methionine.[1,2,23]

Pernicious anemia results from the inability to absorb cobalamins, inability to secrete intrinsic factor results in absorption failure. In addition to megaloblastic anemia, the most significant symptoms of vitamin B_{12} deficiency are weakness, tiredness, pale and smooth tongue, dyspnea, splenomegaly, leukopenia, thrombocytopenia, achlorhydria, paresthesia, neurological changes, loss of appetite and loss of weight. Vitamin B_{12} deficiency also results from insufficient B_{12} intake as may occur with vegetarian diets.

The addition of vitamin B_{12} to food in amounts far in excess of need or absorbability appear to be without hazard. There are no known toxic effects from single oral doses as high as 100 mg, or from doses of 1 mg weekly over 3–5 year periods.[2,3] The USRDA for vitamin B_{12} is 6 mcg per day.

ASCORBIC ACID

Nomenclature

L-ascorbic acid, (1-threo-3 ketohexuronic / acid lactone), vitamin C, cevitamic acids, hexuronic acid, L-xyloascorbic acid, the antiscorbutic vitamin ($C_6H_8O_6$), exists in the reduced form and the reversibly oxidized form, dehydroascorbic acid, both of which are biologically active. Dehydroascorbic acid can be further oxidized to diketogulonic acid, an inactive compound.

Physicochemical Properties and Stability

L-ascorbic acid is a white, crystalline compound which is odorless. It is insoluble in benzene, chloroform, ether, oils; 1 g dissolves in approximately 3 mL of water, 50 mL of absolute alcohol, or 100 mL of glycerol. Crystalline ascorbic acid is stable in dry form but is very susceptible to destruction by oxidation in the presence of moisture, especially if promoted by heat, alkali, or dissolved copper and iron. The vitamin is readily oxidized in the presence of oxygen at a rate increasing with increases in temperature. In the absence of oxygen, heat alone does not destroy ascorbic acid. Ascorbic acid in foods is easily destroyed by enzymatic oxidation and by undue exposure to oxygen.[17]

Function, Deficiency, and Safety

Ascorbic acid has very important metabolic roles such as mixed-function oxidation; and hydroxylating enzymes depend on ascorbic acid as a cofactor. L-ascorbic acid is used metabolically to form and maintain intercellular and skeletal material such as the collagen of fibrous tissues and the matrix of bone, dentine, and cartilage. It is essential for the maintenance of capillary tissue structure.[27] Ascorbic acid is required for the synthesis of the catecholamines, dopamine, norepinephrine, and epinephrine and for the maintenance of the immune system.[28] It also functions as a component of the overall antioxidant protective mechanism in cells and tissues, thus contributing in the maintenance of human health. It can react both directly, by reaction with aqueous peroxyl radicals and indirectly by restoring the antioxidant properties of α-tocopherol.[29] New knowledge about ascorbic acid function indicates a neurohumoral action, a role in male fertility and an effect on airway construction in asthmatics and individuals exposed to air pollution.[30]

In a deficiency of ascorbate, the abnormal effects observed are in collagen formation, fatty acid metabolism, brain function, drug detoxification, infection, and fatigue. In a mild deficiency, symptoms such as weakness, anorexia, and greater susceptibility to infection and stress occur. Scurvy occurs following a prolonged deficiency and is characterized by anemia; alteration of collagenous tissues in bone, cartilage, teeth, and connective tissue; failure of wounds to heal, fatigue and lethargy; rheumatic pains in the legs and degeneration of the muscles; skin lesions; capillary weakness. Clinical symptoms are accompanied by a reduction of the vitamin C concentration of blood plasma, leukocytes, whole blood, and urine.[26]

Currently gram amounts of ascorbic acid are suggested for treatment or prevention of a wide array of health aberrations. A 1987 review concludes that the practice of ingesting large quantities of ascorbic acid will not normally result in calcium oxalate stones, increased uric acid excretion, impaired vitamin B_{12} status, iron overload, systemic conditioning or increased mutagenic activity in healthy individuals.[31] In patients with stone-forming tendency, high-dose ascorbic acid intakes should be monitored or avoided. In rare cases of excessive gastrointestinal absorption of iron, use of high doses of ascorbic acid is contraindicated. Ascorbic acid is considered safe and nontoxic at levels normally consumed.[1-3] The USRDA for ascorbic acid is 60 mg/day.

THIAMIN

Nomenclature

Thiamin was the first recognized water-soluble vitamin, therefore is referred to as vitamin B_1. It has also been referred to as the antiberiberi, antineuritic or polyneuritic vitamin. The complex molecule contains a pyrimidine and a thiazole nucleus joined by a methylene bridge and is chemically known as 3(4-amino-2-methylpyrimidyl-5-methyl)-4-methyl-5, (β-hydroxyethyl) thiazolium chloride. It is manufactured as the hydrochloride ($C_{12}H_{17}ClN_4OSHCl$) and the mononitrate ($C_{12}H_{17}N_5O_4S$).

Physicochemical Properties and Stability

Thiamin hydrochloride and thiamin mononitrate crystallize into colorless or white forms, have a characteristic odor, and a slightly bitter taste. The crystals are stable in atmospheric oxygen. They are soluble in water, much less so in alcohol, and insoluble in ether or other fat solvents. The hydrochloride is more soluble in water, 50% versus 2.7% for the mononitrate. In the absence of light and moisture, thiamin salts are relatively stable towards atmospheric oxygen. Thiamin is destroyed by sulfites and degraded by thiaminase. Acid solutions are also fairly stable; in neutral or alkaline solution, however, decomposition occurs. In solution with a pH less than 5, thiamin is fairly stable to heat and oxidation. At a pH of 5 or higher, thiamin is destroyed by autoclaving, and at a pH of 7 it is more easily destroyed by boiling or merely storing at room temperature.[17]

Function, Deficiency Symptoms, Safety

Thiamin in the active pyrophosphate form (TPP) is required metabolically for the formation of acetylcoenzyme A from pyruvate and the oxidative decarboxylation of ketoglutarate to succinyl-coenzyme A (SCOA). Pentose production is also dependent on TPP (pentose phosphate shunt).

Thiamin deficiency produces disorders in the function of the organs and tissues involved in the metabolism of carbohydrates such as the nervous system, the heart, the liver, gastrointestinal tract and muscle tissue. The classical pathological disease caused is called beriberi. In humans, thiamin depletion leads to mental symptoms which include depression, irritability, inattentiveness, and defective memory. Subjective and objective changes in the peripheral nervous system are encountered including tenderness of the calf muscles, partial anaesthesia, muscle weakness, paresthesia and hyperesthesia, and reduced or absent tendon reflexes. Electrocardiographical changes show the development of a cardiomyopathy. More general complaints included weakness, loss of weight, anorexia, and gastric upsets. Clinical cases of thiamin deficiency may occur frequently in association with chronic alcoholism and can result in Wernicke's encephalopathy.[2]

Very rare transient hypersensitivity has been noted after high oral doses (5–10 g). Normally excess ingested thiamin is readily excreted and is not a potential hazzard. For oral administration the safety factor is large.[1–3] The USRDA for thiamin is 1.5 mg/day.

RIBOFLAVIN

Nomenclature

Riboflavin is also known as vitamin B_2, lactoflavin or vitamin G, or chemically as 7,8-dimethyl-10-ribityliso-alloxazine ($C_{17}H_{20}N_4O_6$).

Physicochemical Properties and Stability

Riboflavin is a crystalline compound, occurring as fine, orange-yellow needles. It has a bitter taste and is odorless. It is soluble in water only to the extent of 10–13 mg/100 mL at 25°C; 230 mg dissolve per 100 mL at 100°C. Riboflavin is slightly soluble in ethyl and benzyl alcohols. Riboflavin phosphate (sodium), riboflavin 5′-phosphate ester monosodium salt ($C_{17}H_{20}O_9N_4PNa$) or flavin mononucleotide is a yellow crystal with water solubility several hundred times greater than that of pure riboflavin. It is fully active biologically, enzymatically and microbiologically. Both riboflavin and the phosphate ester are in commercial production.

Riboflavin is stable to acids, air, and the common oxidizing agents, bromine, and nitrous acid but is sensitive to alkali. Neutral aqueous solutions of riboflavin display an intense yellowish green fluorescence, which decreases on the addition of acid or alkali; optimal fluorescence occurs within a pH range of 3–8. Neutral aqueous solutions of riboflavin are relatively heat-stable if protected from light. They can be sterilized by short-time autoclaving. Riboflavin is destroyed by light, the rate of destruction becoming greater with increasing temperature and pH. It is readily degraded by ultraviolet or sunlight (420–560 nm). Reducing agents can transform riboflavin in alkaline, neutral, or acidic acid solutions directly into the pale yellow dihydroflavin, which is reoxidized on shaking with air.[17]

Functions, Deficiency Symptoms, and Safety

Flavoproteins containing a riboflavin component, flavin adenine denucleotide (FAD) or flavin mononucleotide (FMN) function in oxidation reactions in the metabolism of energy and nitrogen-containing food components. The abilities of the flavins to be varyingly potentiated as redox carriers at differential binding sites, to participate in one and two electron transfers and in reduced form to combine with oxygen, provide a unique and manifold physiological role.[1]

Riboflavin deficiency in man is generally characterized by angular stomatitis, glossitis, seborrheic dermatitis about the nose, vulva and scrotum, amblyopia, and vascularization of the cornea. A normocytic anemia may occur. Soreness and burning of the lips, mouth and tongue are common complaints, and this is usually accompanied by discomfort in eating and swallowing. Clinical signs of riboflavin deficiency are rarely seen among inhabitants of the developed countries.[2]

Riboflavin has a low toxicity. Adverse reaction has not been reported with oral administration of this vitamin. The limited solubility and absorptivity of riboflavin and its ready excretion seem to preclude a health risk in its use as a food additive.[1,3] The USRDA for riboflavin is 1.7 mg/day.

NIACIN

Nomenclature

Niacin (or nicotinic acid or vitamin PP, the pellagra-preventing factor or vitamin B$_3$, also called the antipellagra vitamin) is pyridine-3-carboxylic acid or pyridine-β-carboxylic acid (C$_5$H$_5$NO$_2$), one of the simpler vitamin structures. It is also one of the most stable compounds and the first vitamin to be prepared in crystalline form.

Physicochemical Properties and Stability

Niacin occurs as white, needle-shaped crystals or as a white, crystalline powder, odor-free or with a slight odor, and with a tart taste. Niacin is sparingly soluble in water (1 g/60 mL) and ethanol (1 g/100 mL), readily soluble in alkalies and insoluble in acetone and ethyl ether. It is also soluble in glycerol, propylene glycol and dilute acids. Niacin is nonhygroscopic, very stable in air and resists autoclaving. In an alkaline medium and at high temperature it undergoes decarboxylation. It is stable against oxidation in the presence of the usual oxidizing agents even at elevated temperatures.[17]

Niacinamide is a white crystalline powder, with a bitter taste. It is very soluble in water (100 g/100 mL), in ethanol (66 g/100 mL), and in glycerol (10 g/100 mL). It is less soluble in acetone, and chloroform, and very slightly soluble in ethyl ether. Niacinamide in dry form is stable below 50°C. Aqueous solutions of niacinamide are very stable even when subjected to autoclaving. Niacinamide hydrolyzes easily in acid or alkaline media, forming niacin.[17]

Function, Deficiency Symptoms, Safety

Niacin coenzymes, nicotinamide adenine dinucleotide (NAD) and nicotinamide adenine dinucleotide phosphate (NADP) are essential in oxidation and reduction reactions in the synthesis and degradation of fatty acids, carbohydrates and amino acids. The coenzymes, components of many enzymes, function in diverse reactions as, for example, the conversion of alcohols, sugars and polyols to aldehydes or ketones, hemiacetals to lactones, aldehydes to acids and certain amino acids to keto acids.[1]

Pellagra, is characterized by dermatosis, diarrhea, dementia, anorexia, weight loss, and oral lesions, such as stomatitis, red tongue, and genital and perianal changes. Neurological symptoms include depression, apathy, headache, dizziness, irritability, and confusion.[1,2,18]

A transient flushing skin reaction follows the oral intake of an oral dose (usually more than 75 mg). High oral doses of niacin can produce skin rash, nausea, vomiting, diarrhea, cardiac arrhythmias and abnormal liver function. Niacinamide is usually well tolerated. Oral doses of 200 mg to 10 g of nicotinamide daily has been used therapeutically under medical controls for periods as long as 10 years. Some reactions have occurred at the higher levels but have responded to cessation of therapy.[1-3] The USRDA for niacin is 20 mg/day.

PYRIDOXINE

Nomenclature

Vitamin B_6, adermin, the antiacrodynia factor, rat antidermatitis vitamin, or the yeast eluate factor, includes the complex, pyridoxine, pyridoxal and pyridoxamine (the alcohol, aldehyde, and amine structures of vitamin B_6), all of which occur in mammalian tissue and are biologically active. The physiologically active forms, pyridoxal phosphate (codecarboxylase) and pyridoxamine phosphate, are also present. Pyridoxine, 5-hydroxy-6-methyl-3,4-pyridinedimethanol, the principle form, is manufactured by chemical synthesis as the hydrochloride ($C_8H_{11}NO_3HCl$).

Physicochemical Properties and Stability

Pyridoxine hydrochloride is a white to practically white crystal or crystalline powder. It is soluble in water (1 g/4.5 mL), ethanol, and propylene glycol, sparingly soluble in acetone, and insoluble in ether or chloroform. Crystalline pyridoxine hydrochloride is stable in air but is slowly affected by sunlight if exposed sufficiently. Acidic solutions of pyridoxine hydrochloride are stable and may be heated 30 min at 120°C without decomposition. Likewise pyridoxine hydrochloride solutions are not easily affected by heating with mild alkali. Alkaline or neutral aqueous solutions are sensitive to light, with subsequent destruction of the vitamin after sufficient exposure.[17]

Functions, Deficiency Symptoms and Safety

Many pyridoxal phosphate-dependent enzymes are known. In the form of pyridoxal 5′-phosphate, vitamin B_6 acts as the coenzyme of a series of enzymes which catalyze transamination, decarboxylation, deamination and desulphydration, and cleavage or synthesis of amino acids.[19] The intimate involvement of vitamin B_6 in amino acid metabolism explains why an increase of dietary protein leads to increased vitamin B_6 requirement. Pyridoxal phosphate also is an essential enzyme for energy production, fat metabolism, central nervous system activity, and hemoglobin production. Antagonists interfere with pyridoxine function.[20]

Severe vitamin B_6 deficiency in humans results in seborrheic dermatitis in the areas of the nose, eyes and mouth, erosions of the buccal mucosa and mouth, glossitis and abdominal distress. There may be an incidence of kidney stones with the deficiency. Nervous disorders such as peripheral neuritis, depression and confusion are evident. Nervous disorders are primarily seen during the period of active growth, producing epileptiform convulsions in the infant. Pyridoxine-deficient diets are associated with microcytic hypochromic anemia and loss of ability to convert tryptophan to nicotinic acid. Convincing evidence of the essentiality of vitamin B_6 in human nutrition was the widespread occurrence in the early 1950s of convulsive seizures in infants fed a heat-processed commercial liquid milk formula low in vitamin B_6, symptoms which responded to pyridoxine therapy.[2,19]

Daily intake of pyridoxine up to 50 times the RDA for periods up to 3–4 years have been administered without adverse reactions. Severe sensory nervous system dysfunction was reported in 7 adults who took doses of vitamin B_6 from 2–6 g/day and a similar observation in one adult taking 500 mg daily which were reversible upon cessation of supplementation.[21] The human data suggest that oral daily doses less than 500 mg/day appear to be safe on the basis of literature reports[22] where the compound was administered for periods from 6 months to 6 years. The USRDA for vitamin B_6 is 2 mg/day.

PANTOTHENIC ACID

Nomenclature

Pantothenic acid is the chick antidermatosis factor, anti gray hair factor, vitamin B_5 and chemically is D(+)-N-(2,4-dihydroxy-3,3-dimethylbutyryl)-β-alanine, ($C_9H_{17}NO_5$). It is an optically active organic acid with biological activity residing in the dextroisomer. The vitamin is widely distributed in foods of both animal and plant origin. In both plant and animal tissues the vitamin occurs very largely as coenzyme A, a "bound form." Free pantothenic acid is an unstable, extremely hygroscopic liquid; it is therefore unsuitable for practical application and is used mainly in the form of calcium pantothenate.

Physicochemical Properties and Stability

Pantothenic acid is a pale yellow, viscous liquid, soluble in water and alcohol and insoluble in benzene and chloroform. Since the peptide linkage is not very stable, pantothenic acid is fairly easily destroyed. It is not in commercial production.

Calcium pantothenate ($C_{18}H_{32}CaN_2O_{10}$), the form usually used in the nutrification of food, occurs as a slightly hygroscopic, somewhat bulky, white powder. it is odorless, stable in air and has a slightly bitter taste. Its solutions are neutral or slightly alkaline to litmus. One gram of calcium pantothenate dissolves in about 3 mL of water. It is soluble in glycerin, but is virtually insoluble in alcohol, in chloroform, and in ether. Calcium pantothenate, shows fairly good stability to heat at pH 5-7, but its stability decreases progressively as the pH either decreases or increases from this range.[17]

Functions, Deficiency Symptoms, Safety

Pantothenic acid is an essential component of coenzyme A (CoA) which forms many different acyl-CoA derivatives including acetyl-CoA. Acetyl CoA is formed in the degradation of fat, carbohydrates and a number of amino acids. Biosynthetic pathways dependent on pantothenic acid containing acyl Co-A derivatives include fatty acids, phospholipids, cholesterol, steroid hormones, acetylcholine, and porphyrin rings.

On the basis of studies in human volunteers and of observations on pantothenic acid-deficient animals, deficiency of pantothenic acid may be related to reduced growth or weight loss, fatigue, insomnia, disorders of the nervous system such as impaired motor coordination, paresthesia and burning feet syndrome, gastrointestinal disturbances such as vomiting, distress, and cramps, inhibition of antibody formation, impairment of adrenal function, and effects on muscle, namely tenderness in the heels, leg cramps.[2]

The vitamin is very well tolerated in oral doses 100 times the RDA. Toxicity is minimal; at a dose of 10 g of calcium pantothenate per day no toxic manifestation are known other than occasional diarrhea and minor gastrointestinal disturbances.[1,3] The USRDA for pantothenate is 10 mg/day.

BIOTIN

Nomenclature

Biotin, also known as bios IIB, CoR, and vitamin H, (cis-tetrahydro-2-oxothieno-[3,4-d]imidazoline-4-valeric acid), present in soil, in bacteria, and in nearly all animal and plant food, is one of the water-soluble vitamins. d-Biotin ($C_{10}H_{16}N_2O_3S$) is a monocarboxylic acid containing a cyclic urea structure with sulfur in a thioether linkage. The molecular structure of biotin contains three asymmetric carbon atoms. Eight different steroisomers are therefore possible, of which only the dextro-rotary, so-called d-biotin occurs in nature and possesses vitamin activity. l-Biotin is inactive in animals; the dl form has 50% activity.

Physicochemical Properties and Stability

d-Biotin occurs as colorless needles or white, crystalline powder only slightly soluble in water (about 22 mg/100 mL at 25°C). It is soluble in dilute alkali and hot water, sparingly soluble in dilute acid and practically insoluble in organic solvents. The sodium salt is highly soluble. The vitamin in dry state has a high degree of stability. Dry, crystalline d-biotin is fairly stable in air, daylight and heat; it is gradually destroyed by ultraviolet radiation. Aqueous solutions are relatively stable if weakly acid or weakly alkaline. In strong acid and alkaline solutions the biological activity is destroyed by heating. Neutral solutions are stable at 100°C.[17]

Functions, Deficiency Symptoms, Safety

Biotin functions as a prosthetic group in a number of enzymes, pyruvate carboxylase, acetyl-CoA carboxylase, propionyl-CoA carboxylase and 3-methylcrotonyl-CoA carboxylase which are concerned with the transfer of a carboxyl group.[25]. It is required for a series of carboxylation reactions which are involved in the degradation of amino acids and also in the carboxylation of acetyl-CoA to malonyl-CoA. The biotin-dependent carboxylation of aceytl-CoA is a key reaction for the body in the synthesis of fatty acids. The reversible carboxylation of pyruvate to oxaloacetate, a connecting link in the citric acid cycle, is biotin dependent.[25]

Biotin deficiency has been produced in humans. It is evidenced by a desquamation of skin, loss of hair, accompanied by mild depression, lassitude, muscle pains, somnolence, anorexia with enhanced serum cholesterol, and slight anemia. Biotin deficiency in man has not been identified as a regular pathological entity on normal diets. No adverse reactions to orally administered biotin have been reported.[1,2] The USRDA for biotin is 0.3 mg/day.

VITAMIN A

Nomenclature

Vitamin A, retinol ($C_{20}H_{29}OH$), is the isoprenoid polyene alcohol, [3,7-dimethyl-9-(2'6'6'-trimethyl-1'-cyclohexen-1'-yl)2,4,6,8,-nonatetraene-1-ol], also known as axerophthol, the antixerophthalmic vitamin and the antiinfective vitamin. As an unsaturated cyclic alcohol with 20 carbon atoms and 5 conjugated double bonds, it can exist in different isomeric forms with different biological activities, the all-trans (full bioactivity), the 2-mono-cis (neo) or 13-cis (¾ activity), the 6-mon-cis or 9-cis, and the 2,6-di-cis or the 9,13-di-cis (¼ activity). The all-trans isomer possesses the highest biological activity, namely, 3,333,000 IU/gram. Retinyl esters (acetate or palmitate) are usually used in nutrification of foods.

Vitamin A Activity. Until recently, vitamin A activity has been expressed as international units (IU), one IU being equivalent to 0.3 mcg of retinol, 0.344 mcg vitamin A acetate, 0.358 mcg vitamin A propionate, 0.55 mcg vitamin A palmitate, or 0.6 mcg β-carotene. The carotene-vitamin A relationships were derived from studies on the rat and are assumed to hold for man. Because of the considerably poorer utilization of dietary carotenoid provitamins A as compared to retinol, the expression of the total vitamin A activity of a diet as IU has to be qualified by indicating the percentages of the activity coming from retinol and that coming from provitamins. Currently the term "retinol equivalent" has been introduced.

I retinol equivalent = 1 mcg retinol (vitamin A alcohol)
= 6 mcg β-carotene
= 12 mcg g other provitamin A carotenoids
= 3.33 IU Vitamin A activity from retinol
= 10 IU vitamin A activity from β-carotene

β-carotene and β-apo-8'-carotenal are added to foods as food colorants and simultaneously provide added vitamin A value, thus serving a dual role as a food improver, colorant and a nutrient source.[32]

Physicochemical Properties and Stability

Vitamin A is fairly stable when heated to moderate temperatures in an inert atmosphere in the absence of light, but it is unstable in the presence of oxygen or air or when exposed to ultraviolet light. Mineral acids are known to destroy vitamin A as well as its isomers. In the presence of alkali, vitamin A is quite stable so that alkaline saponification of vitamin A-containing materials may be carried out without serious loss. The presence of metals may also accelerate the oxidation of vitamin A.[17] In handling vitamin A concentrate, the three main precautions necessary are (1) inert atmosphere, (2) subdued light, and (3) avoidance of trace metals and excess acid. Vitamin A may be stabilized by (1) sealing under vacuum or inert gas, (2) storage at low temperatures, (3) addition of antioxidants, (4) formulation in liquid emulsions, (5) sealing with a protective material such as gelatin or vegetable gums and waxes, and (6) complexing with other materials.[33]

Functions, Deficiency Symptoms, Safety

No co-enzyme role has been demonstrated as in the case of the water-soluble B vitamins. Retinol complexed with a protein (retinol-binding protein) is the principal form of transport of the vitamin in blood from the liver. Vitamin A esters are the liver storage form and vitamin A aldehyde (retinal) in the retina combines with protein to form the essential photosensitive pigment, rhodopsin, in the visual process of man and animals.

Outside of the very specific role vitamin A plays in vision, it is necessary for growth, reproduction, the integrity of the mucous-secreting cells of the epithelia, the synthesis of glycoproteins, the prevention of keratinization, and maintenance of the immune system. Nightblindness is an early symptom of vitamin A deficiency. This is followed by progressive conjunctival and corneal degeneration of the eye which can lead to blindness (xerophthalmia). The sense of taste and smell are negatively affected; therefore, food intake and growth are reduced. Susceptibility to infection increases partly due to the loss of ciliated goblet cells in bronchial passages and maintenance of epithelial tissue which becomes dry and keratinized.[1] There is growing evidence of cancers associated with vitamin A deficiency and lower tumor burdens with higher carotenoid status.[34]

Prolonged continuous daily intakes of excessively high levels of vitamin A can cause hypervitaminosis A, symptoms of which in a mild state can be intracorneal pressure, headaches, nausea, malaise, etc., and in more severe conditions joint pains, loss of body hair, crackling and peeling of skin, etc. Hypervitaminosis A results when the retinol binding capacity of the special circulating blood proteins is exceeded and exposure of tissues to unbound vitamin A exceeds their tolerance, thus initiating hypervitaminotic symptoms.[35]

In adults, intakes from over 50,000–1,000,000 IU daily have produced adverse effects within days or several weeks at the higher levels and after 6–10 months at the lower levels.[35] Infants and small children show toxicity at lower levels than adults. High levels of vitamin A intake during pregnancy should be avoided. The degree and timing of hypervitaminosis A is influenced by the amount of vitamin A consumed, the physical form of the vitamin preparation, age and weight of the subject, general health conditions and other factors. Continual daily ingestion of large doses of vitamin A should not be undertaken without medical or nutritional guidance.[2,35,36] The USRDA for vitamin A is 5000 IU/day.

β-CAROTENE

β-Carotene ($C_{40}H_{56}$) is a most important provitamin A form and a member of the natural carotenoids, which now number well over 400 structures. In pure form the chemically synthesized trans isomer appears as red-purple, rhombic crystals. Like vitamin A, β-carotene is insoluble in water, practically insoluble in ethanol and slightly soluble in vegetable oils. Exposed to air, β-carotene absorbs oxygen, giving rise to inactive, colorless oxidation products. In order to employ β-carotene in food applications special market stabilized suspensions, solutions, emulsions, powders, etc., are required, as in the case of vitamin A esters.[32]

In addition to its colorant and vitamin A precursor role, β-carotene also functions as a quencher of singlet oxygen and free radicals and in so doing also has an antioxidant role.[37] β-carotene has been shown to enhance several aspects of immune function; thus, a multi-purpose need for β-carotene is becoming evident in the quest for continued health.[34,37,38] Contrasted with vitamin A, β-carotene, at high intake levels is relatively nontoxic as the body carries on the conversion to vitamin A in a controlled manner.

Toxicity studies in animals have shown that β-carotene is not carcinogenic, mutagenic or teratogenic and does not cause hypervitaminosis A. Daily supplementation of high doses of β-carotene over 15 years at levels approximately 60 times the normal intake level has not been associated with adverse effects other than skin pigmentation which is self-correcting when high intakes are lowered.[39]

VITAMIN D

Nomenclature

The two principal forms of the fat-soluble, antirachitic vitamin are vitamin D_2[9,10-secoergosta-5,7,10(19),22-tetraen-3β-ol] also termed calciferol, ergocalciferol ($C_{28}H_{44}O$), activated ergosterol, and viosterol; and vitamin D_3[(9,10-secocholesta-5,7,10(19)-trien-3β-ol]) also termed activated 7-dehydrocholesterol and cholecalciferol ($C_{27}H_{44}O$). These are white, crystalline compounds formed from the irradiation process of the appropriate sterol followed by purification procedures. Vitamin

D_3 is fully active biologically for man and all animals. It is the naturally occurring antirachitic steroid; it also is produced in the skin by exposing the body to direct sunlight. Vitamin D_2 is also fully effective for humans.

The International Unit (IU) of vitamin D, adopted by WHO as the standard of activity was defined as the biological activity of 1 mg of an oily solution of vitamin D_3 containing 0.025 mcg pure, crystallized vitamin D_3. The USP Unit corresponds with the International Unit.

Physicochemical Properties and Stability

Since vitamin D_2 and D_3 are sensitive to oxygen and moist air, they must be handled as previously described for vitamin A. The presence of antioxidants and physical insulation from contact with air, acids and trace minerals, such as copper and iron which act as prooxidants, promotes stability. Dry stabilized vitamin D supplements retain their potency much longer and can be used in contact with minerals. When kept in stabilized oil away from light, vitamin D retains its potency for long periods.[17]

Function, Deficiency Symptoms, Safety

Vitamin D has a complex role (1) in bone formation and development, (2) in maintaining blood levels of calcium and phosphate, (3) in calcium absorption in the intestinal wall, (4) in mobilizing calcium from bone, and (5) in other mineralizations involved in the prevention of rickets and osteomalacia mechanisms. During the past two decades it was discovered that vitamin D was hydroxylated in the liver, forming 25-OHD_3, and continuing in the kidney with another hydroxylation, forming 1,25-$(OH)_2D_3$. It is generally understood that most of vitamin D physiological functions involves dihydroxy vitamin D_3. With the chemical synthesis of 1,25$(OH)_2D_3$ it is now possible to treat vitamin D resistant rickets, hypoparathyroidism, renal osteodystrophy and osteoporosis. Bone remodeling is also dependent on vitamin D which is essential for normal shaping of the skeleton during growth and development.[40-41]

Ingestion of massive doses of vitamin D has been shown to cause widespread calcification of soft tissues. Doses of vitamin D many times the recommended allowance, if continued over a long period of time, can result in extensive calcification of the kidneys, heart, arteries, stomach, and other soft tissues, accompanied by nausea, weakness, polyuria, polydipsia, hyperlipemia, renal calculi and even death. It is particularly important to avoid the administration of large doses in infants, whose daily intake need not exceed 400 IU. Since excessive amounts of vitamin D are hazardous, only individuals with diseases influencing vitamin D absorption or metabolism are judged to require more than 400 IU/day. prophylactic adult doses greater than 1000 IU/day should be monitored. Doses of 10,000 IU or more may be given, under medical supervision, as specific treatments.[2,3] The USRDA for vitamin D is 400 IU/day.

VITAMIN E

Nomenclature

Vitamin E is a generic term for a series of lipid soluble tocol and trienol compounds of which α-tocopherol is of major importance. The chemical name of α-tocopherol ($C_{29}H_{50}O_2$) is 2,5,7,8,-tetramethyl-2-(4',8',12'-trimethyltridecyl)-6-chromanol.

Vitamin E activity in food is derived from a series of compounds of plant origin, the tocopherols and tocotrienols. These compounds are present in varying amounts in animal tissues. The structure which has the highest vitamin E activity for man and animals is α-tocopherol and is not the one of the tocopheryl series which is always most abundant in foods.

β-, γ-, and δ-Tocopherols and the tocotrienols have lower biological activities, estimated to be 0–40% that of α-tocopherol. One IU of vitamin E is defined as the activity of 1 mg of dl,α-tocopheryl acetate (RS at asymmetric carbon atom positions 2). The dl,α-tocopheryl acetate (also known as all rac-α-tocopheryl acetate) of commerce (RS at asymmetric carbon atoms position 2, 4', and 8') is presently considered to have the same biological activity. On the basis of α-tocopherol equivalents (TE), d, α-tocopherol (also known as RRR-α-tocopherol) would be 1; dl, α-tocopherol, 0.74. 1 TE is equal to 1.5 IU. Vitamin E, in the form of d, α-tocopherol, dl, α-tocopherol and their esters, have been commercially available for several decades.

Physicochemical Properties, Stability

The tocopherols are slightly viscous, pale yellow liquids freely soluble in most organic solvents. Both α-tocopherol and α-tocopheryl acetate are freely soluble in vegetable oils, ethyl alcohol, chloroform, and acetone. They are insoluble in water. They are generally stable to heat, acid and alkali in the absence of oxygen, but they oxidize readily, particularly in the free tocopherol form, in the presence of iron salts to form quinones, dimers and trimers. In order to improve miscibility in aqueous media and stability, vitamin E is converted into beadlet, granular or powder form. α-Tocopheryl acetate is the principal commercial form of vitamin E used as a nutrient in pharmaceuticals, in food nutrification, and as an additive for animal feeds. To retard the development of oxidative rancidity, α- or γ-tocopherols are added to foods with or without ascorbates as antioxidants.[17]

Functions, Deficiency Symptoms, Safety

Vitamin E functions in general as a biological antioxidant. There are claims today for use of vitamin E in noninfectious disease and in promoting general well-being, acting as a preserver of cell membranes, in protecting lipoidal structures, and in porphyrin metabolism, in xanthine oxidase and in selenoenzyme-glutathione peroxidase systems. It is more recently recognized as essential for the maintenance of the structure and function of the human nervous system. Antioxidant compounds such as α-tocopherol may play a role in delaying plaque formation in arteries and thus prevent or retard atherosclerotic heart disease based on reports from the United States and Europe. Concern about undesirable chronic levels of liquid peroxidation in tissue components and related promotion of carcinogenesis and their amelioration by a free radical scavenger leds to a reconsideration of desirable daily intake of α-tocopherol.[42-45] The occurence of vitamin E deficiency of pure dietary origin is not common in developed countries. Premature infants are more susceptible to a vitamin E deficiency, and hemolytic anemia is a vitamin E deficiency abnormality observed.

Toxicity of vitamin E is low; the vitamin is not mutagenic, carcinogenic or teratogenic, and so moderate amounts can be safely consumed. Doses as high as 3000 IU per day have been administered with few side effects in human studies with double blind protocols.[47] High level vitamin intake is contraindicated in individuals with coagulation defects produced by vitamin K deficiency caused by malabsorption or anticoagulant therapy. The USRDA for vitamin E is 30 IU/day.

VITAMIN K

Nomenclature

The general term, vitamin K, is now used to describe not a single chemical entity, but a group of quinone compounds which have characteristic antihemorrhagic effects. They are all related to 2-methyl-1,4-naphthoquinone. Vitamin K occurs in green plant matter in nature as vitamin $K_{1(20)}$ phytomenadione, phytonadione, phylloquinone (2-methyl-3-phytyl-1,4-naphthoquinone) ($CH_{31}H_{46}O_2$); as vitamin $K_{2(20)}$, menaquinone-4 (2-methyl-3-digeranyl-1,4-naphthoquinone) in the body tissues of animals and man; as vitamin $K_{2(30)}$, menaquinone-6 (2-methyl-3-difarnesyl-1,4-naphthoquinone) produced by microbial flora in food and animals; and as vitamin $K_{2(35)}$, menaquinone-7 (2-methyl-3-farnesylgeranylgeranyl-1,4-naphthoquinone), also of microbiological origin; and also others.

Physicochemical Properties, Stability

Vitamin K1 is a yellow liquid; vitamin K_2 a yellow crystal. Most all vitamin K compounds dissolve readily in most of the common organic solvents, such as ether, benzene, hexane, acetone, but are insoluble in water and only sparingly soluble in methanol or ethanol. They are essentially stable to air, to heat and dilute acid, but are sensitive to alkali, strong acid, reducing agents and ultraviolent radiation and even to diffuse daylight.[17]

Function, Deficiency Symptoms, Safety

Vitamin K is indispensable for maintaining the function of the blood-coagulation system.[46] Vitamin K is required for the synthesis of blood clotting proteins, namely prothrombin (factor II), factors, VII, IX and X, and proteins C, M, S and Z. Vitamin K dependent coagulation factors are distributed in the extrinsic system, which is activated by injury, the intrinsic system, which is activated by platelets, and in the final common pathway leading to the conversion of fibrinogen to fibrin. The concerted action of the different factors and the activated thromboplastin transform the precursor prothrombin into the clotting enzyme thrombin, which, in turn, initiates the actual clotting phase by converting the soluble fibrinogen to the insoluble fibrin. Vitamin K is involved in the γ-carboxylation of the specific glutamic acid residues of the clotting factor precursors produced in the liver.[1,2]

Vitamin K deficiency is uncommon in healthy people. Vitamin K deficiency results in a fall in the prothrombin content of the blood, eliciting a hemorrhagic tendency and the incidence of hemorrhages in varied tissues and organs (the subcutaneous tissue, muscles, brain, intestinal tract, abdominal cavity, genital organs, etc.) and which can, especially, give rise to complications in neonatal and premature births in humans. Other symptoms are regarded as consequences of this phenomenon. Vitamin K_1 is generally well tolerated in oral applications. No hazards have been attributed to long-term ingestion of elevated amounts of the natural forms of vitamin K.[2,3]

AMINO ACIDS

Introduction

The primary interest for nutrification of foods with amino acids is their potential use in improving the protein quality of cereal grain products.[48] It is well recognized that all essential amino acids of a given diet should be present in a quantitative relationship to optimally serve for maintenance or/and growth needs.[49] A diet with a missing or an insufficient level of an essential amino acid is limited in overall protein synthesis. L-lysine is a limiting amino acid in corn, millet, oats, rice, rye, sorghum and wheat: L-tryptophan is also limiting in corn. The second limiting amino acid in cereal grain, is L-threonine. When plant protein supplements are added to cereal grain products such as soy protein products, added methionine or methionine analog may be necessary for optimal protein utilization.

Nutrification of human food with amino acids is not in wide commercial practice, although amino acid supplementation with methionine or methionine analog and lysine in animal feeds has been practiced for many years in the United States and some other countries. In future food nutrification with amino acids, more attention will need to be given to potential interactions among food ingredients which may influence flavor, stability and/or availability characteristics of the food product. Additions will also have to meet regulatory limitations.[50]

The amino acid nutrification of cereal grain products has been reviewed by Jansen[51] and by Mitsuda and Yasumoto.[52] Technological and practical aspects of adding amino acid to foods have been discussed by Senti and Pence[53] and Beigler.[54] Most amino acids are prepared by fermentation techniques.[55] The synthesis of the amino acids, methionine, lysine threonine and tryptophan and their application in nutrifying food is presented by Ottenheym and Jenneskens.[56] Clark[57] has examined cereal base diets in meeting the protein requirements of adults; studies with children have been done by Graham et al.[58] and by Bressani.[59] Some global studies with amino acid nutrified cereals have been examined in detail by Austin[60] and further interpreted in the 1984 NAS report.[61] The structures of all of the amino acids are included in Fig. 4.3.

Chemical Properties, Stability, Bioavailability

The amino acids, lysine, methionine, tryptophan and threonine are all soluble in water to varying degrees. These amino acids are relatively stable under dry, cool conditions, but are sensitive to high temperature and high humidity conditions, particularly in the presence of reactive carbonyl groups and oxidizing agents.[62]

Reduction of the biological availability of added amino acids and proteins during processing and storage is brought about by the various reactions, of which browning or the Maillard reaction is probably the most important. In this reaction the amino groups, particularly the epsilon amine of lysine combines with carbonyl groups from reducing sugars or oxidized fats to form N-substituted derivatives, which the body digests and absorbs poorly. The irony is that Maillard browning such as occurs in the crust of bread is desirable from visual appeal but lowers bioavailability of the resultant protein product. Another reaction that may reduce bioavailability is the so-called Strecker degradation in which free amino acids are degraded by carbonyls to form aldehydes and ketones containing one less carbon atom. In the bleaching of flour with benzoyl peroxide, amino acids may be destroyed under these oxidizing conditions. The bioavailability of amino acids in foods and the effects on protein quality assessment has been reviewed by Friedman.[63]

Forms Used As Additives

Methionine is added as either L or DL methionine. Lysine is added as either L-lysine HCL, L-lysine-L-glutamate dihydrate, L-lysine-orotate, or L-lysine-L-aspartate. Threonine and tryptophan are added in the L forms only. Methionine can present potentially serious odor and flavor problems in food fortification projects. This problem can be minimized by the use of N-acetyl-L-methionine (NAM), which is an approved food additive for use as a source of L-methionine to improve

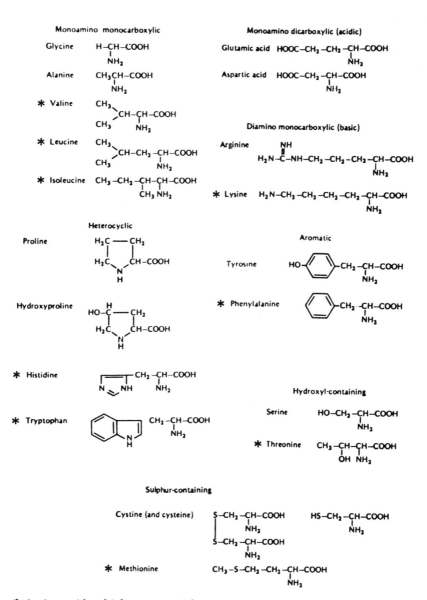

*Amino acids which are essential to man.
Histidine is essential to children only.

From Muller and Tobin 1980

FIG. 4.3. STRUCTURES OF IMPORTANT AMINO ACIDS

significantly the biological quality of the total protein in a food containing naturally occurring, primarily intact vegetable protein. It may not be used in infant foods or foods containing added nitrates or nitrites in order to limit nitrosamine formation. NAM must be used in sufficient concentration to increase the PER of the protein in the finished ready-to-eat food to the equivalent of casein. NAM is much more stable than methionine in model food systems conducive to Maillard browning, but is less stable under oxidative conditions.[64]

Functions, Deficiency, Requirements, Safety

Methionine, lysine, tryptophan, threonine all share the common function of being required for protein synthesis and specific enzymes. In addition, certain metabolic pathways are dependent on these amino acids. For example, tryptophan is required for serotonin and niacin synthesis; methionine is required for lipid metabolism; and lysine is a component of essential cross-linkages in elastin and collagen.

In a deficiency of any of the essential amino acids, impaired growth results and protein synthesis is abnormal. Anemia may result, and, in the case of methionine, a fatty liver may develop. The requirements for protein and the individual amino acids (Table 4.6) vary depending on the age of the individual. For example, the amounts required for young children and adults for methionine, lysine, tryptophan, and threonine are as follows: 27 & 13; 64 & 12; 12.5 & 3.5; and 37 & 7 mg/kg of body weight per day respectively. Balanced amino acid intake taken in excess over requirements is relatively safe; however, in amino acid nutrification projects imbalance and antagonism, which can occur when one amino acid is added in relatively great excess, must be avoided.[65]

Practical experience in field trials would indicate that the most economical intervention to enhance the protein quality of marginal cereal-grain diets results from supplementation of the diet with a soy protein or other oil seed protein products and then addition of lysine and/or other amino acids, if needed, to maximize protein utilization.

CONCLUSION

Past experience indicates that certain foods may be nutrified with added vitamins and/or amino acids without flavor and stability problems and full bioavailability of the incorporated nutrient when properly implemented for specific application. In this chapter, an attempt is made within the allotted space to present some characteristics of the nutrients and their role in nutrition as an aid to the choice of their inclusion in food products in instances where the nutrification technique seems worthy of application. As increased population pressures put greater demands on the supply of more nutritious food and as knowledge expands on nutrient interrela-

TABLE 4.6
ESTIMATES OF AMINO ACID REQUIREMENTS[a]

Amino Acid	Requirements, mg/kg per Day, by Age Group			
	Infants, Age 3–4 mo[b]	Children, Age ~2 yr[c]	Children, Age 10–12 yr[d]	Adults[e]
Histidine	28	?	?	8–12
Isoleucine	70	31	28	10
Leucine	161	73	42	14
Lysine	103	64	44	12
Methionine plus cystine	58	27	22	13
Phenylalanine plus tyrosine	125	69	22	14
Threonine	87	37	28	7
Tryptophan	17	12.5	3.3	3.5
Valine	93	38	25	10
Total without histidine	714	352	214	84

[a]Source: NAS/NRC.[68] From WHO (1985).
[b]Based on amounts of amino acids in human milk or cow's milk formulas fed at levels that supported good growth. Data from Fomon and Filer (1967).
[c]Based on achievement of nitrogen balance sufficient to support adequate lean tissue gain (16 mg N/kg per day). Data from Pineda et al. (1981).
[d]Based on upper range of requirement for positive nitrogen balance. Recalculated by Williams et al. (1974) from data of Nakagawa et al. (1964).
[e]Based on highest estimate of requirement to achieve nitrogen balance. Data from several investigators (reviewed in FAO/WHO, 1973).

tionships and human quantitative needs, there is reason to expect nutrification of foods with added vitamins and amino acids will continue to be one means of dietary improvement.

REFERENCES

1. SHILS, M. E. and YOUNG, V. R. 1988. Modern Nutrition in Health Disease. Lea & Febiger, Philadelphia.
2. MACHLIN, L. J. 1984. Handbook of Vitamins: Nutritional, Biochemical and Clinical Aspects. Marcel Dekker, New York.
3. MARKS, J. 1985. The Vitamins: Their Role in Medical Practice. MTP Press, Hingham, Mass.; 1983. Vitamin Safety: Vitamin Information Status Paper. F. Hoffmann-LaRoche and Co., Basle.
4. ANON. 1986. Use of vitamin as additives in processed foods. Food Technol. 41(11), 163–168.
5. BORENSTEIN, B. 1968. Vitamins and amino acids. In Handbook of Food Additives, T. E. Furia (ed.). Chemical Rubber Co., Cleveland.
6. BORENSTEIN, B. and GORDON, H. T. 1987. Additions of vitamins, minerals and

amino acids to foods. *In* Nutritional Evaluation of Food Processing, 3rd Ed., E. Karmas and R. S. Harris (eds.). Van Nostrand Reinhold Company, New York.
7. BAUERNFEIND, J. C. 1982. Ascorbic acid technology in food applications. *In* Ascorbic Acid, Chemistry, Metabolism and Uses, P. A. Seib and B. Tolbert (eds.). American Chemical Society, Washington, DC.
8. KLAEUI, H. M., HAUSHEER, W. and HUSCHKE, G. 1970. Technological aspects of the use of fat-soluble vitamins and carotenoids and of the development of stabilized and marketable forms. *In* Fat-soluble Vitamins, R. A. Morton (ed.). Pergamon Press, Oxford.
9. LEKLEM, J. E. 1988. Vitamin B_6 bioavailability: Application to human nutrition. Food Technol. *42*(10), 194–197.
10. WALL, J. S. and CARPENTER, K. J. 1988. Variation in availability of niacin in grain products. Food Technol. *42*(10), 198–205.
11. BAILEY, L. 1988. Factors affecting folate bioavailability. Food Technol. *42*(10), 206–213.
12. ERDMAN, J. W., POOR, C. L. and DIETY, J. M. 1988. Food processing and dietary effects on the bioavailability of vitamin A, carotenoids and vitamin E. Food Technol. *42*(10), 214–225.
13. LEVANDER, O. A. and CHENG, L. 1980. Micronutrient Interactions: Vitamins, Minerals and Hazardous Elements. Ann. N.Y. Acad. Sci. *355*.
14. MACHLIN, L. J. and LANGSETH, L. 1988. Vitamin-vitamin interactions. C. E. Bodwell and J. W. Erdman (eds.). Marcel Dekker, New York.
15. SAUBERLICH, H. E. 1985. Bioavailability of vitamins. Prog. Food Nutr. Sci. *9*, 1–33.
16. BORENSTEIN, B., BENDICH, A. and WAYSEK, E. H. 1988. Vitamin bioavailability in fortified foods. Food Technol. *42*(10), 226–228.
17. BAUERNFEIND, J. C. 1978. Vitamins, essential micronutrients for man. *In* Encyclopedia of Food Science, M. S. Peterson and A. H. Johnson (eds.). AVI/Van Nostrand Reinhold, New York.
18. WEINER, M. and VAN EYS, J. 1983. Nicotinic Acid: Nutrient-Cofactor-Drug. Marcel Dekker, New York.
19. REYNOLDS, R. D. AND LEKLEM, J. E. 1984. Vitamin B_6: Its Role in Health and Disease. A. R. Liss, New York.
20. BAUERNFEIND, J. C. and MILLER, D. N. 1978. Vitamin B_6: Nutritional and pharmaceutical usage, stability, bioavailability, antagonists and safety. Proceedings of a Workshop Human Vitamin B_6 Requirements. National Acad. Sciences, Washington, DC.
21. SCHAUMBURG, H., KAPLAN, J., WINDEBANK, A., VICK, N., RASMUS, S., PLEASURE, D. and BROWN, M. 1983. Sensory neuropathy from pyridoxine abuse: A new megavitamin syndrome. N. Engl. J. Med. *309*(8), 445–448.
22. COHEN, M. and BENDICH, A. 1986. Safety of pyridoxine: A review of human and animal studies. Toxicol. Lett. *34*, 129–139.
23. SCHNEIDER, Z. and STROINSKI, A. 1987. Comprehensive B_{12}. Walter De Gruyter and Co., Berlin.
24. HAWKES, J. G. and VILLOTA, R. 1989. Folates in foods: Reactivity, stability during processing, and nutritional implications. Crit. Rev. Food Sci. Nutr. *28*(6), 439–538.
25. DAKSHINAMURTI, K. and CHAUHAN, J. 1989. Biotin. Vitam. Horm. *45*, 337–384.
26. CLEMETSON, C. A. B. 1989. Vitamin C. CRC Press, Boca Raton.

27. EUGLARD, S. and SEIFFER, S. 1986. Biochemical functions of ascorbic acid. Annu. Rev. Nutr. 6, 365–406.
28. BENDICH, A. 1987. Vitamin C and immune responses. Food Technol. 41(11), 112–114.
29. BENDICH, A., MACHLIN, L. J. and SCANDURRA, D. 1986. The antioxidant role of vitamin C. Adv. Free Radical Biol. Med. 2, 419–444.
30. BURNS, J. J., RIVERS, J. M. and MACHLIN, L. J. 1987. 3rd Conference on Vitamin C. Ann. N.Y. Acad. Sci. 498.
31. RIVERS, J. M. 1987. Safety of high-levels vitamin C ingestion. Ann. N.Y. Acad. Sci. 498, 445–454.
32. BAUERNFEIND, J. C. 1981. Carotenoids as colorants and vitamin A precursors: Technological and Nutritional Applications. Academic Press, Orlando.
33. BAUERNFEIND, J. C. 1983. Vitamin A technology and applications. World Rev. Nutr. Diet. 41, 110–199.
34. BENDICH, A. 1989. Carotenoids and the immune response. J. Nutr. 119, 112–115.
35. ANON. 1980. IVACG Report: The Safe Use of Vitamin A. International Vitamin A Consultative Group. The Nutrition Foundation, Washington, DC.
36. BENDICH, A. and LANGSETH, L. 1989. Safety of vitamin A. Am. J. Clin. Nutr. 49, 358–371.
37. BURTON, G. W. 1989. Antioxidant function of carotenoids. J. Nutr. 119, 109–111.
38. HENRYK, D., ERDMAN, J., Jr., KRINSKY, N. I., BENDICH, A. and LACHANCE, P. 1988. Papers from a Symposium on Carotenes in Food and in Health. Clin. Nutr. 7(3), 97–125.
39. BENDICH, A. 1988. The safety of beta-carotene. Nutr. Cancer II, 207–214.
40. NORMAN, A. W., SCHAEFER, K., GRIGOLEIT, H. G. and v. HERRATH, D. 1988. Vitamin D: Molecular, Cellular and Clinical Endocrinology. Walter de Gruyter, Berlin.
41. DELUCA, H. F. 1988. The vitamin D story: A collaborative effort of basic science and clinical medicine. FASEB J. 2P, 224–236.
42. MACHLIN, L. J. 1980. Vitamin E: A Comprehensive Treatise. Marcel Dekker, New York.
43. DIPLOCK, A. T. 1989. Vitamin E: Biochemistry and Health Implications. Ann. N.Y. Acad. Sci. 570.
44. SOKOL, R. J. 1989. Vitamin E and neurological function in man. Free Radical Biol. Med. 6, 189–207.
45. McCAY, P. B. 1985. Vitamin E: Interactions with Free Radical and Ascorbate. Annu. Rev. Nutr. 5, 323–340.
46. SUTTIE, J. W. 1988. Current Advances in Vitamin K Research. Elsevier, New York.
47. BENDICH, A. and MACHLIN, L. J. 1988. Safety of oral intake of vitamin E. Am. J. Clin. Nutr. 48, 612–619; 48, 718–719.
48. SCRIMSHAW, N. S. and ALTSCHUL, A. M. 1971. Amino Acid Fortification of Protein Food. MIT Press, Cambridge, Mass.
49. VISEK, W. J. 1984. An uptake of the concepts of essential amino acids. Annu. Rev. Nutr. 4, 137–155.
50. ALTSCHUL, A. M. 1974. New Protein Foods: Technology, Vol. 1A and 2. Academic Press, New York.
51. JANSEN, G. R. 1974. The amino acid fortification of cereals. In New Protein Foods, Vol. IA, A. Altschul (ed.). Academic Press, New York.

52. MITSUDA, H. and YASUMOTO, K. 1974. The amino acid fortification of intact cereal grains. *In* New Protein Foods, Vol. IA, A. Altschul (ed.). Academic Press, New York.
53. SENTI, F. R. and PENCE, J. W. 1969. Technological aspects of adding amino acids to foods. Presentation Int. Conf. Amino Acid. Fortification of Protein Foods. MIT, Cambridge, Mass.
54. BEIGLER, M. T. 1969. Practical problems in amino acid fortification. *In* Protein-Enriched Cereal Foods for World Needs, M. Milner (ed.). Am. Assoc. Cereal Chem., St. Paul.
55. AIDA, K. 1979. Production of Amino Acids and Nucleotides by Fermentation. H. Chiba, M. Fujimaki, K. Iwai, H. Mitsuda and Y. Morita (eds.). Elsevier Scientific Publ. Co., Amsterdam.
56. OTTENHEYM, H. M. and JENNESKENS, R. 1970. Synthetic amino acids and their use in fortifying foods. Agr. Food Chem. *18*(6), 1010–1014.
57. CLARK, H. E. 1978. Cereal-based diets to meet protein requirements of adult men. World Rev. Nutr. Diet. *21*, 27–48.
58. GRAHAM, G. G., PLACKS, R. P., ACEVEDO, G., MORALES, E. and CORDANO, A. 1969. Lysine enrichment of wheat flour: Evaluation in infants. Am. J. Clin. Nutr. *22*, 1459–1468.
59. BRESSANI, R. 1975. Nutrification of foods: Addition of amino acids to foods. *In* Nutritional Evaluation of Food Processing, 2 Ed. R. S. Harris and E. Karmas (eds.). AVI/Van Nostrand Reinhold, New York.
60. AUSTIN, J. E. 1979. Global Malnutrition and Cereal Fortification. Ballinger Publ. Co., Cambridge.
61. ANON. 1984. NAS Report: The Results and Interpretation of Three Field Trials of Lysine Fortification of Cereals. National Academy Press, National Academy of Sciences, Washington, DC.
62. BARRETT, G. C. 1985. Chemistry and Biochemistry of the Amino Acids. Chapman and Hall, New York.
63. FRIEDMAN, M. 1989. Absorption and Utilization of Amino Acids. CRC Press, Boca Raton.
64. SCHLESKE, K. L. and WARTHESEN, J. J. 1982. Detection and stability of N-acetyl-methionine in model food systems. J. Agr. Food Chem. *30*, 1172–1175.
65. BENDER, D. A. 1985. Amino Acid Metabolism, 2nd Ed. John Wiley & Sons, New York.
66. ANON. 1989. Nutr. Today *24* (Nov./Dec.), 32–33.
67. ANON. 1973. Fed. Reg. *38* (148), 20714.
68. NAS/NRC. 1989. Recommended Dietary Allowances, 10th Ed. National Research Council, Washington, DC.
69. ANON. 1989. Diet & Health. National Academy Press, Washington, DC.
70. ISLER, O. and BRUBACHER, G. 1982. Vitamine I. Thieme, Stuttgart.
71. MULLER, H. G. and TOBIN, G. 1980. Nutrition and Food Processing. AVI/Van Nostrand Reinhold, New York.

CHAPTER 5

Foods Considered For Nutrient Addition: CEREAL GRAIN PRODUCTS

J. C. BAUERNFEIND, Ph.D., and E. DeRITTER

IMPORTANCE OF CEREAL GRAINS

Civilization took giant steps forward when it was discovered, about 10,000 years ago that cereal grains, the seeds of grasses, could be taken from their wild state, cultivated, harvested, improved, and used as reserve foods, thus making possible the expansion of humankind. Even though lifestyles today have changed drastically since those times, the cereal grains still play a dominant role in the food supply.[1] Cereal grains and root and tuber crops are the world's primary sources of food energy. The major cereals are wheat, corn (maize), rice, barley, rye, oats, sorghum and millet. Composition of cereal grains has been tabulated.[1a]

Wheat, first cultivated around 8000 B.C. in the Fertile Crescent east of the Mediterranean Sea, is grown today throughout the world in the producing areas of North and South America, Australia, China, Europe, the Mediterranean countries and the U.S.S.R. It is regarded as the world's largest and most widely cultivated food crop (Table 5.1). Wheat has become prominent because of its pleasant flavor, extensive shelf-life and gluten-forming proteins. Wheat varies by variety and type: hard spring and winter wheat being the bread type; soft winter, the pastry type; and durum, the pasta type.[2-4]

Rice, cultivated originally in India around 3000 B.C., is grown today in Brazil, Burma, China, Egypt, India, Indonesia, Italy, Japan, Pakistan, Philippines, Spain, Thailand, the United States and many other countries. It is consumed by an estimated half of the world's population in main and side dishes, soups, cakes, puddings and sake. Rice, because of it's long history of cultivations, is grown in different environments and with cropping methods ranging from primitive to modern. Wheat and rice are the two most important food cereal grains, worldwide.[2,5]

Corn (maize), a cereal grain indigenous to the Western Hemisphere where it is a dominant food, is consumed in fresh, canned and frozen form, but also in a variety of products following dry or wet milling. The propagation of corn over past centuries has spread to Europe, Asia and Africa.[2,6,7] In the United States, corn is the nation's primary animal feed grain and thus indirectly provides food for humans.

TABLE 5.1
ANNUAL PRODUCTION OF CEREAL GRAIN CROPS BY REGION FOR 1986

Area	Wheat	Rough Rice	Maize (Corn)	Barley	Sorghum	Oats	Millet	Rye
			Million Metric Tons					
Africa	11.5	9.8	30.8	6.2	14.3	0.3	11.7	0.01
North & Central America	93.5	8.3	231.2	28.7	30.5	9.6	0	1.2
South America	16.8	15.3	37.9	0.8	6.1	0.9	0.2	0.1
Asia	188.0	36.6	97.0	18.7	18.4	1.1	16.0	1.4
Europe	116.0	2.2	70.7	70.2	0.4	12.9	0.04	14.0
Oceania	17.8	0.7	0.5	4.3	1.3	1.6	0.03	0.02
USSR	92.3	2.6	12.5	51.4	0.4	21.4	2.8	15.0
Developed world	318.0	26.1	308.1	154.7	26.5	45.6	2.9	30.2
Developing world	218.0	449.4	172.6	25.7	45.0	2.2	28.0	1.6
World	536.0	475.5	480.7	180.4	71.5	47.8	30.9	31.8

Source: Data from FAO (1987).

However, in the southern states of the United States, as in Mexico, Central America, Yugoslavia, consumption of corn as a food is moderate to high. Food uses of dry-milled corn products in the form of grits, meal and flour include breakfast cereals, porridge, snack foods, bread, cakes, muffins, pancakes, tortillas, enchiladas, tacos, and tamales.

Barley, adaptable to a greater range of climate than some other cereals, was a bread cereal of the ancient Egyptians, Greeks, Hebrews and Romans and is believed to have originated in Ethiopia and Southeast Asia thousands of years ago. It is now grown also in North Africa, North America and Western Europe and used in malting, brewing, porridges, soups and flat-type bread.[2,8,9] Rye, like wheat, is used to make leavened bread, is produced in Argentina, Austria, Denmark, France, Germany, Hungary, the Netherlands, Spain, Turkey, the United States and the U.S.S.R.[2,10] Oats, a relatively cold resistant plant, are grown in Australia, Canada, France, New Zealand, Poland, the U.K., the United States, the U.S.S.R. and West Germany, and are used in porridge and baked goods. The wide use of this cereal grain for food was developed in Germany, Scotland and the U.S.S.R.[2,11] Sorghums, also called kafir, jowar, milo, etc., widely grown in Africa, are relatively heat and drought resistant. They are also grown in the United States, Pakistan, Mexico, India, China and Argentina, and are consumed as porridge, in cakes and in flat bread. Millets, an ancient crop cultivated thousands of years ago, are used in cookies, flat breads and porridges, are an important cereal grain for much of Asia, the U.S.S.R. and Western Africa. China, India and Korea are other production countries.[2,12,13]

During 1976-80 cereal grains accounted for more than 4/5th of the total output of major food crops in developing countries.[14] Of this, rice makes up 35% of the total; wheat, 18%; corn, 17%, millets and sorghums about 8%; and roots and tubers 11%.

Cereal grains are a major calorie source for the world's people and account for about 52% of the average intake of calories.[15] The availability and preference for kinds of grain vary from geographical area to area. Asians and Africans obtain 60–75% of their caloric intake from cereals and Latin Americans about 50%. In Mexico corn provides 43% of the total calories. Cereal grain products constitute a significant portion, about 26%, of the daily caloric intake in the U.S. diet.[16] Data from the USDA 1977–78 Nationwide Food Consumption Survey indicated more than 99% of all individuals consumed some grain product.[17] In developing countries 95% of the population consumes cereals as a dietary staple.[15]

Cereal grains are very often the main source of protein, as well as calories, due to the limited consumption of fish, fowl, or meat by low-income groups in developing countries. In general, cereals provide about 47% of the per capita protein intake.[15] It has been reported that bread probably provides 83% of the protein intake in the Middle East; corn 44% in Mexico, and rice 58% in Thailand. Even though the amount of protein in cereal grains is low and the nutritive value of cereal protein is inferior to that of milk, egg, fish and meat products, the protein contribution of the cereal grains is vital for the continuation of human life in many parts of the world.[12,15,18]

Today, cereal grains are favorably perceived in the United States as relatively low in calories, and fat, and high in complex carbohydrates.[19,20] Since the mid-1970s there has been a rise in wheat flour consumption. Rice flour consumption has been increasing since 1960, with a small increase for corn flour and meal. Pasta products, cereal snacks and ready-to-eat breakfast cereals (Table 5.2) have shown dramatic increases in consumption since 1965.[21,22]

MILLING OF CEREAL GRAINS

When humankind began to consume the wheat grain, it was recognized that the interior of the kernel was softer and more pleasant to eat than the outer coverings. In order to get at the inner portion, the endosperm, it was necessary to crack or grind the kernel or grain between two stones and separate the endosperm from the outer layers, the bran and the germ. Stone pounding gave way to the hollow stone hand mills, the earliest recorded about 6700 B.C. followed by the pestle and mortar mill of Egypt about 2000 B.C.[23]

With time, this breaking or grinding action became known as "milling" the grain for the production of flour. Hand milling gave way to progressive adaptations to power from trodding animals, the windmill, the water wheel, the steam, gasoline and diesel engines and finally electricity. Modern milling removes foreign material from the grain, cleans it, adjusts moisture content, breaks up the kernel between rollers, and separates out the bran layers and germ by sifting and air classification. A modern wheat mill may contain 6 or more break rollers, 12 reduction rollers, 16 sifter sections and 8 air classifiers or purifiers.[23]

Cereal grains are dehulled, milled, polished or processed in many ways depending upon the type of grain and separated into fractions some of which are used for feeding animals. The objective of grain processing or milling was to develop products pleasing the eye, the palate and taste buds of humankind. In the past, refined cereal grain and flour products have been associated with wealth and ruling class status. Other reasons for refined cereal products include less phytates, less intestinal irritation, less chewing action, greater digestibility, and better shelf-life. Under present day practices cereal grains are milled to fulfill consumer demands for the production of prepared cereal foods. Milled fractions from grain milling not used in human foods are diverted into formulated animal feeds. In milling the term "percent extraction" is used to denote that percentage of the total whole grain which ends up in the flour.[3]

Wheat in the milling process is converted into flour, (usually 72% extraction) and coarse particles (28%) including the bran and germ. Most of the minerals and vitamins are in these latter parts of the wheat grain (Fig. 5.1 and 5.2). The 72% extraction flour, straight grade usually used for bread, can be further subdivided into patent flour and clear flour for special baking purposes. Patent flour is the purest endosperm portion of the wheat kernel. Farina and semolina are flours in granular form from

TABLE 5.2
U.S. CONSUMPTION OF SOME CEREAL PRODUCTS

	Per Capita Consumption (lb)					
Item	1972	1975	1978	1981	1984	1987
Wheat flour[1]						
White and whole wheat	102.7	107.7	108.5	109.7	111.7	118.3
Durum[2]	7.1	6.8	6.7	6.1	6.4	9.7
Corn products[1]						
Flour and meal	6.2	6.0	5.9	6.2	6.6	6.7
Hominy and grits	1.6	2.7	3.1	2.7	2.8	2.8
Starch	1.9	2.1	2.5	2.2	2.0	2.0
Rice[3]	7.0	7.6	5.7	11.0	8.6	13.4
Pasta products	8.6	9.7	10.3	10.0	11.3	17.1
Breakfast cereals	10.8	12.0	12.8	13.0	14.0	15.2

Source: *Food Consumption, Prices, and Expenditures, 1966–87.* From *National Food Review* (Anon[22]).
[1]Consumption measured at the processing level. Excludes quantities used in alcoholic beverages and fuel.
[2]Semolina and durum flour used in products such as macaroni, spaghetti, and noodles.
[3]Milled basis.

a particular type of wheat.[3,24] Wheat flour or semolina is the major ingredient in biscuits, bread, buns, cakes, chapaties, cookies, crackers, doughnuts, macaroni, muffins, noodles, pancakes, rolls, spaghetti, and waffles. Different flour types are produced which may be treated with chemical agents and/or be made into ready-mixed flours with additives for varied consumer use. Additives, such as maturing agents, bleaching agents and self-rising ingredients are blended frequently into wheat flours at the mill.

Corn is milled both by a wet process, yielding modified starch products, dextrose, syrups, feed products and oil, and by a dry process with separation into hull, germ and endosperm fractions (Fig. 5.3). The endosperm products, grits and meal depending largely on particle size, are for food use. An alternative nondegerming milling process commonly used by small millers simply grinds whole corn grain into meal and grits. Roller milling of barley gives four major products: flour (65% extraction, primarily the endosperm); tailings flour; shorts (mixtures of aleurone, pericarp, some germ and endosperm) and bran (hulls and pericarp). Pot barley (65% extraction) and pearled barley (35% extraction) are manufactured by gradually removing the hull and outer portion of the kernel by abrasive action. Milling of rye is similar to that of wheat. Rye flours (65–70% extraction) and whole rye meal are used in bread production. The use of rye flours adds to the varieties and flavors of breads. Sorghums are milled by a wet or dry process, the latter, an adaptation of wheat milling. By debranning and degerming operations the major products resulting are bran, germ, fines or meal and grits, the latter which can be reduced to a flour. Pearled sorghum is produced by abrasive milling to remove the bran followed by impact degermination. There is limited commercial production of millet flours of different extractions following debranning operations. Oats are dehulled following heating and cooling stages, thus exposing the groat or inner kernel (75% extraction) which, sized and flaked, can be fiber reduced and ground into a white flour.[23,25]

The milling of rice is different from that of the other cereals as the primary objective is not flour but a maximum yield of unbroken milled grains. Milling of the unhulled rice grain, also called paddy or rough rice involves cleaning, removal of the hull, removal of the germ and bran (pericarp and aleurone) layers (Fig. 5.4) and sizing to produce white, uncoated rice, which may be tumbled to add a coating of talc and glucose to improve appearance. Milled or white rice represents 40–76% extraction of rough rice.[5,26]

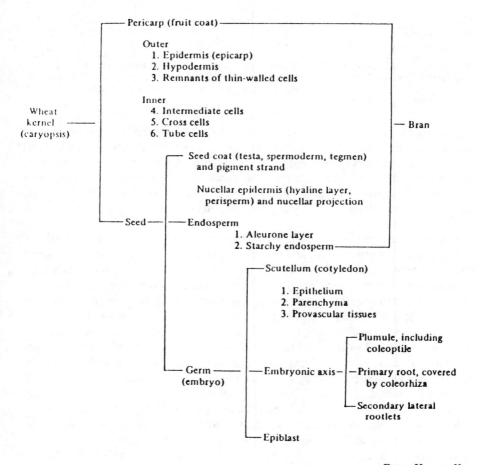

From Hosey[30]

FIG. 5.1. PARTS OF A WHEAT KERNEL

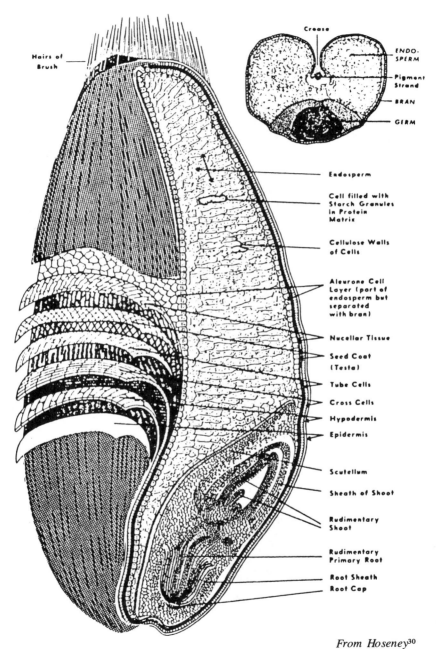

FIG. 5.2. CROSS-SECTIONS OF A WHEAT KERNEL

From Hoseney[30]

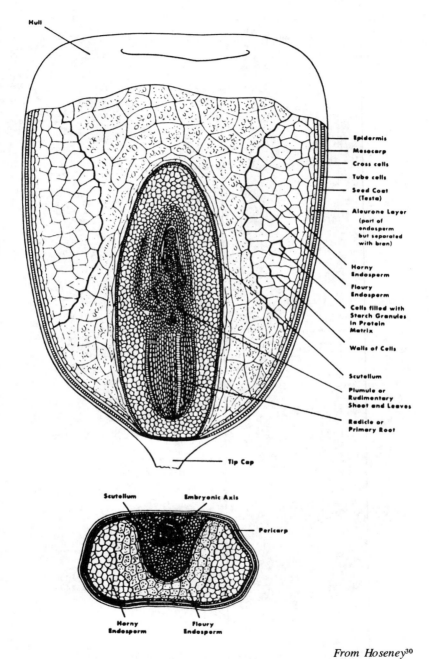

From Hoseney[30]
FIG. 5.3. CROSS-SECTIONS OF A CORN (MAIZE) KERNEL

Loss of Nutrients

The nutrients in any kernel of a given cereal grain have a distribution pattern[3,5,27] among its components, namely endosperm, bran layers, germ, etc. (Fig. 5.1–5.4) and therefore in milling, not only is there a reduction of particle size but also a change in the carbohydrate, fat, fiber, mineral, protein and vitamin content in the milled products. There are losses in nutrient contents of the resulting flour and meals, prepared from the original whole cereal grains.[27–29]

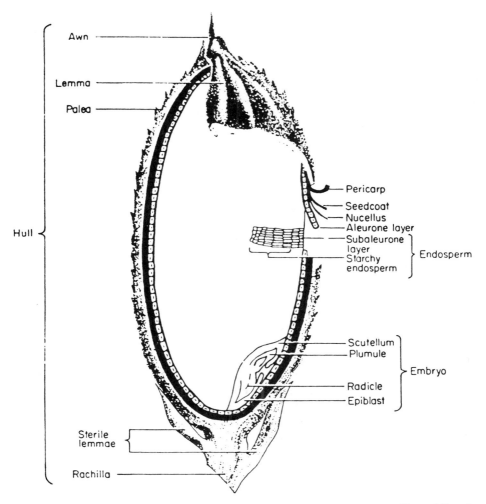

From Juliano[5]

FIG. 5.4. STRUCTURE OF RICE GRAIN

Recent studies of changes (Table 5.3) in nutrient contents were carried out by Peterson and Eggum[31-37] following milling of wheat, rice, corn, barley, sorghum and rye. Hard winter wheat was milled by roller and hammer milling into flours having different extraction rates. Milling of wheat[32] into refined flours resulted in drastic changes in chemical composition: mineral content was reduced by 70%, with similar losses in vitamins and fiber; protein loss approximated 10% with changes in amino acid content. Rough rice was processed[34] by husk removal, abrasive milling, and finally hammer milling to yield products having variable extraction rates. The production of white rice resulted in a marked decrease in the concentration of fat, fiber, ash and certain minerals and vitamins. Yellow corn was processed[35] by dehulling, grinding and sifting, with the resulting dehulled and degermed products. Degerming decreased fat and minerals by about 70% and significantly reduced fiber, lysine and tryptophan content. Barley was milled[33] into flours with different extraction rates. Mineral content was decreased by approximately 60%, with significant decreases in protein and lysine content. Sorghum and rye were also processed by milling[31,36] into flours of variable extraction rates between 100 and 64%. In both instances high mineral losses were again observed in the milled products. On average, with all the above 6 types[37] of cereal grains, 70–80% of the original vitamin content was reduced by the milling operations (Table 5.3). The general relationship between nutrient content and extraction rate for milled wheat taken from Muller and Tobin[23] is depicted as Fig. 5.5.

RATIONALE OF CEREAL-GRAIN NUTRIFICATION

Traditionally, three basic reasons exist for the nutrification of cereal grain products. One is the restoration of nutrients to refined products, these nutrients having been removed by the milling of the whole grain, either at levels originally present or at higher levels judged appropriate under prevailing situations. The second is the use of cereal-grain products as carriers of added nutrients in amounts judged to significantly bolster the dietary intake of specific populations which are at questionable or insufficient levels. The third is a corollary of the second, where nutrification would be widely practiced to provide an economical public measure to insure improved nutritional health for the general population.[38-40]

In the 1974 proposal[16] of the NAS-NRC Food and Nutrition Board, the following criteria were recommended as guides for the selection of a food source as a carrier of supplemental nutrients for the U.S. diet:

(1) The food source should be relatively economical, so as to be within the purchasing power of the majority of the population, and broadly consumed by all groups of the population, particularly by those groups shown to be at the greatest nutritional risk.
(2) The food source should permit fortification at relatively low levels and yet provide a significant level of added nutrients at normal rates of consumption.

(3) The range of consumption of the food source by various segments of the population should be reasonably well defined and not so broad as to provide only insignificant nutritional intake of the added nutrients at the lower range of consumption or to risk excessive intake at the upper range of consumption of any of the added nutrients to the point of potential toxicity.
(4) Uniform distribution of the added nutrients in the carrier should be feasible, and problems introduced through segregation as the food moves through the distribution channel should be minimal.
(5) The food source should not contribute to instability of the nutrients added nor interfere with the utilization of those nutrients.

The addition of micronutrients (amino acids, minerals, vitamins) to processed cereal grain products such as wheat flour possesses considerable merit. Milled cereal products, like wheat flour, are produced in large volume in continuous milling operations. They are relatively inexpensive food staples and are broadly consumed at regular frequencies by most age and income groups nationally and internationally. Micronutrients can be added to cereal grain products without significantly changing their organoleptic, physical or baking properties. The technology for adding micronutrients has been well established as flour mills in Canada, England, United

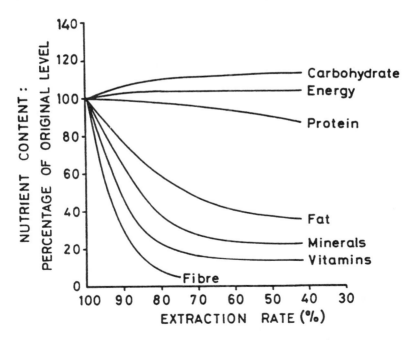

From Muller and Tobin[23]
FIG. 5.5. RELATIONSHIP BETWEEN NUTRIENT CONTENT AND EXTRACTION OF WHEAT FLOUR

TABLE 5.3
INFLUENCE OF MILLING ON NUTRITIVE VALUE OF CEREAL GRAINS

	Wheat				Rice					Corn		
Extraction rate (%)	100	80	75	66	100	82[1]	72[2]	68	64	100[3]	Dehulled[4]	Degermed
Nutrient (%)												
protein (N × 6.25)	14.2	13.4	13.3	12.7	8.6	9.9	9.2	8.8	8.5	9.9	10.1	8.7
starch and sugar	69.9	80.8	82.9	84.0	69.1	85.8	92.5	92.5	92.6	76.0	80.9	89.2
fat	2.7	1.6	1.4	1.1	2.5	3.0	1.2	1.1	1.0	5.2	3.9	1.4
crude fiber	2.4	0.2	0.3	0.2	12.2	0.9	0.1	0.3	0.1	12.8[5]	8.6[5]	4.0[5]
ash	1.8	0.7	0.6	0.5	2.9	1.3	0.6	0.4	0.3	1.4	1.1	0.4
Amino acids (g/16gN)												
cystine	2.1	2.1	2.1	2.2	2.1	2.1	2.1	2.1	2.1	2.2	2.2	2.3
lysine	2.6	2.3	2.2	2.2	3.5	3.5	3.3	3.4	3.3	3.0	2.6	1.9
methionine	1.5	1.5	1.5	1.5	2.3	2.5	2.6	2.5	2.5	2.1	2.2	2.3
tryptophan	1.1	1.1	1.1	1.1	1.2	1.4	1.3	1.3	1.3	0.8	0.7	0.5
threonine	2.6	2.5	2.5	2.5	3.3	3.2	3.2	3.2	3.2	3.5	3.5	3.3
Minerals												
calcium (mg/g)	0.4	0.3	0.3	0.2	0.3	0.1	0.1	0.1	0.1	30.80[6]	14.5[6]	
phosphorus (mg/g)	3.8	1.5	1.3	1.2	3.1	3.2	1.5	1.0	0.9	3.1	2.5	0.8
zinc (ppm)	29.0	12.0	8.0	8.0	24.0	33.0	18.0	17.0	16.0	21.0	17.1	4.4
iron (ppm)	35.0	15.0	13.0	10.0	38.0	8.8	4.1	2.2	2.4	23.3	19.7	10.8
copper (ppm)	4.0	2.4	1.6	1.3	2.8	2.7	2.2	1.9	1.8	1.8	1.4	0.7
Vitamins (μg/g)												
thiamin	5.8	3.4	2.2	1.4	2.8	2.4	1.6	1.0	0.6	4.7	4.4	1.3
riboflavin	1.0	0.5	0.4	0.4	0.5	0.3	0.2	0.2	0.1	0.9	0.7	0.4
niacin	25.2	5.9	5.2	3.4	29.6	29.0	6.0	6.1	3.6	16.2	13.9	9.8
pyridoxine (B₆)	7.5	1.7	1.4	1.3	5.1	5.1	1.9	1.6	1.0	5.4	5.4	1.9
folate	0.6	0.1	0.1	0.1	0.5	0.3	0.1	0.1	0.0	0.3	0.2	0.1
biotin (ηg/g)	116.0	76.0	46.0	25.0	91.0	48.0	43.0	33.0	12.0	73.0	55.0	14.0

	Barley				Sorghum				Rye			
Extraction rate (%)	100	81	75	69	100	80	73	64	100	81	75	68	65
Nutrient (%)													
protein (N × 6.25)	10.8	10.2	9.3	8.9	15.6	16.3	16.3	16.7	11.8	10.4	10.3	9.9	9.6
starch and sugar	67.2	79.8	81.9	84.0	72.9	76.6	79.1	81.5	67.3	72.6	74.9	75.4	74.0
fat	3.3	2.5	1.9	1.7	4.2	2.7	2.2	1.7	2.2	2.0	1.7	1.7	1.2
crude fiber	5.0	1.1	0.9	0.9	2.2	1.6	1.2	0.8	2.2	1.7	1.3	0.9	1.0
ash	2.0	1.2	1.0	0.8	2.0	1.2	1.1	0.9	1.7	1.1	0.9	0.8	0.8
Amino acids (g/16gN)													
cystine	2.1	2.2	2.3	2.2	1.7	1.6	1.6	1.6	2.0	2.2	2.0	2.0	2.1
lysine	3.3	2.9	2.8	2.8	2.0	1.6	1.6	1.3	4.2	3.6	3.8	3.8	3.8
methionine	1.8	1.8	1.7	1.7	1.8	1.8	1.8	1.7	1.6	1.7	1.6	1.6	1.6
tryptophan	1.2	1.2	1.2	1.1	1.0	1.1	1.0	1.0	1.1	1.0	1.0	—	1.0
threonine	3.2	3.2	3.1	3.0	2.9	2.8	2.9	2.8	3.0	3.2	3.0	3.0	3.0
Minerals													
calcium (mg/g)	0.5	0.3	0.3	0.2	0.5	0.4	0.5	0.6	0.4	0.3	0.2	0.2	0.2
phosphorus (mg/g)	3.6	2.6	1.9	1.6	4.0	2.4	1.9	1.5	3.7	2.0	1.7	1.5	1.5
zinc (ppm)	21.0	15.0	11.0	10.0	36.0	21.0	16.0	10.0	33.0	20.0	19.0	15.0	14.0
iron (ppm)	66.0	21.0	16.0	11.0	179.0	83.0	76.0	54.0	41.0	26.0	22.0	20.0	20.0
copper (ppm)	3.8	2.9	2.4	2.4	4.9	5.3	2.8	2.4	4.1	2.9	2.6	2.2	2.2
Vitamins (μg/g)													
thiamine	5.6	1.9	1.0	0.9	4.4	2.0	1.1	0.9	4.2	2.1	1.1	—	0.6
riboflavin	1.0	0.5	0.3	0.3	0.7	0.5	0.4	0.3	1.4	1.1	1.0	—	0.8
niacin	44.6	33.3	21.5	14.4	28.7	29.8	15.3	5.9	8.3	6.3	6.2	—	5.6
pyridoxine	5.3	1.6	1.0	0.8	7.3	3.5	3.0	1.5	3.9	2.2	1.2	—	1.0
folate	0.7	0.5	0.3	0.3	0.3	0.2	0.2	0.1	0.7	0.5	0.3	—	0.1
biotin (ηg/g)	205.0	137.0	112.0	46.0	333.0	125.0	107.0	92.0	145.0	101.0	84.0	—	45.0

Source: Adapted from Pederson and Eggum.[31–37]
[1]Brown rice, [2]milled rice, [3]whole corn, [4]500–1000μ meal, [5]ADF + NDF, [6]ppm.

States and elsewhere have included some type of nutrification practice over many years.

HISTORY OF ENRICHMENT IN THE UNITED STATES, TYPE 4*

Flour and Bread

Attempts had been made in the early 1930s to restore nutrients removed in the processing of cereal grains, but without much success. Manufacturers of processed foods did not have available the economical, pure vitamins from chemical syntheses. When natural products, such as wheat germ, wheat bran, rice polishings, yeast products, etc., were employed as additives in early nutrification efforts, they produced changes in the characteristics of the modified food product. In the mid-1930s to early 1940s a succession of events took place which hastened the cereal grain nutrification movement.[40-43]

In 1936 the AMA Committee on Foods issued a policy statement about enhanced amounts of vitamins in the general food supply. The same year large quantities of pure thiamin were produced by chemical synthesis. Niacin, already available in pure form as a result of chemical synthesis, was identified as the antipellagra factor in 1937. Although riboflavin was synthesized in 1935, unlimited commercial quantities were not produced until several years later. The addition of these pure nutrients to food, such as to white flour without changing the color and flavor of bread, was welcomed, as nutritional improvement became possible without adverse effects on consumer acceptability. In 1938 the AMA joint committees of the Council of Food & Nutrition and Council on Pharmacy & Chemistry reported favorably on the nutrification of certain staple foods with either vitamins or minerals. The following year the Council on Food and Nutrition, as a result of a report prepared by one of its members (Dr. G. Cowgill), adopted a resolution (with qualifications) encouraging the restorative addition of vitamins, minerals and other dietary essentials. An active discussion on food nutrification took place at the 1939 meeting[44] of the American Institute of Nutrition lead by Drs. Morgan, Nelson, Roberts, Sebrell and Taylor. Other significant events were dietary surveys, particularly the 1939 Stiebling-Phipard survey[45] revealing inadequate intakes of certain nutrients by large segments of the U.S. population. Another event was the decision of intent of the British government in 1940 to nutrify flour and bread with thiamin. An NRC subcommittee decision to recommend thiamin nutrification of all white flour purchased by the U.S. Army and Navy and the Food & Drug Administration scheduling of a public hearing to consider a standard for enriched flour also happened in 1940. Personnel from the U.S. Dept. of Public Health Service, the U.S. Dept. of Agriculture, the American

---

*Four nutrient additions: thiamin, riboflavin, niacin and iron.

Medical Association and the National Research Council, including Drs. Wilder, Sebrell, Jolliffe and Williams, testified at the hearing and wanted some action on the addition of nutrients. Following the hearing the NRC Food & Nutrition Board at its first meeting favored the addition of thiamin, riboflavin, niacin and iron to flour.

Actually, nutrification of bread with vitamins was started about 1938 and was in practice before enrichment was officially sanctioned 3 years later. It was made possible in this time period by the addition of a specific yeast to the bread dough. The thiamin content in this yeast had been previously increased by providing the yeast with the component parts of the thiamin molecule, thus stimulating thiamin synthesis. This preliminary practice helped to prepare the baking industry for enrichment when adopted. Around the time of the 1940 Washington flour hearings, the national associations of the millers and bakers held meetings to which physicians and scientists (Drs. Boudreau, Nelson, Roberts, Sebrell, Spies, Stanley, Tisdall and Wilder) were invited to participate. This helped to clarify the objectives of industry, government and scientists in adding nutrients to staple foods such as flour, the major ingredient of bread.

As a results of the FDA hearings, a Standard of Identity for Enriched Flour[46] was established (which became effective January 1, 1942). At the time of the Washington National Nutrition Conference for Defense in May 1941 arranged by the NRC Food and Nutrition Board, flour enrichment was officially launched. Even though there were no standards issued in 1941 for enriched bread, an understanding was reached among the FDA, the NRC and the American Bakers' Association regarding bread, so bread enrichment could be initiated also in May 1941. The War Food Administration issued an order requiring the enrichment of all white bread in 1942; white rolls were added in 1944. In 1943, the standards were amended; calcium and vitamin D were optional ingredients. The term "enriched" was adopted. Proposed standards for enriched bread were also developed in 1943 as a result of further hearings.

With the 1941 launching, the enrichment movement[40] had (1) evidence of need, (2) sponsorship by authoritative bodies, (3) a legal instrument that set established levels and types of nutrients and (4) informed, cooperative industries to put enrichment into practice. In 1973, the FDA proposed revisions of the standard of identity for white flour in which optional vitamin D was deleted, calcium continued optional, and other nutrient levels adjusted from previous ranges to single level values.

The 1942 War Food Administration Order was repealed in October 1946 before the FDA Enriched Bread Standard was issued. In the meantime action had been taken by some states. South Carolina enacted the first flour and bread enrichment law[47] in 1942 as a result of the diligent efforts of Dr. Lease and by 1950, 26 states, Hawaii and Puerto Rico had passed legislation patterned after the levels proposed in the FDA standards.[43] As from the beginning, the baking and milling industries remained supportive in the increasing production of enriched white bread and enriched white flour.

Corn Products

The eating of corn as a major energy food source tends to produce pellagra, as noted in the past in southern United States, unless the diet is rich in other sources of niacin and/or tryptophan or the corn was processed with lime water. In the South, corn is consumed as meal and grits, either from whole, dehulled or degerminated corn. In 1943, the NRC Food and Nutrition Board recommended enrichment standards for corn products. South Carolina enacted the first corn product mandatory state law in 1943 guided again by Lease[48] and the State Nutrition Committee, requiring the enrichment of degerminated corn meal and grits with thiamin, riboflavin, niacin and iron. Later, the South Carolina law was extended to cover whole corn products. Four other southern states, North Carolina, Alabama, Mississippi, and Georgia, enacted similar laws between 1943 and 1948. The federal Standard of Identity for Enriched Corn Meals and Grits for interstate commerce was promulgated in 1955.

Rice

Rice is not a major food for most of the people in the United States, but it is eaten in substantial quantities in some localized areas.[26] South Carolina took the lead again[49] by enacting a law in 1956 permitting enrichment and prohibiting the sale of ordinary white rice. Two types of rice enrichment are involved, (1) packaged enriched rice not requiring water rinsing prior to cooking and (2) bulk enriched rice, usually water rinsed by the consumer, the latter thereby requiring enrichment with rinse resistant nutrients. Both types of enriched rice products require appropriate labeling. In 1958 the FDA Standards of Identity for Enriched Rice were issued for nonrinse and rinse products. The standards for rice are similar to those for flour, except in the case of white rice the requirement for riboflavin is optional. Among countries enriching rice are Columbia, Dominican Republic, Japan and the Philippines.

Pasta

The origin of pasta foods prepared from coarsely ground wheat endosperm (semolina, farina), flour and water is unknown but goes back to prehistoric times, probably at some early stage of domestic wheat production. Pasta is made from durum and other hard wheats and comes in hundreds of different shapes and sizes.[50,51] Pasta was consumed by the ancient Chinese, Greeks and Romans. Commercial pasta production in the U.S.A. began in the mid-19th century, and pasta consumption has continued to grow until it now approximates 15 lb per capita per year. It is consumed in large amounts in Argentina, Chile, Greece, Italy, Libya, Spain, Switzerland, Tunisia and Venezuela. The present day appeal of pasta is its attractive appearance, economy, convenience of preparation, adaptability in recipes and wide acceptance by many age groups. FDA Standards of Identity for Enriched Pasta were issued in 1946 with required levels of thiamin, riboflavin, niacin and iron and optional addition of calcium.

On the basis of what homemakers reported in the 1965 USDA Food Consumption Survey, nearly all white flour and bread (98%) was enriched. Most of the corn meal and grits (93%), macaroni products (94%), and rice (86%) were also reported enriched. Unenriched products that families purchased were other baked goods, such as commercially prepared crackers, rolls, muffins, biscuits, cakes, cookies, coffeecake and doughnuts. Only 30% of these products were reported as enriched by 1965.

RTE Cereals

Ready-to-eat (RTE) cereals, also known as dry breakfast cereals, are processed cereal-grain products comprised of either flaked, gun-puffed, oven-puffed, extruded, shredded, extruded-shredded cereal grains, or in granola form, and related products made from wheat, corn, rice, oats and other grains or mixtures thereof.[52] They are precooked and dried or toasted and are usually consumed with fluid milk. Ready-to-cook or quick-cooking cereals are another form of convenient breakfast foods. In the case of breakfast cereals, there is only one for which a Standard of Identity exists, namely, farina, a granular wheat endosperm product cooked and served hot. Farina supplemented with thiamin, riboflavin, niacin and iron at appropriate levels is listed in the Standards of Identity as Enriched Farina. Farina in dry form is enriched with the same type of premix and in a similar manner as wheat flour.

RTE cereals, were nutrified initially, about 1941, on a basis of restoring nutrient content lost during processing. In 1955, the concept was changed to one providing added nutrients on the basis of a percentage of the daily recommended allowance per serving.[53,54] In 1969, 16% of RTE cereals were nutrified; in 1973, 85%; and in 1979, 92%. A widely used current addition is 25% of the USRDA for thiamin, riboflavin, niacin, pyridoxine, folate, ascorbic acid and vitamin A and at times 10 or 25% for iron per one ounce. With the more popular addition of calcium to foods, some cereals provide up to 20% of the USRDA for calcium; also a few have added vitamin D. RTE cereals consumption has increased greatly over the past 20 years to the 1985 level of 10.6 lb per person annually in the United States. Ready-to-cook cereals consumption figures for 1985 are 3.1 lb per person annually.[52] A breakdown of the breakfast cereals[55] for 1984 is shown as Fig. 5.6.

According to Zabik[56] persons of all ages consuming RTE cereals at breakfast had higher intakes of vitamins and minerals frequently inadequate in the American diet than did nonRTE cereal eaters or breakfast skippers; also reported was the observation that these same individuals (age 5–62+ years) had greater average intake of fiber, complex carbohydrates and lower level of cholesterol and/or percentage of energy from fat.

PL 480 Food for Peace

U.S. Public Law 480 was enacted[57] in 1954 and has been amended since to expand international trade, to develop export markets for U.S. agricultural commodities, to combat malnutrition and hunger in developing countries and to encourage their economic development. Under this Act, food is donated abroad; some is also marketed abroad. In 1966, amendments made possible the nutritional improvement of the shipped cereal-grain products, leading to the development of low-cost nutrified foods to overcome dietary deficiencies in developing countries. Vitamin A and D nutrified nonfat dry milk, and a number of products such as protein fortified wheat flour with added vitamin A, calcium, thiamin, riboflavin, niacin and iron, CSM, a mixture of cornmeal, defatted soy flour, nonfat dry milk, soy oil, vitamins and minerals and WSB, a similar formulated product based on wheat flour are some of the products.

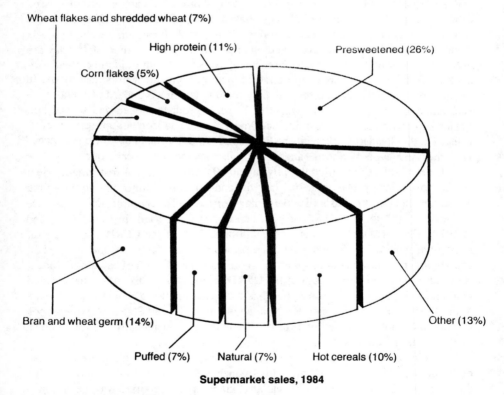

¹Includes cold oats, combination packs of individual servings, and others.
Source: *Progressive Grocer*.

From Bunch and Wendland[55]

FIG. 5.6. BREAKDOWN OF BREAKFAST CEREALS SALES FOR 1984

TABLE 5.4
NUTRIFICATION OF WHEAT FLOUR[1] (mg/kg)

Country	Vitamin B₁ Min.	Vitamin B₁ Max.	Vitamin B₂ Min.	Vitamin B₂ Max.	Niacin Min.	Niacin Max.	Iron Min.	Iron Max.	Calcium Min.	Calcium Max.
Australia	1.5	—	2.2	—	15	—	14	—	1,000	—
Canada[2]	4.4	7.7	2.7	4.8	35	64	29	43	1,100	1,400
Chile	4.3	—	1.3	—	13	—	30	—	—	—
Congo	4	6	2.5	3.5	32	45	26	35	1,000	1,500
Costa Rica	4.4	5.5	2.6	3.3	35	44	28	36	1,100	1,400
Denmark	5	—	5	—	—	—	30	—	2,000	—
Dominican Republic	4.4	5.5	2.6	3.3	35	44	29	38	1,100	1,400
Guatemala	4.4	—	2.6	—	35	—	29	—	1,700	—
Guyana	4.4	5.5	2.7	3.3	35	44	29	36	1,100	1,400
Israel	—	—	2.5	—	—	—	—	—	—	—
Japan	5	8	3	5	—	—	—	—	1,500	3,000
Kenya	4.5	5.5	2.7	3.3	35	44	29	36	—	—
Mexico	4.4	8.8	2.6	5.2	35	70	29	57	—	—
Nigeria	5	—	3.5	—	50	—	35	—	—	—
Panama	4.4	—	2.6	—	35	—	29	—	1,100	—
Peru	4	—	4	—	30	—	20	—	1,000	—
Philippines	4.4	5.5	2.6	3.3	35	44	29	36	1,100	1,400
Portugal	4.4	5.5	2.6	3.3	35	44	28	36	—	—
Puerto Rico	4.4	5.5	2.6	3.3	35	44	28	36	1,100	—
Sweden	4	8	1.5	3	40	80	65	90	—	—
Switzerland	4.4	—	2	—	50	—	29	—	—	—
United Kingdom	2.4	—	—	—	16	—	16.5	—	940	1,560
USA	6.4	—	4	—	55	—	44	—	2,120	—
USSR	2	4	4	—	10	30	—	—	—	—
West Indies	4.4	5.5	2.6	3.3	35	44	28	36	1,100	1,400

Source: Bauernfeind.[62]

Note: This table of values taken from the literature serves as a guide. Up-to-date values need to be confirmed with the regulatory agency of the specific country.
[1] Specifications exist in some countries for other cereal-grain products such as white rice, maize meal, corn grits, pasta products, and breakfast cereals.
[2] Other nutrients permitted are vitamin B_6, 2.5–3.1; folic acid, 0.4–0.5; d-pantothenic acid, 11–13; and magnesium, 1,500–1,900 mg/kg.

Guidelines were developed for the amino acid, vitamin and mineral content of the formulated cereal grain products.[58] See Chapter 6.

Other countries

Flour nutrification was begun in the United Kingdom a year earlier than in the United States. In July 1940, the government adopted the policy of adding thiamin to the 72% extraction flour then in general use at a level of 0.2 mg/100 g (0.91 mg/lb). By March 1942 about 38% of the flour consumed was so nutrified. In 1942, however, supplies of imported wheat were threatened due to the war, and it was decided to raise the extraction rate to 85% to make more flour available for human consumption; thiamin addition then was discontinued. In 1953, the demand for white flour had reached the point where the government permitted both the 80–85% extraction flour and 72% extraction flour, the latter to be nutrified per 100 g with 0.24 mg thiamin (1.09 mg/lb), 1.6 mg niacin (7.25 mg/lb), 1.65 mg iron (7.5 mg lb).[43]

Canada introduced enrichment of white flour in 1953 after considerable discussion and controversy and initially set enrichment levels to be almost identical with those of the United States. Currently, an expanded enrichment program is operational. Enrichment is not compulsory in Canada, except since 1944 in the province of Newfoundland, but is widely carried out. In Chile, mandatory enrichment of white flour according to American standards was initiated in 1954, and various Central American countries, including Costa Rica, El Salvador, Guatemala, Honduras, and Nicaragua and Panama require enrichment. Enrichment of white flour became compulsory in Denmark in 1953 and is widely practiced on a voluntary basis in Sweden. In Germany, Holland, Belgium, Spain and Switzerland enrichment of flour is voluntary. In Japan, flour supplied through the national school lunch program is enriched with thiamin and other nutrients, and "special enriched" wheat products are sold under standards prescribed by the Ministry of Health and Welfare.[43,59–61] Table 5.4 may be consulted for some summarized information.[62]

HISTORY OF ENRICHMENT, TYPE 10*

Cereal Grain Products

The Food and Nutrition Board of the NRC-NAS in 1974 issued a new proposed policy[16] for nutrification of cereal grain products, such as flour, on the basis of information reviewed as evidence of potential risk of deficiency[16] of vitamin A, thiamin, riboflavin, niacin, pyridoxine, folate, iron, calcium, magnesium, and zinc among

---

*Ten nutrient additions: thiamin, riboflavin, niacin, iron, pyridoxine, folate, vitamin A, calcium, magnesium and zinc.

TABLE 5.5
NUTRIFICATION COMPARISONS FOR U.S. FLOUR AND BREAD

Nutrients[1]	Presently Used[2]		Proposed[3]	
	In Flour	In Bread[4]	In Flour	In Bread
Thiamin	2.9	1.8	2.9	1.8
Riboflavin	1.8	1.1	1.8	1.1
Niacin	24.0	15.0	24.0	15.0
Iron	13.0–16.5	8.0–12.5	40.0[5]	—
Calcium	960[8]	600[8]	900	562
Vitamin A[6]	None	None	1.3 (4300 IU)[7]	0.8 (2700 IU)
Pyridoxine	None	None	2.0	1.2
Folic Acid	None	None	0.3	0.18
Magnesium	None	None	200.0	125.0
Zinc	None	None	10.0	6.2

Source: Emodi and Scialpi.[63]
[1]Expressed as mg/lb of flour.
[2]Minimums and maximums in Code of Federal Regulations, Title 21, Parts 136–137.
[3]NAS/NRC (1974).
[4]Bread is considered to contain 62.5% wheat flour based on the conversions of 100 lb of flour to 160 lb of bread.
[5]November 18, 1977, the FDA restored the provision for 13.0–16.5 mg/lb.
[6]Retinol equivalent.
[7]The originally proposed level of 2.2 retinol equivalents (7300 IU) was lowered to 1.3 retinol equivalents (4300 IU).
[8]Optional.

significant segments of the U.S. population. Micronutrient nutrification was proposed with 6 added vitamins and 4 minerals to cereal grain products. Since cereal-grain products adequately meet the criteria for carriers of added nutrients, it was proposed that the 10 nutrients be added to all cereal grain products, wherever technically feasible (Table 5.5), as a means of supplementing dietary intake.[16,63] In the study of the 10 nutrient addition proposal, the report recognized the need to examine (1) dispersion uniformity and segregation potential of added nutrients, (2) stability over normal processing and distribution practice, (3) influence of the enriched products on consumer acceptance, (4) availability of added nutrients and (5) related matters peculiar to specific products.

With the cooperation of the milling and baking industries, an Inter-Industry Committee was formed to acquire data which would determine possible implementation of the NRC proposal. The 5 point investigative program included: (1) a baseline nutrient study of nonenriched flours; (2) effects of nutrient forms on processing and organoleptic properties; (3) stability of added nutrients during processing; (4) bioavailability of added nutrients in products; and (5) interaction effects among nutrients. Because the recommended nutrient levels are intended to be total levels for the enriched products, the natural content of the cereal product had to be determined. With new, added nutrients on which there were little or no previous data, there was a need to select and test compatible nutrient forms. By 1976 the baseline studies[64] were underway, and some added mineral and vitamin studies had been completed relating to stability, bioavailability and baking properties.

In 1977, a workshop[65] on technology of nutrification of cereal grain products was held where further progress was reported. It began to appear technically feasible to fortify cereal-grain products with the vitamins at the levels recommended in the proposed NRC-FNB fortification policy with a few exceptions. Further studies on added vitamin A to corn grits were suggested. Iron addition was not regarded as troublesome if appropriate iron compounds with specifications were chosen for specific grain products. Added zinc did not appear to be troublesome. Further studies were suggested on the additions of calcium and magnesium. Various members of the Inter-Industry Committee agreed to continue the project.[65]

Early in 1979, the Inter-Industry Committee completed its review and released its conclusions and recommendations.[66] The review covered information from laboratory, pilot plant and limited production trials recognizing that extensive full-scale commercial production is the final test. The conclusions of the committee are shown in tabular form (Table 5.6). Additions to wheat flours appear technically feasible. With corn grits and meal, two exceptions were mentioned, a 20% overage for vitamin A addition and for grits, calcium addition should be limited to 300 mg/lb. Additions to rice appear feasible with riboflavin continued as an optional ingredient and ferric orthophosphate used as the iron source. Added calcium and magnesium may not be feasible with current rice grit enrichment practices. It was technically feasible to add the recommended nutrients to bread-type products, if the nutrients already inherent in flour are counted. With cakes, cookies and crackers, nutrient addition appears feasible as long as proper overages are used to compensate for losses during baking and storage. It seemed technically feasible to add all nutrients to pasta except for calcium and magnesium because of insufficient data accumulated at that time period to make a judgment. The committee urged continued evaluation studies.

Another workshop[67] on nutrification was held in 1982 sponsored by the AACC Council on Fortification for the purpose of forming a basis for the development of policies regarding the appropriate addition of nutrients to grain-based foods. There continues to be a strong basis for considering cereal grain products as carriers for added nutrients. While there may be some minor technical problems with individual products in meeting the NRC-FNB 1974 recommendation, in general, it appeared feasible to carry out those recommendations.[67,68] The cereal grain product industry continues as a positive force in providing nutrient intervention strategies, either nationally or internationally. Currently, Enrichment Type 10 still remains in a proposal status in the United States.

CEREAL GRAIN PRODUCT ENRICHMENT STATUS

In 1941, Type 4 enrichment of white flour and bread with 4 nutrients, thiamin, riboflavin, niacin and iron was approved and put into commercial practice with calcium permitted later as an optional ingredient. No additional nutrients for U.S. enriched cereal-grain products have been approved, except vitamin A for some export products (Table 5.7). Meantime, criticism continues on the nutritional inadequacies of milled cereal grain products.

Jansen[69] has declared the 1941 flour enrichment formula greatly outdated and needing revision. The enrichment formula[70] is based on the average diet which people were eating in the 1940 period. It should be determined whether other nutrients should be added to improve the health of the population through better nutrition. Davis[71] recognized refined wheat products to contain significant amounts of protein and energy supplying carbohydrates, but except for the 4 added nutrients (enrichment Type 4) there is a loss of 70-80% of some 20 or more nutrients in the milling of wheat into white flour. He continued to favor consumption of whole grain food products over enriched products because of inadequate nutrient additions. Ranum et al.[61] have tabulated 20 or more nutrients consumed directly by humans which have been reduced by milling whole wheat into flour (Table 5.8) with current extraction rates. The drop of nutrient values in flour ranges from 25-90%. Thus, according to the nutrient restorative concept of the nutrification process, there is a considerable improvement yet to be made in processed cereal grain products such as white flour.

In 1980, Ranum et al.[72] analyzed 95 samples of commercially milled flours collected in 30 different countries with information on extraction rates, flour type, etc. A nutrient score scheme was worked out, reflecting the composition and density of wheat nutrients in flour. Only 11 samples from 9 different countries were nutrified with vitamins and minerals to varying degrees. The investigators concluded that the nutritional quality of a large proportion of flour produced throughout the world is low.

In the United States, white flour and bread enrichment (Type 4) is widely practiced. Bread enrichment properly carried out on a commercial scale in the United States produces quite a uniform loaf as indicated by bread analyses. Kulp et al.[73] analyzed 255 samples of wrapped, sliced, white bread labeled as enriched for thiamin, riboflavin, niacin, calcium, and iron as well as moisture, ash, and lactose (as an indication of milk content). The results for these enriched breads purchased on the open market from 52 cities in 39 states and the District of Columbia were that these breads exceeded the minimum nutrient contents required by federal enrichment standards by 8% for thiamin, 19% for riboflavin, 11% for niacin, and 13% for iron.

In April 1983, the FDA first agreed to permit bakers[74] to market, under the provision of an approved temporary marketing permit, bread nutrified along the lines of the 1974 NRC recommendation (Type 10). Each baker was required to secure a temporary market permit; nutrify the bread to meet the nutrient content of 2700

TABLE 5.6
SUMMARY CHART
TECHNICAL FEASIBILITY OF FORTIFYING CEREAL-GRAIN BASED PRODUCTS AS RECOMMENDED

	Vitamin A	Thiamin	Riboflavin	Niacin	Vitamin B$_6$	Folic Acid	Iron (1)	Calcium	Magnesium	Zinc	
Flour Extended Shelf-Life	A	A	A	A	B	B	A	A	B	B	Consumer acceptance problems indicated from preliminary results of extended storage studies at elevated temperatures and humidities.
Industrial (short shelf-life)	A	A	A	A	A	A	A	A	A	A	
Farina	A	A	A	A	A	A	A	A	A	A	Consumer acceptance problems Indicated from preliminary results of extended storage studies at elevated temperatures and humidities.
Corn Flour	A	A	A	A	A	A	A	A	A	A	
Meal	A	A	A	A	A	A	A	A	A	A	
Grits	A	A	A	A	A	A	A	C	A	A	Calcium addition should be no more than 300 mg/lb.
Rice	A	A		A	A	A	A	C	C	A	Addition of riboflavin may cause consumer acceptance problems. Ferric orthophosphate recommended as iron source. Calcium and magnesium addition might be possible by change in enrichment process to use of "synthetic kernel" technique.

CEREAL GRAIN PRODUCTS 167

										Comments
Bread	A	A	A	A	A	A	A	A	A	Nutrient additions adjusted for level of nutrients inherent in flour.
Soft Sweet Goods Cakes	A	A	A	A	A	A	A	A	A	
All Others	D	D	D	D	D	D	D	D	D	Would appear to be technically feasible based on results obtained on bread cake. Confirmation through testing suggested.
Cookies & Crackers	A	A	A	A	A	A	A	A	A	Iron used at 40 mg/lb.
Pasta	A	A	A	A	A	B	B	A	A	Iron used at 40 mg/lb.
Refrigerated Doughs	A	A	A	D	D	D	D	D	D	
Frozen Products Unbaked	D	A	D	D	A	A	D	D	D	
Baked	D	A	A	A	A	A	D	D	D	
Prepared Mixes	D	A	A	A	A	D	D	D	D	

1. Key:
    A = appears to be technically feasible
    B = insufficient data to evaluate technical feasibility
    C = not technically feasible at present time
    D = no data submitted for committee review

(1) Based on level of 16.5 mg/lb rather than NAS proposal of 40 mg/lb.

Source: Vetter.[66]

TABLE 5.7
U.S. CEREAL ENRICHMENT STANDARDS

This table shows the final nutrient levels required for enriched cereal products as specified by the U.S. Food and Drug Administration and the USDA Agriculture Stabilization and Conservation Service (ASCS). All figures are in milligrams per pound of product except for Vitamin A which is in International Units (IU) per pound. When two figures are shown it indicates a minimum-maximum range. Where one number is shown it indicates the minimum level with overages left to good manufacturing practice. Standards in parentheses are optional.

PRODUCT	THIAMIN	RIBO-FLAVIN	NIACIN	IRON	CALCIUM	VITAMIN A
ENRICHED FLOUR	2.9	1.8	24	20	(960)②	
ENRICHED SELF-RISING FLOUR	2.9	1.8	24	20	960	
ENRICHED FARINA	2.0-2.5	1.2-1.5	16-20	13	(500)②	
ASCS DOMESTIC WHEAT FLOUR	2.9	1.8	24	20		
ASCS EXPORT WHEAT FLOUR	2.9	1.8	24	20	500-625	4000-6000
ASCS SOY FORTIFIED FLOUR	2.9	1.8	24	20	500-625	4000-6000
ENRICHED CORN MEAL and GRITS	2.0-3.0	1.2-1.8	16-24	13-26	(500-750)②	
ENRICHED SELF-RISING CORN MEAL	2.0-3.0	1.2-1.8	16-24	13-26	(500-1750)②	

CEREAL GRAIN PRODUCTS

Product						
ASCS DOMESTIC CORN MEAL	2.0-3.0	1.2-1.8	16-24	13-26		
ASCS DOMESTIC CORN GRITS	2.0-3.0	1.2-1.8	16-24	21-26		
ASCS CORN MASA FLOUR	2.0	1.2	16	13-26		
ASCS EXPORT CORN MEAL and SOY FORTIFIED CORN MEAL	2.0-3.0	1.2-1.8	16-24	13-26	500-750	4000-6000
ENRICHED RICE	2.0-4.0	1.2-2.4①	16-32	13-26	(500-1000)②	
ENRICHED MACARONI and NOODLE PRODUCTS③	4.0-5.0	1.7-2.2	27-34	13.0-16.5	(500-625)②	
ENRICHED BREAD④	1.8	1.1	15	12.5	(600)②	
US RDA (mg or IU per day)	1.5	1.7	20	18	1000	5000

Compliance with the appropriate standards is required: 1) For any ASCS commodity, 2) If any enrichment is used, 3) If the product is labeled or advertised as being "enriched" or containing enriched flour, 4) If the product is sold in States having mandatory enrichment laws. States requiring enrichment of FLOUR and BREAD are: AL, AK, AZ, AR, CA, CO (bread only), CN, FL, GA, HI, ID, IN, KS, KY, LA, ME, MA, MS, MT, NE, NH, NJ, NM, NY, ND, OH, OK, OR, PR, RI, SC, TX, WA, WV, WY; CORN: AL, AK, CA, CT, FL, GA, MS, NY, SC, TX; RICE: AZ, CA, CT, FL, NY, PR, SC; PASTA: AZ, CA, FL, NY, OR, WA, CT (excludes noodles); FARINA: AZ, CA, FL, NY. States with the "25%" rule are AZ, CA, SC, UT. This rule requires that all fabricated foods containing 25% or more of a cereal product ingredient for which a standard of enrichment exists must be made with the enriched form of that product or have the equivalent nutrients added. UT permits the sale of unenriched forms providing they are labeled "unenriched".

①The riboflavin standard for rice has been stayed for many years.

②No claim of calcium enrichment can be made when calcium is present for technological reasons at levels less than the minimum value shown except as required by nutritional labeling (21 CFR 101.9).

③Enriched pasta products are normally made from semolina, durum flour, or wheat flour enriched to these same levels. There are, however, no official standards for enriched cereals used in pasta production.

④Bread containing 62% or more of flour enriched to the standards for enriched flour will meet the standards for enriched bread.

Bread can be additionally fortified to meet the standards proposed by the Food and Nutrition Board of the National Academy of Sciences. In addition to the above, the flour would contain, in mg/lb: 0.3 folic acid, 2.0 pyridoxine, 900 calcium, 200 magnesium, 10 zinc, and 5000 IU/lb. vitamin A. Such bread is to be labeled "Special formula enriched bread."

The above is a condensation of regulations in effect as of JULY 1983.

Used with permission of Pennwalt Corp.

TABLE 5.8
NUTRIENT DENSITY OF MILLED WHEAT FLOUR VERSUS WHOLE WHEAT GRAIN

	Percentage of dietary requirement (USRDA) provided by 2000 calories of the food.		
Nutrient	Whole wheat	Flour	% Drop
Protein	120	90	25
Thiamin	200	50	75
Riboflavin	40	15	65
Niacin	130	30	75
Pyridoxine	100	20	80
Folic Acid	60	15	75
Pantothenic Acid	60	30	50
Biotin	20	5	75
Vitamin E	70	20	70
Ca	20	10	50
Cu	150	30	80
Fe	100	30	70
K	100	20	80
Mg	210	35	85
Mn	460	40	90
P	210	50	75
Zn	120	20	85
Fiber			85
Linoleic Acid			50
Choline			50
Cr			70
F			70
Mo			50
Se			25

Source: Ranum et al.[61]

IU of vitamin A, 1.8 mg of thiamin, 1.1 mg of riboflavin, 1.2 mg of pyridoxine, 15 mg of niacin, 0.19 mg of folate, 6.2 mg of zinc, 12.5 mg of iron, 125 mg of magnesium and 600 mg of calcium per 1-lb loaf; label and market the bread as Enriched Special Formula Bread; and on the bread wrapper compare the composition of Enriched Special Formula Bread contents with enriched bread (Type 4) contents. This special marketing opportunity for improvement of white bread was rescinded January 1988 by the FDA. The nutrient contribution[20] of enrichment Type 10 versus Type 4 for white bread is compared graphically as Fig. 5.7.

In the 1970s and 1980s, several breads were publicized as providing greater nutrient additions to bread than provided by Type 4 enrichment. One developed by International Food Technology[75] provided supplementary quality protein and 15–45% of the USRDA for 20 nutrients in 6 oz of bread. Whole White Bread[76] originated as a U.S. patent by Multimarques, Inc. with nutrient additives claimed to produce bread to more closely match whole wheat bread nutritionally, yet retain a creamy white color and texture of white bread. Marketed Enriched Special Formula Bread (Type 10) was described in several trade publications.[74,77,78] Current expanded Canadian enrichment levels, the proposed expanded U.S. enrichment levels (Type 10) are contrasted with the current standard U.S. enrichment levels (Type 4) for white bread in Table 5.9.

Improved white breads such as those with 10 or more added nutrients can be commercially produced and marketed successfully. At a 1982 hearing[79] before the subcommittee on Natural Resources, Agricultural Research and Environment of the Committee on Science and Technology, U.S. House of Representative 97th Congress, Second Session, Scheuer, White and Sensenbrenner examined the fortification of cereal grains as one economical method of ensuring nutritional adequacy of food and thus favorably contributing to preventive health programs. Personnel from the third largest baker in the country, operating border to border and coast to coast, told the subcommittee of their difficulties since 1978 in marketing a superior white loaf of bread developed with the assistance of Kansas State University and the American Bakers Association, as improved product which met the 1974 NRC 10 nutrient addition recommendations. No problems were encountered in marketing until 1981 when FDA objected to the labeling of the bread, declaring it was outside the standard of identity for enriched bread which should only have 4 nutrients added. The 10 nutrient added bread was sold for the same price as the 4 nutrient added bread. There was no difference in taste. The 10 nutrient added bread could not be labeled Enriched White Bread; it could, however, be called Enriched White Loaf. This experience is illustrative of the limitations of standards of identity for food products which are not easily changed to meet new technological and nutritional advances. The U.S. cereal-grain enrichment policy set in 1941, nearly 50 years ago needs to be reviewed, updated with the objective of providing superior enriched products for consumers in both developed and developing countries.

NUTRIFICATION PROCESS

In nutrifying cereal-grain products, there are a number of general technological and related aspects[15,59,67,80–82] that must be considered, namely:

(1) An accepted nutrification standard prescribing the number and levels of the nutrients in the given product.
(2) The proper application form of the nutrients to be added.
(3) The physical means for nutrient addition, including the use of reliable equipment.
(4) The ease and uniformity of addition of nutrients; such as use of premixes.
(5) The consideration of adequate quality control procedures.

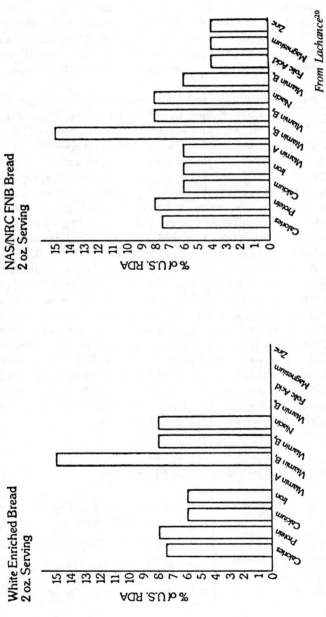

FIG. 5.7. PERCENTAGE OF USRDA FOR ENRICHED BREAD: ENRICHMENT TYPE 4 VERSUS ENRICHMENT TYPE 10
Left graph: Usual USRDA profile for enriched bread.
Right graph: USRDA profile for 1974 NAS/NRC fortified bread.

From Lachance[20]

TABLE 5.9
EXPANDED ENRICHMENT LEVELS FOR WHITE BREAD
Nutrient Levels (mg/kg)

Nutrient	Standard U.S. Enrichment[1]	Expanded Canada Enrichment[2]	Expanded U.S. Enrichment[3]	Expanded Whole White[4]
Thiamin (B_1)	4.0	2.4	4.0	4.0
Riboflavin (B_2)	2.3	1.8	2.4	2.3
Niacin	33.0	22.0	33.0	33.0
Pyridoxine (B_6)	—	1.4	2.6	1.9
Folate	—	0.24	0.4	0.56
Pantothenate	—	6.0	—	4.6
Vitamin A	—	—	6000[5]	—
Iron	28.0	18.0	28.0	28.0
Calcium	—	660.0	1320.0	830.0
Magnesium	—	900.0	275.0	630.0
Zinc	—	—	14	16
Manganese	—	—	—	26
Copper	—	—	—	2.3

Source: Adapted from Ranum *et al.*[61]
[1]Type 4 enrichment used in U.S., 1941 to date.
[2]1987 Current list of allowable nutrients added to enriched flour for enriched bread production in Canada.
[3]Type 10 enrichment for Enriched Special Formula Bread approved by FDA in 1983 under a license arranged with individual bakers with agreements on nutrient contents, labeling and marketing practices. This license arrangement was dissolved by FDA in 1988.
[4]A commercial improved enriched white bread marketed in the early 1980s.
[5]International Units.

(6) The effects of processing, transportation, and storage on nutrient stability.
(7) The effects of added nutrients on consumer acceptability; odor, taste, texture, etc.
(8) Costs.

Standards

An adopted nutrification standard, whether government mandated or not, for a cereal-grain product sets forth the primary goal for nutrient content in the final nutrified product. This standard describes the number of micronutrients to be added and the levels to be claimed in the nutrified product. Levels of nutrients for current enriched cereal grain products prepared in the United States have been tabulated (Table 5.7). The U.S. federal standards do not require enrichment; however, if the product is labeled "enriched," it must contain the types of nutrients and levels set forth for such a product. Since standards may be altered with time, this type of information should be regarded as subject to change.

The natural levels of micronutrients[83-85] in a given product like wheat flour intended to be nutrified must be previously known. Studies have been conducted to determine the mean natural levels of vitamins and minerals ± one standard deviation in wheat flour. The amount of micronutrients to be added[86] makes up the difference between the nutrification standard and the mean natural content. A small additional amount (about 5–20% depending on the nutrient) needs to be included to allow for variations in natural content and to provide for assay variations, thus providing a safety factor to achieve the required claim levels. Addition levels of nutrients to the proposed expanded NRC enriched flour standard (Type 10) either on a basis of milligrams per pound or kilogram are shown in Table 5.10. Canada also has an expanded standard for enriched flour with required nutrients (in mg/100 g): thiamin (0.44–0.77), riboflavin (0.27–0.48), niacin (3.5–6.4) and iron (2.9–4.3) as required additions and vitamin B_6 (0.25–0.31), folate (0.04–0.05), pantothenic acid (1.0–1.3), calcium (110–140) and magnesium (150–190) as optional additives.[87]

Nutrient Form

The judicious use of added nutrients in a nutrification program requires the selection of the proper form of the nutrient and care in the selection of the point of their addition in the food process.[88] Nutrient sources chosen may need a molecular weight adjustment. The form of the vitamin used may be different from the specified vitamin reference in the standard (example: thiamin mononitrate in place of thiamin hydrochloride). Likewise one needs to adjust mineral sources on the basis of their mineral content (example: the iron content of reduced iron versus ferrous sulfate). A tabular presentation (Table 5.11) has been made of the addition rate of actual sources[86] of the nutrients that could be used under the expanded Canadian and U.S. proposed expanded nutrification program (Type 10) for enriched flour, taking into account nutrients naturally present in flour.

Vitamins. After the late 1960s it became more feasible to nutrify wheat flour with vitamin A using dry stabilized vitamin A palmitate (Type 250-SD) powder form.[80,89] The practicality of it as an additive to flour has been verified by more recent investigations.[90-93] Where yellow color is desired in the bakery product, the addition of β-carotene can serve the dual role in providing both color and vitamin A activity.[94,95] The water-soluble vitamins (thiamin, riboflavin, niacin, pyridoxine, folate, and calcium pantothenate) in pure, crystalline form are added directly to flour as is, or in previously prepared premix form. The mononitrate salt of thiamin is the preferred form[96] for cereal grain product nutrification.

Amino Acids. L-lysine is the most limiting essential amino acid in all cereals. L-tryptophan is also limited in corn and L-threonine in rice. Addition of a protein supplement may create a new limiting amino acid, as in the use of soy protein where the limiting acid is methionine. At present L-lysine, dl-methionine and analogue are

TABLE 5.10
SUGGESTED LEVELS OF NUTRIENT ADDITION TO WHEAT FLOUR FOR MEETING PROPOSED NRC NUTRIFICATION STANDARDS

Nutrient	Fortification Standard (mg/lb)	Natural[1] Level (mg/lb)	Addition Level (mg/lb)	Addition Level (mg/kg)
Thiamin	2.9[2]	0.6±0.2	2.65	5.8
Riboflavin	1.8[2]	0.2±0.1	1.8	4.0
Niacin	24.0[2]	5.4±1.4	21.0	46
Folacin	0.3	0.075±0.020	0.26	0.57
Pyridoxine	2.0	0.18±0.07	2.0	4.4
Vitamin A	4,333 IU/lb[3]	0	5,000 IU/lb	11,000 IU/kg
Iron	13–16.5[2]	5.1±1.7	11	24
Calcium	900[4]	62±11	880	1940
Zinc	10			
In Flour Type				
Bread		3.5±0.5	7.5	16.5
Family		2.9±0.6	8	18
Hearth		4.5±1.0	7	15
Cake		2.1±0.5	9	20
Cookie-cracker		3.4±0.9	8	18
All		3.3±0.9	8	18
Magnesium	200			
In Flour Type				
Bread		116±23	110	240
Family		92±29	130	286
Hearth		140±23	80	176
Cake		61±18	160	350
Cookie-cracker		91±18	130	286
All		102±32	110	240

Source: Adapted from Ranum.[86]
[1]Mean natural level ± one standard deviation on an "as is" moisture basis, taken from studies by Keagy et al.[83] and Lorenz et al.[84]
[2]Current U.S. enrichment standards.
[3]Originally proposed as 2.2 retinol equivalents and then revised to 1.3 retinol equivalents = 4,333 IU.
[4]Currently the optional U.S. enrichment standard is 960 mg/lb in flour.

synthetic amino acids which can be considered for food fortification on the basis of price and availability.[88,97]

Minerals. Compounds containing calcium, iron, magnesium, and zinc with acceptable bioavailability, taste and physical properties are suitable for cereal product addition. Two most commonly used iron sources in flour are finely powdered metallic iron and ferrous sulfate.[98] Ferrous sulfate has better bioavailability and solubility, hence more reactivity which can cause food product deterioration. Some color and

TABLE 5.11
SUGGESTED RATES OF NUTRIENT SOURCES TO ADD TO WHEAT FLOUR
FOR MEETING PROPOSED U.S. NRC STANDARDS TYPE 10
AND CANADIAN EXPANDED ENRICHMENT STANDARDS

			Addition Rate	
Nutrient	Source	Nutrient[1] Activity (%)	United States (g/100 lb)	Canada (g/40 kg)
Thiamin	Mononitrate	103	0.257	0.148
Riboflavin	Hydrochloride	100	0.180	0.104
Niacin	Niacin (nicotinic acid)	100	2.10	1.12
Folacin	Folic acid	100	0.026	0.0116
Pyridoxine	Hydrochloride	82.5[2]	0.242	0.096
Pantothenic acid	Calcium pantothenate	92	—	0.357
Vitamin A	Palmitate	250,000 IU/g	2.00	—
Iron	Reduced	98	1.12	0.98
	Ferrous Sulfate	32	3.44	—
Calcium	Sulfate (anhy.)	29	303	—[3]
	Carbonate	40	220	105
Zinc	Oxide	80	1.0[4]	—
	Sulfate	36	2.2[4]	—
Magnesium	Oxide	60	18.3[4]	93
	Carbonate	25	44	224
	Sulfate (dried)	14	79	400

Source: Ranum.[86]

[1]For vitamins, the percent nutrient activity = 100 (molecular weight of the vitamin reference standard/molecular weight of the vitamin source). For minerals, it equals the percent concentration of the element in the source.
[2]The U.S. vitamin reference standard for pyridoxine is pyridoxine with a molecular weight of 169.18. The addition rate for Canda is based on pyridoxine HCl as the standard.
[3]Canadian flour enrichment regulations (1978) allow only calcium carbonate, chalk P.B., or edible bone meal, as the source of calcium. There is no provision for the use of calcium sulfate.
[4]Based on the average addition rate for all flours (8 mg/lb for Zn and 110 mg/lb for Mg).

rancidity problems have developed with ferrous sulfate. Very fine particle iron has improved bioavailability and is used more often in flour with extended storage expectations. Sweden was one of the early countries to adopt iron nutrification of flour. In a 1989 report by Hallberg et al.[99] a microcrystalline, complex ferric orthophosphate [$Fe_3H_6(NH_4) - (PO_4)_6 \cdot 6H_2O$] in labeled wheat rolls was judged acceptable to meet iron fortification needs with regard to both compatibility and bioavailability in humans. Zinc compounds (chloride, oxide, stearate, sulfate) have not been a problem[100] in bread making. A number of compounds of calcium seem satisfactory[101] for nutrification purposes. Magnesium appears to be the mineral additive that could have an adverse effect on bread quality, depending on the compound and amount added,[102] but corrective measures are available. Finely powdered metallic magnesium has performed well in nutrified breads.[103]

Micronutrient premix addition to flour should follow, whenever possible, the treatment with bleaching, maturing or oxidizing agents when such agents are employed.[104]

Methods

Additions of nutrients to any cereal product should be done in a manner to provide uniformity of distribution and good stability without significant alteration in form, appearance, flavor or safety.[105] Each food product poses its own potential technological considerations.[88] In the usual nutrifying operation, as in the case of flour, involving multinutrients, the individual nutrients are not added singularly, which would make for greater costs[106] and be more accident-prone and less amenable to monitoring. All the smaller amounts of nutrients can be incorporated with an appropriate diluent or bulking agent into a premix form and hence introduced into the food product as a single addition in batch or continuous processing.

In case of rice, whole wheat, and corn grits, the enrichment premix may consist of the actual cereal grain kernels with nutrients added at high concentration by impregnation, by a coating process, or a combination of the two.

Tablets, wafers, cubes or soluble packets of nutrients represent another system for addition of nutrients. For example, bread wafers, dispersible in water and containing sufficient vitamins and minerals to nutrify 100 lb of white flour, are added in the water during the dough mixing operation in the bakery.[81]

Concentrated solutions or emulsions or micronized suspensions of micronutrients with edible carrriers are also applicable to spray application onto cereal grain products, for example on RTE cereals[107] or on items after baking or other heat processes.

Equipment

Dry premixes or spray formulations must be metered accurately as they are introduced into the food product. Volumetric feeders are most commonly used to meter a continuous stream of a premix into a food product stream, or a weighted quantity of premix is added to a net weight of the food product in a batch mixing operation. A simple feeder has been described by Lease[48] for addition of vitamins and mineral to corn meal in small mills. In this feeder, an impeller rotates past an adjusted aperture at the base of the hopper to deliver the premix to a spout leading to the product stream. Brooke developed a similar feeder[105] in 1969, but introduced variable speed control, agitation within the hopper and a calibrated aperture slide. A variety of feeders are manufactured around the world (Chapter 17).

Blending of the introduced micronutrients may be achieved by the use of cut-flight conveyors, mixing paddles, or combinations of the two. Both horizontal and vertical blenders are used. Horizontal blenders may be of the ribbon type, the paddle type, or combinations of the two. Vertical mixers have one or more circulating screw agitators (Chapter 17).

Solutions, emulsions, or dispersions of micronutrients may be sprayed onto foods during the last stages of processing. Such solutions or emulsions should be so formulated that the moisture content of the sprayed cereal product is not significantly increased or that most of the water can be evaporated.

Wheat Products

Flour. Wheat flour is enriched efficiently in large commercial mills by metering a premix into blended flour flowing into packing bins. With efficient mixing equipment to ensure uniform distribution, the vitamin-mineral premix is introduced at the rate of 0.25 or 0.50 oz/100 lb of flour. Smaller mills with less sophisticated equipment tend to prefer to add a less concentrated premix, for example, at the rate of 2 oz/100 lb.[81] If 0.2–0.4% lysine is to be added in special formulated products to the premix, the amount of premix added to flour may be increased. In the United States, enrichment can be carried out either at the mill or the bakery. In Canada, all flour is required to be enriched at the mill.

In the United States, thiamin, riboflavin, niacin, and iron have been added to wheat flour since the early 1940s. Since the late 1960s, the U.S. government has approved the addition of dry vitamin A to nutrified wheat flour sent overseas under Public Law 480. The dry vitamin A can be incorporated into the regular vitamin-iron premix for metering into the product.

To nutrify flour with the 6 vitamins and 4 minerals as recommended in the 1974 NRC proposed expanded enrichment (Type 10), Cort et al.[108] developed 2 premixes, a vitamin-iron premix and a calcium-magnesium-zinc mineral premix. These premixes added to flour at the appropriate levels did not discolor the flour and did not contribute undesirable taste or odor. Rubin et al.[109] also described premixes for addition to flour to provide the NRC recommended levels of vitamins and minerals. Two such premixes were prepared, one to provide all of the recommended vitamins and minerals and the second containing all the proposed nutrients except calcium and magnesium.

Nutrification of cereal grain products at small, village mills can be done by blending in a premix, either at the mesh range of semolina or at the mesh range of flour depending on circumstances. An alternative method is to prepare the premix in the form of compressed pellets to be mixed in at a controlled rate to the wheat grain stream just before it enters the attrition rollers of the flour mill. A third method is to prepare a premix in the form of heavily nutrified wheat kernels by procedures specific to the added nutrients, to be mixed in the same manner as pellets. For example, Graham et al.[110] have described a method of producing lysine nutrified whole-wheat kernels. First, the surfaces of the kernels are scored in a very light pearling treatment in a machine fitted with abrasive surfaces. The kernels are then soaked in a 35% solution of L-lysine at 160° F for 3 h. After draining and drying to avoid a powdery, salted appearance, the kernels containing 10–15% L-lysine are ready for use. When blended into ordinary wheat to provide the desired level of added lysine, they are undetectable in appearance and taste. Upon milling, the retention of L-lysine follows the extraction rate of the flour fairly closely.

Bread, Rolls. Enriched flour may be used to make enriched bread, rolls, and other baked goods as a means of nutrification. Another practice in bakeries is to use an enrichment wafer or tablets, or soluble packets of a nutrients mix dispersed in water and added to the flour in the dough mixing operation. Cort et al.[108] baked breads in the laboratory using flour enriched with a vitamin-iron premix and also with flour containing this premix plus the minerals zinc, magnesium and calcium. When these breads were submitted to a taste panel for comparison with regular bread, the panel could not detect any off-flavor and even preferred the bread with the type-10 premix. Rubin et al.[109] reported on bread baking trials in commercial baking equipment using flours nutrified to provide: (1) the NRC recommended levels of 6 vitamins and 4 minerals (Type 10) and (2) the same levels of 6 vitamins, iron, and zinc (magnesium and calcium addition omitted). A panel of 14 experts judged the resulting breads. The initial taste of the breads nutrified both ways was indistinguishable from that of unnutrified or normally enriched bread (Type 4); but, after storage of the bread for a week at room temperature, there was a slight flavor change in the bread nutrified with the complete premix but not in the bread from which calcium and magnesium were omitted in the nutrification. The bread containing the full mineral supplement gave a slightly lower textural score.

Emodi and Scialpi[63] reported significant quantities of magnesium and zinc in normally enriched flour and of calcium in flour plus other bread ingredients. Therefore, to achieve the NRC proposed levels of minerals, they proposed adding the amounts of zinc, magnesium and calcium sufficient to supplement the level already present in the bread ingredients. When the enrichment of flour was made on this basis, the quality of bread containing the full NRC proposed vitamin-mineral (Type 10) supplement was as good as that of bread made today with 3 vitamins and iron (Type 4).

Pasta. Pasta products can be enriched by incorporating an appropriate nutrient premix into semolina in dry blending or by the use of an enrichment powder packet added to the pasta formulation in the mixer at the time of the dough mixing stage before the kneading, extrusion and drying operations. Because of the customary method of home cooking most of the pasta products in a large volume of water, nutrient losses are high following drainage; therefore, these losses must be compensated for by using higher potency nutrient premixes during the enriching process.

Rice

Compared to other cereal-grain meals and flours, white rice represents a different challenge in the technology of nutrification.[26] Not only does white rice, in its most common usage, remain in an unground kernel form, but particularly it may be washed thoroughly before cooking. Rice in the developing countries reaches the market in large cloth bags in bulk form. It is sold to the consumer in in small amounts and a washing step prior to cooking is considered necessary to remove any dust, grit or sand.[81] Where cleaned rice is sold in sealed consumer-size packages, a more common practice in developed countries, the washing practice by the consumer is omitted. Hence, two enrichment premixes are required; nonrinse and rinse-resistant types in rice enrichment.

Rinse-resistant Premix. In the rinse-resistant premix programs, the nutrients are applied with coatings to the rice grain. The coatings are insoluble in cold water, but break down during cooking releasing the nutrients.[110] Other approaches include acid-soaking techniques to absorb the nutrients within the rice grain, the use of fat-soluble forms[111] of thiamin and putting on water-insoluble edible polymers. A number of methods have been reported.

Kondo et al.[112] parboiled white rice in an acetic acid solution containing thiamin hydrochloride, which after sieving, steaming and drying yielded a concentrate containing 1.2 mg/g of thiamin. In a varied process,[113] white rice is soaked in acetic solution containing dibenzoyl thiamin hydrochloride followed by steaming and drying to produce a rice premix (Poly Rice) containing 1.6 mg/g of thiamin. The uniform addition of the rice premix concentrate at 0.5% to regular white rice results in a thiamin nutrified rice produced commercially in Japan. A lysine nutrified rice is prepared in a similar manner; both lysine and threonine additions to rice have been accomplished.[114]

Another nutrified rice premix[113,115] produced in Japan since 1981, called Shingen, contains 8 nutrients (in mg/g): thiamin 1.5; riboflavin, 0.06; niacin, 6.2; pantothenate, 2.3; pyridoxine, 0.08; vitamin E, 1.4; calcium, 8.0; and iron, 1.2. Five nutrients are added by soaking, three by coating. The above rice premix is blended with regular rice at a level of 0.5% making multinutrient enriched rice. This multinutrient nutrified rice (Fig. 5.8) compares favorably[113,114] with brown rice in clinical trials.

The manufacture of the Furter coated rice enrichment premix[116] has been extended by Mickus.[117] The rice premix concentrate is blended with regular white rice (1:199) to produce a multinutrient nutrified rice. LaPierre[118] developed a variation of the Furter process in which the vitamins and minerals in a zein suspension were coated onto rice in special thin layers followed by a shellac coating, a dusting of a whitening agent and a final protective coating. In 1986, Bramall[119] described a process which significantly simplifies the earlier Furter process by reducing the number of steps (Chapter 17).

Because the addition of riboflavin imparts a definite yellow color to some of the premix types which may persist after cooking,[81] the addition of riboflavin has been made optional in the U.S. regulations on enriched rice. One method reported in the literature[120] for the addition of riboflavin to rice employs in the premix stage the much more soluble 5'-phosphate ester, which disperses more quickly and uniformly throughout the nutrified rice during cooking. The process has not been studied by other investigators. A nutrient coating method for rice reported by Fieger and Williams[121] also has not been adopted for commercial development. Peil et al.[122] have proposed placing added nutrients in edible polymers before applying the polymers to the rice grain. Nutrient losses and procedures for nutrification of rice by applying thiamin, niacin and ferric pyrophosphate followed by palmitic acid coating have been examined by Vanossi.[123]

Since 1974, trials have been run with rice to determine the practicality of adding 6 vitamins and 4 minerals (Type 10) enrichment. Vitamin A, thiamin, niacin, pyridoxine, folate, iron and zinc, plus vitamin E were incorporated in one series by Cort et al.[108] into the rice premix concentrate using both the Furter-Mickus coating and the Wright modified coating methods. Both methods gave a satisfactory appearing premix concentrate. Vitamin A, pyridoxine, tocopheryl acetate and folate were found to be stable in the presence of iron (ferric orthophosphate) and zinc (zinc oxide). In another series,[109] five vitamins (no riboflavin) and iron and zinc were again incorporated into rice premix concentrate according to the previously mentioned premix methods on a laboratory scale and on production equipment, confirming the Cort et al.[108] findings. Nutrient retention values of 94–100% after 6 months and 84–100% after 12 months of storage and less than 1% water rinsing losses were observed for the rice premix concentrate. Nutrient retention values after cooking nutrified rice prepared with the premix were 98–100%.

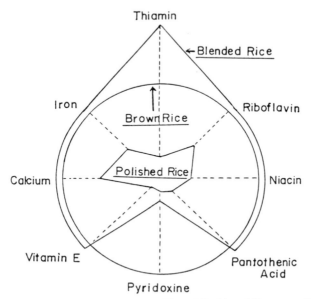

From Misaki and Yasumatsu[113]

FIG. 5.8. COMPARISON OF THE NUTRIENT CONTENT OF WHITE RICE, BROWN RICE AND ENRICHED RICE WITH 8 NUTRIENTS ADDED

Simulated rice kernels premix can be made by extrusion of a stiff dough, containing cereal flours and the nutrification ingredients, through a pasta press, steaming, drying and coating. Formulation is easy, but production can be troublesome. If the kernels are too soft they leach in the water washing and if too hard they are not digested; in addition, in cooked rice they may be detected, hence picked out and discarded.

Nonrinse Premix. The nonrinse rice premix is a powder blend of nutrients with a starch or flour diluent which is dusted onto the rice grains during a blending procedure.[81] Lease et al.[124] used a powdered premix very similar to that used for enriching flour or corn grits to enrich rice. This premix could be made with riboflavin as well as thiamin, niacin, and iron. The riboflavin at a level of at least 1.2 mg/lb imparted a slight cream color to the enriched rice, but the color both before and after cooking was so slight that it was generally acceptable to consumers.[124] The only disadvantage to the powdered premix method of enriching rice is that the rice cannot be rinsed before cooking without high losses of the added nutrients.

Corn Products

Meal. The addition of nutrients to corn meal is made at the mill by metering a powder premix into the stream in the same manner as for wheat flour.[48] To ease and speed the nutrification process of corn products in South Carolina after the enrichment laws were enacted, a long term educational program was sponsored by the State Nutrition Committee and Clemson University. Clemson also produced and distributed to small millers, on a nonprofit basis, the feeder equipment to be attached to the mill and the nutrient premix blend to be added to the corn product during the milling process. With the passage of time, more corn has been processed in fewer and larger mills.

Cort et al.[108] have carried out nutrification trials on corn meal with vitamins and minerals levels suggested by the 1974 proposed expanded NRC enrichment program, using the appropriate vitamin-iron and mineral premixes, with observed acceptable stability and storage performances. Confirmation trials were reported by Rubin et al.[109]

Grits. Corn grits have been nutrified with a powdered vitamin-iron premix (similar to that used for corn meal) when directions are provided for a no water rinse practice for the enriched grit product before cooking. In a trial[109] in 1977, regular and quick-cook grits were enriched with thiamin, riboflavin, niacin, pyridoxine, folate and iron using a nonrinse powder premix. Storage tests for 6 months followed by chemical assay revealed acceptable nutrient retention data for those under test. Added zinc, calcium and magnesium sources were not included in those trials.

When nonrinse directions are not provided, a water-rinse resistant grits premix is required for the nutrification of corn grits. In 1947, degermed corn grits[125] were uniformly enriched with thiamin, riboflavin, niacin and iron by the Furter coating process of first preparing a premix with water-resistant properties and then adding the premix to corn grits in a predetermined ratio to form the enriched grits. Nutrient retention tests, rinsing tests and human bioassays on the enriched grits demonstrated the successful incorporation of the 4 added nutrients (Type 4 enrichment).

RTE Cereals

In the nutrification of RTE cereals, heat-stable nutrients such as the minerals, niacin and riboflavin can be added in the dough phase prior to cooking or extrusion. Heat-labile vitamins, such as thiamin, and vitamins A and C are usually sprayed onto the cereals as they leave the oven or extruder. Vitamin A may be sprayed in the form of an emulsion, but the stability of the vitamin is strongly dependent on the composition of the spray formulation. Sugar in such solutions appears to coat the vitamin A after drying and provides an oxygen barrier. If present in the same phase as vitamin A, vitamin D will normally be at least as stable as the vitamin A. Vitamin E in the form of d- or dl-alpha-tocopheryl acetate is quite stable and can be added to cereals in the same system as vitamin A or in the dough phase as an oil solution or a dry powder.

Another approach is to prepare a single, liquid formulation of all the vitamins to be sprayed at the appropriate processing stage after heat treatment. In any liquid spray, homogeneity, pH and temperature control, use of an antioxidant system and an oxygen barrier, such as sucrose, are considerations in the formulation. Steele[54] discussing cereal nutrification, cites (1) production losses, (2) spray formulation and systems and (3) shelf stability to be sources of potential problems. The cereal industry's ability, over the decades, to nutrify millions of tons of breakfast cereals with nutrients attests to the success of the application methods.[52]

Quality Control

When multinutrient nutrification of food began, each food processor had to purchase the individual nutrients, weigh and add each separately or prepare a blend of the items, more often incorporating an inert diluent to increase the volume of the additives. About 1943, accurately compounded custom manufactured premixes became commercially available. The use of these eases the task of addition and provides greater assurance that the enriched products conform to the desired standard or claim. Analytical control is simplified, as assay of one or two components of the mixture blended into the food product can serve as confirmation of the correct addition of all mixture ingredients. At suitable intervals, qualitative and/or quantitative checks need be made of nutrient content, particularly for the more labile nutrients. A system of record keeping to show the disappearance of the premix in relation to the total production of the enriched product is highly advisable.

Stability

When micronutrients are added to food for the purpose of improved nutrition, it is vital to know whether they are present after market shelf-life and also after any preparatory steps prior to consumption. Trials have been run to put these possibilities to test. Several series were run[63,108,109] during the 1976–80 period. Laboratory or pilot-plant micronutrient stability tests serve as guides to expected performance under commercial operation conditions. Some nutrient stability data for cereal-grain products are listed in Table 5.12. It is good practice to run confirmatory tests under new conditions, new locations, or when special situations are encountered.

Costs

The cost of nutrification of cereal-grain products depends on the nutrients to be added, the overage required to maintain label claims and other equipment, operational and control expenses.[15,61,67,82,89] The contribution of the chemical industry to the practical accomplishment with favorable economy of the nutrification of food has not been widely recognized. One example is the case of thiamin which in 1936, isolated from natural sources, cost $400/g compared to beginning production by chemical synthesis at $10 which by 1940 was reduced to $1/g. Today's cost is a fraction of this. In 1941, cost of 3 enrichment ingredients (Fig.5.9) thiamin, niacin and iron was between 14–17¢/100 lb (cwt) of flour[40,81] with, flour selling at $2.40/cwt, and was further reduced in subsequent years to the present day cost of 5–6¢.

In a consideration of the estimated cost[61,67,82] of nutrifying wheat flour to the NRC proposed levels (10 nutrients added), one must include the possibility of the need of 2 premixes, one containing the 6 vitamins, iron and zinc and another containing calcium and magnesium. Ingredient costs would approximate 25–30¢/cwt, flour selling at $9.60/cwt. Considering the average U.S. per capita flour consumption of about 125lb/yr, it would indicate a supplemental nutrient cost of about 30–35¢ per person annually.

Other Costs. For addition of nutrients to cereal products the equipment (mostly single time purchases) required may vary from simple, on-line feeders for flour streams, etc., to the more complex spraying and drying equipment for fortification of rice kernels. (See Chapter 17.) More detailed cost discussions of cereal-grain products are covered by Austin[15] in his comprehensive volume.

Acceptability

Since wheat flour enriched with 3 vitamins (thiamin, riboflavin, niacin) and iron (Type 4) and enriched, white baked bread have been in commercial and home use

TABLE 5.12
STABILITY OF ADDED NUTRIENTS

Product	Processing and/or Storage Conditions	Nutrient	Loss	Reference
Premix: for flour or corn meal	6 months at room temperature (RT)	Vitamin A palmitate (dry)	0	Cort et al. 1976. Food Technol. 30(4) 52–60.
		Thiamin	1	
		Riboflavin	2	
		Pyridoxine	1	
		Folate	5	
		Tocopheryl acetate (dry)	5	
Rice premix	Enriched rice, 6 months/RT	Vitamin A	1–13	Cort et al. 1976. Food Technol. 30(4), 52–60. Furter et al. 1946. Ind. Eng. Chem. 38, 486–493. Rubin et al. Cereal Chem. 54, 895–904.
		Thiamin	1–4	
		Pyridoxine	0–1	
		Folate	0	
		Tocopheryl acetate (dry)	0	
Rice premix	Simulated rice grains, extrusion cooked and stored 3 months/30°C	Vitamin A acetate (oil)	45–50	Gershoff et al. 1975. Am. J. Clin. Nutr. 28, 170–182.
Corn grits premix	Enriched grits, 6 months/ 45°C	Thiamin	7–13	Furter et al. 1947. Trans. Am. Assoc. Cereal Chem. 5, 26-36.
		Niacin	0–1	
Rice premix	Nutrients added by infusion: washing	Thiamin	7	Kondo et al. 1951. Bull. Res. Inst. Food Sci. 6, 57–69.
	Washing and cooking	Thiamin	12	
Rice premix	Lysine added by infusion: Washing (no steaming)	L-lysine	40	Mitsuda and Yasumato. 1974. In New Protein Foods, Vol. 1A, Academic Press, New York.
	Washing (after 3 min steaming)	L-lysine	20	
	Washing (after 10 min steaming)	L-lysine	10	

TABLE 5.12 (Continued)

Product	Processing and/or Storage Conditions	Nutrient	% Loss	Reference
Whole Wheat	Lysine added by infusion, 13% moisture; 12 months/38°C	L-lysine	<10	Hulse. 1974. In New Protein Foods, Vol. 1A. Academic Press, New York. Ferrell et al. 1970. Cereal Chem. 47, 32-37.
Enriched flour	Nutrified with vitamin-iron and mineral premixes; stored 6 months/RT, 23°C	A palm. (dry) Thiamin Pyridoxine Folate E acet. (dry)	3 0 7 19 0	Cort et al. 1976. Food Technol. 30(4), 52-60.
Enriched flour	Folate added; stored 12 months/ 38°C	Folate	0	Keagy et al. 1975. Cereal Chem. 52, 348-356.
Enriched flour	Gamma irradiation and 3 months/RT 75,000 rads	Thiamin Riboflavin Niacin	1 18 1	Chappel and MacQueen. 1970. Food Irrad. 10, 8-10.
	150,000 rads	Thiamin Riboflavin Niacin	3 17 13	
Enriched flour	Thiamin HCl vs NO_3	Thiamin	NO_3 more stable	Hollenbeck and Obeermeyer. 1952. Cereal Chem. 29, 82-87.
Enriched flour	Enriched with 8 vitamins; treated with bleaching, maturing and oxidizing agents	Thiamin, riboflavin, niacin, E acetate Pantothenate, vit. A, folate Pyridoxine	0 small effect 16	Ranum et al. 1981. Cereal Chem. 58(1), 32-35.

Product	Process	Nutrient	Loss (%)	Reference
Enriched corn and wheat flours	Physical stability to processing, shipping and storage	Vitamin A palmitate (dry)	stable	Parrish et al. 1980. Cereal Chem. 57(4), 284–287.
Enriched flour	Heat treatment of flour products, deep fat frying, baking	Lysine	14–34	Geervani and Devi. 1986. Nutr. Rept. Int. 33(6), 961–966.
Enriched cereal-grain products	Pan bread, corn bread, corn mush, cakes, pancakes, spaghetti preparation	Vitamin A palmitate (dry), Type 250 SD	0–20	Parrish et al. 1980. J. Food Sci. 45(5), 1438–1439.
Doughnuts	Preparation from a mix	Thiamin Riboflavin	35 18–27	Borenstein. 1974. In Wheat Production. AVI/Van Nostrand
Chocolate cake	Baking, pH 8–9, 20–25 min./365–450°C	Thiamin	90	
Enriched cookies and bread	Enriched flour: in bread	Thiamin Riboflavin Niacin	10–12 0–8 3–10	Ranhotra and Gelroth. 1986. Cereal Chem. 63(5), 401–403.
	in cookies (pH 7–8)	Thiamin Riboflavin Niacin	70–80 0–10 0	
Enriched cookies	Made with enriched flour (10 nutrients)	Folate	15	Connor and Keagy. 1981. Cereal Chem. 58(3), 239–244.
Enriched bread	Commercial baking of white bread	Thiamin	21–22	Schultz et al. 1942. Cereal Chem. 19, 532–538.
		Thiamin	16–20	Melnick et al. Am. Baker, Oct., 3–12.
		Thiamin	17–23	Coppock et al. 1956. J. Sci. Food Agr. 7, 457–464.
Enriched bread	Lysine and 4% nonfat dry milk added: baked 20 min/450°F baked 30 min/450°F	L-lysine L-lysine	0–18 30	Jansen et al. 1964. Food Technol. 18, 367–371.

TABLE 5.12 (Continued)

Product	Processing and/or Storage Conditions	Nutrient	% Loss	Reference
Enriched bread	Lysine and 6–14% nonfat dry milk added:			Jansen et al. 1964. Food Technol. 18, 372–375.
	baked 20 min/450°F	L-lysine	36	
	baked 30 min/450°F (no dry milk added)	L-lysine	15	
Enriched bread	Baking	L-lysine	11	Rosenberg and Rohdenburg. 1951. J. Nutr. 45, 593–598.
Enriched bread	Baking	D,L-threonine	20–40	Ericson et al. 1961. Acta Physiol. Scand. 53, 85–88.
Enriched bread	Laboratory baking of yeast-rise bread and storage 5 days/ RT or 2 months/20°C *NS = no significant loss	Vitamin A Vitamin E Pyridoxine Thiamin Riboflavin	NS* NS NS NS NS	Cort et al. 1976. Food Technol. 30(4), 52–60. Emodi and Scialpi. 1978. 6th Int. Cereal Bread Congress Winnipeg, Canada.
Enriched bread	Comparison of conventional vs continuous process	Thiamin Riboflavin and niacin	lower for continuous no difference	Tabekahia and D'Appolonia. 1978. Cereal Chem. 56(2), 79–81.
Enriched bread	Made with enriched flour and baked	Pyridoxine	0–15	Perera et al. 1979. Cereal Chem. 56(6), 577–580.
Enriched bread	0.1–0.5% lysine added to flour, baked	Lysine	11	Saab and Da Silva. 1981. J. Food Sci. 46, 662–663.
Enriched bread	0.48% lysine and 0.3% threonine added; baked 43 min/210°C	L-lysine L-threonine	14 15	Murata et al. 1979. J. Food Sci. 44(1), 271–273.

CEREAL GRAIN PRODUCTS

Enriched bread	Persian type; baked 2 min/ about 204°C	Vit. A acetate Vit. A palmitate	26 32	Vaghefi and Delgotha. 1975. Cereal Chem. 52, 753–756.
Enriched bread	Toasting: white bread whole wheat bread	Thiamin Thiamin	0–24 0–12	Hoffman et al. 1940. Cereal Chem. 17, 737–739.
Enriched bread	Laboratory baking	Folacin	11	Keagy et al. 1975. Cereal Chem. 52, 348-356.
Enriched bread	Toasting of National Bread: 12 mm thick slice 9 mm thick slice 5 mm thick slice	Thiamin Thiamin Thiamin	13 15 31	Coppock et al. 1956. J. Sci. Food Agr. 7, 457–464.
Enriched bread	Up to 5 days of normal, intermittent illumination	Thiamin Riboflavin Niacin	0 0 0	Morgareidge. 1956. Cereal Chem. 33, 213–220.
Enriched bread	Laboratory baking of yeast-rise bread; stored 5 days/23°C	Vitamin A palmitate (dry)	11–13 0–2	Rubin and Cort. 1969. *In* Protein Enriched Foods, Am. Assoc. Cereal Chemists, St. Paul.
Enriched pasta products	Cooking and draining	Pyridoxine	50	Bunting. 1965. Cereal Chem. 42, 569–572.
Enriched pasta products	Stored 1 yr/100°F and 50% rel. humidity	Pyridoxine	0	
Enriched pasta products	Cooking losses of spaghetti, noodles and macaroni	Thiamin Riboflavin Niacin	42–54 30–41 39–50	Ranhotra et al. 1983. Nutr. Rept. Int. 28(2), 423–426. Furuya and Warthesen. 1984. J. Food Sci. 49(4), 984–986.
Enriched pasta	Cooking losses (Fe, Ca, P, Mg, Zn, Cu, Mn)	Minerals	0–20	Ranhotra et al. 1985. Cereal Chem. 62, 117–122.

TABLE 5.12 (Continued)

Product	Processing and/or Storage Conditions	Nutrient	% Loss	Reference
Enriched farina	Quick-cooking, pH 6.9			Lincoln et al. 1944. Cereal Chem. 21, 274–279.
	15 min cooking	Thiamin	9	
	30 min cooking	Thiamin	18	
	60 min cooking	Thiamin	25	
	pH 5.8 after cooking			
	30 min cooking	Thiamin	6	
	60 min cooking	Thiamin	10	
Enriched farina	Cooking trial	Thiamin	1–3	Munsell et al. 1948. J. Am. Dietet. Assoc. 24, 314–316.
		Riboflavin	2–5	
		Niacin	0–6	
Enriched breakfast cereals, ready to eat (RTE)	Average production loss	Vitamin A	29	Steele. 1976. Cereal Foods World 21, 538–540.
		Thiamin	26	
		Riboflavin	12	
		Pyridoxine	32	
		Vitamin B_{12}	17	
		Vitamin C	37	
		Niacin	2	
		Folate	25	
	Average storage loss,			
	3 months/RT	Vitamin A	25	
	6 months/RT	Vitamin A	35	
		Riboflavin	6	
		Vitamin B_{12}	4	
		Vitamin C	10	
	12 months/RT	Vitamin A	50	
		Thiamin	0	

Product	Treatment	Nutrient	Loss (%)	Reference
Enriched RTE cereals	Spray application in sugar solution; stored 6 months	Riboflavin	23	Johnson et al. 1988. Cereal Foods World 33(3), 280–282.
		Vitamin B$_{12}$	17	
		Folate	19	
		Niacin	0	
		Vitamin C	41	
		Vit. A palm.	0–18	
		Na ascorbate	9–20	
		Thiamin NO$_3$	0–10	
Enriched rice	Washing loss by S. Carolina method; coated premix added (1:200)	Thiamin	0.9	Furter et al. 1946. Ind. Eng. Chem. 38, 486–493.
		Niacin	0.3	
		Iron	0.1	
White rice	White rice only no premix added; S.C. washing loss	Thiamin	9	
		Niacin	33	
		Iron	15	
Enriched rice	Cooked in double boiler, not drained	Thiamin	3–6	
		Niacin	2–4	
	Cooked in open vessel, drained	Thiamin	14–49	
		Niacin	18–36	
Enriched rice	Cooked, not drained, vitamin-iron premix added (1:200)	Vitamin A	1	Cort et al. 1976. Food Technol. 30(4), 52–60.
		Vitamin E	0	
		Pyridoxine	0	
		Folate	0	
Enriched rice	Lysine added to parboiled rice; cooked, not drained	L-lysine	0	Bains and Tara. 1970. Progress Rept. CFTRI, Mysore.
Enriched corn grits	Washing loss by S. Carolina method; coated premix (1:800)	Thiamin	8	Furter et al. 1947. Trans. Assoc. Cereal Chemists 5, 26–36.
		Riboflavin	8	
		Niacin	15	
	Cooking loss, no water discarded	Thiamin	8	
		Niacin	0	
		Iron	0	

TABLE 5.12 (Continued)

Product	Processing and/or Storage Conditions	Nutrient	% Loss	Reference
Enriched corn meal	Vitamin-iron premix added; stored 6 months/RT	Vitamin A	2	Rubin et al. 1977. Cereal Chem. 54, 895–904.
		Thiamin	3	
		Pyridoxine	2	
		Folate	18	
		Riboflavin	3	
Enriched corn grits	Vitamin-iron premix added; stored 6 months/RT	Vitamin A	19	
		Thiamin	0	
		Pyridoxine	0	
		Folate	0	
		Riboflavin	8	
	Quick grits with dry vitamin A palmitate:			
	cooked 4 min	Vitamin A	20	
	cooked 6 min	Vitamin A	25	
	cooked 10 min	Vitamin A	30	
	Regular grits with dry Vit. A palmitate: cooked 30 min	Vitamin A	25–34	
Enriched yellow corn meal	Dry vitamin A palmitate added: cooked 5 min	Vitamin A	13	
Corn bread	In corn bread	Pyridoxine	0	Bunting. 1965. Cereal Chem. 42, 568–572.
Enriched corn grits	Thiamin added: extrusion cooked at 300°F and variable screw feed at 380°F	Thiamin	10–39	Beetner et al. 1974. J. Food Sci. 39, 207–208.
		Riboflavin	0–13	
		Thiamin	52–81	
		Riboflavin	0–46	

Enriched corn products	Tortillas baked	Vitamin A	0	Rubin and Cort. 1969. *In* Protein Enriched Food, Am. Assoc. Cereal Chemists, St. Paul.
	Chapatties baked	Vitamin A	8	
Enriched tortillas				Bressani *et al.*, 1976. 2nd Workshop on Fortification, AID, Washington, DC.
	0.3% L-lysine and 0.1% D,L-tryptophan:			
	cooked 3 min	L-lysine	0	
		D,L-tryptophan	6	
	cooked 6 min	L-lysine	1	
		D,L-tryptophan	0	
	0.1% L-lysine and 3% Tortula:			
	cooked 3 min	L-lysine	0	
	cooked 6 min	L-lysine	27	
Enriched corn products	Corn bread baked:			Pace and Whiteacre. 1953. Food Res. *18*, 231–249.
	pH of batter 5.3–5.9			
	pH of bread 6.1–6.4	Thiamin	15–17	
	pH of batter 6.25			
	pH of bread 7.35	Thiamin	27	
	pH of batter 6.4			
	pH of bread 7.97	Thiamin	60	
	pH of batter 6.55			
	pH of bread 8.22	Thiamin	81	
	pH of batter 6.55–6.6			
	pH of bread 8.0–8.5	Thiamin	83–91	
	pH of batter 6.0–6.05	Riboflavin	0	
	pH of bread 6.4–6.5	Niacin	5	
	Corn muffins baked:			
	pH of batter 5.8–5.9			
	pH of bread 6.0–6.1	Thiamin	16–21	

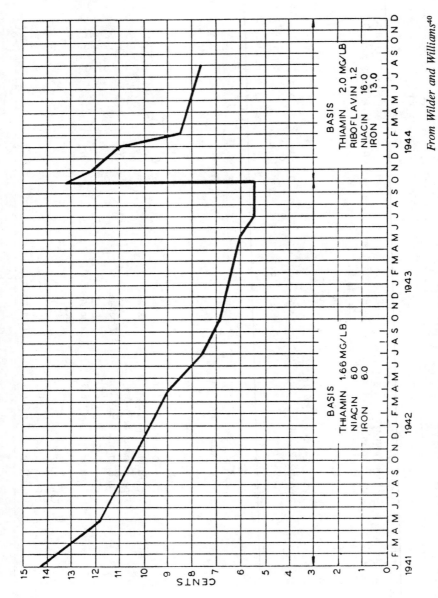

FIG. 5.9. COST OF ENRICHING INGREDIENT PER 100 LB OF FLOUR

From Wilder and Williams[40]

practice for nearly 50 years in the United States and in some other countries, there should be no question about the acceptability of enriched products by consumers. Similar conclusions can be reached about enriched farina, pasta products, corn meal and grits and white rice.

The NRC proposed expanded enrichment proposal calls for 6 vitamins (thiamin, riboflavin, niacin, pyridoxine, folate, vitamin A) and 4 minerals (iron, zinc, magnesium and calcium) to be added to cereal grain products. While some slight flavor or texture differences were noted in early enrichment Type 10 trials, these problems have been resolved by processing or formulation modifications. During the time period the Food & Drug Administration agreed to permit bakers to prepare and market bread of the enrichment Type-10 under the provisions of an approved temporary marketing permit, Enriched Special Formula Bread was marketed successfully with public acceptability.

In a 1980 test study,[63] the quality of bread made with nutrified flour (13.3% moisture) was examined. Data from this study revealed that nutrification of bread with the NRC proposed Type 10 micronutrients was feasible. Bread containing the full vitamin-mineral supplement was acceptable in all characteristics. No off-flavor was noticed by 10 trained taste panelists in nutrified bread stored for 5 days at room temperature or after 4 weeks at freezer temperature. Likewise, in the scoring for aroma, chewability, toastability, characteristics of crust, symmetry, volume and general appearance, none showed significant detrimental effects. Premixes incorporated were formulated to consider the natural nutrient content contributed by flour and the baking ingredients.

Since 1973, ready-to-eat (RTE) breakfast cereals, have been nutrified with 7 vitamins and iron: Some have more added nutrients. The U.S. consumption of these nutrified RTE cereals continues to increase annually[52-56] on a per capita basis, indicating consumer acceptance. Consumer acceptability of nutrified cereal grain products is further indicated by the number of countries which have adopted some earlier form of nutrification for cereal grain products. Studies with some amino acid nutrified cereal-grain products have not indicated consumer acceptance to be a primary concern.[15]

EFFECTS OF CEREAL FORTIFICATION ON HUMAN NUTRITION

Regarding the contribution of nutrified cereal grain products such as flour to the well-being of a population, one can examine conditions before and after the introduction of the program. A partial tabulation of studies dealing with the effect of nutrification of cereal products on humans is given in Table 5.13.

Cereal grain products supply a significant percentage[126] of total intake of nutrients, particularly so for thiamin, riboflavin, niacin and iron (Fig. 5.10) due to the 1940-50 enrichment programs relative to the total dietary energy intake from cereal grain products. If a Type 10 nutrification (NRC 1974 proposal expanded or other updated

TABLE 5.13
INFLUENCE OF CEREAL GRAIN PRODUCT NUTRIFICATION ON HUMAN NUTRITION AND/OR ACCEPTABILITY: GENERAL REFERENCES

Cereal Product	Nutrients	Reference
Cereal-grain products	Vitamins and iron	Figueroa et al. 1950. Rept. 71, Med. Nutr. Lab Surgeon General.
	Thiamin, riboflavin, niacin, iron	Anon. 1949. Nutr. Rev. 7, 101–103. Dickins and Sheets. 1952. J. Home Econ. 44, 433–436. Richardson. 1966. Family Econ. Rev. (June), 10–12.
	Lysine, methionine	Hegsted et al. 1955. J. Nutr. 56, 555–576.
	Pyridoxine	Rubin. 1966. Cereal Sci. Today 11, 234–239.
	Thiamin, riboflavin	Senti. 1971. Cereal Sci. Today 16, 91–102.
	Lysine, tryptophan, leucine, niacin	Kies and Fox. 1972. Cereal Chem. 49, 223–231.
	Amino acids, vitamins, minerals	Rosenfield and Stare. 1973. Bibl. Nutr. Diet. 19, 27–33.
	Amino acids and proteins	Milner. 1974. Cereal Sci. Today 19, 509–512.
	Niacin	Miller. 1978. Food Prod. Dev. 12(4), 30–38. Park et al. 1984. Abstr. Fed. Proc. 43(4), 992.
	Iron	Johnson and Evans. 1976. Abstr. J. Nutr. 106, xxii.
Wheat product	Thiamin, riboflavin, niacin, iron	Williams et al. 1943. JAMA 121, 943–945.
	Thiamin, riboflavin, niacin, iron, vitamin A	Wilder. 1949. Food Ind. (July), 44–48. Aykroyd et al. 1949. Can. Med. J. 60, 328–352. Goldsmith et al. 1950. J. Nutr. 40, 41–69.
	Riboflavin, calcium	Poznanski et al. 1962. J. Am. Dietet. Assoc. 40, 120–124.
	Thiamin, niacin, iron	Kamien et al. 1975. Austr. N.Z. J. Med. 5, 123–133.
	Lysine, other amino acids	Bressani. 1975. In Nutritional Evaluation, Food Processing, 2nd Ed., AVI/Van Nostrand Reinhold, New York.
	Lysine	Bressani et al. 1963. J. Nutr. 79, 333–339. Pereira et al. 1969. Am. J. Clin. Nutr. 22, 606–611. Graham et al. 1969. Am. J. Clin. Nutr. 22, 1459–1468.

TABLE 5.13 (*Continued*)

Cereal Product	Nutrients	Reference
		Graham et al. 1971. Am. J. Clin. Nutr. *24*, 200–206.
		Vaghefi et al. 1974. Am. J. Clin. Nutr. *27*, 1231–1246.
		el Lozy and Kerr. 1976. 2nd workshop on Fortification, AID, Wash. DC.
		Gershoff. 1976. Proc. West. Hemisphere Nutr. Congr. *V*, 41–45.
	Lysine, threonine	Daniel et al. 1968. Ind. J. Nutr. Dietet. *5*, 134–141.
	Lysine	Reddy. 1971. Am. J. Clin. Nutr. *24*, 1246–1249.
		Yasoda and Geervani. 1979. Ind. J. Nutr. Dietet. *16*, 48–51.
		Hoffman and McNeil. 1949. J. Nutr. *38*, 331–334.
		Scrimshaw et al. 1973. Am. J. Clin. Nutr. *26*, 965–972.
	Riboflavin	Guggenheim et al. 1959. Am. J. Clin. Nutr. *7*, 526–531.
Bread	Lysine, vitamin B_{12}	Fukui et al. 1959–60. Tokushima J. Exptl. Med. *6*, 89–97, 269–274; *8*, 1–14.
	Lysine	Krut et al. 1961. S. African J. Lab. Clin. Med. *7*, 1–12.
		King et al. 1963. Am. J. Clin. Nutr. *12*, 36–48.
		Oiso. 1971. *In* Amino Acid Fortification of Protein Foods, MIT Press, Cambridge.
		Rice et al. 1970. J. Nutr. *100*, 847–854.
	Iron sources	Steinkamp et al. 1955. Arch. Internal. Med. *95*, 181–193.
		Elwood et al. 1971. Clin. Sci. *40*, 31–37.
		Cook et al. 1973. Am. J. Clin. Nutr. *26*, 861–872.
Pasta	Thiamin, riboflavin, pantothenate, vitamin A, calcium	Doraisuamy et al. 1968. J. Food Sci. Technol. *5*, 8–11.
Farina	Lysine	Barness et al. 1961. Am. J. Clin. Nutr. *9*, 331–344.
Breakfast cereals (RTE)	Vitamins, minerals	Franta. 1976. Cereal Foods World *21*, 550, 552.
	7 nutrients	Zabik. 1987. Cereal Foods World *32*, 234–239.

TABLE 5.13 (*Continued*)

Cereal Product	Nutrients	Reference
Rice product	Thiamin, niacin, iron	Salcedo et al. 1949. J. Philippines Med. Assoc. 25, 519–534.
		Salcedo et al. 1949; J. Nutr. 38, 443–451; 1950; 42, 501–523.
		Burch et al. 1952. J. Nutr. 46, 239–254.
		Quioque. 1952. Am. J. Pub. Health 42, 1086–1094.
		Sevringhaus. 1952. Int. Rev. Vit. Res. 23, 348–355.
	Lysine, threonine	Bressani. 1975. *In* Nutritional evaluation. Food Processing, 2nd Ed., AVI/Van Nostrand Reinhold, New York.
	others	Hundley et al. 1957. Am. J. Clin. Nutr. 5, 316–326.
	Lysine, threonine, cystine, methionine	Chen et al. 1967. J. Nutr. 92, 429–434.
	Thiamin, riboflavin, pyridoxine, niacin, pantothenate, vitamin E, calcium, iron	Koyanagi et al. 1982. 36th Ann. Meeting Japan Soc. Food Nutr.
		Igarashi et al. 1984. Nipon Eiyo Shokuryo Gakkaishi 37, 145–150.
	Thiamin, riboflavin, vitamin A, iron with or without lysine and threonine	Gershoff. 1976. Proc. West. Hemisphere Nutr. Congr. V, 41–45.
		Gershoff et al. 1977. Am. J. Clin. Nutr. 30, 1185–1195.
	Iron	Hallberg et al. 1978. Am. J. Clin. Nutr. 31, 1403–1408.
Corn product	Lysine, tryptophan, isoleucine	Truswell and Brock. 1958. S. Africa Med. J. 33, 98–105.
	Lysine	Kies et al. 1962. J. Nutr. 92, 377–383.
	Riboflavin, niacin	DuPlessis et al. 1974. S. Africa Med. J. 48, 1641–1649.
	Folate	Colman et al. 1974. Am. J. Clin. Nutr. 27, 339–344.
		Colman et al. 1974. S. Africa Med. J. 48, 1763–1766.
		Colman et al. 1982. Nutr. Rev. 40, 225–233.
	Lysine, thiamin, riboflavin, niacinamide, vitamin A, iron	Urrutia et al. 1976. 2nd Workshop on Fortification, AID, Wash. DC.
	Lysine, tryptophan	Gomez et al. 1957. Acta Paediat. 46, 286–294.

TABLE 5.13 (*Continued*)

Cereal Product	Nutrients	Reference
	Vitamins, minerals, lysine, tryptophan	Bressani *et al.* 1976. 2nd Workshop on Fortification, AID, Wash. DC.
	Lysine, tryptophan, isoleucine, methionine	Scrimshaw *et al.* 1958. J. Nutr. *66*, 485–499.
		Bressani *et al.* 1958. J. Nutr. *66*, 501–513.
	Thiamin, riboflavin, niacin, iron	Lease. 1953. J. Am. Dietet. Assoc. *29*, 866–871.
	Thiamin, riboflavin, vitamin A, iron	Molina *et al.* 1973. INCAP/AID Conf. on Nutr. Improvement of Corn. Guatemala.

proposals) were in effect a more substantial contribution would have been evident in the case of some of the other nutrients charted. Examples of the favorable influence of vitamin nutrification are the dramatic decrease in the incidence of beriberi by addition of thiamin to rice and wheat flour and of pellagra by adding niacin to corn meal or grits. Nutrification of cereal grains with various protein sources or with one or more amino acids has been found in some studies (but not in others) to improve growth and public health. Iron-deficiency anemia has been reported to amenable to regulation by improved iron nutrition. See successful nutrification programs in Chapter 2.

If the objective of a particular nutrification project is not achieved, there may be a variety of underlying causes for such findings.[15] For example, no improvement can be attributed to the study of lysine nutrification of wheat products in Tunisia. Some likely reasons for the lack of effect are that: (1) no nutritional intervention can, in isolation, have any effect without correction of the numerous problems (health, sanitation, ignorance, poverty, etc.) which afflict a developing society; (2) low caloric intakes with the added protein or amino acids may have been used for energy; (3) protein quality may be a less important factor than previously believed in that population sequence; or (4) the presence of a specific, uncorrected, more limiting dietary deficiency masked the effect of nutrient addition under study. With cereal nutrification, as with all nutrition interventions, there are barriers to effective implementation. The identification, understanding, and evaluation of each obstacle is essential to determining the feasibility of a nutrification project. Also, it must be recognized that nutrification of food is not a panacea for all nutritional ills or deficiency situations.

BARRIERS TO IMPLEMENTING CEREAL GRAIN NUTRIFICATION

Austin and Snodgrass[127] mention several categories of potential barriers to the implementation of a cereal nutrification program.

200 NUTRIENT ADDITIONS TO FOOD

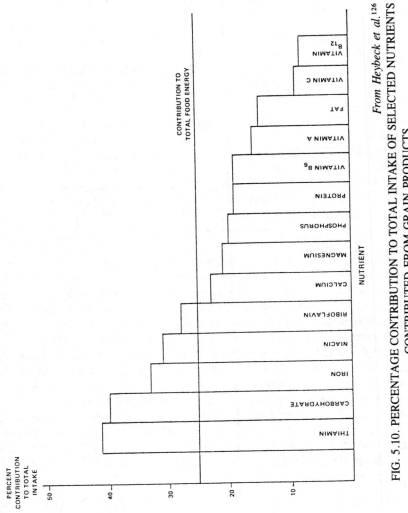

FIG. 5.10. PERCENTAGE CONTRIBUTION TO TOTAL INTAKE OF SELECTED NUTRIENTS CONTRIBUTED FROM GRAIN PRODUCTS

From Heybeck et al.[126]

Diet Adequacy

In the case of protein inadequacy, particularly in growing children, nutrification of cereal grain products with amino acids has been postulated to have little or no value for growth improvement in the face of insufficient calories. In any clinical field study it is advisable to control most, if not all, of the critical nutrients in the nutrification program, as well to control associated health influences.

Technology Concerns

Technical problems may be encountered in the process of introducing the active ingredient(s) in a chosen carrier for a particular cereal food or class of food products. In general, technological problems can be resolved as shown by past experience and data and do not appear to represent a serious impediment to cereal grain nutrification. If new circumstances create technological problems not hitherto encountered, research and development laboratories can probably solve them. Where unacceptable instability problems are encountered, attention need be given to processing variables, temperature, pH, light and oxygen exposure, metal incompatibilities, antioxidant usage, or the use of alternative or coated forms of the added nutrient or added protective compounds. Following are some limitations that may influence nutrified cereal products adversely.

(1) The yellow color of riboflavin included in a white rice premix: Some consumers will object to the presence of colored premix particles either before or after cooking. As previously noted, Lease et al.[124] found only a small percentage of consumers concerned about the color of cooked rice enriched with a powdered premix or with a rinse-resistant premix containing the more soluble riboflavin-5′-phosphate ester, a more expensive form of riboflavin.

(2) Degradation of thiamin may, in some foods, cause an off-odor problem. In high pH bakery products, chocolate cake, soda crackers, etc., thiamin is quite labile. This is a characteristic of thiamin; it becomes unstable as alkaline pH values rise.

(3) Ferrous sulfate added to flour or other cereal products may cause development of objectionable odor after prolonged storage. It can also lead to color changes in flour and cake mixes. Crackers, sprayed with oil but fortified with ferrous sulfate tend to develop rancidity rapidly since iron accelerates oxidation. Ferrous sulfate causes deterioration of flavor and odor of dry-milled corn products such as grits or meal on storage, but reduced iron powder does not. The color of reduced iron may cause slight darkening of white cereal products. Under some circumstances powdered iron could create separation problems due to its high density.

(4) Poor heat stability of L-ascorbic acid occurs in baked goods. A partial remedy, if it applies, is to spray on a formulation containing ascorbic acid after the heating period or include it in an icing or a filling after baking by coating or injection techniques.

(5) Introduced at high levels, certain calcium and magnesium compounds may create textural and/or organoleptic problems. The form and sequence in the process at which these minerals, especially magnesium, are added is critical.

Food Systems

One must examine the flow of the cereal product from production through distribution to consumption. How much of the product passes through centralized mills, and, therefore, can be easily nutrified? In rural areas, many poor families may mill their own grain by hand and be unreachable for various reasons by a nutrification program. What is the likelihood that the nutrified product will reach the nutritionally vulnerable, low income families? Poorer families generally have greater dependence, on cereals, even in the United States, which makes the cereals effective vehicles for nutrification; but the type of product, packaging or distribution practice may limit target use. To reach the needy groups, a decentralized milling structure may allow regional and even village targeting, which can reduce costs dramatically, especially where deficient groups tend to be concentrated in certain developing areas.

Full Acceptance

A desired characteristic of nutrification is that it does not affect the appearance or organoleptic properties of the food carrier. Furthermore, preparation and cooking characteristics and storage stability are also important parameters in determining acceptability of a nutrified product program. When the nutrification is performed at the village level, it is highly visible to all and its acceptance or nonacceptance is easily influenced by the consumers. It is essential if the nutrification program is to be successful that it be fully accepted over time.

Economics

The economic barrier is in some respects the most basic obstacle to nutrification feasibility. For nutrification with synthetic amino acids or natural proteins, the cost of these nutrifying ingredients predominate, while the cost of microingredients (vitamins and minerals) usually represents a much smaller fraction of the total cost of the nutrified product. The nutrients chosen for nutrification must be reconciled with the costs and who is paying for the dietary improvement.

All nutrification costs must be balanced against the cost of not implementing a program, which may arise from such health factors as disease, impaired physical and mental growth, medical costs, dietary imbalances, and decreased productivity.

Legislation

Prior food legislation may exist in a country which prohibits or limits the addition of certain nutrients to a food. Where such decrees may have been established in years past for reasons pertinent to the time, their repeal or modification may be necessary before contemplated food nutrification programs can proceed.

REFERENCES

1. LORENZ, K. and LEE, V. 1977. The nutritional and physiological impact of cereal products in human nutrition. CRC Crit. Rev. Food Sci. Nutr. 8(4), 383–456.
1a. DRAKE, D. L., GEBHARDT, S. E. and MATTHEWS, R. N. 1989. Composition of Foods: Cereal Grains and Pasta: Raw, Processed and Prepared. Agr. Handbook 8-20. U.S.D.A. HNIS, Washington, DC.
2. LOCKHART, H. B. and NESHEIM, R. O. 1978. Nutritional Quality of Cereal Grains. Sixth International Cereal & Bread Congress. Am. Assoc. Cereal Chem., St. Paul.
3. NELSON, J. H. 1985. Wheat: Its processing and utilization. Am. J. Clin. Nutr. 41, 1070–1076.
4. POMERANZ, Y. 1988. Wheat: Chemistry and Technology. Am. Assoc. Cereal Chem., St. Paul.
5. JULIANO, B. D. 1985. Rice: Chemistry and Technology. Am. Assoc. Cereal Chem., St. Paul.
6. SENTI, F. R. and SCHAEFER, W. C. 1972. Corn, its importance in food, feed and industrial uses. Cereal Sci. Today 17(11), 352–356.
7. WATSON, S. A. and RAMSTAD, P. E. 1987. Corn: Chemistry & Technology. Am. Assoc. Cereal Chem., St. Paul.
8. POMERANZ, Y. 1973. Food uses of barley. CRC Crit. Rev. Food Technol. 4(3), 377–394.
9. RASMUSSEN, D. C. 1985. Barley. Am. Soc. Agronomy, Madison.
10. BUSHUK, W. 1976. Rye: Production, Chemistry and Technology. Am. Assoc. Cereal Chem., St. Paul.
11. WEBSTER, F. N. 1986. Oats: Chemistry and Technology, Am. Assoc. Cereal Chem., St. Paul.
12. CASEY, P. and LORENZ, K. 1977. Millet: functional and nutritional properties. Bakers Dig. 51(1), 45–51.
13. HULSE, J. H. 1980. Sorghum and the Millets: Composition and Nutritive Value. Academic Press, New York.
14. PAULINO, L. A. 1986. Food in the Third World: Past Trends and Projections. Res. Rept. 52. International Food Policy Institute, Washington, DC.
15. AUSTIN, J. E. 1979. Global Malnutrition and Cereal Fortification, Ballinger Publishing Co., Cambridge.
16. ANON. 1974. Proposed Fortification Policy for Cereal Grain Products. NRC Rept. National Academy of Sciences, Washington, DC.
17. COOK, D. A. and WELSH, S. O. 1987. The effect of enriched and fortified grain products on nutrient intake. Cereal Foods World 32(2), 191–196.

18. CLARK, H. E. 1978. Cereal-based diets to meet protein requirements of adult man. World Rev. Nutr. Dietet. *32*, 27–48.
19. LACHANCE, P. 1981. Role of cereal grain products in the US diets. Food Technol. *35*(3), 49–60.
20. LACHANCE, P. 1982. Role of grain based food in supplying nutrients. In Adding Nutrients to Foods, J. L. Vetter (ed.). Am. Assoc. Cereal Chem., St. Paul.
21. LEVEILLE, G. A. 1988. Current attitudes and behavior trends regarding consumption of grains. Food Technol. *42*(1), 110–111.
22. ANON. 1989. Food consumption. Natl. Food Rev. *12*(2), 1–9.
23. MULLER, H. G. and TOBIN, G. 1980. Nutrition and Food Processing. AVI/Van Nostrand Reinhold, New York.
24. JOHNSON, A. and PETERSON, M. S. 1974. Encyclopedia of Food Technology. AVI/Van Nostrand Reinhold, New York.
25. WU, Y. V. and INGLETT, C. E. 1987. Effects of agricultural practices, handling. processing and storage of cereals. In Nutritional Evaluation of Food Processing, 3rd Ed., E. Karmas and R. S. Harris (eds.). AVI/Van Nostrand Reinhold, New York.
26. KIK, M. C. and WILLIAMS, R. R. 1945. Nutritional Improvement of White Rice. NRC Bull. No. 112. National Academy of Sciences, Washington, DC.
27. MORAN, R. 1959. Nutritional significance of recent work on wheat, flour and bread. Nutr. Abstr. Rev. *29*, 1–16.
28. THOMAS, B. 1968. Nutritional-physiological views in processing cereal products. Vegetables *15*, 360.
29. SCHROEDER, H. A. 1971. Losses of vitamins and trace minerals resulting from processing and preservation of foods. Am. J. Clin. Nutr. *24*, 562–573.
30. HOSENEY, C. 1986. Principles of Cereal Science and Technology. Am. Assoc. Cereal Chem., St. Paul.
31. PEDERSON, B. and EGGUM, B. O. 1983. Influence of milling on nutritive value of flour from rye. Qual. Plant Plant Foods Hum. Nutr. *32*, 185–196.
32. PEDERSON, B. and EGGUM, B. O. 1983. Influence of milling on nutritive value of wheat. Qual. Plant Plant Foods Hum. Nutr. *33*, 51–61.
33. PEDERSON, B. and EGGUM, B. O. 1983.Influence of milling on nutritive value of barley. Qual. Plant Plant Foods Hum. Nutr. *33*, 99–112.
34. PEDERSON, B. and EGGUM, B. O. 1983. Influence of milling on nutritive value of rice. Qual. Plant Plant Foods Hum. Nutr. *33*, 267–278.
35. PEDERSON, B. and EGGUM, B. O. 1983. Influence of milling on nutritive value of maize. Qual. Plant Plant Foods Hum. Nutr. *33*, 299–311.
36. PEDERSON, G. and EGGUM, B. O. 1983. Influence of milling on nutritive value of sorghum. Qual. Plant Plant Foods Hum. Nutr. *33*, 313–326.
37. HEGEDUS, M., PEDERSON, B. and EGGUM, B. O. 1985. Influence of milling on nutritive value of cereal grains. Qual. Plant Plant Foods Hum. Nutr. *35*, 175–180.
38. LORENZ, K. 1982. Enrichment and fortification of cereal based products in the U.S.A. Lebensm.-Wiss. Technol. *15*, 121–125.
39. SEBRELL, W. H. 1941. Public health aspect of enriched flour and bread. Conference of Bakers and Millers, Chicago; 1953. Public Health Repts. *68*(8), 741–746.
40. WILDER, R. M., WILLIAMS, R. R. 1944. Enrichment of Flour and Bread. NRC Bull. No. 110 National Academy of Sciences, Washington, DC.
41. PARKER, F. M. 1945. Notes on enrichment. Bull. Assoc. Operative Millers, July.

42. BRADLEY, W. B. 1962. Thiamin enrichment in the United States. Ann. N.Y. Acad. Sci. *98*, 602–606.
43. ANON. 1958. Cereal Enrichment in Perspective. NRC Rept. National Academy of Sciences, Washington, DC.
44. Am. Inst. Nutr. 1939. Proceeding of the 6th Annual Meeting. J. Nutr. Suppl. *17*, 22.
45. STIEBLING, N. K. and PHIPARD, E. F. 1939. Diets of families of employed wage earners and clerical workers in cities. Circ. No. 507. U.S. Dept. Agr., Washington, DC.
46. ANON. 1941. Title 21-Foods and drugs. Chapter I: Food and Drug Administration. Part 15: Wheat flour and related products; definitions and standards of identity. Fed. Reg. *6*, May 27, 2574–2582.
47. LEASE, E. J., RINGROSE, R. C. and LEASE, J. G. 1942. Combating dietary deficiencies with enriched and fortified foods. Circ. No. 62., So. Carolina Agr. Expt. Sta., Clemson.
48. LEASE, E. J. 1953. Corn meal enrichment. J. Am. Dietet. Assoc. *19*, 866–871.
49. LEASE, E. J., BRUNSON, J. P. and McDILL, J. 1955. Rice Enrichment in South Carolina. Rice. J. *58*(9), 14–19.
50. DICK, J. W. 1987. Quality aspects of pasta products. *In* Cereals and Legumes in the Food Supply, J. Dupont and E. Osman (eds.). Iowa State University Press, Ames.
51. DOUGLASS, J. S. and MATHEWS, R. N. 1982. Nutrient content of pasta products. Cereal Foods World *27*(11), 558–561.
52. FAST, R. B. and CALDWELL, E. L. 1990. Breakfast Cereals and How They Are Made. Am. Assoc. Cereal Chem., St. Paul.
53. HAYDEN, E. B. 1980. Breakfast cereals: trend foods for the 1980s. Cereal Foods World *25*(4), 141–143.
54. STEELE, C. J. 1976. Cereal fortification: technological problems. Cereal Foods World *21*(4), 538–540.
55. BUNCH, K. and WENDLAND, B. 1986. Grain products regain popularity. Natl. Food Rev. NFR-34 (summer), 1–5.
56. ZABIK, M. E. 1987. Impact of ready-to-eat cereal consumption on nutrient intake. Cereal Foods World *32*(3), 234–238.
57. SHAUGHNESSY, D. E. 1976. Food for Peace Programs and Marketplace. Proc. Meeting of Oregon Wheat Growers League, Portland.
58. HOOVER, S. R. and SENTI, F. R. 1969. Enrichment and fortification of U.S.A. donated foods. Proc. 8th Int. Congress, Nutr., Prague.
59. WILDER, R. M. 1956. A brief history of the enrichment of flour and bread. JAMA *162*(17), 1539–1541.
60. AXFORD, D. W. E. and WILLIAMS, D. A. 1981. Flour enrichment around the world. FMBRA Bull. No. 4. Flour Milling and Baking Res. Assoc., Hartfordshire.
61. RANUM, P., KULP, K. and BARRETT, F. 1982. Cereal fortification programs. Proc. 7th World Cereal and Bread Congress, Prague:1983. Developments in Food Science *5B*, 1055–1063.
62. BAUERNFEIND, J. C. 1988. Nutrification of food. *In* Modern Nutrition in Health & Disease, 7th Ed. M. E. Shils and Y. R. Young (eds.). Lea & Febiger, Philadelphia.
63. EMODI, A. S. and SCIALPI, L. 1980. Quality of bread fortified with ten micronutrients. Cereal Chem. *51*, 1–3.
64. HEPBURN, F. N. 1976. Status report on FNB proposal for cereal fortification. Cereal Foods World *21*(8), 360–362.

65. ANON. 1978. Technology of fortification of cereal grain products. Proc. workshop held May 16–17, 1977. National Research Council, Washington, DC.
66. VETTER, J. L. 1979. Final Report - Inter Industry Committee: Amer. Inst. Baking, Manhattan; 1979. Food Processing. April issue, 38; 1979. Expanded Fortification of Bakery Goods. AIB Tech. Bull. *1*(12), 1–5.
67. VETTER, J. L. 1982. Adding Nutrients to Foods: Where Do We go from Here? Am. Assoc. Cereal Chem., St. Paul.
68. PONTE, J. G. 1982. Expanded flour and bread enrichment and fortification. Proc. 7th World Cereal and Bread Congress, Prague.
69. JANSEN, G. R. 1971. Food fortification and enrichment. *In* Consumer Concerns—Food Proceedings. Colorado State Univ. Dept. Food Sci. & Nutr., Fort Collins.
70. SWAMINATHAN, M. and DANIEL, V. A. 1968. Enrichment and fortification of foods with nutrients as a means for overcoming malnutrition in developing countries. J. Nutr. Dietet. *5*, 316–336.
71. DAVIS, D. R. 1981. Wheat and nutrition. Nutr. Today *16*(4), 16–21;(5), 22–24.
72. RANUM, P. M., BARRETT, F. F., LOEWE, R. J. and KULP, K. 1980. Nutrient levels in internationally milled white flours. Cereal Chem. *57*(5), 361–366.
73. KULP, K., GOLOSINEC, O. C., SHANK, C. W. and BRADLEY, W. B. 1956. Current practices in bread enrichment: nutritive content of enriched bread. J. Am. Dietet. Assoc. *32*(4), 331–33.
74. GAGE, J. D. 1984. Enriched super bread: labeling and production aspects. Bakers Dig. Mar. 13, 25.
75. WOLF, S. K. 1974. Fortified loaf delivers superior nutrition yet retains natural flavor appeal. Food Prod. Dev. *8*(9), 18,24,29.
76. MORRIS, C. E. 1981. Whole white bread matches nutrition of whole wheat. Food Eng. *63*(9), 69.
77. LABELL, F. M. 1984. Bakers can now make bread more nutritious. Food Proc. *45*(4), 64–65.
78. CRAFT, P. J. 1985. This special bread may prove to be a kid's choice. Food Eng. *57*(3), 70–71.
79. ANON. 1983. Fortification of Cereal Grains with Essential Vitamins and Minerals U.S. House of Representative Rep. 179, dated 4/29/82. U.S. Government Printing Office, Washington, DC.
80. BORENSTEIN, B. 1974. Enrichment of wheat food products. *In* Wheat: Production and Utilization, G. E. Inglett (ed.). AVI/Van Nostrand Reinhold, New York.
81. BROOKE, C. L. 1968. Enrichment and fortification of cereal and cereal products with vitamins and minerals. J. Agr. Food Chem. *16*(2), 163–167.
82. RANUM, P. M. 1977. The cost of implementing the NRC proposed fortification policy for cereal-grain products. Proc. Workshop on Technology of Fortification of Cereal-Grain Products. National Research Council, Washington, DC.
83. KEAGY, P. M. *et al.* 1980. Natural levels of nutrients in commercially milled wheat flours: vitamin analysis. Cereal Chem. *57*(1), 59–65.
84. LORENZ, K., LOEWE, R., WEADON, D. and WOLF, W. 1980. Natural levels of nutrients in commercially milled wheat flours: mineral analysis. Cereal Chem. *57*(1), 65–69.
85. KULP, K., RANUM, R. M., WILLIAMS, P. C. and YANSZAKI, W. T. 1980. Natural

levels of nutrients in commercially milled wheat flour: description of samples and approximate analysis. Cereal Chem. 57(1), 54-58.
86. RANUM, P. M. 1980. Note on levels of nutrients to add under expanded flour fortification/enrichment programs. Cereal Chem. 57(1), 70-72.
87. ANON. 1987. Health Protection and Food Laws. Food to which vitamins, minerals, amino acids may be added: flour, p. 38. Canadian Minister of Health and Welfare, Ottawa.
88. BORENSTEIN, B. and GORDON, H. T. 1987. Addition of vitamins, minerals and amino acids to foods. In Nutritional Evaluation of Food Process ing, 3rd Ed., E. Karmas and R. S. Harris (eds.). AVI/Van Nostrand Reinhold, New York.
89. RUBIN, S. H. and CORT, W. M. 1969. Aspects of vitamin and mineral enrichment. In Protein Enriched Foods for World Needs M. Milner (ed.). Am. Assoc. Cereal Chem., St. Paul.
90. LUI, L. I. and PARRISH, D. B. 1979. Biopotency of vitamin A in fortified flour and accelerated storage. J. Agr. Food Chem. 27, 1134-1136.
91. PARRISH, D. B., EUSTACE, W. D., PONTE, J. G. and HEROD, L. 1980. Distribution of vitamin A in fortified flours and effect of processing, simulated shipping and storage. Cereal Chem. 57(4), 284-287.
92. PARRISH, D. B., HEROD, L., PONTE, J. G., SEIB, P. A., TSEN, C. C. and ADAMS, K. A. 1980. Recovery of vitamin A in processed foods made from fortified flours. J. Food Sci. 45(5), 1438-1439.
93. MURPHY, P. A. 1989. Chemical stability of vitamin-fortified wheat for developing countries. 198th ACS National Meeting Abstracts, Sept. 10-15.
94. GORDON, H. T., JOHNSON, L. E. and BORENSTEIN, B. 1985. The use of beta carotene in bakery products. Cereal Foods World 30(40), 274-276.
95. GORDON, H. T. and BAUERNFEIND, J. C. 1982. Carotenoids as food colorants. CRC Crit. Rev. Food Sci. Nutr. 18, 59-97.
96. HOLLENBECK, C. M. and OBERMEYER, H. G. 1952. Relative stability of thiamin mononitrate and thiamin chloride hydrochloride in enriched flour. Cereal Chem. 29, 82-87.
97. OTTENHEIM, H. H. and JENNESKENS, P. J. 1970. Synthetic amino acids and their use in fortifying foods. J. Agr. Food Chem. 18, 1010-1014.
98. CLYDESDALE, F. M. and WIEMER, K. L. 1985. Iron Fortification of Foods. Academic Press, Orlando.
99. HALLBERG, L., ROSSANDER-HULTHÉN, L. and GRAMATHKOVSKI, E. 1989. Iron fortification of flour with a complex ferric orthophosphate. Am. J. Clin. Nutr. 50, 129-135.
100. RANHOTRA, G. S., LOEWE, R. J. and PUYAT, L. v. 1977. Bioavailability and functionality of zinc in various organic and inorganic sources. Cereal Chem. 54, 496-499.
101. RANHOTRA, G. S., LEE, C. and GELROTH, J. A. 1980. Expanded cereal fortification: Bioavailability and functionality (bread-making) of various calcium sources. Nutr. Rep. Int. 22(4), 469-475.
102. RANHOTRA, G. S., LOEWE, R. J., LEHMANN, T. A. and HEPBURN, F. N. 1976. Effect of various magnesium sources on breadmaking characteristics of wheat flour. J. Food Sci. 41, 952-954.
103. RANHOTRA, G. S. and WINTERRINGER, G. L. 1982. Use of magnesium powder in fortified bread. Cereal Chem. 58(6), 446-447.

104. RANUM, P. M., LOEWE, R. J. and GORDON, H. T. 1981. Effect of bleaching, maturing and oxidizing agents on vitamins added to wheat flour. Cereal Chem. 58(1), 32–35.
105. BAUERNFEIND, J. C. and BROOKE, C. L. 1973. Guidelines for nutrifying 41 processed foods. Food Eng. 45(6), 91–97.
106. GAGE, J. 1972. Food fortification, some visible and invisible cost considerations. Food Prod. Develop. 5(7), 20–21.
107. JOHNSON, L., GORDON, H. T. and BORENSTEIN, B. 1988. Vitamin and mineral fortification of breakfast cereals. Cereal Foods World 33(3), 280–283.
108. CORT, W. M., BORENSTEIN, B., HARLEY, J. H., OSADCA, M. and SCHEINER, J. 1976. Nutrient stability of fortified cereal products. Food Technol. 30(4), 52–60.
109. RUBIN, S. H., EMODI, A. and SCIALPI, L. 1977. Micronutrient additions to cereal products. Cereal Chem. 50(4), 895–904.
110. GRAHAM, R. P., MORGAN, A. I. JR., HART, M. R. and PENCE, J. W. 1968. Mechanisms of fortifying cereal grains and products. Cereal Sci. Today 13, 224–227.
111. KAWASAKI, C. 1961. Modified thiamin derivatives. Proc. 10th Pacific Sci. Congr. Univ. Hawaii.
112. KONDO, K., MITSUDA, H. and IWAI, K. 1951. Studies in the enrichment of white rice. Vitamin 4, 203–204.
113. MISAKI, M. and YASUMATSU, K. 1985. Rice enrichment and fortification In Rice: Chemistry and Technology, B. O. Juliano (ed.). Am. Assoc. Cereal Chem., St. Paul.
114. MITSUDA, H. and YASUMOTO, K. 1974. The amino acid fortification of intact cereal grains. In New Protein Foods, A. M. Altschul (ed.). Academic Press, New York.
115. HUNNELL, J. W., YASUMATSU, K. and MORITAKA, S. 1985. Iron enrichment of rice. In Iron Fortification of Foods. F. M. Clydesdale and K. L. Wiemer (eds.). Academic Press, Orlando.
116. FURTER, M. F., LAUTER, W. M., DE RITTER, E. and RUBIN, S. H. 1946. The enrichment of rice with synthetic vitamins and iron. Ind. Eng. Chem. 38, 486–493; also 1949. U.S. Pat. 2,475,133.
117. MICKUS, R. R. 1955. Seals enriching additives on white rice. Food Eng. (27(1) 91–93, 160.
118. LaPIERRE, R. 1955. U. S. Pat. 2,712,499.
119. BRAMALL, L. D. 1986. A novel process for the fortification of rice. Food Technol. (Australia) 38(7), 281–284.
120. LEASE, E. J., WHITE, H., LEASE, J. G. 1962. Enrichment of rice with riboflavin. Food Technol. 16(5), 146–148.
121. FIEGER, E. A. and WILLIAMS, V. R. 1945. U. S. Pat. 2,390,210.
122. PEIL, A., BARRETT, F., RHA, C. and LANGER, R. 1981. Retention of micronutrients by polymer coatings used to fortify rice. J. Food Sci. 47, 260–262.
123. VANOSSI, L. 1978. Vitamin enriched rice. Tecnia Moletoria 29(3), 172–174.
124. LEASE, E. J., MALPHRUS, L. D., MALPHRUS, R. K. and LEASE, J. G. 1958. Consumers reaction to rice enriched with riboflavin. Food Technol. (12(11), 620–622.
125. FURTER, M. F., LAUTER, W. M., RUBIN, S. H. and SIEMERS, G. F. 1947. The enrichment of corn grits with synthetic vitamins and iron. Trans. Am. Assoc. Cereal Chemists 5(1), 26–36.

126. HEYBACK, J. P., COCCODRILLI, G. D. and LEVEILLE, G. A. 1987. The contribution of consumption of processed food to nutrient intake status in the United States. *In* Nutritional Evaluation of Food Processing 3rd Ed., E. Karmas and R. S. Harris (eds.). AVI/Van Nostrand Reinhold, New York.

127. AUSTIN, J. E. and SNODGRASS, D. R. 1976. Cereal fortification: barriers to implementation. *In* Improving the Nutrient Quality of Cereals, H. L. Wilcke (ed.). Agency for International Development, Washington, DC.

CHAPTER 6

Foods Considered for Nutrient Addition: FOOD ANALOGS AND EXTRUDED OR BLENDED FOOD MIXTURES

R. DIXON PHILLIPS, Ph.D.
and
RONALD R. EITENMILLER, Ph.D.

INTRODUCTION

Analogs, blended foods, and extruded foods, like other nutrified products, are characterized by a specific target population, and the intent to accomplish specific nutritional-medical, philosophical or economic goals. Unlike most of the foods considered elsewhere in this volume, they are totally engineered from ingredients rather than being produced by fortifying (adding nutrients to) existing food products or commodities. These foods occupy a continuum from simple mixtures (blends), to blends which are extrusion cooked to impart texture, to sophisticated extrudates which resemble animal products (i.e., analogs). However, our discussion will be simplified by the fact that, most fall into two basic subcategories: Inexpensive blends for feeding undernourished or at-risk persons in developing countries, and relatively expensive, engineered analogs produced for consumers in developed countries who are motivated by health or philosophical reasons.

BLENDS FOR LDC FEEDING

The creation of scientifically crafted blends for feeding undernourished and at-risk persons in the developing countries began following World War II when the success of newly developed drugs in reducing deaths from infectious diseases made nutritional deficiencies more noticeable and prevalent as populations expanded.[1] The rationale underlying the ensuing endeavor was humanitarian, tempered with unease at the prospect of large hungry populations and the social and political instabilities they engender. Widespread awareness of the severity of malnutrition was promoted by the activities of the United Nation's Food and Agriculture Organization (FAO) whose nutrition Committee met first in 1948. In 1949, the Joint FAO/WHO (UN World Health Organization) Expert Committee on Nutrition met and recommended a study be initiated of the "poorly defined nutritional syndrome of the tropics and subtropics."[2] In the early 1950s, a number of surveys and conferences defined the nature of the problem, its causes, contributing circumstances, and likely victims, and began to struggle with counteractive measures.[3]

It became clear that the disease in question had been widely observed and reported in the medical literature under a variety of names since the early part of the century. The consensus emerged that it was due primarily to protein deficiency in the diet. Its victims were usually recently weaned children, although older children and adults might exhibit similar symptoms. The name which gained acceptance, kwashiorkor, is a Ghanaian tribal word which conveys the sense that the disease occurs in a child who is weaned when the next sibling is born,[4] thus this age group became the primary target for intervention efforts.[5] While breast milk from well-nourished mothers comprises the ideal and sufficient food for infants up to approximately 6 months of age, mothers in poor areas are seldom well nourished. An individual lactating female may be capable of producing only 500–600 mL of milk per day while her >5 kg infant requires >850 mL for proper growth.[6] At this time, or somewhat later if the mother has sufficient milk, the infant's increasing nutrient requirements necessitates the introduction of weaning foods. This precipitates an abrupt transition as the food given to weanlings is often of poor nutritional quality consisting of starchy paps or gruels.[6,7] Alternatively, there may be no special weaning foods, and children are shifted from the breast to an adult diet which is so bulky (low nutrient density) that weanlings cannot consume enough to meet their requirements.[6,8] Local customs and nutritional ignorance often forbid the feeding of the very types of food the child needs most.[6,7] Animal-derived foods may not be given due to cultural beliefs, or to the priority given adults, especially men.[8] Additionally, the food is often prepared from contaminated ingredients or is contaminated during preparation or storage.[6] This commonly leads to the development of enteric infections and diarrhea which, coupled with ignorance of disease and its causes, often condemns the child to death. In Central American for example, the belief that diarrhea results from parasites prompts treatment by giving laxatives and an even poorer, watery, low-protein diet.[7]

Given the rapid agreement that kwashiorkor is essentially protein malnutrition, it is logical that the early emphasis was heavily on protein deficiency, maldistribution and malnutrition. In later years it became popular to deemphasize protein while accentuating the lack of calories and other nutrients in developing country diets. The tension between these emphases was reflected by the Protein Advisory Group (PAG) of the UN which defended the emphasis on protein while stressing its broader interest in other nutrients.[9] Other, closely reasoned and detailed arguments on the unique problems of sufficient protein in actual diets of persons living under the less than ideal conditions of developing countries[10] may have served to moderate excessive "antiprotein" revisionism. Some research findings over the years have called into question the exclusive or even predominant role of protein deficiency in the development of kwashiorkor. For example, a recent hypothesis relates the disease symptoms to proliferation of free radicals in the body due to malnutrition, bacterial disease, or dietary toxins (e.g., aflatoxin).[11] At the same time, others have observed that the increasing consumption of cereals at the expense of higher-protein legumes arising from the "Green Revolution" have resulted in a return of kwashiorkor to some populations from which it had previously disappeared.[10] It seems certain that the etiology of the disease is complex, including an entire range of interacting social ills from malnutrition to hygiene, and that the immediate cause of particular manifestations depend on the stage of the syndrome being observed.

In the latter half of the 19th century, researchers in Europe and the United States set adult humans requirements for protein at about 1 g/day/kg of body weight to maintain N balance.[12] Following pioneering work on protein composition, studies in the mid 1900s established the first reliable values for amino acid requirements.[12] The third leg of this requirement triad, protein digestibility/amino acid availability, also has long roots, its variability among proteins being measured for over 100 years,[13] with steadily increasing emphasis. The most widely cited guidelines for protein and amino acid requirements and protein quality in terms of amino acid profile have been those published by FAO beginning in 1957 and continuing with updated versions in 1973 and 1985. Other groups, such as the Food and Nutrition Board and National Research Council of the United States have suggested similar profiles (Table 6.1).[14-17]

As an adduct or alternative to such guidelines, high-quality animal proteins such as egg or milk have served as standards for protein quality comparison. The abundance of milk on world markets in the 1950s meant that milk proteins were not only a standard of protein quality but, as nonfat dry milk (NFDM), became the currency of relief donations. Large quantities of NFDM were distributed by agencies such as UNICEF and by government agencies.[18] The use of milk for supplementing diets was limited, however, by its lack of acceptability in some cultues, the unlikelihood in many places (especially in the tropics) that indigenous production could be established on a scale sufficient to replace the donated material, and the shortage of NFDM in the United States and other donor countries which developed in the 1960s.[18,19] These factors spurred existing efforts to develop nutritious blended foods, principally from plant sources.[18]

The original authorization for food donations to needy countries by the United States was in the Agricultural Act of 1949 which was amended by the passage of Public Law 480, the Agricultural Trade Development and Assistance Act in 1954. These laws provided for both the sale and donation of surplus agricultural commodities to developing, at-need countries in an attempt to relieve hunger in and build trade relationships with developing countries, while reducing surpluses and supporting domestic prices in the United States. This program, administered by the U.S. Department of Agriculture, oversaw the export of 265 million tons of food worth more than $26 thousand million (U.S. billion) between 1955 and 1966. This comprised about 20% fo all food aid in that period.[20] In 1966, these donations reached about

TABLE 6.1
UN FOOD AND AGRICULTURE ORGANIZATION (FAO) AND U.S. FOOD AND
NUTRITION BOARD OR THE NATIONAL ACADEMY OF SCIENCES (FNB)
AMINO ACID REFERENCE PATTERNS FOR HUMANS
(mg Amino Acid/g Protein)

Amino Acid	FAO Pattern					FNB Pattern
	1957	1973	1985			1980
			2–5 Yr	10–12 Yr	Adult	
Histidine			19	19	16	17
Isoleucine	42	40	28	28	13	42
Leucine	48	70	66	44	19	70
Lysine	42	55	58	44	16	50
Methionine + Cystine	42	35	25	22	17	26
Phenylalanine + Tyrosine	56	60	63	22	19	73
Threonine	28	40	34	28	9	35
Tryptophan	14	10	11	9	5	11
Valine	42	50	35	25	13	48

Source: Taken from FAO;[14] FAO/WHO;[15,16] Food and Nutrition Board.[17]

100 million people in 112 countries. Seventy million of these were children, 40 million of which being reached in school lunch type programs and 10 million in maternal and child health programs. In 1979, over $1 (U.S.) billion worth of food was distributed.[21] The major commodities in this program were wheat, feed grains, rice, NFDM and edible oil. Of these, only NFDM was suitable for infant/child feeding per se. However about half of the corn and wheat was shipped as milled products, fortified at the same levels as specified by FDA for sale in the United States.[22]

It had been observed from the time of the earliest studies on protein quality that animal-derived proteins in flesh, milk or egg are superior to plant-derived proteins. These differences can be explained by the differing amino acid contents and availabilities in the various proteins. Table 6.2 contains values for protein content, amino acid profile and digestibility of selected protein sources.[13,23–27] Human requirements for specific nutrients suggests the principles by which blended foods were designed. Four approaches for arriving at satisfactory blends have been suggested.[28,29] These are: (1) supplementation of a deficient protein with pure amino acids; (2) supplementation with higher biological value-proteins; (3) the combination of two or more proteins which are deficient in different amino acids such that the resulting blend is superior to the components; (4) combinations of the previous three methods. Each of these approaches has been proven in both theoretical and applied studies. The fortification of lysine-deficient cereals with L-lysine has been shown to improve the overall protein quality; supplementation with a superior (usually animal-derived) protein has improved the quality of a poorer (usually plant) protein; and blends of complementary proteins have demonstrated superior quality to

TABLE 6.2
PROTEIN CONTENT AND DIGESTIBILITY AND ESSENTIAL AMINO ACID PROFILE OF SELECTED PROTEIN SOURCES

	Egg (Whole)	Beef (Average Cut)	Milk (NonFat Dry)	Corn (Whole Ground)	Wheat (Whole Ground)	Sorghum (Whole Ground)	Soybean (Defatted Meal)	Cottonseed (Defatted Meal)	Peanut (Defatted Meal)
% Protein[1] (as is)	12.9	13.6	35.9	8.9	13.3	11.0	47.0	48.1	47.9
% Protein[2] Digestibility	93–100	91–99	90–99	70–95	80–92	67–96	75–92[3]	78–98	91–98
Amino Acid[4] Profile (g/100 protein)									
Histidine	2.4	3.5	2.6	2.1	2.0	1.9	2.6	3.1	2.8
Isoleucine	6.6	5.2	6.4	4.6	4.4	5.4	5.8	4.5	4.7
Leucine	8.8	8.2	9.8	13.0	6.7	16.1	8.3	7.4	7.0
Lysine	6.4	8.7	7.8	2.9	2.8	2.7	6.8	5.1	4.1
Methionine + Cystine	5.5	3.7	3.3	3.2	3.7	3.4	3.4	3.6	2.7
Phenylalanine + Tyrosine	10.1	7.5	10.0	10.7	8.7	7.7	8.7	9.4	9.9
Threonine	5.0	4.4	4.6	4.0	2.9	3.6	4.2	4.2	3.1
Tryptophan	1.7	1.2	1.4	0.6	1.2	1.1	1.5	1.4	1.3
Valine	7.4	5.6	6.9	5.1		5.7	5.6	5.8	5.7

[1]Taken from Watt and Merrill.[26]
[2]Taken from Hopkins.[13]
[3]Taken from Kirby et al.;[23] Ilori and Conrad;[24] Pedersen and Eggum.[25]
[4]Taken from Orr and Watt.[27]

their ingredients.[28,29] However, when actual food proteins are blended, four types of products, not all of which are superior to the individual components, can be formed. The way in which nutritional quality varies with composition in these combinations is shown in Fig. 6.1. Type I represents the blending of protein sources with similar

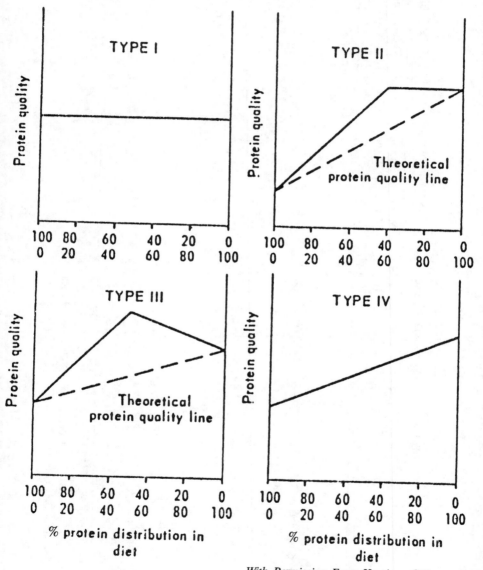

FIG. 6.1. TYPES OF RESPONSE LINES OBTAINED WHEN MIXING TWO PROTEIN SOURCES

With Permission From Harris and Karmas[45]

quality and similar amino acid limitations. An example given[28] is the combination of corn with peanut flour. No improvement in protein efficiency ratio (PER) was found because both proteins are limiting in lysine. Similarly, the addition of a purified form of protein to its source, e.g., addition of wheat protein concentration to wheat flour, increases the protein content but not the quality, providing the concentration process had not altered the amino acid profile. Type II behavior is observed when a balanced, superior protein (e.g., fish flour) is added to an inferior one (e.g., corn). Similar behavior would be expected upon supplementation with pure amino acid within the range likely to be practiced. Type III is the complementation pattern observed when cereal and legume proteins are blended. The cereal is usually limiting in lysine but with a slight excess of sulfur amino acids, while the legume is low in sulfur amino acids but contains ample lysine. The fourth type of behavior occurs when there is no supplementation and one protein is superior to the other. The example given was blends of sesame and cottonseed flours. Based on amino acid profile, it should be straightforward both to predict the specific type of behavior particular protein blends would exhibit and to design optimal blends from the amino acid profiles. However, variations in digestibility-availability often produce unexpected results.[28] Beyond the protein content and amino acid profile of plant-based blends, the proper level of calories, fat, vitamins and minerals must also be assured.[30] Thus, the formulation of plant protein-based mixtures becomes a matter of blending wholesome, available ingredients to meet the nutritional and sociological (cost, palatability) requirements of the target population.

In 1966, UNICEF collaborated with the U.S. food industry to develop formulas meeting the above requirements. Guidelines which evolved from this effort specified that such mixtures contain 18–20% protein and levels of vitamins and minerals comparable to (or as in the case of iron greater than) those in skim milk.[18] Specific PAG guidelines on high-protein mixtures followed[31] (Table 6.3). Guidelines which evolved in donor countries, such as the United States, revealed the complexity of the agendas which their governments were attempting to meet. Shortages of NFDM occurred in the United States (major source) in the early 1960s and prompted development of plant protein blends. In 1965 the USDA in cooperation with the U.S. Agency for International Development (USAID) and the U.S. National Institutes of Health (NIH) developed "Guidelines for Food Formulations for Infants and Children" and "Permissible Ranges in Composition and Nutrient Content for the Food Formulations."[20] The nutrient content guidelines are summarized in Table 6.4.[19] Compositions of two of the earliest and most important blends are given in Table 6.5.[19] Other general specifications included the requirement that blends were to be partially precooked so as to be ready for eating after 1–2 min of boiling. This provided a mechanism for reducing deteriorative enzyme activity and saving fuel in developing countries while assuring sterilization prior to consumption. As PL 480 was still in effect, the use of corn or wheat as the cereal component and soy flour and NFDM as protein supplements were specified.[19] In 1966, U.S. policy underwent a significant change with the passage of the Food for Peace Act. There was a greater em-

TABLE 6.3
PAG GUIDELINES FOR PROTEIN-RICH SUPPLEMENTARY FOOD MIXTURES

	Units/10 Calories[1]	Units/100 g
Protein	5.4	Not less than 20 g[2]
Fat		As much as feasible, up to 10 g
Crude fiber		Not more than 5 g[3]
Moisture		Preferably 5–10 g
Total ash		Not more than 5 g
Acid-insoluble ash		Not more than 0.05 g
Vitamin A, retinol equivalent	108 mcg	400 mcg[4]
Thiamin	80 mcg	0.3 mg
Riboflavin	108 mcg	0.4 mg
Niacin	1330 mcg	5.0 mg
Folate	54 mcg	0.2 mg
Vitamin B_{12}	0.54 mcg	2.0 mcg[5]
Ascorbic acid	5400 mcg	20 mg
Vitamin D	108 IU	400 IU[6]
Calcium	80 mg	300 mg (as phosphate or carbonate)
Iron	2.7 mg	10 mg (as food-grade compound of adequate iron availability)
Iodine	28 mcg	100 mcg (as idodate or iodide)

Source: Anon.[31]

[1]Calculated on the basis of 370 kcal/100 g

[2]This protein level assumes an NPU not less than 60 and a PER not less than 2.1. If these values are higher, the level of protein may be reduced as follows: NPU = 80, 15 g; NPU = 75, 16 g; NPU = 70, 17.1 g; NPU = 65, 18.5 g.

[3]Crude fiber higher than this may be acceptable, although it would require clinical testing.

[4]1300 IU as vitamin A palmitate.

[5]Under certain local conditions, the addition of vitamin B6 (to approximately the level of thiamin) and of alpha-tocopherol should be considered.

[6]The values for vitamins and minerals are considered minimal, except in the case of vitamin D, where no further increase is desirable. The excess of each vitamin added during processing should be no greater than that needed to maintain label requirements over the expected shelf-life of the product.

phasis on nutrition and the requirement that only surplus commodities be distributed was dropped. While the well-being of U.S. agriculture and consumers was still carefully considered, there was also greater sensitivity to the needs of recipient countries.[32]

If the laws, policies and guidelines of international agencies, donor and receptor governments provide the strategy for attacking malnutrition, specific projects which design, produce, distribute and evaluate products and their impact comprise the tactics. Undergirding every project of this type are substantial research efforts in nutrition and food science, economics and sociology. In developing countries, such projects are often conducted at regional research centers such as the Institute of Nutrition of Central America and Panama (INCAP), and supported by international donor

TABLE 6.4
USAID/NIH GUIDELINES FOR FOOD FORMULATIONS
FOR INFANTS AND CHILDREN

Constituent	Minimum	Maximum
Energy (kcal)	350	
Protein (g)	18	22
Fat (g)	2	
Linoleic acid (g)	1	
Essential amino acids		
Lysine	0.95	
Methionine (g)	0.3	
Total S amino acids (g)	0.6	
Tryptophan (g)	0.22	
Threonine (g)	0.65	
Apparent NPU (%)	60.0	
PER	2.1	
Minerals		
Calcium (g)	0.5	0.6
Phosphorus	0.42	0.6
Sodium (g)	0.3	0.45
Iron (mg)	5.0	15
Copper (mg)	0.5	1
Iodine (mcg)	60.0	100
Zinc (mg)	2.5	5
Vitamins		
A (units)	1500	2250
D (USP units)	200	250
C (mg)	20	
Alpha-tocopheral acetate (IU)	1.5	
Thiamin (mg)	0.5	
Riboflavin (mg)	0.5	
Niacin (mg)	6.0	
Pantothenic acid (mg)	3.0	
Pyridoxine (B_6) (mg)	0.35	
B_{12} (mcg)	3.0	
Folacin (mg)	0.1	

Source: Senti.[19]

and voluntary agencies. In developed countries, government laboratories, universities and commercial food industry have each played a major role. The key steps of projects built around rationally designed blends are: (1) Formulation: setting the desired level of nutrients and choosing the ingredients to provide them; (2) Processing: choosing the appropriate level of sophistication and specific processes leading to the desired form; (3) Product evaluation: safety, nutritional, and acceptability/tolerance testing of the resulting product; (4) Storage, marketing and distribution approaches; (5) Impact: assessing the degree of success of the intervention.[8] The choice of major ingredients depend on availability, cost and acceptability in the location where production is taking place. It should be noted that, while the macro components, cereals and legumes, may be available in both developing and industrialized countries, synthetic vitamins and isolated minerals are high-tech ingredients and may have to be supplied by donors to developing country programs. Alternatively, local sources of vitamins, such as specific green leaves, have been incorporated.

One of the earliest sustained efforts to design and produce plant protein-based blends was at INCAP where work began in the late 1950s and continued over more than a generation. The first blends were based on partially defatted sesame meal, cottonseed flour, skim milk, lime-treated and nonlime treated corn, kikuyu leaf meal (a local high-vitamin A source), torula yeast, L-lysine, plus added vitamins and minerals. INCAP vegetable mixture 8 was comprised of 50% lime treated corn (masa), 35% sesame flour, 9% cottonseed flour, 3% kikiyu leaf meal and 3% torula yeast. It gave a feed efficiency of 2.15, which was not improved by substitution of cottonseed by dry milk, nor by addition of 0.45% lysine.[33] Buckwheat proved superior to the true cereals while sorghum was inferior to corn and rice in the formulations.[34] The cost of sesame flour prompted development of INCAP mixture 9 containing equal parts of corn and sorghum plus cottonseed flour, yeast and leaf meal. INCAP mixtures 8 and 9 were utilized in human clinical trials with children who were recently recovered from, recovering from the acute phase of, and those admitted with the acute phase of malnutrition.[35,36] Experiments with recovered subjects revealed no problems of tolerance. In postacute-phase patients both mixtures promoted nitrogen retention similar to that from milk at protein intakes of 2 g/kg and above, although milk was better at lower intakes. In acute-phase patients, recovery was equivalent for milk-fed and mixture-fed patients.[37] Multigenerational studies to assess toxicological effects (due to gossypol or other toxins) of Incaparina were carried out in rats with negative results.[38] The increasing importance and availability of soy protein materials in the United States and elsewhere prompted the investigation of soy flour as a substitute for cottonseed flour in INCAP mixtures. This blend (mixture 14) contained 58% corn flour, 38% soybean flour, 3% torula yeast, 1% calcium phosphate, and 4500 IU of vitamin A/100 g. It proved to be superior to the cottonseed-based blends and almost equivalent to milk in rat studies, although it was deficient in sulfur amino acids at low protein levels.[39]

INCAP's policy was that Incaparina should be produced and distributed by private industry, but to assure the desired cost, quality and safety, cooperation between government, industry and INCAP would be required. This led to formal agreements between the Institute and companies considered competent to plan and execute market research as well as produce the product under INCAP guidelines. Marketability of the product was demonstrated in field acceptability trials in several Central American countries. Guatemala, the most populous country in the region and the home of

INCAP, was the site of the most extensive and successful effort to commercialize Incarparina. Cerveceria Centroamerican, S.A., a company with quality control, marketing and distribution capabilities, was chosen to produce and market the product. The operation started small and gradually expanded with numerous adjustments of marketing and distribution strategy. The product was sold for $0.24, then $0.20/lb. Sales expanded steadily in the first year reaching 100,000 lb. They were nearly 2 million lb in 1967. Surveys on consumption of Incaparina were conducted in 1965 and 1968. In the first, 389 families were sampled: 67% were familiar with the product; 45% were using it; 79% of those served it to all family members while 12% served it to children only. In the 1968 survey, 92% were familiar with Incaparina, 37% used it regularly and an additional 29% reported occasional use. Nonusers cited nonproduct reasons for not using it and had a favorable opinion of the price, preparation and availability. Of consumers, 64% gave Incaparina to children under 1 year, 89% to those 1–2 years, and 91% to 2–5 year olds. Interestingly, the reason given for the failure of these blends to penetrate the institutional market was the donation of other blends by the U.S.[40] Distribution of Incaparina in Colombia was undertaken by the Subsidiary of Quaker Oats in that country. The "model" for consumption of the blend was a thin grain-based gruel called coladas. The formulations chosen included corn, soy and cottonseed flours (Mixture 9), practically all ingredients being produced locally. The price was kept low, $0.12/500 g bag, which is competitive with beans and rice. While alternative ingredients were investigated, improvements in milling and mixing were responsible for increasing consumer acceptance. At the time of the report, Incaparina equivalent to 60 million glasses (at a protein cost of 0.002 pesos/g versus 0.02 for milk) were being marketed annually.[41] Incaparina in Nicaragua and El Salvador was not as successful as in Guatemala and Colombia due to the small size of the markets and the lack of expertise of the firms which attempted to commercialize it. However, a regional marketing scheme for those areas as well as small, government-subsidized effort in Panama were cited as future efforts.[40]

The development of guidelines for composition of blended foods promulgated in the mid 1960s led directly to the design and production of such foods for donation to needy countries by U.S. agencies. Ranges of various components were specified. A cereal:soy:NFDM ratio of 70:15:15 was optimal based on amino acid profile, but a 70:25:5 blend provided a satisfactory balance and was adopted by USDA for the first 2 products due to its lower cost and to the shortage of NFDM.[19] The first of these products, officially known as Blended Food Product, Child Food Supplement, Formula No. 1, was developed by the American Corn Millers Expert Institute as "CEPLAPRO." It foreshadowed future developments, an extruded rice analog made from degermed corn meal, durum wheat flour, soy flour and NFDM (58:10:25:5) supplemented with vitamins and minerals. It was first used for family feeding programs in Vietnam, where 713,000 lb costs $0.133/lb packaged in 50 lb bags and delivered to port.[19,42] It was reported to be acceptable, but its relatively high cost led to the development of the second product, corn-soy-milk. CSM is probably the best known of the products to be developed in the United States during this period. Extrusion was eliminated for this product to lower cost and because it was designed for feeding children as a gruel. CSM was developed by the American Corn Millers Federation in cooperation with USDA and was formulated to contain 64% precooked degerminated corn meal, 24% toasted soy flour, 5% NFDM, 5% soybean oil, and 2% of a mineral-vitamin premix. Alternative formulations utilizing full fat soy flour and corn germ fraction were permitted to achieve the desired fat content. Fat level of 2% was originally specified, but this was later raised to 6% (Table 6.5) as research eliminated anticipated problems with rancidity.[20] Animal feeding studies with CSM revealed a PER of 2.5, equivalent to that of casein. Human feeding studies on CSM were conducted in Peru, Taiwan and Algeria. In all cases the formulation was well tolerated and accepted (especially when sweetened) and produced satisfactory weight gain and nitrogen balance.[19] The availability of wheat in many areas of the world as well as recognition of the needs of the U.S. wheat industry prompted the development of mixture 3, wheat-soy blend (WSB). This product (Table 6.5) differed from CSM in the variety of cereal-derived ingredients it contained. Possible variations utilized straight-grade flour and wheat protein concentrate, bulgur flour and wheat protein concentrate, as well as soy flour, soy oil and mineral-vitamin mix. There was considerable variation in amino acid profile and nutritive quality among the various wheat components with white flour exhibiting a PER of 0.6–0.8 while wheat protein concentrate (derived from middlings by grinding and sieving) had a value of about 2.0. The final blends had PER values of about 2.1. It was found necessary to precook all the ingredients in this blend to inactivate enzymes associated with fat rancidity.[19] Satisfactory storage stability of CSM blends has been confirmed in both laboratory and field settings when appropriate conditions were employed. However, deterioration due to nonenzymatic browning becomes a problem when dextrose is added to the mix or when the blends are stored under abusive conditions.[20] These blends were designed for distribution through U.S. foreign aid channels, annual distribution reaching nearly 200,000 metric tons in 1979.[43] The programs at INCAP and in the United States and their products are only examples of the hundreds of similar efforts and blended foods around the world. An extensive compilation of active and terminated projects and products was published in 1981.[8] This list includes one hundred products from 41 countries in Africa, Asia, North and South America. In addition, in depth descriptions of projects and products in Sri Lanka, India, The Phillipines and Thailand may be found in Austin.[44]

EXTRUDED BLENDS

Although they were generally made of precooked ingredients and were cooked into thin gruels or beverages prior to consumption, the emphasis of most of the blends discussed previously was composition rather than processing. The need for thermal

TABLE 6.5
FORMULATION AND COMPOSITION OF U.S. FOOD FOR PEACE BLENDS[1]

Ingredient	Content (%)	Composition	Maximum (%)	Minimum (%)
Blended Food Product, Formula No. 2: Corn-Soy-Milk (CSM)				
Corn meal, processed	63.8	Moisture		10.0
Soy flour, defatted, toasted	24.2	Protein	19.0	
Nonfat dry milk	5.0	(N * 6.25)		
Soy oil, refined, stabilized	5.0	Fat	6.0	
Mineral-vitamin premix	2.0	Crude fiber		2.0
Blended Food Product, Formula No. 3 Wheat-Soy Blend (WSB)				
Wheat fractions, total	73.4	Protein	20.0	
(a) Straight-grade flour	38.4	(N * 6.25)		
(b) Wheat protein concentrate	35.0	Lysine	0.95	
or		Fat	6.0	
(a) Bulgur flour	53.4	Crude fiber		2.5
(b) Wheat protein concentrate	20.0	Ash		6.6
Soy flour, defatted	20.0	Moisture		11.0
Soy oil, refined, stabilized	4.0			
Minerals and vitamins	2.6			
providing the following levels of nutrients[2]				
Vitamin A (IU)	1658			
Vitamin D (USP units)	200			
Vitamin E (IU)	9.6			
Thiamin (mg)	1.49			
Riboflavin (mg)	0.59			
Niacin (mg)	9.1			
Vitamin B_6 (mg)	0.52			
Vitamin B_{12} (mg)	0.004			
Pantothenic acid (mg)	3.7			
Folacin (mg)	0.33			
Ascorbic acid (mg)	40			
Calcium (mg)	685			
Iron (mg)	20.8			
Phosphorus (mg)	562			
Magnesium (mg)	202			
Sodium (mg)	296			
Potassium (mg)	624			
Iodine (mg)	0.05			
Zinc (mg)	4.6			

[1] Taken from Senti.[19]
[2] Taken from Hover and Senti.[76]

processing in the production of high-protein blends arises from the nature of the ingredients and is further indicated by social and sanitary concerns. High-protein oilseeds and legumes generally contain a variety of toxic and antinutritional factors such as enzyme inhibitors and lectins which are heat labile. Protein and starch which have been denatured from their highly ordered native configurations have improved digestibility. Enzymes which produce rancidity in fat-containing foods are destroyed by heat. Cooking reduces the microbial load inherent to raw ingredients lowering the risks of enteric infections in the consumer.[45] The toasting of defatted soy flour or precooking of corn grits is a straightforward process in industrialized countries, where it is often an integral part of production of such materials. Necessary processing infrastructures often do not exist in developing countries. This fact leads to the need for careful consideration of the various options and scales of processes. A systematic analysis of the possibilities is presented in Heimendinger.[8] The lowest technology approach to producing nutritious blends features home processing. The costs and difficulties inherent in this approach depend on whether customary or new food ingredients are being utilized. A major cost/problem is that of information dissemination. For example, a project in Upper Volta (Burkina Faso) required the continuous effort of 300 village workers and 20 nurses to educate villagers and maintain the preparation of a weaning food for about 8,000 preschool children. At the next level, village-scale processing, there is need to organize a cooperative effort, purchase raw materials and to capitalize equipment. This is usually comprised of simple milling and mixing devices, although more sophisticated equipment such as extruders may be feasible. Industrial processing is the most ambitious technologically and requires markets of a sufficient size. Costs include raw materials, facilities, energy, packaging, advertising/education, labor and equipment capitalization. The more sophisticated the process, the larger the required scale. An analysis of possible industrial production of formulated food in the North Africa-Middle East region concluded that only in countries of more than 5 million would large scale production be economical. It was estimated that in such a country, the under-5 year old population is 10% of the total and that only 10–20% of them would be reached by the food. These would consume 300 g/week. This works out to an annual production of 600–1200 tons, anything less than which would not be profitable. Further, only 20–30% of production would be sold through commercial channels with the rest requiring government subsidy. The cost of a facility which would mill and blend a cereal-legume mix was estimated as $100,000 for startup and $0.028/kg for operating. Total costs of a 19–25% protein product would be $0.30/kg, of which 35% are attributed to raw materials and 28% for promotion.[46]

The desire to use indigenous crops for production of designed blends coupled with the lack of indigenous processing capability prompted investigation into appropriate technology which was transferable to developing countries. Much of this effort has centered around low cost extrusion cooking. The food extruder has been defined as "a flighted Archimedes screw which rotates in a tightly fitting cylindrical barrel."[47] This definition could be modified today to include the twin-screw extruder in which co- or counter-rotating screws fit into a figure 8 shaped barrel. Twin-screw machines have become very popular in the Western food industry, but are too complex and costly to fit into the low-cost category. An extruder operates by conveying raw ingredients down the barrel where they are cooked by the frictional dissipation of energy and/or externally applied heat. The extrusion process is attractive because of its versatility and low cost and because it is a high temperature-short time process. Thus, many of the traditional unit operations of food processing are integrated into a single process in extrusion. Because of the varying rates at which desirable and undesirable processes occur, ingredients can be processed so as to destroy undesirable factors while minimizing nutrient loss.[47] The feasibility and utility of low-cost extrusion cooking in the production of nutritious blends was studied in a major USAID-sponsored project (1974–80) conducted by Colorado State University in conjunction with other agencies.[48,49] Alternative processing equipment such as direct fired roasters were also examined, however it was concluded that drum cookers, which are often considered "lower technology" than extruders were unacceptable because of the cost and complexity of ancillary equipment (e.g., boilers). The characterization of low-cost extruders (LECs) was among the first activities of this project. The desired characteristics of such machines included low cost (< $50,000/ton/h extrusion costs), moderate production rate (250–2000 kg/h), simple operation (requiring minimal know-how), minimal auxiliary equipment (boilers, dryers, etc.), versatility (should handle a variety of cereals, legumes and oilseeds), low maintenance (by local personnel and parts as far as possible), sanitation (easily cleanable and suitable for human food). Three specific machines, the Brady crop cooker, the Insta-Pro Extruder and the Anderson Extruder were examined. It was concluded that the Brady was best for small-scale operations for producing precooked composites for gruels, weaning foods and the like. The Insta-Pro was found able to handle higher fat/moisture feeds than the other two and could make simple shaped products. The Anderson could make the broadest range of products, but was the most expensive, becoming competitive at production of over 2 metric tons (M.T.)/h. The first extrusion trials were on blends of corn and soy (CSB) to determine if co-extrusion of these ingredients produced a material comparable to that previously made under Title II guidelines. Blends containing 70% corn/30% soy were successfully extruded on Brady and Insta-Pro machines. They exhibited PER values of 2.5–2.9 (corrected) depending on whether either or both grains were decorticated, and microbial plate counts of < 1000. The same products made in Sri Lanka, Tanzania and Costa Rica had PERs of 2.0–2.3. Clinical trials confirmed the high nutritional quality of LEC-CSB. Other blends, 50–50 blends of chickpea with wheat, sorghum or rice supplemented with 10% NFDM after extrusion exhibited PERs greater than casein. Glanded cottonseed presents a different problem from other oilseed/legume ingredients due to the presence of gossypol, a toxic pigment. Unlike enzyme inhibitors and lectins, gossypol is heat denatured by reaction with available nucleophiles, often the epsilon amino group of lysine. Nonetheless, extrusion of cottonseed and cottonseed-cereal blends produced good protein quality when supplemented with lysine. In storage studies on extruded corn-soy blends which had been fortified with vitamins, minerals, and antioxidants after extrusion, the extrusion process was shown to greatly improve retention of vitamins and reduce production of free fatty acids and rancidity compared to raw controls stored up to 6 months.

The pioneering studies discussed above have resulted in much additional investigation into use of extrusion in producing nutritious blends.[50] Table 6.6 summarizes many of these efforts. Most have concentrated on cooked blends which are remilled for use as gruels, weaning foods, etc., however some effort has also gone into producing snacks and other textured items.[51]

ANALOGS

Analogs are products which resemble a traditional food in flavor, color, texture, appearance and use.[52] The general category includes such foods as margarine, whipped toppings and textured protein foods. In terms of nutritional impact, the most important analogs are those designed to simulate and/or extend traditional proteinaceous foods. Most of these are based on vegetable protein, however, more recently, restructured animal-based (e.g., surimi based) foods encompass a new category (in the West) of proteinaceous analogs. The first plant protein based meat analogs were produced more than 100 years ago, when J. H. Kellogg made veal steak-like product from fresh wheat gluten.[53] In 1954 Robert Boyer received the seminal patent in the field of protein texturization which described the production of vegetable protein fibers by a spinning process similar to that used for textile fibers. Since that time there have been hundreds of patents which modify and extend Boyer's process as well as those which strike out in totally new directions.[54]

The development of textured protein products was prompted by the desire of some to avoid meat and other animal products for health or religious reasons, and the potential cost advantages from the direct consumption of plant proteins. Pioneers, like Kellogg and the founders of companies like Worthington Foods in Ohio and Loma Linda Foods in California, were apparently prompted by the first consideration. Consumers who are not "motivated" by religious or philosophical beliefs are likely to purchase analogs to replace or extend traditional animal foods when the price differential is perceived to justify it. In addition, the desire to reduce fat and cholesterol, and increase fiber intake is sufficient to encourage some consumers to include analogs in their diets. Less publicized but of interest is the possibility that consumption of plant rather than animal proteins may in itself reduce serum cholesterol.[55] The relative costs of producing meat analogs compared to meat itself has been estimated in various ways. The length of time for which one acre's production can support the dietary protein needs of an individual may be computed for various protein sources. These figures range from 77 days for beef cattle to 527 days for wheat flour to 2224 days for soybeans.[56] Likewise if the cost per kilogram

TABLE 6.6
VEGETABLE MIXTURES PROCESSED BY LOW-COST EXTRUSION

Location	Ingredients	Formula (%)
INCAP	Corn/soybeans	81/15, 82/15, 70/30
	Rice/soybeans	81/18
	Oats/soybeans	82/18
	Sorghum/soybeans	70/30
	Cassava/soybeans	54/30
	Cowpea/corn + methionine	65/25, 72/28
	Cowpea/cassava + methionine	81/19
	Soybean/sesame	50/50
	Corn/soybean/sesame	72/14/14, 72/21/7
	Rice/soybean/sesame	72/14/14, 72/21/7
	Wheat/soybean/sesame	72/14/14, 72/21/7
	Corn/pigeon peas/soybeans	60/24/6
	Corn/redbeans/pigeon peas/soybeans	60/10/10/20
Thailand	Rice/soy/fish	75/20/5
	Rice/soy/sesame	65/25/10
	Rice/peanut/fish	75/15/10
	Corn/peanut/fish	75/15/10
	Cassava/peanut/fish	55/30/15
Indonesia	Rice/soybean	70/30
	Rice polish/soybean	70/30
	Corn/soybean	70/30
	Cassava/soybean	70/30
Philippines	Corn/pigeon pea/peanut	62/25/13
	Corn/mungbean/peanut	70/20/10
	Corn/rice/winged bean	35/35/30
	Corn/rice/cowpea/coconut (defat.)	10/10/70/20
	Rice/coconut (defat.)	60/40

Source: Taken from Akniyele.[50]

of "net utilizable protein" is calculated, it ranges from $7.19 for beef to $0.90 for wheat flour to $0.68 for soybean flour (early 1970s prices).[53] Considered from another perspective, the total energy requirements for production of ground beef, spun soy protein, and extruded soy pieces have been estimated at 37,000; 13,900; and 5,680 kcal/kg respectively.[57] These figures suggest that it should be possible to manufacture meat analogs at a lower cost than required to produce meat itself.

Of the attributes necessary to meat analogs, texture is uniquely important, and processes for producing it have received the most technological effort.[57] In animal flesh, texture-producing proteins are organized into fibrous bundles which extend over distances many times the length of individual molecules. Plant materials lack the texture of meats because proteins are present in discrete bodies and in three-dimensional networks into which are dispersed fat or starch-containing organelles. Thus, it is logical to attempt to mimic animal proteins by removing plant proteins from their matrices and reorganizing them into fibers. The most abundant source of concentrated plant proteins has been oilseed meals from edible vegetable oil production, especially from soybeans (Fig. 6.2). Older defatting technology which featured high temperature, high pressure expelling, resulted in residues in which proteins were severely damaged and suitable only for animal feed or fertilizer. However, modern solvent extraction processes not only produces a higher yield of superior oil, but also proteinaceous meals suitable for texturization.

In order to convert the globulins, prolamins and glutelins of plants into ordered arrays, the native proteins must be mobilized and oriented into arrangements possessing directional structure (anisotropy), then immobilized so that those structures are maintained throughout future processing steps up to the point of consumption.[54] The mobilization step is effected by altering the hydration, pH, ion strength or temperature of protein dispersions. These processes result in effects ranging from solvating to solubilizing to dissociating the protein molecules. Orientation of molecules or groups of molecules is achieved by subjecting mobilized proteins to directional flow (shear stress). Finally protein arrays are immobilized by heating or changes in pH-ion strength which caused protein chains to bind together via hydrophobic and disulfide linkages.[54] As crucial as texturization of protein is to analog production, the texturized proteins do not in themselves comprise complete analogs. They are the base to which is added binders, flavors, colors, nutrients and other ingredients.[58] A further distinction may be drawn between products which are complete simulators of meats and are commonly known as analogs, and less sophisticated "extenders" which are small textured and flavored pieces and which are designed to be blended with real meat.[57] For our purposes we shall include both in the general category of analogs.

Producing textured protein analogs began by taking advantage of the unique native texture of purified wheat gluten,[53] but was subsequently expanded by technology which could impart texture to plant proteins which did not possess the desired texture in their native forms. A recent summary of vegetable protein texturization processes listed eight techniques for texturizing proteins.[54] These include wet spinning, extrusion, gel texturization, tear texturization, melt spinning solvent texturization, texturization by surface deformation and texturization by freezing. Of these, wet spinning and extrusion are the most important commercial processes to date.

Boyer's original patent (U.S. Patent 2,682,466; 1954) described a process in which vegetable, animal or a combination of proteins were texturized to a product which "closely resembles natural meat as to its appearance, as to its fibrous qualities, as to its flavor, as to its nutritive value, and as to its chewiness."[59] This is done by dispersing isolated (85-98%) oilseed protein in an alkaline medium (1-15% NaOH) to form a viscous, concentrated (10-30%) spinning dope. These conditions cause native proteins to become denatured and dissociated, with the breakage of disulfide bonds. This dope (pH 9-13.5, viscosity 10-20 thousand c.p.) is forced through a spinneret containing 5-16 thousand holes, approximately 20 microns in diameter, into a coagulating bath containing acid and salt. Proteins are aligned by shear stress and insolubilized by reduction of the pH to their isoelectric point and salting out. Disulfide cross-links may also reform. Simultaneously, the coagulated fibers are

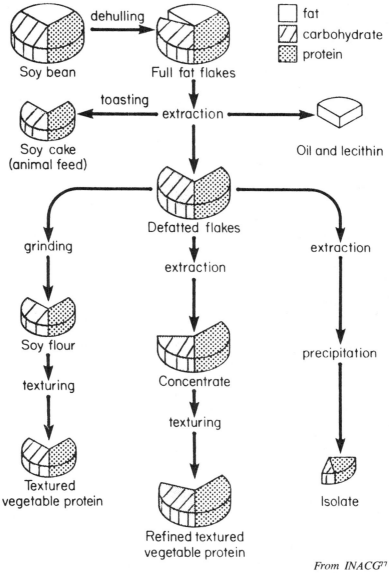

From INACG[77]
Courtesy of L. Schutte
FIG. 6.2. SCHEMATIC DIAGRAM OF THE CHANGES IN THE COMPOSITION OF SOY BEANS AS A RESULT OF PROCESSING

stretched to further align proteins and increase strength and elasticity, then partially desalted by soaking and compressing.[53] The basic Boyer technology has been extensively modified by its originator (U.S. Patents 2,730,447 and 2,730,448; 1956) and by others.[53,52,59] Protein fibers are chopped and oriented randomly or anisotropically, depending on the desired product, and binder, colors, flavors, nutrients added to produce final products.[53]

The second major texturization technology is extrusion cooking. Extrusion enjoys several advantages over spinning technology. It is able to use raw materials of lower protein content (less costly), is technologically less demanding, and produces little chemical/biological waste.[60] As a result of these advantages, most commercial protein texturization processes since the late 1970s have featured extrusion. The production of meat analogs and extenders in the United States and other developed countries is not constrained by considerations particular to low-cost extrusion, so various simple-to-sophisticated approaches have been developed. As with wet spinning, early processes for protein extrusion were described in the patent literature. Patents by Wilding (U.S. 3,488,770; 1970), Flier (3,940,495; 1976) and Wilding (4,044,157; 1977) described textured protein products and extrusion processes for making them. The most common starting material for textured plant protein (TPP) made by extrusion is defatted soy flour, although many other protein sources such as defatted peanut, cottonseed, sunflower and similar meals have been investigated. These materials should contain at least 50% protein with a protein dispersibility/nitrogen solubility index of 50-70% and contain less than 1% fat and 3% fiber. Moisture content of feed dough should be 20-40%; pH may be adjusted to 5.5 to produce a tougher, or to 8.5 for a more tender product. The range is commonly 6.5-7.5. Sodium chloride may be added to increase firmness, calcium salts or elemental sulfur to enhance crosslinking, and lecithin to improve flow characteristics during extrusion. Conditions in the extruder barrel include temperatures of 120-200°C and pressures of 16-60 atm. Screws typically have compression ratios (ratio of the screw volume at the discharge end over that at the feed end) of 1.5:1-4:1. The combination of forces in the extruder barrel (temperature, pressure and shear) cause the dough to become plasticised, and the proteins to become unfolded and aligned. Residence time in the barrel ranges from less than 30 s to several minutes. At the end of the barrel, the dough flows through a die in which shear/aligning forces increase further. Upon exiting the die, the dough is forced to expand by vaporizing water and forms a porous, rigid product with a laminar, fibrous, crosslinked structure. Such extrudates are cut to the desired size during or after extrusion and dried. This product is capable of absorbing 2-6 times its weight of water, broth or other liquid containing desired additives. It may also be enrobed with fat, flavors, colors or nutrients at the end of the drying step. The expanded pieces may also be leached in warm water to remove undesirable carbohydrates and increases protein content as the latter are now largely insoluble.[53,57,58,60,61] This process produces expanded chunks which may be flavored and colored and which have a chewy, meat-like texture upon rehydration and even following autoclaving. Products which more nearly resemble meats can be produced by more involved extrusion processes. These include the use of an elongated tempering die in which the melt cools and steam bubbles, which form in the falling pressure of the dough, cause fiber formation as the entire mass flows in one direction. The problem with preventing moisture flashing is that the flavor improvement which accompanies it is lost. This is obviated by the use of double extrusion where the dough (30–45% moisture) is first extruded at a temperature of about 100°C to flash off moisture and undesirable flavors, and then fed into a second extruder which heats and cools the dough and orients the proteins into layered sheets resembling meat.[57,58,60,65]

The nutritional quality of meat analogs made from the textured proteins described above depend on the composition of the starting ingredients, the effects of the various processing steps and for micronutrients, on deliberately added nutrients. The nutritional quality of textured soy meal, concentrate and isolate has been extensively studied due to their economic importance. The amino acid profile of soybean meal was presented in Table 6.2. Sulfur amino acids are limiting and their content is known to decline as soy proteins are increasingly purified.[62] However, the evolving estimates of amino acid requirements (Table 6.1) has made plant proteins like soy increasingly attractive. Earlier estimates assign an FAO amino acid score of 65–90, depending on the particular soy product, but current human requirements would conclude soy protein to be adequate for human needs. Biological testing has supported these conclusions. Rat PER values for soy proteins vary from 2.16–2.48 for flour, 2.02–2.48 for concentrate, and 1.08–2.1 for isolate versus 2.50 for casein.[57] In contrast, in studies with human children and adults, even soy isolate performed as well as beef and milk.[63,64]

The processing steps applied to soy and other proteins during texturization and subsequent operations are not unique in themselves, but may be applied in unique combinations and for specific intervals.[65] Exposure of proteins to very high pH is known to result in racemization of amino acids and formation of dehydroalanine and subsequently of lysinoalanine (LAL) and nonphysiological cross-links within the treated protein.[66] These changes result in proteins which are toxic to rats. Heating protein result first in denaturation and finally, if too severe, in destruction of amino acids and formation of LAL-type cross-links. Judicious heating has long been known to improve the digestibility of native proteins, and in the case of legume flours to destroy various antinutritional factors (trypsin inhibitor, lectins) which are present in raw seed and flours. Breaking disulfide bonds allows more complete denaturation of protein, improving their digestibility. Heating protein in the presence of reducing sugars may lead to loss of available lysine via the Maillard reaction; however, lysine availability has been shown to increase at some stages of extrusion, and decrease at others. Lysine loss during extrusion is dependent on both temperature and moisture, and at increasing severe conditions, availability other amino acids are also lowered.[67] Thus, the conditions used in texturization of protein foods have the potential of either improving or decreasing their nutritional quality. Wet spun soy fibers have better nutritional quality than the original isolate which was interpreted to mean that the isolate contained residual antinutritional factors which were destroyed or eluted by the spinning process.[57] However, fibers are never consumed alone, rather in a matrix of other protein and nonprotein ingredients. A beef-like product made from soy fiber, egg albumin, wheat gluten and soy flour had a PER of 2.3 versus 2.5 for casein. At an intake of 2 g/kg/day in children, the analog was equivalent to milk in protein quality, but in terms of minimum intake for N balance was 80% as good.[68] Kinsella[57] has reviewed numerous studies of nutritional quality of spun and extruded analogs, the results of which indicate that complete analogs and extender-meat blends are equivalent to good quality animal proteins when consumed at adequate levels. Other results indicate that at marginal intakes textured soy-meat blends are inferior to all meat diets, and may be improved by methionine supplementation.[58]

Fortification of analogs is an innate part of their production and use. The inclusion of animal protein binders in the production of spun fiber analogs raises their protein quality to that of animal products. Likewise, extenders are specifically made to be combined with meats[69] and these blends typify the Type II supplementation discusses earlier (Fig. 6.1). As with protein, vitamins in analogs may be derived from the major protein ingredient or from supplementation. Soybeans have reasonable levels of B-vitamins and their fate during extrusion has been most thoroughly characterized. Generally, thiamin is most labile to heat while riboflavin is relatively stable, but in different studies, extrusion conditions were found to have varying effects on B-vitamin retention.[67] Increasing temperature generally resulted in greater losses of thiamin, but the opposite was sometimes observed with riboflavin. Thiamin loss was generally greater at lower moisture contents. Total losses of B-vitamin ranged from 0-90% in the various studies cited. Similar results were reported for ascorbic acid and fat soluble vitamins. Losses ranged from less than 25% to greater than 80%, making generalizations very difficult. Because of the uncertain fate of vitamins during extrusion, fortification often takes place after that component of analog production. Camire *et al.*[67a] have recently reviewed chemical and nutritional changes in foods during extrusion.

Government Regulations and Analogs

Intertwined with the marketing of analog products in the U.S. market is the development of the Food and Drug Administration regulations on their use and on their labeling including use of the term "imitation." The first major boost for texturized plant proteins came in 1971 when they were approved for use in the National School Lunch Program.[53,70] The regulations controlling their use in child feeding programs specified that products with a composition and protein quality summarized in Table 6.7[57] must be hydrated to a moisture content of 60-65% and blended with cooked meat at a ratio no greater than 30% TPP:70% meat.[57,69] In January 1973, the FDA proposed a regulation which defined the term "imitation."[71] The use of "imitation" for labeling purposes was originally defined in Section 403 (C) of the Federal

TABLE 6.7
THE SPECIFICATIONS OF TEXTURED VEGETABLE PROTEINS
FOR USE AS MEAT EXTENDERS IN SCHOOL LUNCH PROGRAMS

Component	Minimum amount
Protein[1]	50.0 wt %
Fat[2]	2.0 wt %
Magnesium	70.0 mg/100 g
Iron	10.0 mg/100 g
Thiamin	0.30 mg/100 g
Riboflavin	0.60 mg/100 g
Niacin	16.0 mg/100 g
Vitamin B_6	1.4 mg/100 g
Vitamin B_{12}	5.7 mcg/100 g
Pantothenic acid	2.0 mg/100 g

Source: Kinsella.[57] From Anon. 1971. Food and Nutrition Notice No. 219, U.S. Department of Agriculture, Washington, DC.
Note: Biological value of protein: the PER of the textured vegetable protein shall not be less than 1.8 on basis of PER = 2.5 for casein. PER of a meat-textured vegetable protein combination shall not be less than 2.5 PER. Moisture content of the hydrated form shall not exceed 65.0%, or be less than 60.0%.
[1]Nitrogen times 6.25 (dry weight basis).
[2]Must not exceed 30%.

Food Drug and Cosmetic Act which states that a food which resembles and is intended to substitute for another food shall be deemed to be misbranded "unless its label bears in type of uniform size and prominence, the word imitation and immediately thereafter the name of the food imitated." In 1938 when the Act was adopted, Congress sought to protect consumers from uniformed purchase of an inferior substitute product which could be mistaken for a traditional food product.[71] The 1973 document stated that, with the significant advances in food technology, substitute foods were not necessarily nutritionally inferior to the traditional foods for which they substitute. Therefore, the FDA proposed to narrow the scope of the term. The nutritional equivalency portion of the FDA final rule (August 1973) provides that a food which is not nutritionally inferior to the food for which it substitutes and which it resembles is not deemed to be an imitation. Nutritional inferiority is determined using 20 nutrients (protein and 19 vitamins and minerals) for which U.S. Recommended Daily Allowances (USRDAs) have been established. Nutritional inferiority is defined as any reduction ($>2\%$ per serving) in the content of any of these 20 nutrients that are present in the traditional food.

FDA guidelines formulated in 1980 clearly state that nutrients may appropriately be added to a food that replaces traditional food in the diet to avoid nutritional inferiority in accordance with 21 CFR 101.3(e). Since these rulings do not pertain to calories, cholesterol or fat content, new products have proliferated that are lower in cholesterol that substitute for traditional products but do not have to bear the burden of the term "imitation." These include the fatty spreads and whipped products which do not convey appreciable nutrients other than calories. Protein analog products have generally not been able to take advantage of the ruling because the 20 nutrients required by FDA to be in equal or greater concentration for nutritional equivalency pose both technological and sometimes philosophical problems to the industry. In order to meet the nutritional equivalency requirements, plant protein-based analogs would have to be substantially fortified to match the traditional animal products. For example, a plant protein product would be required to contain 10 mg phosphorus per gram protein since this element is found in meats, even though the U.S. diet has an almost four-fold surplus of phosphorus.[72] Surimi-based products, because of the mincing and washing steps involved in the manufacture have been shown to have lower protein and potassium contents than their real counterparts.[73] Other nutrients, such as water-soluble vitamins and minerals, are also likely to be lost to a significant extent during surimi manufacture because of their leachability and sensitivity to oxygen, heat, etc., associated with various processing steps.

Tentative final regulations concerning the names for protein foods prepared predominantly form plant proteins and used to replace meat, poultry, seafood, eggs and cheese include the following points: If the product contains less than 65% protein by weight (dry basis) excluding flavors, colors and other added substances, it should inclulde the name of the source and the term "flour" and/or a term denoting the physical form of the plant protein ingredient such as "soy granules" or "soy flour granules." If the product contains 65-90% protein the name shall include ". . . protein concentrate" with the name of the source specified. If the product contains 90% or more protein the name shall include ". . . protein isolate" or "isolated . . . protein" with the source likewise noted. The regulations also specified the required levels of vitamins and minerals in these products and required level of protein quality as previously noted. Textured plant proteins blended with meat, poultry, seafood, eggs or cheese at levels of 30% or less are considered to be nutritionally equivalent to the food with which they are mixed if they have a PER 80% that of casein or better. Vegetable protein products capable of 100% substitution for animal protein products must have a PER equivalent to that of casein to avoid nutritional inferiority.[70]

Utilization of Analogs

By far, the major use of textured protein products has been as meat extenders, much of it used in the school lunch program. Consumption in the 1971-73 period ranged from 10-24 thousand metric tons.[53,58] This was projected to grow to 51,000 M.T. by 1975 and 100,000 M.T. by 1985.[57] At the same time, total textured protein production was expected to reach over 800,000 M.T. by 1980 and over 2 million M.T. by 1985.[53,58] By the late 1970s these numbers were seen to have been extremely optimistic. The economic pressures in the early part of the decade which encouraged consumers to buy analogs also prompted the marketing of many inferior products with predictable long-term results.[57] The results of a survey, reviewed in Duda[53] and interpreted as supportive of future growth in analog consumption, showed that blends of textured soy and meat ranged in consumer acceptability from 18–20%, with 61–70% finding them unacceptable. According to Kinsella,[57] the major determinants of growth in analog consumption are interrelated factors such as protein availability, price, manufacturer and consumer attitudes, developing technologies and government regulations. Price considerations include relative costs of traditional animal-based foods compared to analogs. Consumer attitudes depend on evolving health and nutrition information (whether true or false), perceived value, and sensory quality compared to traditional products. Sellers et al.[74] analyzed the success/failure of several analogs and blends. Blends of ground beef and textured soy flour marketed in Minneapolis failed to achieve stable retail sales, due primarily to low sensory quality, while a blend of soy isolate and ground beef achieved a stable 25% market share in Jewel Food Stores because they were indistinguishable from whole ground beef. Analog marketing has passed through several stages: (1) the original targeting of religiously motivated consumers by Worthington Foods and Loma Linda Foods in the 1960s; (2) an attempt to build much broader markets in the early 1970s by companies such as Miles Laboratories (via Worthington Foods and Morningstar Farms) and General Mills; (3) a subsequent retrenchment and divestiture of analog manufacturing facilities by mainstream food producers; (4) stabilization of a smaller market directed toward ethically and health motivated consumers. The failure of analogs to be accepted by the general consumer was again due mainly to poor sensory characteristics which touted health considerations could not overcome.

Despite the need for a more modest assessment of future developments in the field, it should be remembered that analogs must still enjoy a level of acceptance and are available in most supermarkets. Table 6.8[75] lists companies which produced soy ingredients and analogs in the United States in 1988. Composition information for the Morningstar Farms® line of meat analogs is presented in Table 6.9.

CONCLUSIONS

Analogs and blends represent a major intervention in human food customs in the 20th century. They are a product of our rapidly increasing knowledge in nutrition, food science, and technology. As such, they are undoubtedly the precursors of a great array of products which could be specifically designed to deliver optimum nutrition and maximum safety and convenience to future consumers in all parts of the world. That consumers will accept analogs cannot be questioned, as experience with margarine, whipped toppings, and coffee creamers attest. However, the challenges are greater with more complex foods which, used as entire meals, carry important social and emotional significance. Basic staples on which we depend for survival

TABLE 6.8
U.S. PRODUCERS OF EDIBLE SOYBEAN PROTEIN PRODUCTS

Company[1]	Flours[2]	Concentrates	Isolates	Flours	Concentrates	Isolates
AP	•					
ADM	•	•	•	•		
Cargill	•				•	
CS	•	•			•	
GPC			•			
HP	•					
LG	•					
PMS					•	
RP			•			•
AES			•[3]			
WF					•[4]	•[5]

Source: Wolf.[75]

[1] AP = AG Processing, Inc.
ADM = Archer Daniels Midland, Co.
LG = Lauhoff Grain, Co.
AES = A. E. Staley Manufacturing, Co.
CS = Central Soya
GP = Grain Processing Corp.
HP = Honeymead Products
PMS = PMS Foods, Inc.
RP = Ralston Purina
WF = Worthington Foods, Inc.

[2] Includes grits and flakes.
[3] Protease modified forms.
[4] Meat analogs containing soy protein concentrate plus isolate.
[5] Meat analogs containing spun soy protein isolate.

and foods with symbolic as well as nutritional value will not be displaced but may be dramatically extended and new products made possible from otherwise underutilized food sources. Nevertheless, as progress continues from the first, rather crude approximations toward both better analogs and perhaps entirely new food forms, increasing benefits in food economy, nutrition, and equity will be realized.

REFERENCES

1. ALYWARD, F. and JUL, M. 1975. Protein and Nutrition Policy in Low-Income Countries. Charles Knight & Co., London.
2. Joint FAO/WHO Expert Committee on Nutrition. 1950. Report on the First Session, World Health Org. Tech. Rept. Ser. No. 16. WHO, Geneva.
3. KAPISIOTIS, G. D. 1969. History and status of specific protein-rich foods FAO/WHO/UNICEF protein food program and products. In Protein-Enriched Cereal Foods for World Needs, M. Milner (ed.). Am. Assoc. Cereal Chem., St. Paul.
4. WILLIAMS, C. D. 1935. Cited by N. S. Scrimshaw and M. Behar, 1959. World-wide occurrence of protein malnutrition. Fed. Proc. *18* (Suppl.) *3*, 82–88.
5. ANON. 1975. Pre-School Child Malnutrition Primary Deterrent to Human Progress. A Summary of an International Conference on Prevention of Malnutrition in the Pre-School Child. In PAG Compendium, Vol. 6, pp. E41–E49.

TABLE 6.9
COMPOSITION OF MORNINGSTAR FARMS FROZEN ANALOGS

Product Name		Grillers[1]	Links[2]	Patties[3]	Scramblers[4]	Strips[5]
Code		2520	2512	2514	2518	2516
Net weight	g	100	100	100	100	100
Water	g	46.8	52.3	48.9	78.2	42.7
Calories		290	237	240	105	333
Protein	g	22.2	18.7	21.3	10.3	11.9
Carbohydrates	g	8.1	7.7	8.95	4.89	15.7
Dietary fiber	g	2.91	1.79	3.3		1.4
Total fat	g	18.7	18	17.2	4.89	24.8
Saturated fat	g					
Monoglycerides	g					
Polyunsaturated	g					
Cholesterol	mg	1.76	1.21	1.53	3.21	1.27
Vitamin A—Carotene	RE					
Vitamin A—Preformed	RE					
Vitamin A—Total	RE	—[7]	—[7]	—[7]	177	—[7]
Thiamin—B_1	mg	6.56	3.15	2.53	0.374	11.9
Riboflavin—B_2	mg	0.33	0.25	0.26	0.86	0.258
Niacin—B_3	mg	7.94	8.38	9.48	—[7]	7.81
Pyridoxine—B_6	mg	0.514	0.34	0.4	0.16	0.336
Cobalamin—B_{12}	mcg	6.19	6.71	6.62	2.34	3.69
Folacin	mcg					
Pantothenic	mg				2.23	
Vitamin C	mg	—[7]	—[7]	—[7]	—[7]	—[7]
Vitamin E	mg					
Calcium	mg	81.3	20.2	30.3	66.3	37.6
Copper	mg					
Iron	mg	4.2	3.95	4.17	1.45	1.95
Magnesium	mg					
Phosphorus	mg					
Potassium	mg	184	103	138	121	107
Selenium	mcg					
Sodium	mg	508	710	1146	226	1317
Zinc	mg				0.94	
Cals. from protein	%	31	28	31	39	14
Cals. from carbohydrate	%	11	12	13	19	19
Cals. from fat	%	58	61	56	42	67
Polyunsat./Saturated		0.0:1	0.0:1	0.0:1	0.0:1	0.0:1
Sodium/Potassium		2.8:1	6.9:1	8.3:1	1.9:1	12.3:1
Calcium/Phosphorus		0.0:1	0.0:1	0.0:1	0.0:1	0.0:1
CSI		−0.9	−0.9	−0.9	−0.8	−0.9

Source: Information kindly provided by Dr. Richard Leiss, Director R&D Worthington Foods, Inc.
[1]Hamburger patty analog.
[2]Sausage link analog.
[3]Sausage patty analog.
[4]Scrambled egg analog.
[5]Bacon strip analog.
[6]Contains less than 2% USRDA.

6. BROWN, R. E. 1978. Weaning foods in developing countries. Am. J. Clin. Nutr. *31*, 2066–2072.
7. PEREZ, C. 1958. Progress in understanding and preventing protein malnutrition in Central America. In Adv. Hum. Nutr. p. 89–93, INCAP.
8. HEIMENDINGER, J., ZEITLIN, M. and AUSTIN, J. E. 1981. Nutrition Intervention in Developing Countries. Study IV. Formulated Foods. Office of Nutrition, Development Support Bureau, U.S. Agency for International Development.
9. ALYWARD, F. and JUL, M. 1975. Appendices 1 (Extract from Statement No. 20 of the Protein Advisory Group) and 2 (PAG Statement No. 25 On The Global Maldistribution of Protein). In Protein Nutrition Policy in Low-Income Countries, F. Alyward and M. Jul (eds.). Charles Knight & Co. Ltd., London.
10. SCRIMSHAW, N. S. 1981. Nutritional significance of protein quality. In A Global View in Protein Quality in Humans: Assessment and In Vitro Estimation, C. E. Bodwell, J. S. Adkins and D. T. Hopkins (eds.). AVI/Van Nostrand Reinhold, New York.
11. GOLDEN, M. H. N. and RAMDATH, D. 1987. Free radicals in the pathogenesis of kwashiorkor, Proc. Nutr. Soc. *46*, 53–68.
12. BIGWOOD, E. J. 1962. Protein deficiency in underdeveloped countries with special reference to sulphur deficiency and aminoaciduria in kwashiorkor, in central Africa. In PAG Compendium, Vol. E1, John Wiley & Sons, New York.
13. HOPKINS, D. T. 1981. Effects of variation in protein digestibility. In A Global View in Protein Quality In Humans: Assessment and In Vitro Estimation, C. E. Bodwell, J. S. Adkins and D. T. Hopkins (eds.). AVI/Van Nostrand Reinhold, New York.
14. FAO. 1957. Report No. 16. FAO Committee meeting in October in Rome on "Protein requirements." (In English)
15. FAO/WHO. 1973. Energy and Protein Requirement. Report of a Joint FAO/WHO Ad Hoc Expert Committee. WHO Technical Report Series No. 522. WHO, Geneva.
16. FAO/WHO. 1985. Energy and Protein Requirements. Report of a Joint Expert Consultation. WHO Technical Report Series No. 724. WHO, Geneva.
17. Food and Nutrition Board. 1989. Recommended Dietary Allowances, 10th Ed. National Research Council/National Academy of Sciences, Washington, DC.
18. ALLAN, D. M. 1972. Focus on food mixtures. UNICEF News *71*, 23–28.
19. SENTI, F. R. 1968. Formulated cereal foods in the U.S. Food For Peace Program. Presentation AACC/AOCS Joint Meeting.
20. BOOKWALTER, G. N. 1981. Requirements for foods containing soy protein in the Food For Peace program. J. Am. Oil Chem. Soc. *58*, 455–460.
21. AUSTIN, J. E. 1981. International network of nutrition institutions. In Nutrition Programs in the Third World Cases and Readings. Oelgeschlager, Gunn & Hain Publishers, Cambridge.
22. FORMAN, M. J. 1966. Enrichment and Food For Peace. Cereal Sci. Today *11*, 231–232.
23. KIRBY, L. K., NELSON, T. S., JOHNSON, Z. B. and YORK, J. O. 1983. the effect of seed coat color of hybrid sorghum grain on the ability of chicks to digest dry matter and amino acids and to utilize energy. Nutr. Rep. Int. *27*, 831–836.
24. ILORI, J. O. and CONRAD, J. H. 1976. The nutritive alue of protein in selected sorghum lines as measured by rat performance. Nutr. Rep. Int. *13*, 307–313.
25. PEDERSEN, B. and EGGUM, B. O. 1983. The influence of milling on the nutritive value of flour from cereal grains. 6. Sorghum. Plant Foods Hum. Nutr. *33*, 313–326.

26. WATT, B. K. and MERRILL, A. L. 1975. Composition of Foods, Agriculture Handbook 8. U.S. Department of Agriculture, Washington, DC.
27. ORR, M. L. and WATT, B. K. 1968. Amino Acid Content of Foods, Home Economics Research Report No. 4. U.S. Department of Agriculture, Washington, DC.
28. BRESSANI, R. 1965. Formulated vegetable mixtures. W. Hemisp. Nutr. Cong., pp. 86–90.
29. BRESSANI, R. 1988. Protein complementation of foods. *In* Nutritional Evaluation of Food Processing, 3rd Ed., R. S. Harris and E. Karmas (eds.). AVI/Van Nostrand Reinhold, New York.
30. STEINKE, F. H. and HOPKINS, D. T. 1983. Complementary and supplementary effects of vegetable proteins. Cereal Foods World 28, 338–341.
31. ANON. 1972. PAG Guideline On Protein-Rich Mixtures for use as Supplementary Foods. PAG Guideline No. 8. *In* PAG Compendium, Vol. 6., pp. E631–E636.
32. SENTI, F. R., COPLEY, J. J. and PENCE, J. W. 1967. Protein-fortified grain products for world uses. Cereal Sci. Today *11*, 426–430, 441.
33. SQUIBB, R. L., WYLD, M. K., SCRIMSHAW, N. S. and BRESSANI, R. 1959. All-vegetable protein mixtures for human feeding. I. Use of rats and baby chicks for evaluating corn-based vegetable mixtures. J. Nutr. *69*, 343–350.
34. BRESSANI, R., AGUIRRE, A. and SCRIMSHAW, N. S. 1959. All-vegetable protein mixtures for human feeding. II. The nutritive value of corn, sorghum, rice and buckwheat substituted for lime-treated corn in INCAP vegetable mixture eight. J. Nutr. *69*, 351–355.
35. BRESSANI, R., ELIAS, L. G., AGUIRRE, A. and SCRIMSHAW, N. S. 1961. All-vegetable protein mixtures for human feeding. III. The development of INCAP vegetable mixture nine. J. Nutr. *74*, 201–208.
36. BRESSANI, R., AGUIRRE, A., ELIAS, L. G., ARROYAVE, R., JARQUIN, R. and SCRIMSHAW, N. S. 1961. All-vegetable protein mixtures for human feeding. IV. Biological testing of INCAP vegetable mixture nine in chicks. J. Nutr. *74*, 209–216.
37. SCRIMSHAW, N. S., BEHAR, M., WILSON, D., VITERI, F., ARROYAVE, G. and BRESSANI, R. 1961. All-vegetable protein mixtures for human feeding. V. Clinical trials with INCAP mixtures 8 and 9 and with corn and beans. Am. J. Clin. Nutr. *9*, 196–205.
38. BRESSANI, R., ELIAS, L. G., BRAHAM, E. and ERALES, M. 1969. Long term rat feeding studies with vegetable protein mixtures containing cottonseed flour produced by different methods. J. Agr. Food Chem. *17*, 1135–1138.
39. BRESSANI, R. and ELIAS, L. G. 1966. All-vegetable protein mixtures for human feeding. The development of INCAP vegetable mixture 14 based on soybean flour. J. Food Sci. *31*, 626–631.
40. SHAW, R. L. 1969. Incaparina in Central America. *In* Protein-Enriched Cereal Foods for World Needs, M. Milner (ed.). Am. Assoc. Cereal Chem., St. Paul.
41. DIMINO, A. 1969. Incaparina in Colombia. *In* Protein-Enriched Cereal Foods for World Needs, M. Milner (ed.). Am. Assoc. Cereal Chem., St. Paul.
42. TOLLEFSON, B. 1967. New milled corn products, including CSM. Cereal Sci. Today *11*, 438–441.
43. CROWLEY, P. R. 1982. World food and nutrition problems. Cereal Foods World *27*, 564–565.
44. AUSTIN, J. E. 1981. Supplementary feeding and formulated foods.'' *In* Nutrition Pro-

grams in the Third World Cases and Readings, Oelgeschlager, Gunn & Hain Publishers, Cambridge.
45. HARRIS, R. S. and KARMAS, E. 1988. Nutritional Evaluation of Food Processing, 3rd Ed. AVI/Van Nostrand Reinhold, New York.
46. BUFFA, A. 1971. Food, technology and development. Part I—Processing low-cost nutritious native foods for world's hungry children. Factors, formulas, processes. A special UNICEF report. Food Eng. (Nov.) 79–106.
47. HARPER, J.M. 1981. Extrusion of Foods, Vol. 1. CRC Press, Boca Raton, Fla.
48. HARPER, J. M. and JANSEN, G. R. 1981. Nutritious Foods Produced by Low-Cost Technology. Summary Report of Cooperative Activities Between Colorado State University and the Office of International Cooperation and Development, USDA 1974–1980. Depts. Agricultural and Chemical Engineering, Colorado State University, Ft. Collins.
49. HARPER, J. M. and JANSEN, G. R. 1985. Production of nutritious precooked foods in developing countries by low-cost extrusion technology. Food Rev. Int. *1*, 27–97.
50. AKNIYELE, I. O. 1987. Combinations of cereals, legumes and meat products in extrusion products. *In* Cereals and Legumes in the Food Supply, J. Dupont and E. E. M. Osman (eds.). Iowa State Univ. Press, Ames.
51. SIEGEL, A. and LINEBACK, D. R. 1976. Development, acceptability and proximate analyses of high-protein, rice-based snacks for Thai children. J. Food Sci. *41*, 1184–1188.
52. ROSENFIELD, D. 1978. Nutritional optimization of new foods. J. Am. Diet. Assoc. *72*, 475–477.
53. DUDA, Z. 1974. Vegetable Protein Meat Extenders and Analogues. AGA/MISC/74/7 FAO UN, pp. 1–89.
54. GIDDEY, C. 1983. Phenomena involved in the "texturization" of vegetable proteins and various technological processes used. *In* Plant Proteins for Human Food, C. E. Bodwell and L. Petit (eds.). Martinus Nijhoff/Dr. W. Junk Publishers, The Hague.
55. CARROLL, K. K., HUFF, M. W. and ROBERTS, D. C. K. 1979. Vegetable protein and lipid metabolism. *In* Soy Protein and Human Nutrition, H. L. Wilcke, D. T. Hopkins and D. H. Waggle (eds.). Academic Press, New York.
56. WILDING, M. D. 1970. Oilseed protein. Present utilization pattern. J. Am. Oil Chem. Soc. *47*, 398–401.
57. KINSELLA, J. E. 1978. Texturized proteins: fabrication, flavoring, and nutrition. CRC Rev. Food Sci. Nutr. *10*, 147–207.
58. HORAN, F. E. and WOLFF, H. 1976. Mean Analogs—A Supplement. *In* New Protein Foods, Vol. 2, Technology, Part B, A.M. Altschul (ed.). Academic Press, New York.
59. HANSON, L. P. 1974. Vegetable Protein Processing, Noyes Data Corp. Park Ridge, N.J.
60. HARPER, J. M. 1981. Extrusion of Foods, Vol. II. CRC Press, Boca Raton, Fla.
61. SMITH, O. B. 1976. Extrusion Cooking in New Protein Foods, Vol 2, Technology, Part B, A.M. Altschul (ed.). Academic Press, New York.
62. WOLF, W. J. 1970. Soybean proteins: their functional, chemical, and physical properties. J. Agr. Food Chem. *18*, 969–976.
63. TORUN, B. 1979. Nutritional quality of soybean protein isolates: studies in children of preschool age. *In* Soy Protein and Human Nutrition, H. L. Wilcke, D. T. Hopkins and D. H. Waggle (eds.). Academic Press, New York.
64. SCRIMSHAW, N. S. and YOUNG, V. R. 1979. Soy protein in adult human nutrition: a review with new data. *In* Soy Protein and Human Nutrition, H. L. Wilcke, D. T. Hopkins and D. H. Waggle (eds.). Academic Press, New York.

65. PHILLIPS, R. D. 1989. Effect of extrusion cooking on the nutritional quality of plant protein. *In* Protein Quality and the Effects of Processing, R. D. Phillips and J. W. Finley (eds.). Marcell Dekker, New York.
66. FRIEDMAN, M., GUMBMANN, M. R. and MASTERS, P. M. 1984. Protein-alkali reactions: Chemistry, toxicology, and nutritional consequences. *In* Nutritional and Toxicological Aspects of Food Safety, M. Friedman (ed.). Plenum Press, New York.
67. BJORCK, I. and ASP, N.-G. 1984. The effects of extrusion cooking on nutritional value—a literature review. *In* Extrusion Cooking Technology, R. Jowitt (ed.). Elsevier Applied Science Publishers, New York.
67a. CAMIRE, M. E., CAMIRE, A. AND KRUMHAR, K. 1990. Chemical and nutritional changes in foods during extrusion. Crit. Rev. Food Sci. Nutr. *29*(1), 35–57.
68. BRESSANI, R., VITERI, F., ELIAS, L. G., DE ZAGHI, S., ALVARDO, J. and ODELL, A. D. 1967. Protein quality of a soybean protein textured food in experimental animals and children. J. Nutr. *93*, 349–360.
69. KIES, C. and FOX, H. M. 1973. Effect of varying the ratio of beef and textured vegetable protein nitrogen on protein nutritive value for humans. J. Food Sci. *38*, 1211–1213.
70. ANON. 1987. Soy Protein Products Characteristics, Nutritional Aspects and Utilization. Soy Protein Council, Washington, DC.
71. VANDERVEEN, J. E. 1987. Nutritional equivalency from a regulatory perspective. Food Technol. *41*, 131–140.
72. ROSENFIELD, D. 1976. Fortification philosophy for protein food analogs. Food Prod. Dev. *10*, 67–71.
73. ANON. 1988. Surimi update. *In* Foodways to Better Health, A Food, Nutrition and Health Newsletter 2, 3. Cooperative Extension Service, The University of Georgia, Athens.
74. SELLERS, S. G., BENNETT, J. W. and COLE, W. 1988. The importance of traditional quality for foods containing vegetable protein ingredients. *In* Soy Protein and National Food Policy, F. H. Schwarz (ed.). Westview Press, Boulder, Col.
75. WOLF, W. J. 1988. The relative merits of various protein food ingredients. *In* Soy Protein and National Food Policy, F. H. Schwarz (ed.). Westview Press, Boulder, CO.
76. HOVER, S. R. and SENTI, F. R. 1969. Enrichment and fortification of U.S. donated foods. (Presentation) VII Int. Congr. Nutr., Prague. Aug. 28–Sept. 5.
77. INACG. 1982. The Effects of Cereals and Legumes on Iron Availability. Nutrition Foundation, Washington, DC.

CHAPTER 7

Foods Considered for Nutrient Addition: ROOTS AND TUBERS

J. CHRISTOPHER BAUERNFEIND, Ph.D.

INTRODUCTION

Tuberous plants, with underground food storage tissues, are quite adaptable, accumulating carbohydrates under favorable weather conditions for growth and maturation, lying dormant under unfavorable conditions, and withstanding such cycles until harvested. These foods are valued for their abundant yield of nutrients with a low labor input in their root cropping pattern.

POTATOES

Potatoes, tubers of good nutritional qualities, are abundantly and economically produced in the temperate zones. They have been traced back in early history, about 200 A.D., as a food of the Indians of Peru.[1] In the past, nutritional deficiencies have been little known in countries whose populations have consumed the white potato as a major energy food.

An approximate average composition of white or Irish potatoes is 17% carbohydrates, 2% protein, 2% fiber, 1% ash, 0.1% fat, 78% water plus some minerals and vitamins.[2,3] They are a fair-to-good source of iron, potassium, magnesium and phosphorus. Among the water-soluble vitamins present (ascorbic acid, thiamin, pyridoxine, niacin, folate), ascorbic acid is furnished in the greatest amount relative to daily needs. One medium-sized potato, baked, yields about 20 mg of L-ascorbic acid, ⅓ of the 60 mg NRC 1989 recommended daily allowance. The potato as a vitamin C source has a legendary claim: In the American Civil War, those prisons having access to potatoes were relatively free of scurvy.[3] White potatoes are very low in total carotenoid content (3 mg/g dry wt). Small amounts or traces of individual carotenoids have been identified.[2,4]

The downward trend in the United States of the white potato since 1910 has stabilized and slightly turned up due to the progressing development[4a] of new and convenient processed potato foods (Fig. 7.1) of the canned, chipped, dehydrated and frozen types. Currently, over ⅔ of the total U.S. annual potato production, about 35 billion pounds (between 100–150 lb/person) are marketed and consumed in processed forms. Other significant potato-producing countries are Australia, France, Germany, Netherlands, U.K. and U.S.S.R.[2,3] Production is being expanded in some developing countries. Potatoes are second only to maize in terms of number of producer countries and fourth after wheat, maize and rice in global tonnage.

With the continuing trend of more potatoes in processed form, substantial amounts of the natural vitamin C content have been lost. Ascorbic acid losses (Table 7.1) during the manufacture of potato flakes, granules and dehydrated slices and dices generally are the greatest whenever the surface area of the cut potato is increased and exposed to both oxygen and high temperatures for prolonged time periods.[2] In the flaking operation, water blanching and drum drying result in significant loss, while in granule production, vitamin losses are high during the mashing and mixing stages.[2,3] Other vitamins (Table 7.1) are also lost during processing. Myers and Roehm[5] reported that freshly cooked potatoes contained from 2½–5 times more vitamin C than any tested dehydrated product. As a solution to nutrient loss, they proposed that processed potato products should be nutrified with ascorbic acid. The same proposal was offered by Bring and Raab.[6]

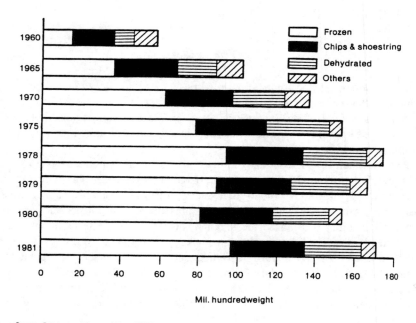

Source: Potatoes and Sweetpotatoes, USDA

From Jones and Zepp[4a]

FIG. 7.1. RAW POTATOES USED FOR PROCESSED POTATO PRODUCTS

TABLE 7.1
APPROXIMATE LOSSES OF VITAMINS DURING PREPARATION
AND PROCESSING OF POTATOES

Method of Preparation or Processing	% Total Loss of Vitamins				
	Ascorbic Acid	Thiamin	Niacin	Folic Acid	Pyridoxine
Boiled, unpeeled[1]	20	10	0	20	0
Boiled, peeled[1]	20–50	0–40	0–30	10–40	15–20
Oven-baked[1]	25	15	5	30	10
Raw, fried[1]	30–50	10	5	20	—
Peeled, boiled, fried[1]	40	40	40	—	—
Mashed[1]	30–80	—	—	—	—
Hash-browned[1]	30–80	—	—	—	—
Salad[1]	65	—	—	—	—
Dumplings[1]	85	—	—	—	—
Prepeeled, sulphited, boiled[2]	30	30	—	—	—
Prepeeled, sulphited, fried[2]	—	45	—	—	—
French fries[2]	25–35	20–40	20	35	25
Chips[2]	30–85	—	—	—	—
Flakes[2]	50	>90	25	50	40
Granules[2]	55	>90	25	50	20
Canned[2,3]	10–70	50	50	30	30

Source: Woolfe.[2] Figures taken from various authors.
[1]Domestic preparation.
[2]Processing.
[3]Losses to consumer are less if can liquid is also consumed.

Nutrification of processed potatoes with vitamins and minerals may not be a simple process, but, depending on particle size and the nature of ingredients, a varied technology exists for their addition to food.[7–12] Mere mixing of the dry potato flakes or granules with crystalline or powder L-ascorbic acid frequently will not yield a uniform product for bulk or small serve packaging; also, the mechanical mixing breaks up potato particles, causing further loss. Alternative interventions include spray application of ascorbic acid formulations. If discolorations are encountered,[7] adaptations such as a spray formulation of ascorbic acid, a sulfite salt and a film-forming soluble gum, or a powder ascorbic acid suspension in an antioxidant treated vegetable oil may be considered and carried out in a manner not to impair physical properties of the product. One successful approach is the patented process whereby a nutrient flake premix of minerals and vitamins is prepared (approximately the same size and shape of the potato product to be nutrified) and blended uniformly into the potato flow stream prior to packaging.[12] There is also the alternative of mixing ascorbic acid into the cooked product just before drum drying, followed by cooling and packaging of the flaked product. In one study of the flake process[10] retention of ascorbic acid after processing was about 72%. After storage for 28 weeks at 26°C in air, the flakes retained 70–76% of the amount remaining after processing.

Nutrified, dehydrated potatoes have been added to food recommended for federally reimbursed school lunches under the National School Lunch Program. A ½ cup serving of reconstituted potatoes containing the industry ascorbic acid nutrification standard (20 mg) is included in the USDA listed foods of good sources of vitamin C meeting the children's daily need for this vitamin.[3]

Various forms of vitamin A exist for the nutrification of foods,[11] including potato products. The availability of dry, stabilized vitamin A palmitate, in varied particle sizes, has added to the options to nutrify dehydrated potato products, even though the white potato is a minor source of natural vitamin A as compared to the yellow sweet potato. As an option beyond dry blending with a selected particle-sized potato product, vitamin A may have to be incorporated within the composition of the potato product before the dehydration stage or by a spray or a coating technique on to the dry potato form, similar to nutrifying ready-to-eat breakfast cereals. Early trials[10] on incorporating vitamin A into dehydrated potato flakes were quite good when properly processed and packaged (Table 7.2). Maintaining a low moisture level in the final nutrified product minimizes vitamin losses and assures better product quality; nitrogen packaging adds further support for attaining these objectives.

The USDA has distributed dehydrated potatoes nutrified with 800 mg of vitamin C and 16,000 IU of vitamin A/lb to eligible needy families under the commodity distribution program since 1968. Families are authorized to receive one pound of dehydrated product per person per month, providing 54% of the recommended daily allowance of vitamin C for a family of 4 persons.[7]

Potato chip production significantly alters and lowers nutrient value. Nutrification would, of course, increase nutrient value and consumer interest, as it does for any other processed potato product.[13] Vitamins and minerals may be added to potato chips by the salt premix approach. Several manufacturers now can offer a nutrified salt premix containing vitamins A, B_1, B_2, B_6, C, E, and niacin. It is technologically feasible for the chip manufacturer to add a designated nutrified salt, physically standardized with predetermined nutrient levels, at a prescribed rate to chips to meet salting and nutrifying objectives simultaneously.

To provide vitamin A value and also improve the color of frozen fried potato sticks, β-carotene can be added to the antioxidant-containing frying oil, or alternatively after normal frying procedures by a dip or spray applied to the potato sticks with a liquid carotene formulation prior to packaging and freezing. Choice of application depends on which gives the desired controlled coloring results and carotene storage retention values.[3,4]

In potato processing, significant losses of amino acids occur due to leachng action[14] as a result of slicing and hot water blanching, with additional losses caused by sugar-amino acid reactions in heat treatment.[2,3] Kies and Fox[15] reported methionine to

TABLE 7.2
VITAMIN A CONTENT OF NUTRIFIED POTATO FLAKE PACKED IN AIR
AND UNDER NITROGEN AT DIFFERENT STORAGE TEMPERATURES[1]

Storage Weeks	Air Pack			N_2 Pack		
	75°F	98°F	113°F	75°F	98°F	113°F
0	10,900	—	—	10,900	—	—
4	9,900	—	—	10,900	—	—
7	—	—	7,600	—	—	7,900
10	—	—	7,100	—	—	7,500
12	—	8,350	—	—	9,250	—
16	8,000	7,000	6,050	10,600	8,150	7,400
28	7,420	—	—	10,600	—	—

Source: Cording et al.[10]
[1]Initial value of 10,900 IU/3 oz represents a recovery of 10,900 IU/3 oz; or 91% of 12,000 IU/3 oz added before drying.

be the first limiting amino acid in dehydrated potato flakes for human nutrition. In nitrogen balance studies with adults, subjects showed an increase in nitrogen retention when methionine was added to the potato product diet. The addition of 0.37% methionine to potato flakes could significantly improve the protein of the flakes without affecting product palatability. There is also loss of minerals by leaching action in frozen potato stick, chip and dehydrated potato production.[2] To date, nutrification of dehydrated potato products with iron has not been successful because of subsequent discolorations.[7]

CASSAVA

In many tropical countries cassava, as an economical and primary source of carbohydrates, occupies much the same position in the diet as potatoes in parts of the temperate zone. Cassava (also called mandioca, tapioca and yuca) is consumed as a staple food by an estimated 400 million people in Africa, Asia and South America (Table 7.3) with a 1982 world production of about 128 million tons of fresh roots. It is an ancient crop of flexible characteristics, easily propagated, high yielding, able to grow in marginal moist soil, drought resistant, relatively inexpensive to produce, and can be harvested 6–24 months after planting, thus adding to its ground storage value as a protective food against famine. How cassava has been processed depends on how the product fits into local use[16] and the export potential of countries like Brazil, China, Columbia, India, Indonesia, Mozambique, Nigeria, Tanzania, Thailand, Uganda, Vietnam, West Indies and Zaire.[16–19]

The developing world is short of calories; cassava is a high calorie food.[17] It is a food of the poor, but other classes consume it, too, but at a lower percentage.[18]

TABLE 7.3
1986 CASSAVA PRODUCTION IN DIFFERENT COUNTRIES

Country	Area (Million Hectares)	Yield (Tons/Hectare)	Production (Million Tons)
Africa	7.69	7.9	60.8
Zaire	2.20	7.1	15.6
Nigeria	1.30	11.3	14.7
Tanzania	0.45	12.2	5.5
Mozambique	0.57	5.8	3.3
Asia	3.80	11.6	44.2
Thailand	1.20	12.6	15.2
Indonesia	1.21	11.0	13.3
India	0.30	19.7	6.0
Vietnam	0.50	6.0	3.0
South America	2.55	12.2	31.2
Brazil	2.07	12.5	25.5
Paraguay	0.20	14.4	2.9
Columbia	0.15	8.9	1.3
Central America	0.16	5.4	0.9
World	13.51	9.7	137.4

Source: FAO Production Yearbook, 1986.

An approximate composition of the fresh cassava root is 34% carbohydrate (starch and sugars), 1% protein, 1% fiber, 0.5% fat, 0.5% ash and 63% water, plus some minerals and vitamins. In the processing of the cassava root, ascorbic acid, thiamin and niacin and much of the mineral content are lost. Cassava products are low in protein content and also poor in protein quality by being deficient in the sulfur amino acids and tryptophan.[20] Protein malnutrition in the absence of caloric malnutrition is apparent in cassava eating countries. Since fresh cassava roots are quite perishable, it is imperative to convert the roots to dry products for wide acceptance and expanded usage. Use of cassava in the human diet involves boiling, frying or roasting and baking to prepare mushes, pastes, soups, gruels, fried and roasted snacks, cookies, cakes, breads and local dishes.[16-21] Food use of cassava should double its present rate before the year 2000.[19]

Initially, cassava meal or flour manufacturing was a backyard industry. However, with people moving from rural to urban centers, more demand has grown for prepared cassava products.[22] The increasing population of the cassava producing countries increased the demand for more product volume, an improvement in product quality and lower costs.[16,23] Where sufficient demand has been confirmed, production sites and processing technology development, relative to output and costs, need to be followed by pilot plant trials before commitment to large scale operations.[18]

A cassava flour for partial incorporation into local bread would decrease imports of more expensive wheat flour.[18] Breads have been prepared with as much as 30% cassava flour (more often 10-20%) or cassava starch, wheat flour and some oilseed flour, such as soybean, with added calcium stearoyl lactate as a dough strengthener. Experiments using mechanical leavening with a cassava-soy-wheat formulation have provided bread of good volume and eating quality and higher protein quality compared to all wheat flour breads.[16] Nonwheat breads can be prepared from sorghum plus cassava flour and xanthan gum.[24] Further technology is needed to produce high quality cassava flours, improved milling to produce the composite flour, and baker technology to optimize baking procedures. Ongoing studies have these objectives.[25]

Cassava flour nutrification has been under consideration for some time.[18] Commercial production should be monitored for situations whereby cassava flour, cassava flour/cereal grain blends or cassava starch blends as high calorie type foods might be nutrified with added nutrients, protein, vitamin A, iron, iodine, other nutrients, when warranted, to overcome deficiency disorders.[17] Supplementation of cassava with a soybean product, be it soybean isolate[21] or isolate plus methionine[22] or soy flour[26] may be attractive with favorable costs. The preferred soy additive will be dictated by the local production of soy and its processing. Potential nutrification of appropriate cassava products is promising and is closer to reality than decades past.[18,21,22] Greater and more immediate returns can result from research on the nutrification, marketing and soy processing practices than research on the genetic improvement of cassava,[21] but both types of research need to be continued.

REFERENCES

1. TALBURT, W. F. and SMITH, O. 1987. Potato Processing, 4th Ed. Van Nostrand Reinhold Co., New York.
2. WOOLFE, J. A. 1987. The Potato in the Human Diet. Cambridge University Press, London.
3. McCAY, C. M., McCAY, J. B. and SMITH, O. 1987. The nutritive value of potatoes. In Potato Processing, 4th Ed., W. F. Talburt and O. Smith (eds.). Van Nostrand Reinhold Co., New York.
4. BAUERNFEIND, J. C. 1981. Carotenoids as Colorants and Vitamin A Precursors: Technological and Nutritional Applications. Academic Press, Orlando, Fla.
4a. JONES, E. and ZEPP, G. 1983. U.S. potato industry shifts towards processed products. Natl. Food Rev. NFR-23 (summer), 5-8.
5. MYERS, P. W. and ROEHM, G. H. 1963. Ascorbic acid in dehydrated potatoes. J. Am. Diet. Assoc. 42, 325-327.
6. BRING, S. V. and RAAB, F. P. 1964. Total ascorbic acid in potatoes. J. Am. Diet. Assoc. 45, 149-152.
7. WILLARD, M. J., HIX, V. M. and KLUGE, G. 1987. Dehydrated mashed potatoes, potato granules. In Potato Processing, 4th Ed., W. F. Talburt and O. Smith (eds.). Van Nostrand Reinhold Co., New York.

8. BAUERNFEIND, J. C. 1982. Ascorbic acid technology in agricultural, pharmaceutical, food and industrial applications. *In* Ascorbic Acid: Chemistry, Metabolism and Uses, P. A. Seib and B. M. Tolbert (eds.). Advances in Chemical Series 200. American Chemical Society, Washington, DC.
9. SAUER, F. 1971. Vitamin fortification of dehydrated products. ARS Serv. Circ. 74-55. U.S. Dept. Agriculture, Washington, DC.
10. CORDING, J., JR., ESKEW, R. J., SALINARD, G. J. and SULLIVAN, J. 1961: Vitamin stability in fortified potato flakes. Food Technol. *15*(6), 279–282.
11. BAUERNFEIND, J. C. 1983. Vitamin A: Technology and applications. World Rev. Nutr. Diet. *41*, 110–199.
12. BORENSTEIN, B. and GORDON, H. T. 1987. Addition of vitamins, minerals and amino acids to foods. *In* Nutritional Evaluation of Food Processing, 3rd Ed., E. Karmas and R. S. Harris (eds.). Van Nostrand Reinhold Co., New York.
13. SMITH, O. 1987. Potato chips. *In* Potato Processing, 4th Ed., W. F. Talburt and O. Smith (eds.). Van Nostrand Reinhold Co., New York.
14. SULLIVAN, J. P., KOZEMPEL, M. F., EGOVILLE, M. J. and TALLEY, E. A. 1985. Loss of amino acids and water-soluble vitamins during potato processing. J. Food Sci. *50*(5), 1249–1253.
15. KIES, C. and FOX, H. M. 1972. Effect of amino-acid supplementation of dehydrated potato flakes on protein-nutritive value for human subjects. Food Technol. *21*(6), 865–870.
16. GRACE, M. R. 1977. Cassava Processing. FAO Plant Series No. 3. UN Food & Agriculture Organization, Rome.
17. FALCON, W. P., JONES, W. D., PEARSON, S. R., DIXSON, J. A., NELSON, G. C., ROCHE, F. C. and UNNEVEHR, L. J. 1984. The Cassava Economy of Java. Stanford University Press, Stanford.
18. COCK, J. H. 1985. Cassava, New Potential for a Neglected Crop. Westview Press Inc., Boulder.
19. OKEZIE, B. O. and KOSIKOWSKI, F. U. 1982. Cassava as a food. CRC Crit. Rev. Food Sci. Technol. *17*(3), 259–275.
20. LANCASTER, P. A., INGRAM, J. S., LIM, M. Y. AND COURSEY, D. G. 1982. Traditional cassava-based foods: Survey of processing techniques. Econ. Bot. *36*(1), 12–45.
21. PHILLIPS, T. P. 1973. Cassava Utilization and Potential Markets. International Development Research Center, Box 8500, Ottawa, Canada KIG 3H9.
22. FRAZAO, M. 1972. Fortification of Cassava—Brazil. Presentation: Workshop on Food Fortification. Agency of International Development, Washington, DC.
23. INGRAM, J. S. 1975. Standards, Specifications and Quality Requirements for Processed Cassava Products. G102. Tropical Products Institutes, London.
24. MARSERO, M. 1989. Cassava flour in breadmaking. Tecnica Molitoria *40*(3), 182–184.
25. ANNUAL REPT. 1984. Cassava Program. Working Document No. 1, 1985. Centre Internacional de Agricultura Tropical, Columbia, SA.
26. COLLINS, J. L. and TEMALILWA, C. R. 1981. Cassava flour fortification with soy flour. J. Food Sci. *46*, 1025–1028.

CHAPTER 8

Foods Considered for Nutrient Addition: SUGARS

MARIO R. MOLINA, Ph.D.

INTRODUCTION

The most important food and nutrition problems around the world have been identified as protein-energy malnutrition, anemias associated with iron and folate deficiencies, hypovitaminosis A and iodine deficiency.[12,17,32,46,49,50] Of problems, protein-energy malnutrition can be recognized mainly as a food problem, while the other deficiencies (vitamin A, iodine and iron and folate) are micronutrient deficiencies. Micronutrient deficiencies can be corrected through several alternatives, such as: increasing consumption of the food items which contain them in the desirable concentrations and in a bioavailable form; or by supplying them periodically in a therapeutic dose; or by nutrifying suitable food carriers to assure an adequate intake of the micronutrients. Among the aforementioned alternatives, the public health nutrification of a suitable food carrier with the desired micronutrient has proved to be the most economical and practical alternative to ameliorate and/or prevent the principal micronutrient deficiencies cited. It is generally recognized that food nutrifying action is taken to fulfill a public health objective (to overcome micronutrient deficiency or insufficiency) and should be looked upon as a measure to be adopted in conjunction with other longer range interventions (agricultural production programs, food and nutrition education activities, and other effective social and economic approaches), which will assure adequate nutrition and optimal health for all vulnerable population groups.

In public health fortification programs the carrier or vehicle should have several desirable characteristics: first, it should be consumed regularly and in relatively constant amounts by the target population. The acceptability and/or quality of the carrier food or ingredient should not be affected by the micronutrient added, and, perhaps more importantly, the carrier should not affect the bioavailability of the added micronutrient. Also, the method of addition of the micronutrient should be technologically simple and should represent a low cost operation which, if possible, should be comparable with the production process of the carrier. The final product mixture obtained (micronutrient and carrier), should be stable and homogeneous and the bioavailability of the micronutrient should not be compromised under the recommended storage conditions of the mixture. Sugar and common salt have proved to have most of the desired characteristics mentioned above, and this is the reason why they have been used as public health carriers in nutrification programs. Efficient salt fortification programs have eradicated iodine deficiency,[16] and sugar fortification programs have been effective in eradicating vitamin A deficiency.[10] The 1975–77 field studies demonstrated the effectiveness of vitamin A nutrified sugar in improving vitamin A status (Table 8.1) in Guatemala. Since most forms of iron adversely affect the storage properties of common salt,[43] sugar has also been examined as a carrier for either iron alone or iron and ascorbic acid.[18,35,36,40,47]

The present chapter reviews the studies using sugars as carriers of micronutrients, with special reference to the vitamin A nutrification program developed originally for the Central American region.[5]

CHARACTERISTICS OF SUGARS AS CARRIERS OF SUPPLEMENTARY NUTRIENTS

Sugar (sucrose) is a food ingredient that provides a source of carbohydrates and a desirable sweet taste. The production and/or refining of sugar in most countries is a centralized operation. This fact facilitates the use of sucrose as a carrier of nutrients, since its fortification could be controlled with relative ease. Because sucrose can be selectively handled, only the portion of the production destined for direct consumption could be fortified and not that going for industrial purposes.

In the USA, reports indicate that from 1925–1970 the average per capita intake of sugar remained relatively constant at about 45 kg/yr.[40,44] In Guatemala, the average direct sugar intake by the rural population has been calculated as 36g/day.[23,30,37] Based on these Guatemalan data, the vitamin A to be supplied by the fortification program in Guatemala could be initially calculated. Similar data for other Central American countries indicate that the direct sugar consumption in rural areas is relatively constant,[24–28] thus Central American guidelines for vitamin A fortification of table sugar could be prepared.[7] The same data on table sugar intake in Central America served as a basis for considering sugar as a possible vehicle or carrier for iron in the form of NaFeEDTA.[48] The reported increased sugar consumption patterns in the world seem to be associated with increased income. Also, more sugar is being utilized in manufactured products rather than in expanded direct household use.[40]

The behavior and stability of micronutrients in nutrified sugar used in heated beverages (coffee or tea or cocoa), heated meals or baked goods prepared at home with the table sugar should be known. The possible implications of sugar in cardiovascular disease,[22] obesity,[15] diabetes and blood lipids[13] should be considered as possible limitations that could affect sugar consumption and therefore the intake of

TABLE 8.1
INTAKE OF RETINOL EQUIVALENT[1] PER CAPITA PER DAY

Survey Period	From Natural Food Sources	From Fortified Sugar	Total
October–November 1975 (baseline)	221	0	221
April–May 1976	178	336	514
October–November 1976	198	425	623
April–May 1977	251	419	670
October–November 1977	182	445	627

Source: Arroyave.[11a]
[1] In micrograms.

any added micronutrient. It is recognized that with increased consumption of sugar containing foods, reduced consumption of nutritionally superior foods (such as fruits and meat) might occur; however, fortification of sugar would help to counter such changes.[40] Nutrification of sugar with phosphates and calcium has been suggested to minimize dental decay.[40]

EXISTING KNOWLEDGE OF THE NUTRIFICATION OF SUGARS: VITAMIN A AS A MODEL

Operational Aspects

The eventual purpose of the vitamin A fortification of table sugar in Guatemala, as defined by Pineda,[42] has been to supply the recommended daily required amount of retinol (250–400 μg/day) to preschool children whose table sugar intake averages 20 g/day. Thus, the fortification level was established as 15 μg of retinol per gram of table sugar. This amount is considered safe for adults, who also ingest part of their daily recommended consumption of vitamin A (2500 IU according to FAO/WHO) from food items in their otherwise deficient diet.

Preliminary studies at Hoffmann-LaRoche, showed that vitamin A palmitate 250-SD, a powder form, could be used in the fortification process.[3] Later, it also became evident that retinyl palmitate 250-CWS, a beadlet product, could be used as indicated by laboratory tests (Table 8.2). Presently, this latter product is used in the nutrification process.[42]

Preparation of the Premix. Initially, the fortification process involves the preparation of a premix. At present the premix has the formulation stated in Table 8.3. To prepare such a premix the sugar and the stabilized vitamin A palmitate beadlet product (250-CWS) are first mixed in a revolving drum mixer or other proven equipment. The oil containing the dissolved stabilizer (Ronoxan A) is then added stepwise to the mixture while mixing until all is added and uniformity is obtained (Fig. 8.1). This premix is packed in double polyethylene bags which in turn are put into

TABLE 8.2
STABILITY OF ADDED VITAMIN A IN NUTRIFIED SUGAR

			Percentage Retention of Vitamin A						
			45°C (Months)			23–25°C (Months)			
Product	Trial	Vitamin A Type	1	2	3	1	2	3	6
Premix[1]									
A	1	250-CWS	92	83	—	99	98	—	99
B	1	250-SD	87	79	—	97	95	—	96
C	2	250-CWS	—	—	86	—	—	92	94
D	2	250-SD	—	—	77	—	—	93	89
E	3	250-CWS	93	—	81	97	—	90	90
F	3	250-SD	92	—	74	100	—	95	93
Nutrified sugar[2]									
G	4	250-CWS	91	—	76	96	—	96	92
H	4	250-SD	90	—	73	100	—	88	85

Source: Bauernfeind and Arroyave.[12a]
[1]Vitamin A-sugar premix (50,000 IU/g).
[2]Vitamin-nutrified sugar (50–70 IU/g).

heavy paper bags and stored in a clean, dry and dark place. Special care should be taken to ensure proper storage conditions for the premix, as the bags are initially closed and then later reopened for use.[42]

As a practical example in the preparation of 100 kg of premix, 50 kg of sugar are mixed with 22 kg of retinyl palmitate 250-CWS until a uniform mix is obtained (approximately 10 minutes in a blender). Then, 26 kg more of sugar are added and the mixing is continued. Separately, 1.65 kg of the oil is placed in a stainless steel reservoir bubbling N_2 gas continuously. The oil is then heated to 60°C and 8.2 g of the stabilizer are added, mixing until the paste is dissolved (approximately 5 minutes). Nitrogen is bubbled continuously during this time to prevent any possible oxidation of the oil. It has been found that other vegetable oils (soybean, maize or cottonseed oil) could be substituted for the original peanut oil.[38] As a third step, the warmed oil containing the stabilizer (Ronoxan A) is slowly added to the vitamin A/sugar mixture. The mixing is continued for about 10 minutes after the addition of all the oil to assure uniformity. A uniform color is indicative of a good quality, well-prepared premix. A V-shaped, solid-liquid mixer is a good alternative apparatus for the mixing operation.

The process summarized above and presently used for the preparation of the premix[42] differs somewhat from the original work carried out at INCAP.[3,4] The differences are found primarily in the fact that originally vitamin A palmitate 250-SD was used to attain a final concentration of 0.021 mg of retinol per gram of sugar, rather than the presently used 0.015 mg/g concentration. The former, original concentration (0.021 mg/g) was based on the calculation of an amount of sugar which

TABLE 8.3
FORMULATION OF THE VITAMIN A FORTIFIED PREMIX
(Per metric ton, with 10% excess)

Ingredient	Concentration (kg)
Retinyl palmitate 250-CWS	220.00
Peanut oil (peroxide free)[1]	16.50
Stabilizing mixture[2]	0.08
Sugar	763.42

Source: Data from Pineda.[42]
[1]Other vegetable oils as those of soybean, maize, cottonseed or african palm may be used according to availability (Mejía and Pineda.[38]).
[2]Ronoxan A from Hoffmann-LaRoche, Switzerland.

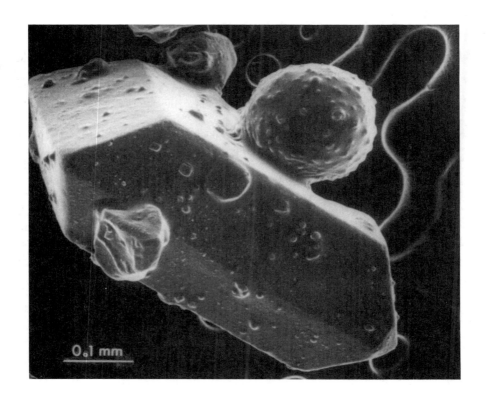

Courtesy of John Gmünder
FIG. 8.1. MAGNIFIED PHOTOGRAPH OF VITAMIN A BEADLETS ADHERING TO SUCROSE CRYSTAL

would supply the daily recommended intake of vitamin A (0.75 mg of retinol) for adults as stated by FAO/WHO.[20] The rationale for modifying the vitamin A fortification level was the recognition that the primary goal of the program should be adequate vitamin A intakes of preschool children, not adults, since the latter derive part of their vitamin A requirements from dietary sources other than fortified sugar.[42]

In the preparation of the premix the work of Lacera[31] et al. should be mentioned. These researchers investigated the possibility of substituting part of the added vegetable oil with shark's liver oil (rich in natural vitamin A) and increasing the oil content of the premix. Lacera et al.[31] reported that an acceptable, good quality premix could be prepared by adding 6.4 ml of shark's liver oil per 100 g of premix, rather than the standard 1.65 ml of vegetable oil. The added shark's liver oil supplied between 10-12% of the vitamin A activity desired in the final premix. Considering that sharks are a marine resource found off the coasts of various Central American countries with people suffering from vitamin A deficiency, this modification seems worthy in the quest to lower the need for imported pure vitamin A (such as retinyl palmitate). If adopted, the stability of the fish oil vitamin A addition in the sugar mixture would need to be examined.

Fortification Process. The process involves blending the premix with regular white sugar to produce vitamin A nutrified sugar. The operation can presently be affected either (1) in the centrifuge at the end of the sugar washing cycle or (2) during the transportation of the sugar (on transporting belts), either before or after drying and prior to final packaging.[42]

When fortification of the crystallized sugar is carried out on the transporting belts, an adjustable precision feeder mechanism is synchronized with the propulsion system rate of the belt; thus, the flow of the premix is synchronized with the flow of the sugar stream. A thorough mixing is accomplished during the drying process.

When the fortification process is conducted in the centrifuge at the end of the sugar washing cycle, the weight of the centrifuge charge must be first obtained. The weight of the charge is calculated from the physical constants of the centrifuge (height and large and small radius) corrected by the pi value and the density of the product being centrifuged, according to the following general expression:

$$p = \pi d (R^2 - r^2) h$$

Where: p = weight of the charge of the centrifuge (kg)

$Pi = 3.1415 = \pi$

d = density of product being centrifuged (kg/m³)

R and r = large and small radius of the centrifuge, respectively (m)

h = height of the centrifuge (m)

In Guatemala the average density of the product being centrifuged is 880 kg/m³ (Pineda[42]).

Once the weight of the charge of the centrifuge is known, the amount of premix needed per lot being centrifuged is relatively easy to establish and to program in repeated cycles. Here again, the mixing of the premix and the sugar is accomplished during the drying and packing operations.

The vitamin A nutrified sugar is generally packed in cloth bags and stored for marketing. During the fortification process and storage of the nutrified sugar, moisture exposure should be kept at a minimum for maximum stability of the incorporated vitamin A.

Quality Control

Homogeneity. One of the first concerns of the entire fortification operation of table sugar with vitamin A is the attainment of an even distribution of the micronutrient in the sugar.

In the studies carried out using vitamin A palmitate 250-SD, even distribution of vitamin A has been reported in the nutrified sugar.[2,4,19,30] This work has also resulted in a rapid, quantitative method for determining the vitamin A in the nutrified sugar,[1,6,9] based on the Carr-Price procedure.[45] Two easy-to-read publications were prepared by INCAP[1,8] with the intent of educating sugar manufacturers and thus assuring satisfactory quality control procedures for the program. These goals are reflected in the latest easy-to-read publication.[42] One colorimetric test is illustrated as Table 8.4.

Even distribution of the vitamin A in the final fortified product is assured by preparing a good quality premix. The even distribution of retinyl palmitate in the premix is verified by chemical assay, although an empirical judgment can be obtained by visually observing for uniform color and a granular, homogeneously "lightly greasy" texture.[42]

Acceptability. Welfare institutions and the INCAP dining facilities were used to test the acceptability of the vitamin A fortified sugar over a four-month period.[29] Results of this "blind test" showed that consumers could detect no difference between regular sugar and the vitamin A nutrified sugar. In a second study, vitamin A fortified sugar was distributed through regular channels to a rural community.[3] Again, the results showed that the acceptability of the nutrified sugar was not appreciably different from that of the regular sugar.

In addition, triangle tests were performed on drinks prepared with vitamin A fortified sugar. The samples tested included coffee, Incaparina, pineapple refreshment, tea, orangeade, lemonade and horchata (a rice flour cold drink). The panelists were able to detect the fortified sugar in coffee, pineapple refreshment and orangeade, but they considered the flavor imparted by the vitamin A containing sugar to be acceptable.

Bioavailability. Studies of the bioavailability of vitamin A in the enriched sugar carried out on rats demonstrated that the product contained 100% of the expected biological activity.[29]

TABLE 8.4
RAPID COLORIMETRIC METHOD FOR THE CONTROL OF THE FORTIFICATION OF SUGAR WITH VITAMIN A

A. *Description of the method*

1) Reagents

   a) Chromogen reagent. To prepare this reagent weigh in a beaker 60 g of trichloroacetic acid and 40 g of methylene dichloride (CH_2Cl_2) or ethylene dichloride ($CH_2Cl\text{-}CH_2Cl$). To dissolve completely, warm mixture in a water bath at 60-70°C with constant stirring. Store the reagent in an amber glass container with glass stopper.

   b) Distilled water.

B. *Materials*

1) Test tubes 13 x 100 mm.
2) A measuring scoop (plastic or glass) which, when leveled, should contain approximately 500 mg (1/2 g) of sugar.
3) A small glass funnel to introduce the sugar into the test tube.
4) A dropper.
5) A 10 ml graduated syringe (glass or polyethylene) to measure the chromogen reagent. It is convenient to attach a length of polyethylene tubing to the tip of the syringe to facilitate delivery of the reagent into the test tube.
6) Color scale. In 13 x 100 mm test tubes place 4 ml of the following concentrations of copper sulfate water solution ($CuSO_4$, $5H_2O$) per 100 ml: 0.0, 1.0, 2.5, 5.0, 7.5, 10.0, 12.5, 20.0, and 25.0. Cover tubes with a rubber stopper sealing them airtight to prevent any evaporation. Label tubes from 1 to 9.

C. *Procedure*

With the measuring scoop place 500 mg of the sugar into a 13 x 100 mm test tube. Add 3 drops of distilled water and warm in a water bath at a temperature of 60-70°C for 1 minute; shake occasionally. Cool at room temperature in a cold water bath (±20°C). Add with the measuring syringe 3 ml of the chromogen reagent and mix immediately. Compare against the color scale the blue color developed, which reaches its peak between 5-10 seconds. After 10 seconds the color begins to fade.

In our experience, using white sugar fortified within the limits recommended by the fortification program in Guatemala (43 to 57 IU per gram), the readings fall between tubes 6 and 9.

When the sugar being fortified is not completely white, but is instead yellow due to impurities, the color reaction tends to give a greenish color.

The colorimetric method permits rapid determination of whether a sample of sugar is or is not fortified with vitamin A, as well as the approximate level of fortification. For this reason it can be employed as a field method. For this purpose, the necessary reagents and materials can be placed in a portable box and transported directly to the places where one would wish to check the presence of vitamin A in the sugar.

Source: Arroyave et al.[10]

In a study of lactating mothers supplied with fortified sugar, Arroyave et al.[11] reported that their blood serum retinol level increased significantly over the course of the study. Thus, the results indicated that the vitamin A was biologically available to the mothers. Furthermore, the authors found that after the fourth month of lactation the babies from mothers consuming nutrified sugar showed a higher serum retinol level than the babies of the control mothers. A similar relationship was noted in studies of the maternal milk retinol content. Since mother's milk was the sole dietary source of vitamin A for the babies, the finding on their serum values again confirm the bioavailability of vitamin A from the ingestion of nutrified sugar.

Toro et al.[45] working with sugar fortified with retinyl acetate 325L (Hoffman-LaRoche) in Chile failed to decrease the clinical signs of vitamin A deficiency in 160 school children and 60 adults in a 3-month period. The authors attributed this finding to the short period of ingestion of the enriched sugar. Assays of fortified sugar taken at consumption locations at time intervals would have revealed the presence or absence of the expected vitamin A content.

Economic Aspects

Since the original studies, it has been determined that the cost of the vitamin A added to the sugar is relatively low. In fact, Arroyave[3] stated that such a cost was equivalent to US$0.03 per person per year. This relatively low cost (around US$2.25 per metric ton of sugar) was a major factor in the decision by the Central American sugar manufacturers to absorb the cost of the nutrification program. For these types of intervention programs to proceed successfully, the operational costs should be kept at a minimum, as accomplished in the present Central American case.

Legal and Political Aspects

The legal and political aspects are an important part in any fortification program, such as the vitamin A addition to table sugar. Each must be considered and regulations should support their public health value and thus assure that the program will be implemented properly and monitored adequately. The responsibilities of all concerned should be clearly defined, indicating who will carry out each component in the program, as well as to delineate what sanctions are to be imposed if the program is not operated properly. In Central America the fortification of sugar with vitamin A has been legislated in Costa Rica, Guatemala, Honduras and Panama. The regulation applies to refined white table sugar rather than to sugar for industrial purposes.[2,7,19]

POTENTIAL FOR THE NUTRIFICATION OF SUGARS WITH OTHER NUTRIENTS

Iron

Sugar has also been evaluated as a carrier of iron. At INCAP Viteri and García-Ibáñez[47] reported the possible fortification of sugar with ferric-sodium-EDTA. The operation could be effected in a similar fashion to that for vitamin A, as previously described, or both nutrients could be added in the same mixture. When the iron fortified sugar (13 mg of iron as ferric-sodium-EDTA/100 g sugar) was consumed by 31 normal subjects mixed in a corn-bean-bread and coffee diet, a mean iron absorption value of 6.4% was observed. The absorption value compared well with the 2.8% value obtained when ferric sulfate was used in a similar trial.

Disler et al.[18] added iron in a variety of compounds to a commercial white cane sugar at two levels (100 and 200 mg/kg). In several cases, ascorbic acid was also added to the sugar at a concentration of either 1 or 2 g/kg. The authors reported two methods of fortification; (1) dissolving the iron and ascorbic acid in water and spraying the solution onto the sugar; (2) dampening the sugar in water (1 g/kg) before mixing the sugar with each of the finely ground dry supplements. The latter method was preferred, since when the former was used a discoloration (purple/brown color) of the sugar resulted. After fortification, the sugar was air dried and could be stored between 22–27 °C in a mean relative humidity of 55% without problems. The same authors (Disler et al.[18]) reported that when ferric orthophosphate was used with ascorbic acid in the fortification of sugar the absorption value was much better when the fortified sugar was added to a maize porridge before cooking (12.7%) than when it was added after cooking (1.8%). This finding suggests that an absorbable iron complex may be formed between the insoluble ferric orthophosphate and ascorbic acid during cooking. Jams prepared with sugar fortified with ferric orthophosphate and ascorbic acid provided a relatively high iron absorption value (13.8%). But this was not the case when the sugar was fortified only with ferric orthophosphate (absorption value 2.3%), indicating the benefit of added ascorbic acid. In biscuits prepared with ferric orthophosphate and ascorbic acid, the relatively high absorption value mentioned in the other products was not obtained and can be attributed to destruction of ascorbic acid by the high baking temperture.[18]

Layrisse[33] and Layrisse et al.[35] indicate that a benefit of using sugar as a carrier for iron is that the sugar acts as a reducer and maintains the iron salts in a ferrous form. At a concentration of 1 mg of iron per gram of sugar, the fortification does not affect the color nor the taste of sugar.

When iron fortified sugar is ingested with a diet of wheat and black beans the addition of ascorbic acid increases the absorption of both the extrinsic and the intrinsic iron in the diet, thus lowering the negative effect of the absorption-inhibiting substances in the vegetable product.[18,33,35,36]

One major problem reported with iron fortified sugar is the marked discoloration developed when coffee or tea are prepared with it. The discoloration develops almost immediately as the sugar is added.[18] Layrisse et al.,[36] however, noted that when Fe-(III)-EDTA was used as the fortifying compound the discoloration in tea was produced very slowly for the first 2 h and the iron itself resisted precipitation for at least 24 h. Although the discoloration problem may be reduced using Fe-(III)-EDTA, the question remains whether or not such a compound can prevent the formation of nonabsorbable tannin-iron complexes. The addition of Fe-(III)-EDTA to maize appears to favor the absorption of both extrinsic and intrinsic iron.[34]

Other Micronutrients

The nutrification of sugar with phosphates and calcium has been examined primarily to minimize the possible negative effect of sugar on dental decay.[21,40] The fortification of sugar with fluorides has also been examined with a similar purpose.[39] A comprehensive review on the subject was published by Navia.[41]

Patents have been obtained for the production and marketing of multinutrient fortified sugar.[14] Industrial efforts[41] have been made to produce a sugar fortified with both vitamins and minerals, but the producers mention problems of odor, taste and discoloration with the fortified product. However, considering the advantages of sugars as a universal carrier and emerging technological advances, there is hope that the sensory limitations of marketed multinutrient sucrose products will be overcome.

SUMMARY

The Central American experiences with vitamin A nutrification of crystalline sugar as a successful intervention strategy in the alleviation of vitamin A deficiency in the Central American population is an outstanding achievement in the history of public health, brought about by the creative efforts of organic chemists, nutritionists, food technologists and food engineers, as well as the support of the food industry, government and the general public. Hopefully, through this accomplishment, sugar may become more universally recognized as a potentially practical carrier of other micronutrients where merit exists for its consideration.

REFERENCES

1. AGUILAR, J. R., ARROYAVE, G. and GALLARDO, I. C. 1977. Manual de Supervisión y control de programas de fortificatión de Azúcar con vitamina "A." Instituto de Nutrición de Centro América y Panamá (INCAP). Publicación INCAP E-913. Guatemala Centro América.

2. AGUILAR, J. R., ARROYAVE, G. and PORTELA, E. 1975. Rapid method for adding vitamin A to sugar at an industrial level. 10th Int. Congr. Nutr., Kyoto, Japan.
3. ARROYAVE, G. 1971. Distribution of vitamin A to population groups. Proc. West. Hemisphere Nutr. Congr. *III*, 68–77.
4. ARROYAVE, G. 1977. Control of vitamin A deficiency fortification of sugar with vitamin A. Part II. Sugar Azúcar *72*, 36–40.
5. ARROYAVE, G. and BRENES, E. A. 1972. Control de la deficiencia de vitamina A en Guatemala. Rev. Col. Médico (Guatemala) *23*, 66–80.
6. ARROYAVE, G. and DE FUNES, C. 1974. Enriquecimiento de azúcar con vitamina A. Método para la determinación cuantitativa de retinol en azúcar blanca de mesa. Arch. Latinoam. Nutr. *24*, 147–153.
7. ARROYAVE, G., AGUILAR, J. R. and FLORES, L. M. 1978. Evaluation of programs to control vitamin A deficiency. Proc. West. Hemisphere Nutr. Congr. *V*, 46–56.
8. ARROYAVE, G. AGUILAR, J. R. and PORTELA, E. 1975. Manual de Operaciones Para la Fortification de Azúcar Con Vitamina "A." Instituto de Nutrición de Centro América y Panamá (INCAP), Publicación INCAP E-853. Guatemala, Centro América.
9. ARROYAVE, G., PINEDA, O. and DE FUNES, C. 1974a. Enriquecimiento de Azúcar con vitamina A. Método rápido para la fácil inspección del proceso. Arch. Latinoam. Nutr. *24*, 155–159.
10. ARROYAVE, G., AGUILAR, J. R., FLORES, M. and GUZMÁN, M. A. 1979. Evaluation of sugar fortification with vitamin A at the national level. Scientific Publ. No. 384. Pan Am Health Organization, Washington, DC.
11. ARROYAVE, G., BEGHIN, I., FLORES, M., SOTO DE GUÍDO, C. and TICAS, J. M. 1974b. Efectos del consumo de azúcar fortificada con retinol, por la madre embarazada y lactante cuya dieta habitual es baja en vitamina "A." Estudio de la madre y del niño. Arch. Latinoam. Nutr. *24*, 485–512.
11a. ARROYAVE, G. 1986. Vitamin A deficiency control in Central America. *In* Vitamin A Deficiency and Its Control, J. C. Bauernfeind (ed.). Academic Press, Orlando.
12. AYKROYD, W. R. 1970. Eliminación de las enfermedades carenciales. Resultados y perspectivas. World Health Organization (WHO), Geneva, Switzerland. Estudio Básico No. 24.
12a. BAUERNFEIND, J. C. and ARROYAVE, G. 1986. Control of vitamin A deficiency by the nutrification of food approach. *In* Vitamin A Deficiency and Its Control, J. C. Bauernfeind (ed.). Academic Press, Orlando.
13. BIERMAN, E. L. and NELSON, R. 1975. Carbohydrates diabetes, and blood lipids. World Rev. Nutr. Diet. *22*, 280–287.
14. CARTER, J. F. 1971. Production of fortified sugar. U.S. Patent No. 3,607,310. Sept. 21.
15. DANOWSKI, T. S., NOLAN, S. and STEPHAN, T. 1975. Obesity. World Rev. Nutr. Diet. *22*, 270–279.
16. DeMAEYER, E. M., LOWENSTEIN, F. W. and THILLY, C. H. 1979. The control of endemic goitre. World Health Organization (WHO), Geneva, Switzerland.
17. DIEZ-EWALD, M. and MOLINA, R. A. 1972. Iron and folic acid deficiency during pregnancy in Western Venezuela. Am. J. Trop. Med. Hyg. *21*, 587–591.
18. DISLER, P. B., LYNCH, S. R., CHARLETON, R. W., BOTHWELL, T. H., WALTER, R. B. and MAYET, F. 1975. Studies on the fortification of cane sugar with iron and ascorbic acid. Br. J. Nutr. *34*, 141–152.

19. DORIÓN, R. C. 1977. Control of vitamin A deficiency. Fortification of sugar with vitamin A. Part I. Sugar Azúcar, 72, 33-36.
20. FAO/WHO Joint Expert Group. 1967. Requirements of vitamin A, thiamine, riboflavine and niacin. WHO Tech. Rep. Ser. No. 362. Geneva, Switzerland.
21. FINN, S. B. and GLASS, R. B. 1975. Sugar and dental decay. World Rev. Nutr. Diet. 22, 304-326.
22. GRANDE, F. 1975. Sugar and cardiovascular disease. World Rev. Nutr. Diet. 22, 248-269.
23. Instituto de Nutrición de Centro América y Panamá. 1969a. Evaluación nutricional de la poblacion de Centroamérica y Panamá. INCAP, Guatemala.
24. Instituto de Nutrición de Centro América y Panamá. 1969b. Evaluación nutricional de la poblacion de Centroamérica y Panamá. INCAP, El Salvador.
25. Instituto de Nutrición de Centro América y Panamá. 1969c. Evaluación nutricional de la poblacion de Centroamérica y Panamá. INCAP, Honduras.
26. Instituto de Nutrición de Centro América y Panamá. 1969d. Evaluación nutricional de la poblacion de Centroamérica y Panamá. INCAP, Nicaragua.
27. Instituto de Nutrición de Centro América y Panamá. 1969e. Evaluación nutricional de la poblacion de Centroamérica y Panamá. INCAP, Costa Rica.
28. Instituto de Nutrición de Centro América y Panamá. 1969f. Evaluación nutricional de la poblacion de Centroamérica y Panamá. INCAP, Panamá.
29. Instituto de Nutrición de Centro América y Panamá. 1974. Fortification of sugar with vitamin A in Central America and Panama. INCAP.
30. Instituto de Nutrición de Centro América y Panamá (INCAP). 1975. Evaluation of sugar fortification with vitamin A at the national level. Proposal submitted to U.S.A.I.D. in Nov. 1975. INCAP.
31. LACERA, A., MEJÍA, L. A., MOLINA, M. R. and BRESSANI, R. 1983. Fortificatión de azúcar con aceite de hígado de tiburón, para alimentación humana. In Proc. Int. Conf. "Marine Resources of the Pacific." P. M. Arana, (ed.). Viña del Mar, Chile.
32. LAYRISSE, M. 1966. The aetiology and geographic incidence of iron deficiency. Plenary Sessions. XI Congr. Int. Soc. Haematol.
33. LAYRISSE, M. 1975. Iron nutriture. Proc. West. Hemisphere Congr. IV, 148-154.
34. LAYRISSE, M. and MARTÍNEZ-TORRES, C. 1977. Fe-(III)-EDTA complex as iron fortification. Am. J. Clin. Nutr. 30, 1166-1174.
35. LAYRISSE, M., MARTÍNEZ-TORRES, C., RENZÍ, M., VÉLEZ, F. and GONZÁLEZ, M. 1976a. Sugar as a vehicle for iron fortification. Am. J. Clin. Nutr. 29, 8-18.
36. LAYRISSE, M., MARTÍNEZ-TORRES, C. and RENZI, M. 1976b. Sugar as a vehicle for iron fortification: further studies. Am. J. Clin. Nutr. 29, 274-279.
37. LEE, J. E. and RUÍZ, C. 1982. La canasta mínima de alimentos dentro de la economía familiar. Resumen de la Semana Técnico-Científica sobre Alimentación y Nutrición. INCAP.
38. MEJÍA, L. A. and PINEDA, O. 1986. Substitución del aceite de maní usado para la fortificacion de azucar con vitamina "A" por otros aceites vegetales de azúcar con vitamina "A" por otros aceites vegetales disponibles en Centroamérica. Arch. Latinoam. Nutr. 36, 127-134.
39. MERNAKER, L., NAVIA, J. M. and TAYLOR, R. E. 1978. Rat molar incorporation and cariostatic effect of fluoride consumed together with sucrose. Proc. Int. Assoc. Dentr. Res. 146, A-111. (Abstr.)

40. NAVIA, J. M. 1968. Enrichment of sugar and sugar products. J. Agr. Food Chem. *16*, 172–176.
41. NAVIA, J. M. 1983. Fortification of sugar. *In* Handbook of Nutritional Supplements, Vol. I: Human Use, M. Rechcigl, Jr. (ed.). CRC Series in Nutrition and Food. CRC Press, Boca Raton, Fla.
42. PINEDA, O. 1989. Fortificación de Azúcar con vitamina A. Manual de Operaciones. Instituto de Nutrición de Centro América y Panamá (INCAP), Guatemala.
43. SAYERS, M. H., LYNCH, S. R., CHARLTON, R. W., ROTHWELL, H., WALKER, R. B. and MAYER, F. 1974. The fortification of common salt with ascorbic acid and iron. Br. J. Haematol. *28*, 483–495.
44. STARE, F. J. 1975. Role of sugar in modern nutrition. World Rev. Nutr. Diet. *22*, 239–247.
45. TORO, O. DE PABLO, S., AGUAYO, M., GATTAN, V., CONTRERAS, I. and MONCKEBERG, F. 1976. Prevention of vitamin A deficiency by fortification of sugar: A field study. Arch. Lationoam. Nutr. *26*, 169–179.
46. VALVERDE, V., DELGADO, H., NOGUERA, A. and FLORES, R. 1984. Malnutrition in tropical America. *In* Malnutrition: Determinants and Consequences, P. L. White and N. Selvey (eds.). Alan R. Liss, New York; 1983. Proc. West. Hemisphere Nutr. Congr. *VII*, Aug. 7–11.
47. VITERI, F. E. and GARCÍA-IBÁÑEZ, R. 1977. Prevention of iron deficiency in Central America by means of sugar fortification with Na-Fe-EDTA. West. Hemisphere Nutr. Congr. *V*, 419. (Abstr.)
48. VITERI, F. E., GARCÍA-IBÁÑEZ, R. and TORÚN, B. 1978. Sodium iron Na-Fe-EDTA as an iron fortification compound in Central America. Absorption studies. Am. J. Clin. Nutr. *31*, 961–971.
49. VITERI, F. E., GUZMÁN, M. A. and MATA, L. 1973. Anemias nutricionales en Centro América, influencia de infección por uncinaria. Arch. Latinoam. Nutr. *23*, 33–53.
50. World Health Organization (WHO). Vitamin A Deficiency and Xerophthalmia. Report of a Joint WHO/USAID meeting. WHO Tech. Rep. Ser. *590*. Geneva, Switzerland.

CHAPTER 9

Foods Considered for Nutrient Addition: FATS AND OILS

J. CHRISTOPHER BAUERNFEIND, Ph.D.

INTRODUCTION

Fats and oils in the chemical class of compounds called lipids, perform many desirable biological, nutritional, organoleptic, and physical, functions (Table 9.1) in the maintenance of health and life. Hence, when reducing the fat content of the diet, because of the current negative image of food fat, one should not overlook the positive contributions of lipids and the need to examine the optimal composition of dietary fat which can exert a variety of metabolic effects.[1] Three food groups (fats and oils; meat, poultry and fish; and dairy products) provided about 90% of the fat in the U.S. food supply throughout the past 75 years. The amount of fat in the U.S. food supply increased ⅓ between 1909–13 and 1984, from 124 to 166 g per capita per day.[2] The U.S. consumption pattern of fats and oils[3] for 1986 versus 1936 are contrasted in Fig. 9.1.

Several important developments in the past influenced changes in fats and oils consumption, two of which are technological and one which has a nutritional basis. The Wesson process, developed at the turn of the century, provided a pattern for other oils to follow. This method refined and deodorized cottonseed oil, turning it into a bland product with a delicate flavor. The invention of hydrogenation which converts vegetable oils into semisolid fats, made modern shortenings and margarine industries possible. These two processes enabled the vegetable oil industry to compete with fats from animal sources. The third development was the mid-20th century evidence and association of the incidence of arterial disease with consumption of diets high in saturated fats and cholesterol, and also the subsequent concern of cancer associated with high consumption of fats.[4] The per capita (U.S.) consumption of various fats and oil products[4] over the past 25 years are plotted as Fig. 9.2. What percentage of daily calories should come from fats and oils for good health expectancy continues to be debated; however, U.S. opinion favors a reduction from the current level of approximately 40% to 30% or less as a future goal.[5]

Fats (butter, lard, shortenings, margarine, ghee, tallow, vanaspati) and oils (canola, corn, cottonseed, coconut, olive, palm, peanut, safflower, soybean, sunflower) are

TABLE 9.1
IMPORTANT FUNCTIONS OF FOOD LIPIDS

Food quality
   Color—carotenoids
   Texture, structure—cocoa butter
   Flavor, aroma—carbonyl compounds
   Lubricity—mouthfeel
   Satiety

Nutritional
   Source of energy via β oxidation
   Carriers of fat-soluble vitamins
   Source of essential fatty acids
   Physical functions—micelle formation/bile; facilitate absorption of fat-soluble vitamins

Biological
   Vitamins A, D, E, and K—numerous effects
   Cholesterol—precursor of vitamin D_3, corticosteroids, bile acids
   Linoleic acid—Component of skin acylglucoceramides
   Inositol phospholipids—receptor signaling, signal transduction
   Arachidonic acid—eicosanoids and lipoxins
   Docosahexaenoic acid—specific membrane functions
   n-3 Polyunsaturated fatty acids—modulators of eicosanoid synthesis?
   Acetyl ether phospholipids—platelet-aggregating factor; antitumor agent

Source: Kinsella.[1] Copyright © Institute of Food Technologists.

consumed directly or are used as food ingredients[3,6] in the preparation or manufacture of edible products (Table 9.2.). While liquid products are termed oils and solid products, fats, both terms refer to triglycerides representing more than 90% of the fatty components of their composition. Oils used in light cooking or consumed with cut-vegetables as salad oil, as well as certain other fats, may serve as carriers of added nutrients; primarily fat soluble vitamins and/or carotenoids having provitamin A activity, depending on the use of the nutrified fat or oil product. Processed fats and oils may be inadequate sources of vitamins because of nutrient losses during refining or insufficiencies in their natural state.

General processing procedures[7] involving lipids are briefly described in Table 9.3. As currently developed and approved, fat substitutes[7] may replace added butter, margarine and other lipids in processed foods in an effort to lower calorie content, but nutrient content of the food could be simultaneously lowered unless corrected by nutrient addition.

CAROTENOIDS

Carotenoids are usually added to fats and oils to provide a pleasing yellow-to-red shade of color and in fewer instances for improved vitamin A value claims. For shortening or lard products primarily used as cooking and baking fats, a dual color benefit is conferred on the consumer, namely the pleasing color in the bulk fat after purchase and upon presentation for eating. The secondary benefit of enhanced color[8] of the baked item, such as pie crust, evokes pride in the preparer and appetite in the consumer. In coloring fats such as hydrogenated oil or shortening, the selected carotenoid application form has been a 20–30% β-carotene suspension (micronized β-carotene crystals in a lipid base) at a range of 7.5–15.0 mg of pure carotene per kilogram of fat. β-Carotene suspension, at a predetermined amount, is added to warm, clarified, deodorized oil with sufficient agitation and time to dissolve the carotene and produce a uniform color before the product moves on to the chilling and packaging operations. When shortening colored at 3 different added carotene levels (9.2, 19.8, and 26.2 mg/kg) was used to prepare cookies, cake, pie crust and frosting, respectively, and then was examined and assayed, carotene retention values of 75–95% were observed as well as even coloring throughout the products.[8]

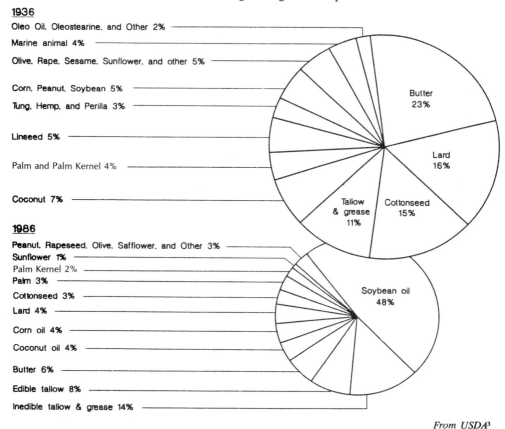

From USDA[3]

FIG. 9.1. U.S. CONSUMPTION OF FATS AND OILS, 1936 and 1986

β-Carotene and other carotenoids are subject to thermal degradation when sufficient heat is applied[9] If designated oils such as popping or deep-frying oils are to have carotene added as the means of coloring popcorn, french fries, fish sticks or other breaded foods, it may be advisable to employ a high-stress β-carotene suspension containing antioxidants to retard carotene losses. Less oil volume is required for popping versus deep frying. However, about 5–15 g of pure β-carotene are used per 100 kg of popping oil, while about 1.5–3.0 g/100 kg is needed for frying oils used to cook potato or fish stick products. An alternative approach for color improvement is to employ the usual oil cooking procedure for potato or fish sticks and follow up the cooking step by applying a carotene spray or dip before freezing.[8]

Vegetable oils used in light cooking and salad oils are easily colored with added β-carotene. There are two purposes for added color: (1) to provide and control a predetermined yellow hue for the product; and (2) to serve as a deterrent to flavor deterioration activated by exposure to light. Current research indicates that, under specific conditions, the addition of small amounts of β-carotene to purified vegetable oils, such as soybean[10] or olive[11] can delay oxidative changes. Carotenoid addition for improved fat stabilization needs further investigation, as β-carotene is an unusual type of lipid antioxidant.[12] Several modes of the antioxidant action of carotenoids

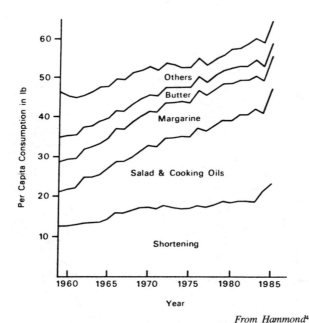

From Hammond[4]

FIG. 9.2. PER CAPITA CONSUMPTION OF VARIOUS FATS AND OIL PRODUCTS IN THE UNITED STATES BY YEAR

Copyright © by Institute of Food Technologists.

have been reviewed by Burton.[13] β-Carotene suspensions can be added to warm, deodorized oil, returned to the production batch and mixed to provide the anticipated coloration desired before cooling and bottling.[8] Other antioxidants may be added to protect the oil if needed.

The so-called "French and Russian" dressings have an orange or red hue which cannot be duplicated with the use of β-carotene. French dressings are readily colored with β-apo-carotenal in the form of apo-carotenal suspension or carotenal solution to be dispersed evenly in the oil phase of the dressing prior to the addition of other ingredients. About 10–30 mg of pure β-apo-carotenal per kilogram of dressing are used. In the preparation of Russian dressing, the water, the vinegar, alginate, and gum are mixed and the oil phase gradually added with constant agitation. Canthaxanthin (a nonvitamin A precursor), in the form of colloidal canthaxanthin in a spray powder formulation and in the amount of 15–30 mg of pure canthaxanthin per kilogram, is dispersed in warm water and added to the dressing with continued mixing. Good color stability has been experienced with both types of dressings.[14] Toppings, coffee whiteners, confectioner's coatings and other fat formulated foods are also candidates for carotenoid addition.

β-Carotene, prepared by industrial syntheses, in the year of its introduction (1954) was first used experimentally to color margarine and winter butter.[8] The yellow color of summer butter is primarily due to the natural carotenes and has been associated with vitamin A activity the past 75 years. The natural color of butter varies with the feeding practices of the dairy cow and the season of the year. Under winter conditions the diary cow, without access to fresh green grass or carotene containing ration ingredients, produces butter which is very light or nearly white in color (if not artificially colored). For many decades winter or light colored butter has been colored primarily with noncarotene colorants.

Light colored butter can be colored successfully with β-carotene in both the batch or continuous butter making processes. In the continuous process 20–30% β-carotene suspension is added to and dissolved in warm butter fat and monitored into the production stream with the continuation of normal processing. β-Carotene in the form, of water-dispersible β-carotene granules, beadlets or powders is dispersed in a small amount of warm water and added to the batch process of churning butter. About 4–7 mg of pure β-carotene per kilogram are needed to return winter or light colored butter to its traditional yellow color. This amount of carotene supplies about 3000–5000 IU of vitamin A activity per pound. In the United States, color added to winter butter is not declared on the label; neither does the label show vitamin A content. Butter colored with β-carotene is well accepted for flavor, keeping qualities and color stability.[8]

Margarine is a yellow water-in-oil emulsion of partially hydrogenated vegetable oils and nonfat fluid milk with flavors and with or without salt. As a table spread, like butter, margarine requires a rich yellow-color for ready consumer acceptance. The addition of β-carotene to margarine is widely practiced around the world. About 3–8 mg of pure β-carotene per kilogram may be added depending on the shade of

TABLE 9.2
FATS AND OILS USED IN EDIBLE PRODUCTS, BY USES

Year beginning October 1	Aug	Sept	Oct 1985 Sept 1986	Oct	Nov	Dec	Jan	Cumulative Oct 1986 Jan 1987
			Thousand lb					
Coconut Oil								
Total edible	25,312	27,098	332,821	33,760	27,913	22,918	20,779	105,370
Corn oil								
Salad or cooking oil	40,452	39,571	524,014	45,161	40,009	43,607	37,702	166,479
Margarine	13,923	21,229	199,938	14,537	18,486	31,903	16,535	81,461
Cottonseed oil								
Baking or frying fats	14,380	11,859	202,317	15,786	10,575	9,869	9,439	45,669
Margarine	2,203	D	D	3,388	2,898	1,862	2,420	10,568
Salad or cooking oil	31,940	30,647	372,723	36,040	37,800	39,993	37,710	151,543
Other edible	1,292	D	D	1,588	1,399	1,238	1,105	5,330
Total edible	49,815	47,670	627,182	56,802	52,672	52,962	50,674	213,110
Lard								
Baking or frying fats	18,357	20,237	299,466	22,289	22,921	19,303	13,469	77,982
Margarine[1]	2,806	2,547	58,995	2,007	2,397	2,771	2,158	9,333
Total edible	20,876	22,548	354,919	23,752	25,151	21,904	15,704	86,511
Palm oil								
Baking or frying fats	27,841	32,647	304,053	30,507	27,048	23,911	19,702	101,168
Total edible	32,677	39,371	363,944	37,510	33,274	30,165	24,945	125,894
Peanut oil								
Salad or cooking oil	11,207	11,523	D	12,355	11,594	9,192	10,123	43,264
Total edible	11,486	11,594	137,383	12,446	11,756	9,298	10,328	43,828

Soybean oil								
Baking or frying fats	276,192	282,038	3,440,173	310,147	289,259	279,592	250,716	1,129,714
Margarine	132,196	148,797	1,735,188	167,852	153,243	169,688	138,848	629,631
Salad or cooking oil	404,095	424,839	4,685,502	413,800	370,354	413,030	376,536	1,573,720
Other edible	8,375	9,406	138,295	12,990	7,889	8,732	11,052	40,670
Total edible	820,858	865,080	10,003,753	904,789	820,745	871,042	777,159	3,373,735
Sunflower oil								
Total edible	2,134	2,962	85,990	4,759	3,992	5,844	6,152	20,677
Tallow edible								
Baking or frying fats	72,664	78,446	1,015,671	96,206	76,602	74,491	66,721	314,020
Total edible	73,135	78,909	1,021,062	96,816	77,084	74,989	66,972	315,871
Total fats and oils used in edible products								
Baking or frying fats	432,260	456,782	5,563,408	512,380	451,256	440,464	390,046	1,794,146
Margarine	151,919	177,244	2,044,568	188,752	177,720	206,852	160,963	734,287
Salad or cooking oil	560,220	527,218	5,971,669	527,673	477,988	525,110	491,249	2,022,020
Other edible	28,154	291,711	392,866	48,037	29,197	31,574	28,558	137,366
Total edible	1,124,005	1,190,955	13,972,488	1,276,842	1,136,161	1,204,000	1,070,816	4,687,819

Source: USDA.[3]
[1]Includes lard and edible tallow.
D = Withheld to avoid disclosing figures for individual companies.

TABLE 9.3
DEFINITIONS OF TERMS CONCERNING THE EXTRACTION AND PROCESSING OF FATS AND OILS

Term	Definition
Extraction of fats and oils	Recovery of fats and oils from their natural sources; involves different techniques depending on the type of source
Oil from oilseeds	Cleaned, dehulled oilseeds are cooked under steam and pressed into cakes with screw presses, expressing the oil; residual oil is extracted from the flaked meal with solvent
Oil from fruit pulps, e.g. olive and palm	Olive oil is recovered by milling olives into a paste which is pressed to yield the oil. Palm oil is recovered by various means; one involves pressing palms which have been sterilized to prevent free fatty acid formation
Fat from animal sources	Tallow, which comes from cattle and sheep, and lard, from hogs, are recovered from specific fatty tissues by a process called rendering. Dry rendering involves heating the fatty tissues in tanks and draining off the liquefied fat. Wet rendering involves application of steam or hot water to liberate the fat which is recovered by skimming and centrifugation
Processing and purification	
Bleaching	Process for removing color-producing substances and other impurities from fats and oils; involves the use of an acid- or heat-activated adsorbent material and/or activated charcoal
Degumming	Process for eliminating phosphatides or lecithin from oil; involves blending the oil with water or injecting it with steam at elevated tempertures. The oil is separated from hydrated lecithin by centrifugation
Deodorization	Steam distillation process for removing volatile substances that contribute to undesirable flavors and aromas; involves blowing steam through hot oil under high temperatures and vacuum
Fractionation	Process for removing solids at specific temperatures; e.g., winterization
Refining	Process for removing free fatty acids and other impurities from fats and oils; involves treating the fat or oil with an alkaline solution
Winterization	Process for removing from the oil triglycerides with high melting points which crystallize out and cause the oil to cloud when chilled; involves filtering out crystalized material from the chilled oil

TABLE 9.3 (*Continued*)

Term	Definition
Modification	
Hydrogenation	Process for improving the oxidative and thermal stability of fats and oils, and for converting vegetable oils to plastic fats with a desired level of hardness; involves the catalytic addition of hydrogen to double bonds of fatty acids
Interesterification	Process for modifying the triglyceride structure by rearranging the acyl groups among triglycerides; involves a catalytic method done at low temperatures. Lard is commonly esterified before it is used in shortening manufacture to improve its baking characteristics

Source: Anon.[7] Adapted from ISEO (1980) and Weiss (1970). Copyright © Institute of Food Technolgists.

color desired and the type of margarine product. Of the 33,000 IU of vitamin A activity per kilogram of margarine, about 6–12,000 IU comes from added β-carotene, the remainder from added preformed vitamin A which is colorless.[8] In commercial practice, a 20–30% β-carotene suspension is dissolved in warm margarine oil in large bulk holding tanks which have built-in mixing facilities for uniform distribution before being passed on to the emulsification phase in margarine production. Storage tests and animal bioassay studies demonstrate good color retention and full bioavailability of the added carotene.[15]

VITAMIN A

An association of vitamin A with oils goes back to the time when certain fish and/or fish liver oils were the only high potency sources of the vitamin; however, there was a possible disadvantage of fishy off-flavors. When a chemically synthesized, pure vitamin A was developed and offered at economical prices, it became feasible to nutrify other oils and fats.

Vitamin A nutrification of light-cooking and salad oils is not practiced in commerce, although it has been considered from time to time and is feasible if the nutrified product is packaged in opaque or dark color containers. The nutrification process is quite simple wherein a liquid vitamin A ester concentrate in an appropriate amount is added to clarified, degassed oil, mixed for uniformity and packaged in light-protected containers. Antioxidants are added to retard oxidative processes acting on the oil and the added vitamin. Inert gas replacement of headspace air is suggested for maximum retention of product quality.

Fader nutrified vegetable oils and shortenings following the refining process[16] and reported a 2–6% loss of vitamin A following nutrification and a later 5–10% loss after 4 months of storage at 25°C. In simulated consumer recipie testing, use of the nutrified oil was found equally acceptable to regular oil when incorporated in mayonnaise, soup and fried and cooked foods. The qualities of frying fat were best preserved at 160–180°C, with 60–80% of added vitamin A being retained after 30 minutes of heating. Vitamin A retention of baked goods containing nutrified shortening, namely pastry rings (37% fat), puffed pastries (40% fat) and grilled tortillas (18% fat) was 94, 87, and 71% respectively.[16] Stability of vitamin A added to vegetable oil (3400 IU/100 g) packaged in containers was studied by Hellstrom *et al.*[17] When packaged in light brown bottles and exposed to sunlight, significant destruction was noted, but not when stored in the refrigerator or packaged in black bottles.

Margarine, a bread spread and cooking aid, interchangeable with butter, has been nutrified with vitamin A acetate or palmitate ester at 20,000–50,000 IU/kg (about 15,000 IU/lb) for some time (Table 9.4). When β-carotene is added to provide color, a common practice, it simultaneously provides about ⅓ of the claimed vitamin A activity, the remainder being supplied by the vitamin A ester-additives.[18] Most margarines are nutrified also with vitamin D. Williams[19] details the early history of nutrification of margarine and vanaspati.

In the commercial practice of nutrifying margarine there can be some variation in the manner in which the vitamin ingredients are incorporated. Where vitamin A, vitamin D and β-carotene[15] are to be added simultaneously, it is possible for the margarine manufacturer to have premeasured amounts of the three ingredients custom packaged in single sealed containers to be opened and added to a given volume or weight of warm, clarified and deodorized vegetable oil in a tank outfitted with agitators for mixing. The addition occurs before the nutrified oil is passed on to the emulsifying equipment. Where this custom service is not available, the three ingredients must be weighed out separately and added.

Biological assays of nutrified margarine have demonstrated full bioavailability of added vitamin A and chemical assays have verified good retention of the added vitamin A under varying storage conditions.[20–22]

Peanut butter, a bread spread and popular sandwich filler can be nutrified[23] by (1) mixing an oil dilution of vitamin A ester into the butter after grinding or (2) adding a metered premix of dry, stabilized vitamin A granules with the salt during the grinding operation. Added vitamin A is quite stable in peanut butter. Since the natural vitamin B_1 content of peanuts is destroyed during the roasting process, it is quite appropriate to add thiamin mononitrate during or after the grinding process to restore vitamin content.

VITAMIN E

Vitamin E (α-tocopherol) is an essential nutrient having a vast interplay with other nutrients and enzymes in maintaining the body's defenses against disease and the

TABLE 9.4
VITAMINS A AND D COMMONLY ADDED TO MARGARINE

Country	Vitamin A, IU/kg	Vitamin D, IU/kg
Australia	30,000	4,000
Austria	20,000	1,000
Belgium	20,000	1,000
Brazil	15,000–50,000	500–2,000
Canada	33,000	
Chile	14,000–18,000	1,000
Columbia	20,000–30,000	2,000–4,000
Denmark	20,000	625
Finland	20,000	2,500–3,500
Germany	20,000–30,000	1,000
Greece	25,000	1,500
Israel	30,000	3,000
Japan	30,000–40,000	
Mexico	20,000	2,000
Netherlands	20,000	2,000
Norway	20,000	2,500
Philippines	22,000	1,100[1]
Portugal	20,000–35,000	875–1,000
South Africa	20,000	1,000
Sweden	30,000	1,500
Switzerland	30,000	3,000
Turkey	20,000	1,000
United Kingdom	30,000–33,000	2,900–3,500
United States	33,000	4,400

Source: Morton.[18]
[1] 100 mg vitamin B_1 also added.

environment. Its addition to foods can be considered to have a dual purpose: (1) as a nutrient; and/or (2) as an antioxidant exerting a protective action on food components susceptible to oxidation.

In contrast with animal fats, plant or vegetable oils[24] are richer but variable sources of α-tocopherol and γ-tocopherol (10% α-tocopherol equivalent activity). Crude vegetable oils removed from the plant source by pressure or solvent extraction go through a series of processes before they can serve as refined salad oils or oils to be manufactured into margarine. Refining, bleaching, deacidifying, deodorizing and hydrogenating contribute to tocopherol losses.[25] The range in α-tocopherol content (mg/100 g) for oils as tabulated in 1980[24] were as follows: corn, 2.3–29.4; cottonseed, 32–56; olive, 0.8–24; palm, 18.8–25.6; peanut, 10.7–33.9; safflower, 34–45.8 and soybean, 3.4–11.5. Carpenter et al.[26] analyzed 14 liquid oils, some blended, from a Washington D.C. retail store and reported a content range of 1–60 mg/100 g for α-tocopherol and 15–102 mg for γ-tocopherol.

Liquid vegetable oils and margarines[27] are both visible fat contributors to the U.S. diet, the latter supplying 99–117 calories daily. They are also sources of the essential fatty acids. Since margarines are made from vegetable oils with additional processing, they too are variable sources of the tocopherols. A study, made on the tocopherol composition of margarines purchased from stores in selected locations in the United States, revealed an α-tocopherol range of 0.3–24.3 mg/100 g; a γ-tocopherol range of 3–55 mg.

In animal and some human studies, a relationship has been proposed between α-tocopherol and polyunsaturated fatty acids (PUFA): The more PUFA consumed the greater the need for dietary α-tocopherol.[28] This concept continues to be debated[29] but is a recognized factor (RDA, 1980) and may become a greater concern as consumption of omega-3 fatty acid foods increase, since they are very sensitive to oxidation. Some vegetable oils and margarines have a low α-tocopherol PUFA/ratio[30] which has stimulated some consideration toward the nutrification of margarines,[31] and possibly light cooking and salad oils, with added vitamin E.

Vitamin E has been added to some European margarines for over a decade.[18,31] α-Tocopheryl acetate or α-tocopherol have been added prior to the emulsifying step in the margarine process. Margarines with a natural low α-tocopherol/PUFA ratio of 0.1 might be raised to a more acceptable value of 0.4. Since margarines contain a vitamin A level of 15,000 IU/lb, equivalent to three times the US RDA vitamin A allowance and vitamin D at a level of 400 IU/lb, equivalent to the US RDA allowance, it may be appropriate to have margarines contain vitamin E at a level of 30 or 90 mg/lb, that is equivalent to one or three times the US RDA allowance.[31]

Frying is a common food preparation method throughout the food industry. Vitamin E loss in vegetable frying oils increases significantly with increasing fatty acid oxidation which occurs during prolonged heating. Furthermore, the natural or added tocopherols, such as α-tocopherol in fried foods, deep fried in oil, are subject to further destruction by hydroperoxides formed during fatty acid breakdown, even in freezer storage. Bunnell et al.[32] reports 68–74% tocopherol losses in french fried potatoes stored for 1–2 months at −12°C. If the frying oils and the stored fried foods prepared therein are to have a better sustained vitamin E content, a form of vitamin E which is more stable to heat and oxidation needs to be added to the frying oil. When α-tocopheryl acetate was added to a series of cooking oils and exposed to high temperatures, 96–99% of the natural α-tocopherol was destroyed versus losses of 6–19% of added dl, α-tocopheryl acetate under the same conditions.

OMEGA-3 FATTY ACIDS

Because of the espoused beneficial effects of the omega-3 unsaturated fatty acids on the vascular system, providing protection effect against coronary heart disease, there is now a new challenge for the oil technologist to find a way to incorporate long chain omega-3 polyunsaturated fatty acid[33] or an appropriate precursor acid into margarines with their nutritional qualities intact, assuming such nutritional benefits continue to be supported by further investigations. These unsaturated fatty acids would have to be incorporated following hydrogenation of oils used for margarine production. Budowski[34] notes the long chain omega-3 fatty acids associated with marine oils to be the most unsaturated fatty acids known and are extremely susceptible to free-radical attack. He further considers it prudent to have adequate α-tocopherol present to act as free radical scavenger and antioxidant in the presence of these fatty acids unless they are protected from oxygen exposure.

Apparently the level of consumption of omega-3 fatty acids has decreased and omega-6 fatty acids has increased over the past century[35-37] as a result of technological and agricultural influences on foods consumed over that period (Fig. 9.3). Metabolic aspects[1] of omega-3 and 6 fatty acids are contrasted in Fig. 9.4. Important advances have been made in the relationship of the omega-3 fatty acids to health and disease and efforts to strike a better balance among the types of fatty acids consumed is under consideration.[37-39] Evidence is accumulating for the effectiveness of dietary omega-3 fatty acids in ameliorating arthritis, atherosclerosis, cancer, perturbed immune function and thrombosis.[1] This new knowledge will pro-

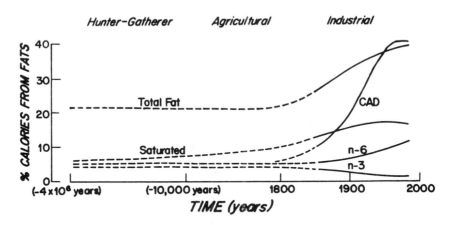

From Leaf and Webber[35]
and data of Eaton and Konner and Kinsella

FIG. 9.3. HYPOTHETICAL SCHEME OF THE RELATIVE PERCENTAGES OF FAT AND DIFFERENT FATTY ACID FAMILIES IN HUMAN NUTRITION AS EXTRAPOLATED FROM CROSS-SECTIONAL ANALYSES OF CONTEMPORARY HUNTER-GATHERER POPULATIONS AND FROM LONGITUDINAL OBSERVATIONS AND THEIR PUTATIVE CHANGES DURING THE PRECEDING 100 YR IN RELATION TO THE RECENT INCREASE IN THE FREQUENCY OF CORONARY ARTERY DISEASE (CAD)

vide a rationale for a consideration of modifying the lipid profiles of present and new food products to improve human health.

Researchers have been interested for some time in reducing the caloric value of lipid substances or finding a substitute for them. Different approaches have been pursued and some substitutes are in advanced studies.[40–42] When one or more of these have proven safe, without side effects, will function properly in varied food technologies now using conventional fats and oils, be approved by the FDA and put into commercial practice, the nutritional and biological contribution of dietary lipids will again warrant careful reevaluation.[43]

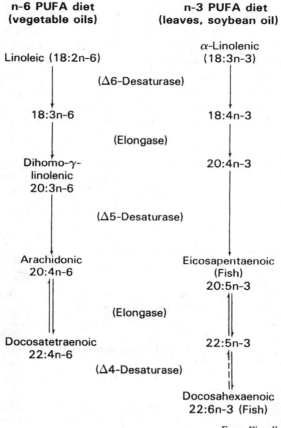

From Kinsella[1]

FIG. 9.4. METABOLISM, DESATURATION, AND ELONGATION OF DIETARY LINOLEIC AND LINOLENIC ACIDS IN HUMANS

Copyright © by Institute of Food Technologists.

REFERENCES

1. KINSELLA, J. E. 1988. Food lipids and fatty acids: importance in food quality, nutrition and health. Food Technol. 42(10), 124–144.
2. RAPER, N.R. and MARSTON, R. M. 1986. Levels and sources of fat in the U.S. food supply. In Dietary Fat and Cancer, I. Clement, D. F. Birt, A. E. Rogers, and C. Mettlin (eds.). Alan R. Liss, New York.
3. USDA. 1987. Oil Crops Situation and Outlook Report. USDA-ERS Rep. OCS-13. USDA, Washington, DC.
4. HAMMOND, E. G. 1988. Trends in fats and oils consumption and the potential effect of new technology. Food Technol. 42(1), 117–120.
5. O'CONNOR, R. P. and CAMPBELL, T. C. 1986. Dietary guidelines. In Dietary Fat and Cancer, I. Clement, D. F. Birt, A. E. Rogers and C. Mettlin (eds.). Alan R. Liss, New York.
6. WEISS, T. J. 1983. Food Oils and Their Uses. AVI/Van Nostrand Reinhold, New York.
7. ANON. 1989. Fats, oils and fat substitutes. Food Technol. 43(7), 66–74.
8. KLAEUI, H. and BAUERNFEIND, J. C. 1981. Carotenoids as food colors. In Carotenoids as Colorants and Vitamin A Precursors: Technological and Nutritional Applications, J. C. Bauernfeind (ed.). Academic Press, Orlando.
9. ONYEWU, P. N., HO, C-T. and DAUN, H. 1986. Characterization of β-carotene thermal degradation production in a model food system. JAOCS 63(11), 1437–1441.
10. WARNER, K. and FRANKEL, E. N. 1987. Effects of β-carotene on light stability in soybean oil. JAOCS 64(2), 213–218.
11. FAKOURELIS, N., LEE, E. C. and MIN, D. B. 1987. Effects of chlorophyl and β-carotene on the oxidative stability of olive oil. J. Food Sci 52(1), 234–235.
12. BURTON, G. W. and INGOLD, K. U. 1984. β-Carotene; an unusual type of lipid antioxidant. Science USA 224(4649), 569–573.
13. BURTON, G. W. 1989. Antioxidant action of carotenoids. J. Nutr. 119, 109–111.
14. GORDON, H. T. and BAUERNFEIND, J. C. 1982. Carotenoids as food colorants. CRC Crit. Rev. Food Sci. Nutr. 18(1), 59–97.
15. MARUSICH, W., DeRITTER, E. and BAUERNFEIND, J. C. 1957. Provitamin A activity and stability of β-carotene in margarine. JAOCS 34, 217–221.
16. PADEN, C. A., WOLINSKY, I., HOSKINS, J. C., LEWIS, K. C., LINEBACK, D. R. and McCARTHY, R. D. 1979. Fortification of accessory food items with vitamin A. Lebensm.-Wiss. u.-Technol. 12, 183–188.
17. HELLSTROM, P., ANDERSON, R. and HEGEDUS, L. 1964. Stability of vitamin A, tocopherol and unsaturated fatty acids in vitaminized vegetable oil exposed to sunlight. Var. Foda 8, 57–61.
18. MORTON, R. A. 1970. The vitaminization of margarine. Roy. Soc. Health J. 90, 21–28.
19. WILLIAMS, P. N. 1956. Nutritional requirements and food fortification. Chem. Ind. London 49, 1469–1473.
20. DEUEL, H. J. Jr., GREENBERG, S. M. 1953. A comparison of the retention of vitamin A in margarine and in butters based on bioassays. J. Food Res. 18, 497–503.
21. MELNICK, D., LUCKMANN, F. H. and VAHLTEICH, H. W. 1953. Retention of preformed vitamin A and carotene in margarine based on physiochemical assays. J. Food Res. 18, 504–510.

22. AMES, S. R., LUDWIG, M. I., SWANSON, W. J. and HARRIS, P. L. 1952. Biochemical studies on vitamin A: nutritional investigation of synthetic vitamin A in margarine. JAOCS 29(4), 151–153.
23. BAUERNFEIND, J. C., ROKOSNY, D. and SIEMERS, G. F. 1953. Synthetic vitamin A aids food fortification. Food Technol. 25(6), 81, 82, 85, 87.
24. BAUERNFEIND, J. C. 1980. Tocopherols in foods. In Vitamin E: A Comprehensive Treatise, L. J. Machlin (ed.). Marcel Dekker, New York.
25. HUNTER, L. E. 1981. Nutritional consequences of processing soybean oil. JAOCS 58, 283–286.
26. CARPENTER, D. L., LEHMANN, J., MASON, B. S. and SLOVER, H. T. 1976. Lipid composition of selected vegetable oils. JAOCS 53, 713–718.
27. SLOVER, H. T., THOMPSON, R. H. Jr., DAVIS, C. S. and MEROLA, G. V. 1985. Lipids in margarines and margarine-like foods. JAOCS 62(4), 775–786.
28. MACHLIN, L. J. 1984. Handbook of Vitamins: Nutritional, Biochemical and Clinical Aspects. Marcel Dekker, New York.
29. JAGER, F. C. 1975. Linoleic acid intake and vitamin E requirement. In The Role of Fats in Human Nutrition, H. J. Vergroseten (ed.). Academic Press, London.
30. CARPENTER, D. L. and SLOVER, H. T. 1973. Lipid composition of selected margarines. JAOCS 50, 372–376.
31. BUNNELL, R. H., BORENSTEIN, B. and SCHUTT, G. W. 1971. Future considerations in margarine fortification. JAOCS 48, 175A-176A.
32. BUNNELL, R. H., KEATING, J., QUARESIMO, A. and PARMAN, G. 1965. Alpha-tocopherol content of foods. Am. J. Clin. Nutr. 17 (1), 1–9.
33. ANON. 1986. Modern fats and oils technology: nutritional complications. JAOCS 63, 718–722.
34. BUDOWSKI, P. 1988. Omega-3 fatty acids in health and disease. World Rev. Nutr. Diet. 57, 214–274.
35. LEAF, A. and WEBER, P. C. 1987. A new era for science in nutrition. Am. J. Clin. Nutr. 45, 1048–1053.
36. EATON, S. B. and KONNER, M. 1985. Paleolithic nutrition: a consideration of its nature and current implications. N. Engl. J. Med. 312, 283–289.
37. KINSELLA, J. E. 1986. Food components with potential therapeutic benefits: the omega-3 polyunsaturated fatty acids of fish oils. Food Technol. 40(2), 89–97.
38. SIMOPOULOS, A. P. 1988. Omega-3 fatty acids in growth and development and in health and disease. Nutr. Today 23(2), 10–16; 23(3), 12–18.
39. DILLON, J. C. 1987. Essential fatty acid metabolism in the elderly: effects of dietary manipulation. In Lipids in Modern Nutrition, M. Horisberger and U. Bracco (eds.). Raven Press, New York.
40. LaBARGE, R. G. 1988. The search for a low-calorie oil. Food Technol. 42(1), 84–90.
41. HARRIGAN, K. A. and BREENE, W. M. 1989. Fat substitutes. Cereal Foods World 34(3), 261–269.
42. JACKEL, S. S. 1989. High-density sweeteners and fat substitutes are on the horizon. Cereal Foods World 34(10), 887–888.
43. SEGAL, M. 1990. Fat substitutes: A taste of the future? FDA Consumer 24(10), 25–27.

CHAPTER 10

Foods Considered for Nutrient Addition: JUICES AND BEVERAGES

ELMER DeRITTER

and

J. CHRISTOPHER BAUERNFEIND, Ph.D.

INTRODUCTION

Regular consumption of water is vital for the continuation of human life. Whether to consume it in its native form or as the major component of some type of beverage product is a choice of the consumer. In earlier times beverages were few in number, namely, coffee, tea, milk, beer and soda water. The beverage industry has grown in diversity[1] over the past 100 years to the point where the necessary daily liquid intake, once primarily water, now to a great extent may consist of a variety of beverages, such as fruit juices (straight or blended), fruit drinks (5-50% juice), carbonated beverages (flavored and unflavored), carbonated beverages with fruit juice, reconstituted fruit flavored beverages, frozen fruit juice bars, and reconstitutable fruit concentrates. In addition to milk there are flavored milks,[2] cocoa, milk and fruit juice mixtures, whey and fruit juice blends[3] and even carbonated milk. In the vegetable beverage category, tomato juice and a few blended vegetable juices make up the major items.[4] There are beer and low-alcohol beer-lemonade or ginger ale mixtures,[5,6] as well as tea, flavored teas, herbal teas, regular coffees, decaffeinated coffee and flavored coffees. Beverage terminology has multiplied; in addition to colas, nectars, ades, punches, and squashes, there are sport drinks,[7] tonics, shandies and coolers. Beverages may be carbonated, canned, refrigerated, frozen, pasteurized, sterilized or preserved chemically. They may be in single strength, concentrate, or reconstitutable dry form.

Some beverages are taken for their nutritive value, some for their stimulating effects, some for weight loss, some for relaxation and sociability but largely as thirst quenchers. Special situations for processed beverages include safety,[8] when and where water supplies are contaminated and clinical use.[9] The interest in dieting, fitness and health is a prime reason for the growth of the beverage industry and is aided by the entrance of noncaloric sweeteners.[10] A history of the progress[1,4] of the beverage industry also shows the influence of ingredient development, technologies in processing, commercial plant design, packaging alternatives, nutritive considerations, and modern distribution practices, each contributing to the current popular choices of beverages over water and their ease of availability in the home, school, workplace, recreation centers and eating-out facilities.

Changes in beverage choices with time have been published. Consumers are drinking more soft drinks than ever before, particularly low-calorie and low-caffeine types.[11] Decaffeinated coffee consumption is also increasing, even though total coffee consumption is down. Iced tea is favored over hot tea. Citrus fruit juice intake has doubled since 1964, and plateaued in 1986; consumption of nectars and other juices is increasing slowly. Consumption volume for carbonated soft drinks, fruit juices and mineral waters in 1985, in Australia, France, Japan, U.K., Germany, the United States, Italy and Spain have been compiled.[12] Beverage consumption (million liters) for 1985 show for fruit juices and drinks; U.K., 700; France, 751; Japan, 1,798; West Germany, 1,860 and U.S.A, 9,568; for soft drinks; France, 946; U.K. 2,620; Japan, 2,907; West Germany, 4,563 and for U.S.A., 39,118. These statistics show a trend toward more healthy drinks, some with exotic flavors, and that the worldwide beverage market is growing.

The use of more fruit juices in drinks has caused an increased demand for these horticultural crops and should become a boon to fruit producers.[13,14] The increasing world consumption of fruit juice beverage products in general has put bulk frozen straight and blended juice concentrates on a year-round international basis[15] with transportation in specially designed refrigerated shipping vessels. Over the past 70 years there has been a changing fruit product use in the United States (Table 10.1).

Since fruits represent a primary source of vitamin C, the main nutritional emphasis in the case of fruit juices has been their adequacy of ascorbic acid content. Fresh citrus juices or frozen citrus concentrates diluted to use levels will normally provide the recommended daily allowance (RDA) of ascorbic acid in a 4–8 ounce serving. Many other fruit juices require nutrification with ascorbic acid to provide a comparable level of this important nutrient. Juices often deliver other nutrients such as provitamin A, vitamin B_1, B_2, B_6, niacin and folate, but these are rarely given attention in terms of nutrification. The trend of adding 10% fruit juice to fruit drinks, has not added significantly to the nutritional value of the beverage; hence, while nutrification practices with added ascorbic acid are commendable, restoration of other nutrients is overlooked.

The U.S. per capita consumption of beverages (gallons) over the years 1965–85 has been tabulated[16] and also shows the growing preference (Table 10.2) of the public for certain products. Americans are drinking[17] more commercially produced beverages: soft drinks greatest (Table 10.3) among 12–34 year-olds, male and female; alcoholic beverages more by 19–50 year-olds; both beverages more associated with leisure activities. There is lowered consumption of milk and coffee and an increase in soft drinks and beer over the 1962–83 period (Fig. 10.1). In 1983 the average daily per capita intake of beverages was an estimated 47 ounces, not including water

TABLE 10.1
U.S. CHANGING PATTERNS OF FRUIT PRODUCT CONSUMPTION
Pounds Per Capita Per Year

Year	Fresh Fruit	Canned Fruit	Canned Juice	Frozen Fruit	Frozen Juice	Chilled	Dried Fruit	All Fruit
1915	154.5	7.4	0.9	0.0	0.0	0.0	17.9	180.7
1925	132.2	12.8	0.2	0.2	0.0	0.0	23.7	169.1
1935	133.2	16.7	4.2	0.6	0.0	0.0	19.5	174.2
1945	139.9	15.4	26.0	2.7	0.0	0.0	22.1	206.1
1955	99.4	26.9	23.2	3.9	30.9	1.7	13.3	199.3
1965	81.1	26.0	18.1	4.1	29.6	4.4	11.1	174.4
1975	84.5	12.9	13.9	3.5	67.4	11.3	10.3	203.8
1985	89.6	9.3	6.9	3.6	74.6	6.5	10.9	201.4

Sources: Fruit Situations—TFS-164, 1967; TFS-176, 1970; TFS-195, 1975; TFS-246, 1988 ERS, USDA.

or reconstituted drink mixes.[17] Children 10 years and younger consumed a greater percentage of soft drinks at the evening meal or between meals, while for most other age groups it was between meals. Sources were the home, public eating places and the school.[18] Data from the 1977–78 Nationwide Food Consumption Survey were analyzed[19] to determine consumption of beverages (7 kinds) by teenagers (13–18 years). The negative part correlation between soft drinks and milk intakes, and the negative part correlations of soft drink intakes with intakes of calcium, magnesium, riboflavin, vitamin A and ascorbic acid, indicate that soft drinks may be contributing to low intakes of those nutrients by some teenagers.

NUTRIENT CONTENT OF RAW FRUITS

Data on the vitamin content of raw fruits[20] assembled by USDA personnel, are summarized in Handbook No. 8-9. It may be noted that the fruits having high vitamin A value due to the higher content of carotenoids are mangos (3900 IU/100 g), apricots (2600 IU), papayas (2000 IU), peaches (500 IU), sour cherries (1200 IU), and tomatoes (900 IU). Thiamin and riboflavin contents of raw fruits fall within relatively narrow ranges, with tangerines, and pineapple being higher in thiamin and passion fruit, bananas, plums and strawberries higher in riboflavin. Passion fruit, common guava, and peaches represent the richer sources of niacin. Acerola cherries (1700 mg/100 g) have by far the highest content of ascorbic acid, followed by the common guava (180 mg), black currants (180 mg), papayas (60 mg), strawberries (55 mg), citrus fruits (35–75 mg), and tomatoes (20 mg). Black currants, strawberries, currants, and tomatoes contain the higher levels of pantothenic acid. Vitamin B_6 levels are greater in bananas, common guavas, mangos, grapes, and tomatoes. Citrus fruits, bananas and blueberries are the better sources of folate. Prunes

TABLE 10.2
BEVERAGES: PER U.S. CAPITA CONSUMPTION, 1965-85[1]

Year	Milk Whole	Milk Other	Milk Total	Tea [2]	Coffee [3]	Soft drinks	Juices Citrus	Juices Noncitrus	Juices Total	Total, excluding alcohol
						Gallons				
1965	28.6	4.3	33.1	6.3	36.3	19.2	2.4	0.8	3.2	98.1
1966	28.2	4.7	32.9	6.3	35.7	20.8	2.5	.8	3.3	99.3
1967	26.9	5.1	32.0	6.4	36.0	21.1	3.5	.7	4.2	100.0
1968	26.2	5.8	32.0	6.7	36.3	23.0	3.4	.8	4.2	102.2
1969	25.4	6.3	31.7	6.7	34.9	23.4	3.2	.9	4.1	100.9
1970	24.8	6.7	31.4	6.7	33.4	23.7	3.7	.9	4.6	99.9
1971	23.9	7.3	31.1	7.1	31.7	24.8	4.1	1.0	5.1	99.9
1972	23.3	7.9	31.2	7.1	34.0	25.4	4.6	.8	5.4	103.3
1973	22.2	8.5	30.7	7.3	33.5	26.8	4.5	.9	5.4	103.8
1974	20.9	8.7	29.6	7.4	33.0	26.7	4.8	.8	5.6	102.4
1975	20.6	9.5	30.1	7.5	31.3	27.3	5.3	.8	6.1	102.3
1976	19.8	0	29.8	7.7	32.4	30.6	5.4	.9	6.2	106.7
1977	18.7	.5	29.2	7.5	24.2	33.1	5.5	.9	6.3	100.4
1978	18.1	.8	28.9	7.2	27.0	35.4	4.8	1.1	5.9	104.5
1979	17.4	1.0	28.4	6.9	29.3	36.8	5.1	1.1	6.2	107.7
1980	16.7	11.4	28.0	7.3	27.0	37.8	5.2	1.1	6.3	106.4
1981	16.0	11.5	27.5	7.2	26.9	38.8	4.9	1.3	6.2	106.6
1982	15.5	11.6	27.1	6.9	26.6	39.5	5.1	1.4	6.5	106.6
1983	15.1	11.9	27.0	6.9	25.6	41.1	5.6	1.5	7.2	107.8
1984	14.5	12.5	27.0	6.8	26.3	44.2	4.9	1.6	6.4	110.7
1985	14.0	13.1	27.1	6.8	25.9	45.6	5.7	1.6	7.3	112.7

TABLE 10.1
U.S. CHANGING PATTERNS OF FRUIT PRODUCT CONSUMPTION
Pounds Per Capita Per Year

Year	Fresh Fruit	Canned Fruit	Canned Juice	Frozen Fruit	Frozen Juice	Chilled	Dried Fruit	All Fruit
1915	154.5	7.4	0.9	0.0	0.0	0.0	17.9	180.7
1925	132.2	12.8	0.2	0.2	0.0	0.0	23.7	169.1
1935	133.2	16.7	4.2	0.6	0.0	0.0	19.5	174.2
1945	139.9	15.4	26.0	2.7	0.0	0.0	22.1	206.1
1955	99.4	26.9	23.2	3.9	30.9	1.7	13.3	199.3
1965	81.1	26.0	18.1	4.1	29.6	4.4	11.1	174.4
1975	84.5	12.9	13.9	3.5	67.4	11.3	10.3	203.8
1985	89.6	9.3	6.9	3.6	74.6	6.5	10.9	201.4

Sources: Fruit Situations—TFS-164, 1967; TFS-176, 1970; TFS-195, 1975; TFS-246, 1988 ERS, USDA.

or reconstituted drink mixes.[17] Children 10 years and younger consumed a greater percentage of soft drinks at the evening meal or between meals, while for most other age groups it was between meals. Sources were the home, public eating places and the school.[18] Data from the 1977–78 Nationwide Food Consumption Survey were analyzed[19] to determine consumption of beverages (7 kinds) by teenagers (13–18 years). The negative part correlation between soft drinks and milk intakes, and the negative part correlations of soft drink intakes with intakes of calcium, magnesium, riboflavin, vitamin A and ascorbic acid, indicate that soft drinks may be contributing to low intakes of those nutrients by some teenagers.

NUTRIENT CONTENT OF RAW FRUITS

Data on the vitamin content of raw fruits[20] assembled by USDA personnel, are summarized in Handbook No. 8-9. It may be noted that the fruits having high vitamin A value due to the higher content of carotenoids are mangos (3900 IU/100 g), apricots (2600 IU), papayas (2000 IU), peaches (500 IU), sour cherries (1200 IU), and tomatoes (900 IU). Thiamin and riboflavin contents of raw fruits fall within relatively narrow ranges, with tangerines, and pineapple being higher in thiamin and passion fruit, bananas, plums and strawberries higher in riboflavin. Passion fruit, common guava, and peaches represent the richer sources of niacin. Acerola cherries (1700 mg/100 g) have by far the highest content of ascorbic acid, followed by the common guava (180 mg), black currants (180 mg), papayas (60 mg), strawberries (55 mg), citrus fruits (35–75 mg), and tomatoes (20 mg). Black currants, strawberries, currants, and tomatoes contain the higher levels of pantothenic acid. Vitamin B_6 levels are greater in bananas, common guavas, mangos, grapes, and tomatoes. Citrus fruits, bananas and blueberries are the better sources of folate. Prunes

TABLE 10.2
BEVERAGES: PER U.S. CAPITA CONSUMPTION, 1965-85[1]

Year	Milk			Tea [2]	Coffee [3]	Soft drinks	Juices			Total, excluding alcohol
	Whole	Other	Total				Citrus	Noncitrus	Total	
						Gallons				
1965	28.6	4.3	33.1	6.3	36.3	19.2	2.4	0.8	3.2	98.1
1966	28.2	4.7	32.9	6.3	35.7	20.8	2.5	.8	3.3	99.3
1967	26.9	5.1	32.0	6.4	36.0	21.1	3.5	.7	4.2	100.0
1968	26.2	5.8	32.0	6.7	36.3	23.0	3.4	.8	4.2	102.2
1969	25.4	6.3	31.7	6.7	34.9	23.4	3.2	.9	4.1	100.9
1970	24.8	6.7	31.4	6.7	33.4	23.7	3.7	.9	4.6	99.9
1971	23.9	7.3	31.1	7.1	31.7	24.8	4.1	1.0	5.1	99.9
1972	23.3	7.9	31.2	7.1	34.0	25.4	4.6	.8	5.4	103.3
1973	22.2	8.5	30.7	7.3	33.5	26.8	4.5	.9	5.4	103.8
1974	20.9	8.7	29.6	7.4	33.0	26.7	4.8	.8	5.6	102.4
1975	20.6	9.5	30.1	7.5	31.3	27.3	5.3	.8	6.1	102.3
1976	19.8	0	29.8	7.7	32.4	30.6	5.4	.9	6.2	106.7
1977	18.7	.5	29.2	7.5	24.2	33.1	5.5	.9	6.3	100.4
1978	18.1	.8	28.9	7.2	27.0	35.4	4.8	1.1	5.9	104.5
1979	17.4	1.0	28.4	6.9	29.3	36.8	5.1	1.1	6.2	107.7
1980	16.7	11.4	28.0	7.3	27.0	37.8	5.2	1.1	6.3	106.4
1981	16.0	11.5	27.5	7.2	26.9	38.8	4.9	1.3	6.2	106.6
1982	15.5	11.6	27.1	6.9	26.6	39.5	5.1	1.4	6.5	106.6
1983	15.1	11.9	27.0	6.9	25.6	41.1	5.6	1.5	7.2	107.8
1984	14.5	12.5	27.0	6.8	26.3	44.2	4.9	1.6	6.4	110.7
1985	14.0	13.1	27.1	6.8	25.9	45.6	5.7	1.6	7.3	112.7

JUICES AND BEVERAGES

	Alcoholic beverages								Total, including alcohol 5/
	Resident population				Adult population 4/				
	Beer	Wine	Distilled spirits	Total		Beer	Wine	Distilled spirits	Total	
	Gallons									
1965	16.6	1.0	1.5	19.1		28.0	1.7	2.6	32.2	117.3
1966	17.1	1.0	1.6	19.7		28.9	1.7	2.7	33.3	119.1
1967	17.5	1.0	1.6	20.1		29.5	1.7	2.8	34.0	120.2
1968	18.0	1.1	1.7	20.8		30.1	1.8	2.9	34.8	123.1
1969	18.5	1.2	1.8	21.5		30.9	1.9	3.0	35.8	122.5
1970	19.2	1.3	1.8	22.4		31.6	2.2	3.0	36.7	122.4
1971	19.7	1.5	1.8	23.1		32.3	2.4	3.1	37.7	123.1
1972	20.1	1.6	1.9	23.6		32.6	2.6	3.1	38.3	127.0
1973	20.9	1.7	1.9	24.5		33.7	2.7	3.1	39.5	128.3
1974	21.8	1.7	2.0	25.4		34.8	2.6	3.1	40.6	127.9
1975	22.2	1.7	2.0	25.9		35.1	2.7	3.1	41.0	128.2
1976	22.4	1.7	2.0	26.1		35.0	2.7	3.1	40.8	132.7
1977	23.3	1.8	2.0	27.0		36.1	2.8	3.0	41.9	127.4
1978	23.9	2.0	2.0	27.9		36.7	3.0	3.1	42.8	132.3
1979	24.7	2.0	2.0	28.7		37.6	3.0	3.0	43.6	136.4
1980	25.2	2.1	2.0	29.3		38.3	3.2	3.0	44.5	135.7
1981	25.6	2.2	2.0	29.8		38.4	3.3	2.9	44.6	136.4
1982	25.4	2.2	1.9	29.5		37.7	3.3	2.8	43.8	136.1
1983	25.2	2.2	1.8	29.3		37.2	3.3	2.7	43.2	137.1
1984	24.9	2.3	1.8	29.1		36.5	3.4	2.6	42.5	139.8
1985	23.4	2.5	1.7	27.6		34.5	3.8	2.5	40.8	140.3

1/ Soft drink and alcoholic beverage per capita figures are constructed by ERS based on industry data. Milk, soft drinks and alcoholic beverages are based on resident population. Coffee and tea are based on total population, and fruit juices are based on civilian population. 2/ Fluid equivalent conversion factor is 200 6-oz. cups per pound of tea, leaf equivalent. 3/ Includes instant and decaffeinated coffee. Converted to fluid equivalent on the basis of 60 6-oz. cups per pound of roasted coffee. 4/ Adult population includes all those 21 years old and older. 5/ Total includes alcoholic consumption based on resident population. Source: Bunch.[16]

TABLE 10.3
BEVERAGE USE VARIES BY AGE

Age group	Milk	Soft drinks[1]	Coffee	Beer	Total alcohol[2]
			Percent of individuals		
6-11	97.1	64.1	2.9	0	.4
12-18					
males	93.0	70.6	11.8	2.2	2.7
females	87.8	74.2	12.3	.9	2.3
19-34					
males	78.7	72.5	49.7	24.9	30.4
females	75.3	69.9	53.9	7.7	18.8
35-50					
males	72.0	52.9	83.0	25.1	34.1
females	68.1	57.2	81.0	5.7	17.4
51-64					
males	77.4	37.2	87.2	7.0	27.0
females	75.3	38.9	86.3	5.2	15.5
Over 65					
males	82.1	21.6	86.5	9.6	16.6
females	79.9	21.4	85.4	1.7	8.3

[1]Includes noncarbonated soft drinks made from powdered mixes. [2]Includes distilled liquor, wine, beer, and ale.
Source: Bunch and Kurland.[17] Nationwide Food Consumption Survey, 1977–78.

are high in most nutrients. The better sources for calcium are currants, oranges, blackberries, limes, lemons and papayas; for iron, passion fruit, currants, lemons, limes and apricots; for potassium, bananas, passion fruit, currants, apricots, guavas and papayas; and for magnesium, bananas, passion fruit, black currants and blackberries.

Numerous factors must be considered in establishing the levels of vitamins to be added to a fruit juice or fruit beverage product in order to assure the desired potencies at the time of consumption. Factors which affect the natural vitamin content of fresh fruits include species, variety, season and environmental conditions, stage of picking at harvesting time, use of herbicides or plant regulators, and storage losses of the fruit. When fruits are converted to juice or juice products, there are losses during manufacturing and storage, which may be further influenced by temperature and pH, exposure to air or light, type of container and presence of antioxidants or preservatives.

NUTRIENT CONTENT OF JUICES AND BEVERAGES

Values compiled by USDA personnel for the vitamin content of some fruit juices[20] are listed in Table 10.4; of some beverages[21,22] in Table 10.5. Citrus fruit juices,

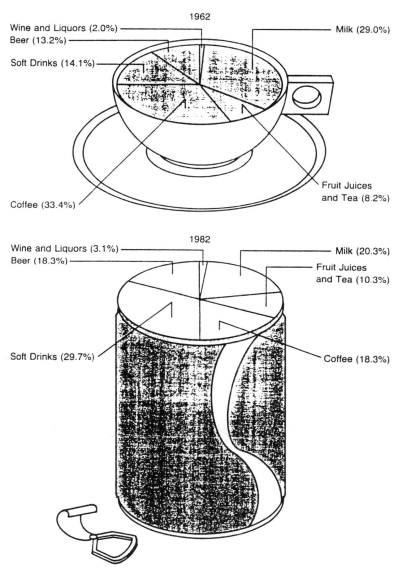

From Duxbury[15] and Bunch and Kurland[17]
FIG. 10.1. BEVERAGE MARKET SHIFTS TO SOFT DRINKS

and passion fruit juices are good sources of vitamin C; tomato and pineapple juices contain intermediate amounts; apricot, cranberry, grape, papaya, peach, pear, and prune juices or nectars have low levels. In general, the fruits having orange to red colors due to provitamin carotenoids are good sources of provitamin A whereas ap-

TABLE 10.4
NUTRIENT CONTENT OF FRUIT JUICES
(Per 100 g, Edible Portion)

Fruit Juice	Vitamin A (IU)	Thiamin (Mg)	Riboflavin (Mg)	Niacin (Mg)	Ascorbic Acid (Mg)	Pantothenic Acid (Mg)	Vitamin B_6 (Mg)	Folacin (Mcg)	Calcium (Mg)	Iron (Mg)	Potassium (Mg)	Magnesium (Mg)
Acerola	509	0.020	0.060	0.400	1,600.0	0.205	0.004	—	10	0.50	97	12
Apple												
Canned or bottled	1	0.021	0.017	0.100	0.9	—	0.030	0.1	7	0.37	118	3
Frozen concentrate Diluted 1 + 3[1]	—	0.003	0.015	0.038	0.6	0.063	0.033	0.3	6	0.26	126	5
Apricot nectar, canned	1,316	0.009	0.014	0.260	0.6	—	—	1.3	7	0.38	114	5
Cranberry, cocktail	—	0.005	0.016	0.050	42.6[2]	0.067	—	0.2	3	0.16	24	3
Grapefruit												
Raw, white/red	10/440	0.040	0.020	0.200	38.0	—	—	—	9	0.20	162	12
Canned, unsweetened	7	0.042	0.020	0.231	29.2	0.130	0.020	10.4	7	0.20	153	10
Canned, sweetened	0	0.040	0.023	0.319	26.9	0.130	0.020	10.4	8	0.36	162	10
Frozen concentrate, Diluted 1 + 3[1]	9	0.041	0.022	0.217	33.7	0.189	0.044	3.6	8	0.14	136	11
Grape												
Canned or bottled	8	0.026	0.037	0.262	0.1	0.041	0.065	2.6	9	0.24	132	10
Frozen concentrate, Sweetened, Diluted 1 + 3	8	0.015	0.026	0.124	23.9[2]	0.024	0.042	1.3	4	0.10	21	4
Lemon												
Raw	20	0.030	0.010	0.100	46.0	0.103	0.051	12.9	7	0.03	124	6
Canned or bottled	15	0.041	0.009	0.197	24.8	0.091	0.043	10.1	11	0.13	102	8
Frozen, single-strength	13	0.059	0.013	0.137	31.5	0.121	0.060	9.5	8	0.12	89	8
Lime												
Raw	0	0.020	0.010	0.100	29.3	0.138	0.043	—	9	0.03	109	6
Canned or bottled	16	0.033	0.003	0.163	6.4	0.066	0.027	7.9	12	0.23	75	7

Orange											
Raw	200	0.090	0.030	0.400	50.0	0.190	0.040	—	11	0.20	200	11
Canned	175	0.060	0.028	0.314	34.4	0.150	0.088	—	8	0.44	175	11
Chilled	78	0.111	0.021	0.280	32.9	0.191	0.054	18.1	10	0.17	190	11
Frozen concentrate,											
Diluted 1 + 3[1]	78	0.079	0.018	0.202	38.9	0.158	0.044	43.8	9	0.10	190	10
Orange-grapefruit, canned	119	0.056	0.030	0.336	29.1	0.140	0.023	—	8	0.46	158	10
Papaya nectar, canned	111	0.006	0.004	0.150	3.0	0.054	0.009	2.1	10	0.34	31	3
Passion fruit											
Purple, raw	717	—	0.131	1.460	29.8	—	—	—	4	0.24	—	—
Yellow, raw	2,410	—	0.101	2.240	18.2	—	—	—	4	0.36	278	17
Peach nectar, canned	258	0.003	0.014	0.288	5.3	—	—	—	5	0.18	40	4
Pear nectar, canned	1	0.002	0.013	0.128	1.1	—	—	—	5	0.26	13	3
Pineapple											
Canned	5	0.055	0.022	0.257	10.7	0.100	0.096	23.1	17	0.26	134	13
Frozen concentrate,											
Diluted 1 + 3[1]	10	0.070	0.020	0.200	12.0	0.125	0.074	—	11	0.30	136	9
Prune, canned	3	0.016	0.070	0.785	4.1	—	—	0.4	12	1.18	276	8
Tangerine											
Raw	420	0.060	0.020	0.100	31.0	—	—	—	18	0.20	178	8
Canned, sweetened	420	0.060	0.020	0.100	22.0	—	0.032	—	18	0.20	178	14
Frozen concentrate,											
Sweetened,											
Diluted 1 + 3[1]	573	0.052	0.019	0.093	24.2	0.125	0.042	4.6	8	0.10	113	8
Tomato											
Canned or bottled	800	0.050	0.030	0.800	16.0	0.250	0.192	—	7	0.80	227	—
Canned concentrate,											
Diluted 1 + 3[1]	900	0.050	0.030	0.800	13.0	—	—	—	7	0.90	235	—
Dehydrated, diluted											
1 lb to 1.75 gal	860	0.030	0.030	0.900	16.0	—	—	—	6	0.50	231	—

Source: Gebhard et al.[20]
[1]Denotes dilution of 1 part with 3 parts H_2O.
[2]Enriched with ascorbic acid.

TABLE 10.5
NUTRIENT CONTENT OF BEVERAGES
(Per 100 g, Edible Portion)

	Vitamin A (IU)	Thiamin (Mg)	Riboflavin (Mg)	Niacin (Mg)	Ascorbic Acid (Mg)	Pantothenic Acid (Mg)	Vitamin B_6 (Mg)	Folacin (Mcg)	Vitamin B_{12} (Mcg)	Calcium (Mg)	Iron (Mg)	Potassium (Mg)	Magnesium (Mg)
Fruit Juice													
Beer, 4.5% alcohol	0	0.006	0.026	0.453	0	0.058	0.050	6.0	0.02	5	0.03	25	6
Beer, light	0	0.009	0.030	0.392	0	0.036	0.034	4.1	0.01	5	0.04	18	5
Cocktail													
Martini	—	0.001	0.003	0.015	0	0.006	0.005	0.2	0	2	0.09	18	2
Bloody Mary	343	0.034	0.022	0.434	13.8	0.163	0.012	13.3	0	7	0.37	146	8
Pina Colada	2	0.028	0.014	0.118	4.7	—	—	10.2	0	8	0.22	71	—
Screwdriver	63	0.064	0.015	0.162	31.2	0.127	0.035	35.1	0	7	0.06	153	8
Tequila Sunrise	97	0.038	0.016	0.190	19.3	—	0.050	—	0	6	0.28	104	10
Wine, table	0	0.004	0.016	0.074	0	0.028	0.024	1.1	0.01	8	0.41	89	10
Distilled spirits[1]	0	0.006	0.004	0.013	0	0.001	0	0	0	0	0.04	4	0
Carbonated drink													
Cola	0	0	0	0	0	0	0	0	0	3	0.03	1	1
Ginger ale	0	0	0	0	0		0	0	0	3	0.18	1	1
Orange	0	0	0	0	0	0	0	0	0	3	0.06	2	1
Milk													
3.3% fat	126	0.038	0.162	0.084	0.94	0.314	0.042	5.0	0.36	119	0.05	152	13
Skim	204[2]	0.036	0.140	0.088	0.980	0.329	0.040	5.3	0.38	123	0.04	166	11
Citrus fruit juice drink Frozen conc., diluted with water, 1 + 2	42	0.014	—	0.180	27.1[2]	0.132	0.024	2.0	0	9	1.12	112	6
Clam and tomato	215	0.040	0.030	0.190	4.1	—	—	—	—	12	0.60	90	—
Coffee, brewed	0	0	0	0.222	0	0	0	0.1	0	2	0.41	54	5
Cranberry juice Cocktail, bottled	4	0.009	0.009	0.035	35.4[2]	0.056	0.019	0.2	0	3	0.15	18	2
Fruit punch drink, canned	14	0.022	0.023	0.021	29.6[2]	0.014	0	1.3	0	8	0.21	25	2

Hot chocolate	2	0.013	0.078	0.081	0.2	0.123	0.016	0	0.18	47	0.17	98	12
Grapedrink, canned	1	0.003	0.004	0.026	34.1[2]	0.004	0.006	0.3	0	—	0.17	5	—
Grape juice drink, canned	2	0.010	0.10	0.100	16[2]	0.012	0.020	0.8	0	3	0.10	35	—
Orange flavor drink, powder diluted	740[2]	0.001	0.015	0	48.8[2]	0	0	57.6[2]	0	25[2]	0.08	20[2]	1
Orange drink, canned	18	0.006	0.003	0.031	34.1[2]	0.015	0.009	—	0	6	0.28	18	2
Pineapple and orange juice drink, canned	531[2]	0.030	0.019	0.207	22.5[2]	0.057	0.047	10.9	0	5	0.27	46	6
Shake, fast food, vanilla	130	0.045	0.182	0.185	0.8	0.418	0.052	3.3	0.36	122	0.09	174	12
Tea, brewed	0	0.000	0.014	0	0	—	0	5.2	0	0	0.02	37	3
Tea, herb, brewed	0	0.010	0.004	0	0	0.011	0	0	0	2	0.08	9	1
Thirst quencher drink, bottled	0	0.005	0	0	0	0	0	0	0	0	0.05	11	1

Source: Cutrufelli and Matthews[21] and Dickey and Weihrauch.[22]
[1]Gin, rum, vodka, whiskey.
[2]Enriched.

ples, grapes, lemons, pears, and pineapple provide juices with low provitamin A levels. The B-vitamins show rather wide ranges in the various juices, none of which contain vitamin B_{12}. By comparing nutrient contents of juices and milk in Tables 10.4 and 10.5 against other beverages one can determine the significance or lack of significance of these beverages as contributors of nutrients and also contrast them with other standard drinks such as beer, coffee, tea, and wine.

Reviews on the vitamin content of beer have been published by Scriban.[23] Blondeau[24] found that vitamin B_{12} occurs in beer primarily as free cyanocobalamin. Duda et al.[25] determined the following ranges of vitamins in 12 Polish beers: thiamin, 0.0014–0.0090 mg %; riboflavin, 0.010–0.042 mg %; niacin, 0.62–2.1 mg %. Ockhuizen[26] and Piendl[27] discuss beer consumption practices and health issues. The nutritional value, including vitamins, of wines has been listed by Puisais and Guiller,[28] Amerine,[29] and Masquelier.[30] Ournac and Flanzy[31] studied the thiamin content of three wines and concluded that thiamin is synthesized by yeasts during fermentation and is slowly released during storage with the lees. Others have reported on the multivitamin content of wine.[32–34]

NUTRIFICATION OF JUICES AND BEVERAGES

Rationale

The rationale for adding nutrients to beverage products includes the concept of product improvement by limiting the seasonal and varietal ranges of natural nutrient content of ingredients (such as fruit juice) used in their manufacture. Vitamin C has been associated with fruit juices since the 18th century when citrus juice was demonstrated to be the successful prophylaxis and treatment for scurvy. The acid-type fruit and vegetable beverages provide a relatively stable medium for ascorbic acid, making these products good carriers or vehicles for nutrification. There is another role that ascorbic acid plays in beverages, namely one of inhibiting oxidation by acting as an oxygen acceptor. Dissolved ascorbic acid in sealed containers[35] of liquid formulations will remove dissolved oxygen and headspace oxygen with time, thus preventing the destructive action of oxygen on other beverage components. Because ascorbic acid in sealed containers of liquids creates an anaerobic or deoxygenated environment it has been mentioned as a possible aid in preventing specific types of microbial growth.[36] Ascorbic acid, however, is not a general preservative. Ascorbic acid is a desirable addition to canned soft drinks because it removes or neutralizes the air corrosion of the container and extends product shelf-life. Oxygen dissolved in an aqueous acid medium, such as carbonated beverages (pH 2.5–4.0), acts as a depolarizer and promotes metal corrosion which in turn causes flavor changes, discoloration, and other objectionable effects.[37] Lastly, the presence of ascorbic acid in nutritionally significant quantities in beverages containing natural iron or added iron improves iron bioavailability.

Commercially prepared fruit juices, fruit juice blends, and fruit drinks containing one or more fruit juice components are widely consumed and can serve as useful sources of vitamin C. Modern processing and canning techniques of both single-strength and frozen concentrate fruit juices are effective in preserving the natural content of ascorbic acid. However, even in fruits considered good sources of ascorbic acid there can be considerable specie, varietal and seasonal variability.[38] In view of the consumer's desire for a varied diet and because of concern of dislikes, intolerances and allergies, the availability of a wide selection of juices and drinks with standardized levels of ascorbic acid and other fruit associated nutrients, to be used interchangeably is laudable. Consequently, commercial juice and drink producers have produced such beverages or have undertaken trial runs of nutrified products. Vitamin C enriched instant coffee as a U.S. ration item[36] was used in World War II and in subsequent military engagements in Korea and Vietnam, conditions which may not have provided ready access to usual fruit and vegetable products.

Fruit and fruit products are variable sources also of the carotenoid provitamin A structures.[39] Fruits naturally contain 1–60% of their total carotenoids as beta-carotene.[40] Since pure beta-carotene and/or beta-apo-8′carotenal when added to beverages provide pleasing colors as well as improved vitamin A value, merit exists for their addition. Where improved color is not at issue, added retinol esters provide vitamin A value without color change.[41]

There is the rationale of adding nutrients to improve a public health situation. The technology of vitamin A nutrification of tea was developed by Brooke and Cort[42] and discussed by Paden et al.[43] as an intervention strategy of conveying meaningful quantities of vitamin A to entire populations at risk of vitamin A deficiency. Tea nutrification, while a promising endeavor (Chapter 17), was never widely adopted. In small scale/short time studies Wills and Dwyer[44] indicated that it is possible to nutrify tea leaves and produce a tea infusion with sufficient thiamin to be of nutritional significance for populations at risk of thiamin deficiency. If a need arose for this approach, a scaled-up investigation would be required.

Thiamin is a limiting nutrient in the Australian diet.[45] The increasing number of cases of Korsakoff's psychosis in Queensland mental hospitals prompted some action for prophylaxis. Supplementing alcoholic beverages with thiamin has been proposed.[46] Wood and Breen[47] have studied the size of the problem, the approaches to the Australian problem and the legal concern of adding a nutrient to an alcoholic beverage. While the technical aspects[48,49] of adding thiamin to beer and other alcoholic beverages have already been examined, Australia must decide whether the adoption of thiamin enrichment of flour and bread or thiamin addition to alcoholic beverages is the solution to their thiamin deficient population segment, which is more severe in drinkers, or whether both measures should be adopted.[45,50–54] Fortification of sorghum beer with thiamin in African studies has been shown to be a feasible endeavor.[55]

There are clinical aspects of public health issues to be considered. Van der Horst et al.[9] analyzed beverages and fruit juices recording pH (2.4–3.6) and content of sodium (30–108 ppm), potassium (0.2–1000 ppm), calcium (13–108 ppm), phosphorus (1–345 ppm), also glucose, fructose and sucrose levels. Concern about lack of information on the nutrient and nonnutrient composition of some of these beverages could affect public health and would provide potential assistance to clinicians when prescribing their use in diets involving disease, weight control, and sports programs. In one peculiar case, thiamin deficiency (beriberi) was reported in a man consuming excessive carbonated beverages and high calorie food.[56]

When the issue of iron addition to a beverage or beverage concentrate arises, one is reminded of the voluminous literature on trying to remove iron or complex it so the influence of this highly reactive mineral would not catalyse oxidative rancidity, discolorations or nutrient destruction. Yet, iron is a dietary essential, often in short supply in the diet and so iron nutrification of food including beverages is a continuing challenge.[57] Calcium is receiving increased attention as an additive to beverages[58] because of the osteoporosis problem and the possibility that ascorbic acid might influence calcium utilization. It may be a questionable nutrification practice, as such sources may not contain significant amounts of calcium or that technological aspects may pose limitations. With hurdles such as these overcome, succes with calcium nutrification could lead to interest in nutrification with other minerals as well.

Multinutrient nutrification of some beverage products has been achieved successfully. Such products[59] include soy-based or casein-based liquids, fruit drinks, frozen fruit concentrates, and dry, fruit-flavored powders. Benk[60] has briefly reviewed the composition of fruit juice based, multivitamin and "fitness" beverages containing vitamins in relation to their nutritive value and legal provisions and also the addition of minerals to nonalcoholic beverages promoting physical fitness.[61]

Nutrient Forms

Vitamins and amino acids as additives are subjects covered in earlier chapters. The water-soluble vitamins, ascorbic acid, biotin, cyanocobalamin, folate, niacin, niacinamide, calcium pantothenate, pyridoxine, riboflavin, and thiamin hydrochloride are available in pure, crystalline form for nutrification purposes. The physical properties of the various vitamins, including solubility and stability, have been tabulated by Bauernfeind and DeRitter.[62]

Vitamin A palmitate for use in water-based foods is commercially available in the form of gelatin-sugar or acacia beadlets which contain the vitamin A in the form of finely emulsified droplets sealed in the dry matrix. These can be reconstituted in water to yield an emulsion. Also available is a liquid emulsion of vitamin A in a gum acacia base, or emulsions can be prepared by the food processor to suit his own needs. All these market forms[63] contain food-acceptable antioxidants to protect the vitamin A against oxidation. They also are suitable to use in beverage powder mixes which are reconstituted in water for consumption. Vitamin A palmitate provides 1820 IU of vitamin A activity per milligram.

Because the pure oil-soluble crystalline carotenoids, like vitamin A, are unstable and difficult to handle, special dry and liquid market forms (Table 10.6) are commercially available which simplify their use in water-based food products such as beverages.[41] In the manufacture of dry beadlet forms, trans beta-carotene is isomerized to a mixture of cis and trans isomers; however, USP rat curative growth assays have yielded practically the same vitamin A potency for the beadlets as for trans beta-carotene in vegetable oil.[40] Beta-carotene provides 1667 IU of vitamin A activity per milligram; beta-apocarotenal, 1200 IU per milligram. In the United States, beta-carotene was approved for food use in 1956, the amount to be added depending on good manufacturing practice. Beta-apocarotenal was approved in 1963 in quantities which may not exceed 15 mg/lb of solid or pint of liquid food. Utilization of carotenoid preparations for foods and beverage uses has been reviewed by Borenstein and Bunnell,[64] Klaeui and Bauernfeind,[65] and Gordon and Bauernfeind.[66]

Iron nutrification of beverages has been reviewed by Coccodrilli and Shah[67] covering whole milk, evaporated, skim, powdered milk, milk-based beverages, coffee, fruit and vegetable-flavored beverages and soft drinks. Ferric compounds (sodium ferric pyrophosphate, ferripolyphosphate and ferripolyphosphate/whey protein complex), in short time tests, performed well in chocolate milk. In a long-term study of iron nutrified, canned, milk-based product, electrolytic iron or carbonyl iron showed appreciable solubilization in the ferrous form. Instant soluble coffee can be nutrified with iron when ferric phosphate is added during the liquid state and then processed and dried in a prescribed manner. Anhydrous ferrous sulfate or ferrous gluconate added to powdered drink mix also containing added vitamins A and C were encouraging technologies; likewise use of Fe(III) EDTA in sweetened carbonated soft drinks is a potential development. Johnson and Evans[68] reported that ground coffee could be nutrified with ferrous fumarate.

Pasteurized or thermally processed soy beverages can be successfully nutrified using a mixture of calcium citrate and tricalcium phosphate with acceptable sensory properties and with physical stability after a 6 month storage period.[69] With the employment of a polyphosphate and a bioavailable calcium source, soymilk was fortified with calcium at levels equal to or greater than those found in cow's milk.[70] Supplementation of orange juice or orange juice concentrate with calcium is technically feasible using a premix of citric and malic acid with calcium carbonate, oxide or hydroxide to yield a soluble calcium concentrate.[71] A clear, storage-stable calcium-fortified acidic beverage has been prepared containing calcium gluconate which is pleasant tasting and can be carbonated or not and flavored with cola or fruit concentrates.[72] Currently there are cola drinks with added calcium, calcium-fortified orange and grapefruit juices in ready-to-serve forms; also calcium-fortified soft drink mix is in marketing programs.[58]

PROCESSING ASPECTS

Books dealing with the technology of juice and beverage production have been published.[1,4,73–76] Losses of nutrients during processing are recorded by Karmas

TABLE 10.6
APPLICATION FORMS OF CAROTENOIDS APPROVED IN USA
FOR JUICES AND BEVERAGES

Form	Description	Uses	Stock Solution[1]
Beta-carotene			
10% dry beadlets	Colloidal beta-carotene in a gelatin-carbohydrate matrix; stabilized with antioxidants; readily dispersible with stirring in warm water, 140°F (60°C)	For coloring beverages and dry products to be reconstituted in warm water	1 g of beadlets to 100 mL of warm water with stirring to disperse. 1 mL = 1 mg of beta-carotene
3.6% liquid emulsion	Soluble beta-carotene in orange and brominated vegetable oil emulsified in a hydrolyzed protein base; pourable at 75°F; sp. gr. of oil phase 1.052 ±0.003 (12.5 to 13.6° Brix); stabilized with antioxidants	Especially for coloring carbonated and noncarbon-orange-flavored drinks and fruit juice blends adjusted for specific gravity and filled in clear glass or opaque containers	3 g of emulsion to 108 mL of water with stirring to disperse. 1 mL = 1 mg of beta-carotene
2.4% dry beadlets	Soluble beta-carotene in vegetable oil emulsified in a gelatin-carbohydrate matrix; stabilized with antioxidants; readily dispersible in water (75°F)	For coloring juices, juice drinks, and dry beverage bases to be reconstituted in water	4 g of beadlets to 96 mL of warm water with stirring to disperse. 1 mL = 1 mg of beta-carotene
2.5 and 5.0% spray-dried powders	Microcolloidal dispersions of beta-carotene in a gelatin-carbohydrate matrix	For coloring beverages and dry products for reconstitution where optical clarity is desired	4 or 2 g of powder to 100 mL with water with stirring. 1 mL = 1 mg of beta-carotene
Apocarotenal			
10% dry beadlets	Colloidal apocarotenal in a matrix similar to that of 10% dry beta-carotene	For coloring beverages and dry products to be reconstituted in warm water	1 g of beadlets to 100 mL of warm water with stirring to disperse. 1 mL = 1 mg of apocarotenal

TABLE 10.6 (*Continued*)

Form	Description	Uses	Stock Solution[1]
2.5 and 5.0% spray-dried powders	Microcolloidal dispersions of apocarotenal in a gelatin-carbohydrate matrix	For coloring beverages and dry products for reconstitution where optical clarity is desired	4 or 2 g of powder to 100 mL with water with stirring; 1 mL = 1 mg of apocarotenal

[1] A suggested convenience for small-scale laboratory coloring trials.

and Harris.[77] Fruit juice production facilities have been examined in respect to design and equipment including aseptic bulk packaging.[78] The manufacture of beverages with fruit juice is described by Kohnstamm including the importance of hygiene, raw material quality and color stabilization.[79] Prendergast[80] discusses production of whey drinks including carbonation, shelf-life and packaging.

Precautions

Mechanisms involved in the destruction of ascorbic acid in juices and beverages have been summarized by Henshall,[81] as well as production steps that might be taken to thwart or delay such mechanisms as oxidative enzyme inactivation, anaerobic environment, and metal complexing, etc. Production of vitamin nutrified beverages, particularly those with added ascorbic acid, necessitates that the following precautions[82] be taken when practical to insure maximum nutrient retention.

(1) All stainless steel equipment is recommended. If stainless steel is not available, aluminum, enamel, glass, or plastic-lined tanks, pasteurizers, etc., should be used. Copper, nickel, plain steel, iron, or brass equipment should be avoided since traces of these metals can accelerate destruction, especially of vitamin C, in a very short time.

(2) The vitamins should be added just prior to flash pasteurization or as late in the processing as possible. In regular juice production the vitamin or a vitamin premix, in weighed amounts, may be added to the entire batch, or may be first dissolved or dispersed in water or juice before addition. Alternatively, a concentrated solution of the vitamin may be added in continuous processing operations by means of a proportioning pump or by direct injection into each packaging unit just before filling.

(3) All stages of the processing operation should be conducted as quickly as possible.

(4) During mixing, emulsification, homogenization, and the like, oxygen or air should not be reintroduced into the product. Agitation to insure uniform distribution of the vitamins throughout the batch may be accomplished by gentle submerged mixing. This may be done with bubbling inert gas through the batch. Where possible, food product should be protected from light and other radiant energy in the presence of oxygen during processing.

(5) Deaeration of the beverage prior to packaging will help to minimize losses during storage of the product.

(6) Containers should be filled to maximum capacity; i.e., the headspace should be kept as small as possible. Headspace air can be reduced further by the use of nitrogen, carbon dioxide, or steam flush prior to sealing the containers. In some instances the addition of glucose oxidase and catalase is useful in removing dissolved and headspace oxygen, which minimizes the amount of ascorbic acid added.

(7) After the filling operation, the beverage should be cooled as rapidly as possible, then stored at or below 70°F.

(8) All autoxidizable ingredients, such as flavoring oils, added to the food product should have a low peroxide value.

(9) Whenever feasible, a short-time heat treatment of fresh fruit products may be employed to inactivate enzymes before or during crushing.

(10) Where practicable, sequestering or stabilizing agents such as phosphates, citrates, EDTA, or cysteine may be considered. Use of minimum amounts of sulfur dioxide (insufficient to cause flavor changes) can be helpful in some products for better ascorbic acid retention values.

Observations

In the production of conventional, clarified apple juice, ascorbic acid is usually added near the end of processing, prior to canning. At this stage of addition, a good portion of the fruit browning mechanism is already at the irreversible stage and only a partial color reversal effect is possible. If sufficient ascorbic acid was added, a nutritional improvement can also be indicated by making a claim content on the label. It is usually anticipated that beverages,[41] to which 40–50 mg of ascorbic acid per fluid volume are present after packaging and processing, will contain 30 mg after a normal market-life storage. A claim of 35 mg/100 mL in apple juice would require that an initial level of 50 mg be present. Much of the canned apple juice marketed in Canada is standardized with added ascorbic acid. A history of ascorbic acid fortification of conventionally produced apple juice prior to canning and bottling has been published by Aitken.[83] If a more natural and lighter colored (opalescent) juice is desired, some ascorbic acid can be sprayed on the fruit during the crushing or grinding operations and more added to the juice prior to the packaging.[84]

One of the earlier group of investigators, Esselen et al.,[85] found added ascorbic acid to be quite stable in processed apple, cranberry and grape juices when these products were fortified at a rate of 50 mg/100 mL. Furthermore, a favorable effect was noted on beverage color retention during storage in apple and cranberry juice. Budrenene[86] reported favorable stability results on vitamin C processed apple juice. The effects of processing conditions on the stability of ascorbic acid in a mixture of apple and pear juices were investigated by Schobinger.[87]

Some fruit juices tend to undergo a flavor change on pasteurization, the magnitude depending on the juice and the process. Birch et al.[88] examined this phenomenon and found the change to be related to the processed fructose and glucose component. Deaeration and added ascorbic acid decreased this flavor development, the amount of retained ascorbic acid being effective ranging from 30–60 mg/100 g for various juices.

Initial losses of ascorbic acid reported by Espada[89] on canning root beer, cola, lime-lemon, orange, ginger ale, strawberry, and black cherry drinks with 50 mg of ascorbic acid added per can or bottle were 10–15%. The oxygen content of the beverage and the residual air in the container influenced the stability of ascorbic acid, which was better in 12-oz cans than in 32-oz bottles. Mrozewski[90] prepared carbonated and noncarbonated beverages with 10–15 mg % vitamin C from natural juices, pomaces, and concentrates of apples, plums, berries, and currants. Addition of CO_2 (4 g/L at 17°C) stabilized the vitamin C content. Full stability of vitamin C was observed when pasteurization of the beverages was carried out in bottles with crown caps at 67°C for 30 minutes. Apple juice concentrate[91] diluted with carbonated water, ascorbic acid added (40 mg/100 mL), was subjected to taste panel evaluation and reported to be preferred over noncarbonated apple juice. Bender[92] reported on the stability performance of natural and synthetic ascorbic acid in an orangeade or orange squash type of beverage under commercial production practices and noted no difference in their behavior.

While adequate additions of ascorbic acid[41] to juice and drink products with good manufacturing practices will usually yield packaged products which will meet label claims, Pelletier and Morrison[93] some time ago reported that beverages picked up on the retail market in Ottawa, Canada, were below label claim. When findings of this type are noted, the manufacturing stages, storage, and distribution patterns of the product must be checked and the cause remedied. Reviews on the technology of ascorbic acid addition to beverages are those of Diemair and Postel;[94] Henshall;[81] Bauernfeind and Pinkert;[95] and Bauernfeind.[36]

Brooke and Cort[42] described two methods for adding vitamin A to tea. Tea dust was nutrified by dry mixing with a spray-dried, stabilized vitamin A palmitate powder, type 250 SD (250,000 IU/g). Tea leaves were nutrified most successfully using an emulsion of vitamin A palmitate (500,000 IU/g) in thick acacia or dextrin solution, which was diluted (2–100 g) with 50% sucrose solution before spraying onto the hot tea leaves as they emerge from the drying chamber. Samples of commercially nutrified and unnutrified tea were submitted to tasters at the point of manufacture and at major marketing centers. In no instances were the tasters able to detect any difference in taste, odor, color, clarity, or other characteristics of the tea infusions. Experiences on the processing aspects of fruit juices with added vitamin A, thiamin, riboflavin, and niacin are related by Fenton-May in his 1975 report.[59]

Dispersion of emulsion or dry preparations of carotenoids in water frequently yields colors that differ from the colors obtained with an equivalent concentration of the carotenoids in vegetable oil. Water-dispersible carotenoid preparations yield a slightly cloudy solution, imparting a pulp-like appearance in some products. At times, homogenizing the carotenoid addition with the flavoring and fruit concentrate is of importance in obtaining a physically stable product with good color.[65] Most water-dispersible carotenoid preparations do not produce the sparkling clarity of water-soluble colors and, hence, have been limited in applications where clarity is necessary. Experimental preparations of the carotenoids yielding greater clarity have been developed by Emodi et al.[96] but are not in general usage. Potential levels of emulsion or beadlet preparations suggested in terms of milligrams of pure carotenoid compound per quart are as follows: beta-carotene[97] for juices, drinks, or carbonated beverages, 1–10; apocarotenal[98] for drinks and beverages, 3–15.

STORAGE ASPECTS

The general stability characteristics of the individual vitamins per se and in processing foods have been described by DeRitter.[99]

Vitamin C

Although the main cause of vitamin C loss is oxidation under aerobic conditions, anaerobic decomposition can also occur. Aerobic oxidation is significantly increased by trace contamination with metal ions, especially copper and, to a lesser extent, iron. Reducing the oxygen content of the juice or beverage by vacuum deaeration or using a blanket of carbon dioxide or nitrogen to displace air in processing can be very useful in improving the retention of vitamin C during processing, as well as on subsequent storage. Oxidative enzymes, such as those present in apple juice, also play a role in promoting the oxidation of vitamin C. Black currant juice is rich in flavonoids which exert a protective effect on the vitamin C content. Temperature of storage is an important factor, since losses of vitamin C increase with increasing temperature. The nature of the container, the amount of oxygen in the headspace, and the presence of stabilizing agents, are factors influencing vitamin C stability.

A summary of stability data generated in E. DeRitter's laboratory for vitamin C in juice products stored at room temperature for 6 and 12 months is shown in Table 10.7. A similar compilation of data on fruit drinks and carbonated, fruit-flavored beverages is given in Table 10.8. These represent commercial trial runs on prod-

TABLE 10.7
STABILITY OF ADDED VITAMIN C[1] IN JUICES

Juice Product	Packaging	Initial Vitamin C	% Retention at 70-75°F (Months)	
			6	12
Apple	glass, 1 qt	49 mg/10 fl oz	—	76
Apple	glass, 24 oz	47 mg/8 fl oz	72	68
Apple	can, 20 oz	41 mg/100 mL	—	76
Apple-cherry	glass, 1 qt	53 mg/10 fl oz	82	63
Apple-orange	glass, amber	63 mg/100 fl oz	76	64
Apple-orange	can	62 mg/100 fl oz	85	77
Apricot nectar	can, 4 oz	59 mg/4 fl oz	100	84
Apricot-pineapple nectar	can	70 mg/100 mL	79	84
Pineapple	can, 6 oz	51 mg/8 fl oz	92	90
Pineapple	can, 11 oz	48 mg/4 fl oz	90	—
Pineapple-grapefruit	can	39 mg/6 fl oz	92	90
Tomato	can, 46 oz	44 mg/4 fl oz	100	80
Tomato	can, 18 oz	54 mg/100 mL	83	81
Tomato	glass	59 mg/6 fl oz	95	80
Tomato-vegetable	can, 46 oz	58 mg/6 fl oz	74	66
Tomato-vegetable	can, 6 oz	42 mg/4 fl oz	81	69

[1]Vitamin C includes ascorbic acid plus dehydroascorbic acid.

ucts containing added ascorbic acid. The processing was done with the prevailing equipment and processing variables in the particular plant at the time and, hence, can serve as a guide to expected performance. Experience in such plant trials can indicate the overages of ascorbic acid needed in the particular product to meet label claim after processing and storage.

In the 1970s, one of the first groups[100] to add vitamin C to tomato juice (60 mg/16 fl oz) conducted 24-month shelf-life studies under a variety of processing and storage conditions to prove that an ascorbic acid label claim was feasible with no impairment of flavor. The effect of time, temperature, and nutrification level on the retention of ascorbic acid in nutrified tomato juice was also reported by Pope.[101]

Smoot and Nagy[102] determined the effects of temperature and time of storage on the vitamin C content of canned, single-strength grapefruit juice. After 12 weeks, the loss of ascorbic acid (AA) plus dehydroascorbic acid (DHAA) ranged from less than 3% at 10°C to more than 68% at 50°C. The loss of AA was continuous and increased with temperature. The levels of DHAA and diketogulonic acid remained essentially unchanged during the 12-week storage period.

In a study of reconstituted beverage products with and without added vitamin C, Beston and Henderson[103] found no serious loss of vitamin C in the first 96 h after reconstitution and also that the stability characteristics of vitamin C are independent

TABLE 10.8
STABILITY OF ADDED VITAMIN C[1] IN FRUIT DRINKS AND BEVERAGES

Juice Product	Packaging	Initial Vitamin C (Mg/Fl Oz)	% Retention at 70–75°F (Months)	
			6	12
Fruit Drinks				
Apple	glass, 2 qt	43/6	82	—
Apricot	can, 6 oz	48/6	95	83
Apricot	can, 12 oz	53/4	92	77
Cherry	can, 46 oz	27/6	77	—
Cranberry	glass, 16 oz	41/6	86	83
Cranberry-apricot	glass, 1 qt	49/6	82	82
Cranberry-orange	glass, 1 qt	61/6	87	72
Cranberry-prune	glass, 1 qt	52/6	85	75
Grape	can, 46 oz	44/6	83	70
Grape	can, 46 oz	22/8	100	100
Grape	glass, 2 qt	39/4	90	—
Grape	glass, 1 qt	35/8	97	89
Lemonade	can, 46 oz	78/8	99	86
Orange	glass, 1 qt	56/8	96	82
Orange, low calorie	glass, 1 qt	44/8	91	73
Orange	can, 46 oz	40/8	95	95
Orange	can, 46 oz	44/8	84	77
Orange-pineapple	can, 46 oz	38/6	92	79
Peach	can, 46 oz	119/6	87	—
Pineapple-grapefruit	can, 46 oz	60/6	90	77
Pineapple-grapefruit	can, 46 oz	40/8	95	—
Pineapple-orange	can, 46 oz	37/8	100	—
Punch	can, 46 oz	38/6	89	69
Punch, low calorie	glass, ½ gal	68/10	85	71
Fruit Drink Conc. [to be diluted in H_2O (1 + 6)]				
Cherry	glass	11.4	81	—
Grape	glass	14.9	82	—
Lemon-lime	glass	10.7	71	—
Orange	glass	11.7	85	—
Raspberry	glass	12.0	90	—
Strawberry	glass	11.2	81	—
Fruit Carbonated Beverages				
Grape	can, 12 oz	46/12	76	61
Orange	can, 12 oz	46/12	76	54
Root beer	can, 12 oz	50/12	82	64
Black cherry	can, 12 oz	51/12	73	53

[1] Vitamin C includes ascorbic acid plus dehydroascorbic acid.

of its origin. The stability of vitamin C in orange drink and soft drinks was reported, respectively, by Davidek et al.[104] and Robertson and Sibley.[105] Ammu et al.[106] found that addition of sugar to single-strength fruit juices prior to freeze drying improved the vitamin C stability of the dried products at 24–28° and at 37°C.

Vitamin A

In observations of the authors, a fruit-flavored drink containing 600 IU of added vitamin A palmitate per fluid ounce was stored in 46 oz cans at 75°F for 12 months with a loss of vitamin A over that period of 20%. A dry orange drink powder containing 9200 IU of vitamin A palmitate was stored in sealed envelopes for 12 months at 75°F; the loss of vitamin A was 22% after 3 months, but no further loss occurred in the remainder of the 12-month storage period. A canned soy protein beverage retain 90% of the added vitamin A on storage for 12 months at room temperature (70–75°F). At 6 months at room temperature, the retention of vitamin A in a meal replacement liquid was 99% and in a dry meal replacement powder for reconstitution, 92%. Other observations are compiled in Table 10.9.

A frozen orange juice concentrate nutrified with thiamin and ascorbic acid in addition to vitamin A showed no loss of vitamin A in 12 months at $-10°F$. Frozen orange drink concentrates containing the same 3 vitamins showed a 12% loss of vitamin A in 6 months and 17% loss in 12 months at $-10°F$. Multivitamin frozen orange drink concentrates containing from 5–9 vitamins showed comparable stability of vitamin A at $-10°F$.

The stability of vitamin A in nutrified tea was reported by Brooke and Cort.[42] Tea dust fortified by dry mixing with vitamin A palmitate powder, Type 250 SD, retained 85% of the vitamin A in 12 months at room temperature. Tea leaves sprayed with an emulsion of vitamin A palmitate in 50% sucrose solution retained 90% of the vitamin A in 6 months at 98°F. When brewed into tea, 3 g of dust or leaves nutrified as above to provide 375 IU of vitamin A per cup yielded 100% recovery of the vitamin A with periods of either 5 minutes or 1 h.

Carotenoids

Storage stability data for various carotenoid products added to juices or beverages are listed in Table 10.10. Beta-carotene and apocarotenal show good stability when added to these products and stored at room temperature for 3–12 months with protection from light. The effect of exposure to direct sunlight at 75°F on carotene in a carbonated orange beverage containing 2.10 mg of beta-carotene and about 30 mg of ascorbic acid per 8 fl oz was reported by Bunnell.[41] Retention of carotene was 89% after 1 month and 82% after 2 months. Apocarotenal is less stable than carotene when exposed to light in a carbonated beverage. Borenstein and Bunnell[64] found complete loss of apocarotenal when such product containing 3.59 mg/qt of

TABLE 10.9
STABILITY OF ADDED VITAMIN A IN BEVERAGE PRODUCTS

Product	Packaging	Product Used	Initial Assay	% Retention, 70–75°F (23°C) (Months)			
				3	6	12
Chocolate drink powder, instant type	liner box	palmitate, 250-S	2670 IU/qt (reconstituted)	100	90	90
Chocolate drink, liquid	bottle	palmitate, 250-S	382 IU/100 g	93	93	92
Fruit punch	can	palmitate, 250-cws	5370 IU/9 fl oz	100	98	80
Grapefruit drink concentrate (frozen)	can	palmitate, 250-S	6250 IU/6 fl oz	100	89	—
Liquid diet food	can	palmitate, 250-S	7100 IU/qt	98	97	95
Low-calorie milk drink	can	palmitate, 250-S	7000 IU/qt	100	100	93
Low-calorie, diet mix dry	film packet	palmitate, 250-cws	2065 IU/2 oz	88	86	84
Pineapple juice	can	palmitate, 250-cws	525 IU/4 fl oz	97	75	—
Pineapple-grape fruit drink	bottle	palmitate emulsion	5200 IU/8 fl oz	78	67	—
Pineapple-grape fruit drink	bottle	palmitate, 250-cws	4400 IU/8 fl oz	80	68	—

TABLE 10.10
STABILITY OF ADDED CAROTENOIDS IN JUICE AND BEVERAGE PRODUCTS

Product	Packaging	Carotenoid Product Used	Initial Assay (Mg/8 Fl Oz)	% Retention at 23°C (Months)		
				3	6	12
Beta-carotene						
Juices						
Orange	can	beadlets	1.04	—	83	—
Blend	can	emulsion	1.32	—	100	90
Juice Drinks						
Apricot	can	beadlets	1.61	—	100	96
Orange	can	beadlets	1.07	—	95	98
Orange	can	emulsion	1.02	—	100	96
Orangeade	can	beadlets	2.20	—	—	96
Pineapple	can	beadlets	0.31	—	100	100
Pineapple-orange	can	beadlets	0.63	—	84	—
Concentrates						
Orangeade base	can	beadlets	7.80	—	93	—
Orange juice	can	beadlets	9.99	—	104	—
Carbonated beverage[1]						
Orange		beadlets	1.40	95	—	—
Apocarotenal						
Drink						
Apricot-orange	can	beadlets	0.59	94	98	—
Carbonated beverage[1]						
Orange	glass	beadlets	1.02	90	—	—

[1]Ascorbic acid added at 100 mg/qt.

apocarotenal and no ascorbic acid was exposed to direct sunlight for 1 month at 75°F. When ascorbic acid was added to the same product at 100 mg/qt, the retention of apocarotenal in 1 month of exposure to sunlight was 16%. In contrast, in the dark for 3 months at 75°F, the retention of apocarotenal without ascorbic acid was 78% and with ascorbic acid 90%. The comparable values for beta-carotene (5.7/mg/qt) in a similar carbonated beverage were 68% and 78% in 1 month in direct sunlight without and with 100 mg/qt of ascorbic acid, respectively, and for 3 months in the dark 85% and 90% without and with added ascorbic acid.

Multinutrients

Stability data obtained by E. DeRitter on multivitamin-nutrified beverage products stored at room temperature for 6 or 12 months and a frozen orange concentrate stored at −10°F for 6 months are given in Table 10.11. All of these products also

TABLE 10.11
B-VITAMIN STABILITY IN MULTIVITAMIN-NUTRIFIED BEVERAGE PRODUCTS

Product	Thiamin	Riboflavin	Pyridoxine	Vitamin B_{12}	Niacin	Folacin	Ca Pantothenate
				% Retention on Storage			
				12 months at 70–75°F			
Soy protein, liquid	68	94	100	75	100	98	—
				6 months at 70–75°F			
Meal replacement, liquid	95	100	74	75	—	—	100
Meal replacement, dry	100	92	96	—	—	—	—
				6 months at −10°F			
Frozen orange concentrate	100	100	99	88	98	—	—

contained vitamins A and C. Stability of the B-vitamins was excellent, except for thiamin and vitamin B_{12} in the soy protein liquid and pyridoxine and vitamin B_{12} in the meal replacement liquid.

Fenton-May[59] reported successful marketing of carbonated fruit juice beverages (10% juice) nutrified with ascorbic acid and a 35% juice product in test marketing to contain 60 mg of vitamin C per 6 fl oz. Vitamin A palmitate can be incorporated with proper overages. Experiences with soy-milk and casein-based sterilized, noncarbonated drinks containing added A, D, B_1, B_2, B_6, B_{12} and niacin are detailed. Dark glass or full-depth case packaging protects against light-exposure loss of vitamin A and B_2. If not preserved by pasteurization, chemical preservation is another option with good pH control and strict sanitary procedures. In a multivitamin (9 vitamins) nutrified beverage, 7-month losses ranged from 0-48%. One way to avoid liquid beverage problems is to substitute a reconstitutable beverage powder. One such product with 10 vitamins, calcium, phosphorus and iron stored for 5 months (110°F, 50% RH) showed vitamin losses of 0-35%.

More recently[107] ascorbic acid, niacinamide, vitamins B_6 and B_{12}, folate, biotin, riboflavin, calcium pantothenate and beta-carotene were added to a series of diet-type and sweetened carbonated beverages and with appropriate care and attention to vitamin chemical characteristics, stability performance (Table 10.12) was found to be good to excellent over a period of a few months. Preet et al.[108] report soft drinks fortified with ascorbic acid (50 mg/90 mL) and iron (12.5 mg) to be highly acceptable in India.

Kinetic Studies

In studies on the stability at elevated temperatures of juices and aqueous vehicles, Uprety and Davis[109] found the stability of ascorbic acid to be a function of pH, temperature, vehicle, and headspace in the container. A prediction of the stability at normal temperatures could be made on the basis of these elevated temperature studies. Saguy et al.[110] reported on the kinetics of ascorbic acid loss in grapefruit juice in thermal and concentration processes, which indicated an apparent first order anaerobic reaction dependent on temperature and degree of product concentration but not on the initial ascorbic acid content. The effect of temperature on the rate of reaction followed the Arrhenius equation with an energy of activation of 5–11.3 kcal/mol for solids content of 11–62° Brix. The authors established an empirical kinetic equation to correlate rate of reaction with temperature and degree of concentration.

Lee et al.[111] studied the kinetics of destruction of ascorbic acid in tomato juice under anaerobic conditions and found it to be first order with respect to ascorbic acid concentration. The effect of storage temperature on the rate of destruction was accounted for by the Arrhenius equation with an activation energy of 3.3 kcal/mol at pH 4.06 and a dependency on pH. The maximum rate of destruction was found

TABLE 10.12
VITAMIN STABILITY IN NUTRIFIED SODA[1] DIET ORANGE

	10 Oz. Glass Initial	1 Month	2 Months
Ascorbic acid	23 mg	22	20
Niacinamide	3.10 mg	2.96	3.00
Vitamin B_6 HCl	0.46 mg	0.43	0.46
Vitamin B_{12}	0.69 mcg	0.44	0.53
Folic acid	62 mcg	61	58
Biotin	47 mcg	42	41
Riboflavin (B_2)	0.27 mg	0.26	0.22
Cal pan	1.74 mg	1.50	1.46
Vitamin A (as beta-carotene)	2680 IU	2400	2470

Source: Gordon et al.[107]
[1]All assays/10 fl oz.

near the pK_a of ascorbic acid. A mathematical model and a computer simulation program were developed to predict stability of ascorbic acid. The rate of copper-catalyzed destruction increased with increasing copper content and was influenced by pH. Gould[112] reported that nutrified tomato juice retains ascorbic acid well if stored at low temperature, but at 31°C or above, ⅓ of the vitamin was lost after 9 months. The effect of temperature on the rate of change of ascorbic acid concentration was claimed to be a logarithmic function. Riemer and Karel[113,114] conducted shelf-life studies on ascorbic acid in dehydrated tomato juice. Degradation of vitamin C followed first-order reaction kinetics. The effect of temperature on the reaction rate could be described by the Arrhenius equation. Water activity had a strong effect on the reaction rate constant and on the activation energy. The effects of oxygen on this dehydrated system were negligible. The rates of deterioration of dehydroascorbic acid were similar to those of ascorbic acid.

Effect of Light, Oxygen and Air

The stability of ascorbic acid in commercially bottled orange juice in clear glass bottles with metal caps stored at 22°C in the dark or under constant illumination at 3500 lux was studied by Granzer.[115] In 37 days, the losses of ascorbic acid were 5–6% with light exposure and 3–4% in the dark. Andrews and Driscoll[116] stored three brands of single-strength orange juice from frozen concentrate in one-liter bottles of either brown or clear glass closed with foil and exposed to light. After 8 days, the retention of ascorbic acid was 82–85% in brown bottles and 75% in clear glass bottles. Rother[117] noted injurious effects of light on ascorbic acid in soft drinks containing orange juice.

Kitagawa[118] found high losses of vitamin C, especially the reduced form, when vegetable and fruit juices were exposed to ultraviolet light. With visible light, the losses of vitamin C were less severe. Proctor and O'Meara[119] reported that irradiation of orange juice with high-voltage cathode rays caused considerable los of ascorbic acid, but the loss of total vitamin C was much less (dehydroascorbic acid retains activity). In the frozen state, ascorbic acid in orange juice is stable to irradiation.

The effects of oxygen at levels of 0.002–3.5% on the retention of ascorbic acid in canned and frozen orange juices was studied by Kefford et al.[120] In frozen juices stored at 0°F for 1 year the presence of free oxygen in the cans permitted slow oxidative losses of ascorbic acid. In pasteurized juices stored at 86°F, oxidative destruction of ascorbic acid occurred only during the first few day since free oxygen disappeared rapidly from the cans; throughout subsequent storage, anaerobic loss continued at a rate about 1/10 of that in the early period. Chogovadze and Bakuradz[121] reported that glucose oxidase, with or without catalase, reduced losses of ascorbic acid in orange juice stored 40 days at 20°C.

Mathe[122] reported greater stability of carotenoids in orange beverages after dark storage than after exposure to light at room temperature for a similar period of time. Addition of ascorbic acid partially inhibited the degradation of carotenoids in the light. Granzer[115] found no significant loss of total carotenoids in orange juice stored for 45 weeks at 22°C under constant illumination with 3500 lux and attributed the stability of the carotenoids to the antioxidant action of ascorbic acid.

Certain types of bottled soft drinks, especially orange and grapefruit flavored products with unsaturated terpenes in their flavor component are subject to oxidative rancidity induced by light exposure. The addition of 5–15 mg of ascorbic acid per fluid ounce produces a marked stabilizing effect on the flavor.[123] However, if artificial colors are employed, color fading is possible and one can choose to use less ascorbic acid or add a color like beta-carotene, which is more light stable in the presence of ascorbic acid. Although beta-carotene is sensitive to light in the presence of oxygen, if dissolved and headspace oxygen is removed by the use of ascorbic acid, exposure to sunlight has little destructive effect. Strictly from a color viewpoint, beta-carotene has advantages over some of the FDC colors in that it is not affected by the reducing action of ascorbic acid as occurs with the color dyes.[41] Decolorization of FD&C colors (the so-called azo or coal tar dyes) can occur in carbonated beverages in the presence of ascorbic acid depending on (1) the specific FD&C color's reaction to reducing agents, (2) the oxygen and dissolved metal content, and (3) exposure of the bottled beverages to sunlight.

Effect of Metal Ions and Stabilizing Agents

Johnsson and Hessel[124] studied the stability of ascorbic acid in ready-to-drink juices and found Cu^{2+} and Fe^{3+} ions to accelerate oxidative loss of ascorbic acid. With a Cu^{2+} ion concentration of 15 mg/L, little loss of ascorbic acid occurred in 24-h storage. These authors reported little effect of pH on ascorbic acid stability in the acid pH range normally occurring in juices. Timberlake[125] studied the stability of ascorbic acid in black currant juice and in model systems resembling black currant juice. Oxidation of ascorbic acid in the presence of copper was increased significantly by addition of small amounts of iron, and increasing the copper level greatly increased ascorbic acid oxidation. Sawtell[126] commented also that literature data support the exceptional stability of vitamin C in black currant juice. The fact that vitamin C is better preserved in juices with a high anthocyanin content was mentioned by Saburov and Ul'yanova.[127]

Ethylenediaminetetraacetic acid (EDTA) improved the stability of added ascorbic acid in wine,[128] and the di-NaCa salt of EDTA added to tomato juice helped to preserve the original ascorbic acid present.[129] Timberlake[125] noted the effect of EDTA and other metal-chelating agents in stabilizing ascorbic acid in black currant juice with added copper and iron.

When 30 mg of ascorbic acid were added per 100 g of heat-extract or raw cranberry juice and the juices held at 27°C for 1 h, there was a 15% destruction of ascorbic acid in the raw juice, while the loss in the heated juice was negligible.[130] The addition of 0.5 or 1% Sequestrene to the raw cranberry juice as it was pressed did not result in a higher retention of ascorbic acid in cranberry cocktail, indicating that enzymic oxidation rather than metal-catalyzed oxidation is the likely destructive agent. Johnson and Toledo[131] studied the storage stability of ascorbic acid in 55° Brix orange juice concentrate packaged aseptically in plastic and glass containers. The presence of H_2O_2 in the headspace greatly accelerated the degradation of ascorbic acid. SO_2 at 500 ppm aided the retention of ascorbic acid, but gave a detectable off-flavor to the product. Levels of SO_2 below 500 ppm were ineffective. Pribela and Danisova[132] studied the effect of SO_2, oxalic acid, Na benzoate, and sorbic acid on the stability of vitamin C during storage of fruit juices, including orange, lemon, grapefruit, strawberry, cherry, and currant. Daily loss of vitamin C with SO_2 was 0.6%, with oxalic acid and Na Benozate 1.0% and with sorbic acid 2%.

Other additives shown to be useful in stabilizing ascorbic acid in beverages include cysteine,[133] histidine, glycine, or methionine,[134] tartrazine,[135] and peptides obtained by protein hydrolysis.[136] The addition of 100 mg % of various polyphosphates to lemon juice was shown by Hirata[137] to protect vitamin C in the juice. Morse and Hammes[138] found better stability of vitamin C in orange juice and grape juice containing $FeSO_4$ when cysteine was added at a level of 0.084 mg/mL. The stabilizing influence of cysteine and sodium metabisulfite on ascorbic acid nutrified, bottled orange drink (80% juice) stored at room temperature was investigated; in descending order of effectiveness was 400 ppm, 200 ppm cysteine, 400 ppm and 200 ppm, sodium metabisulfite.[139]

The well-known effect of sulfite in destroying thiamin was demonstrated by DiGiacomo et al.[140] in a stability test of orange juice. Preservatives such as K benzoate, ethyl paraben, or K sorbate had no effect on the thiamin content, whereas SO_2 at 1 ppm decreased the thiamin to 12% of the original content after 9 days.

Effect of Container

The type of container in which juices and beverages are packaged has a significant effect on the stability of ascorbic acid. Packaging can be in metal, glass, or containers with a plastic component in contact with the product. Glass bottles frequently have a large headspace, particularly if the product is pasteurized in the bottle, where room for expansion must be allowed. Even with the usual deaeration of the product, the headspace will usually contain oxygen. In carbonated beverages, the problem is less acute due to the high partial pressure of CO_2 which reduces the oxygen content of the product.

Metal cans for juice or drink packing are usually lacquered internally to minimize metal contamination, but losses of ascorbic acid still occur, presumably by reaction with headspace oxygen. After an initial loss, the stability of ascorbic acid on storage is usually good. Klein et al.[141] studied the stability of vitamin C in 6 commercial fruit juice products after opening lacquered or nonlacquered tin cans and storing for 12 days. With the lacquered cans, the vitamin C dropped in 12 days to about 50% in the refrigerator and to about 10% at room temperature. In the nonlacquered cans, the tin content was higher and rose slightly on storage after opening, and the vitamin C content of the juices was only 25-33% of that in the lacquered cans and decreased further on storage.

Drinks packed in plastic containers can present a problem with vitamin C stability if the diffusion of air through the wall of the container is a factor. Blow-molded or laminated bottles provide protection approaching that of glass. Berry et al.[142] and Bisset and Berry[143] reported good stability of vitamin C in orange juice or concentrate frozen for 12 months packed in various commercial containers. Chilled, single-strength orange juice retained vitamin C much better packed in glass than in plastic containers. Massaioli and Haddad[144] studied the stability of vitamin C in various orange juices which were placed in sealed glass or PVC containers and refrigerated for 14 days with a daily treatment of vigorous shaking for 5 seconds or swirling gently and inverting twice. The orange juices had been packaged originally in tinplated cans, PVC containers, or coated paperboard cartons and contained either no preservative or various combinations of sorbic acid, Ca sorbate, SO_2, benzoic acid, and Na benzoate. In the refrigerated 14-day test, most juices showed satisfactory vitamin C retention with total losses of 3.3-13.7%. Losses of vitamin C were greater with vigorous shaking and were linear with time. In studies of vitamin C stability in tomato juice, both Cerutti[145] and Jurkovic et al.[146] found better stability in metal cans than in glass bottles. Suckewer et al.[147] reported a 7% loss of folic acid in either cans or jars of tomato juice stored in darkness for 12 months.

Dry beverage powder to be reconstituted prior to consumption may be nutrified with added ascorbic acid and other vitamins, but the successful storage life is dependent on having a low moisture content in the marketed product initially and so maintained by humidity-resistant packaging.[36] Packaging aspects of nutrified beverages are included in reviews by Henshall[81] and Gresswell.[123]

Future Trends

With the trends of increased consumption of beverages and the concern of the public for nutritious foods which meet current health guides, it would seem that nutrients will continue to be added to beverages. Hopefully, more consideration might be given to the choice of nutrients added and the levels chosen. Replacement beverages for milk and juices, such as soft drinks, must be examined more closely for appropriate nutrient content.

REFERENCES

1. WOODROOF, J. G. and PHILLIPS, G. F. 1981. Beverages: Carbonated and Non-Carbonated. AVI/Van Nostrand Reinhold, New York.
2. MANN, E. J. 1987. Lactic beverages. Dairy Ind. Int. 52 (2), 13–14; (3), 9–10.
3. CANTARELLI, C. and BENEA, F. 1984. New beverages based on fruit juices with milk or milk products. Ind. Bevande 13(70), 73–78.
4. NELSON, P. E. and TRESSLER, D. K. 1980. Fruit and Vegetable Juice Processing Technology, 3rd Ed. AVI/Van Nostrand Reinhold, New York.
5. RUPPEL, G. 1987. Mixed drinks based on beer: Taboo or opportunity? Brauwelt 127(32), 1411–1414.
6. HANNIGAN, K. 1984. Premium drink with distinctive style: shandy beverage. Food Eng. 56(1), 52–53.
7. BLENFORD, D. E. 1987. Drink your health. Food Flavor. Ingred. Packag. Proc. 9(11), 11.
8. GRACEY, M. et al. 1985. Use of carbonated soft drinks to provide safe drinking water. Ann. Trop. Paediatr. 5(1), 3–6.
9. VAN DER HORST, G., WESSO, I., BURGER, A. P., DIETRICH, D. L. L., and GROBLER, S. R. 1984. Chemical analysis of cool drinks and pure fruit juices: some clinical implications. S.A. Med. J. 66, 755–758.
10. JACKEL, S. S. 1989. High-density sweeteners and fat substitutes are on the horizon. Cereal Foods World 34(10), 887–888.
11. ANON. 1986. Beverage choices are changing. NRA News 6 (April), 38.
12. ANON. 1987. Attitudes and economics make for a transitional soft drink market. Food Eng. Int. 12 (Oct), 27–28.
13. LEVI, A. E. and FOLWELL, R. J. 1987. Demand analysis for beverages with emphasis on horticultural crops. Acta Hortic. 203, 227–234.
14. ANON. 1989. New beverages, frozen desserts benefit from fruit's appeal. Food Eng. 60(7), 25; (8), 36–37.
15. DUXBURY, D. D. 1988. Imported bulk frozen fruit juice concentrates supplied year-around. Food Proc. 49(7), 73–76.
16. BUNCH, K. L. 1987. Food Consumption, Prices, & Expenditures 1985. Statist. Bull. 749. USDA-ERS-Nat. Econ. Div., Washington, DC.
17. BUNCH, K. and KURLAND, J. 1984. How America quenches its thirst. Nat. Food Rev. NFR-27 (summer), 14–17.

18. MORGAN, K. J., STULTS, V. J. and STAMPLEY, M. S. 1985. Soft drink consumption patterns in the U.S. population. J. Am. Diet. Assoc. 85(3), 352–354.
19. GUENTHER, P. M. 1986. Beverages in the diets of American teenagers. J. Am. Diet. Assoc. 86(4), 493–499.
20. GEBHARDT, S. E., CUTRUFELLI, R. and MATTHEWS, R. H. 1982. Composition of Foods, Fruits and Fruit Juices, Raw—Processed—Prepared. Agr. Handbook No. 8-9. USDA, Washington, DC.
21. CUTRUFELLI, R. and MATTHEWS, R. H. 1986. Composition of Foods: Beverages. Agr. Handbook No. 8-14 USDA. Washington, DC.
22. DICKEY, L. E. and WEIHRAUUCH, J. L. 1988. Composition of Foods: Fast Foods. Agr. Handbook 8-21. USDA, Washington, DC.
23. SCRIBAN, R. 1970. Barley, malt and beer vitamins. Ann. Nutr. Aliment. 24, B377–B399.
24. BLONDEAU, R. 1975. Vitamin B_{12} in French beers. Cah. Nutr. Diet. 10, 59–62.
25. DUDA, G. et al. 1981. Vitamin content in Polish beers. Zywienie Czlowieka 8, 63–68.
26. OCKHUIZEN, T. 1988. How wholesome is beer? Voedingsmiddelentechnologie 21(5), 13–16.
27. PIENDL, A. 1989. The importance of beer in nutrition today. Brauwelt 129(14), 546–552.
28. PUISAIS, J. and GUILLER, A. 1975. Observations concerning the nutritional value of wine. C. R. Congr. Natl. Soc. Savantes, Sect. Sci. 1970, 95, 315–325.
29. AMERINE, M. A. 1977. Wine in human nutrition. Bull. OIV (Numero Special), 137–151.
30. MASQUELIER, J. 1978. Wine and nutrition. Ann. Technol. Agr. 27, 427–439.
31. OURNAC, A. and FLANZY, M. 1967. The increase in vitamin B_1 in wine stored with its lees. Ann. Technol. Agr. 16, 41–54.
32. AVAKYAN, B. P. and SARKISYAN, M. T. 1971. Vitamins in Armenian fruit and berry wines. Biol. Zh. Arm. 24, 84–86.
33. AVAKYAN, B. P. and BAGDASARYAN, E. O. 1975. B group vitamins of table wines treated by different processes. Biol. Zh. Arm. 28, 76–79.
34. VOIGHT, M. N., EITENMILLER, R. R., POWERS, J. J. and WARE, G. O. 1978. Water-soluble vitamin content of some California wines. J. Food Sci. 43, 1071–1073.
35. BAUERNFEIND, J. C. 1985. Antioxidant function of L-ascorbic acid in food technology. Int. J. Vit. Nutr. Res. Suppl. 27, 307–333.
36. BAUERNFEIND, J. C. 1982. Ascorbic acid technology in agricultural, pharmaceutical, food and industrial applications. In Ascorbic Acid: Chemistry, Metabolism and Uses, P. A. Seib and B. M. Tolbert (eds.). American Chemical Society, Washington, DC.
37. JOHNSON, H. T., McALPINE, A. W. and SCHENEK, A. M. 1955. Some aspects of canning soft drinks. Food Technol. 9, 643–647.
38. MULLOR, J. B., VIGIL, J. B. and MIGUEZ, M. A. 1968. Vitamin C content of fruits and fruit products. Variations in species, varieties, seasons, and industrial techniques. Rev. Fac. Ing. Quim. Univ. Nac. Litoral 37 (pt 1), 165–182.
39. BAUERNFEIND, J. C. 1958. Carotenoids in fruits, juices and concentrates. Symp. Frucht-Konzentrate, Bristol, 265–290, Juris Zurich.
40. BAUERNFEIND, J. C., OSADCA, M. and BUNNELL, R. H. 1962. Beta-carotene, color and nutrient for juices and beverages. Food Technol. 16(8), 101–108.

41. BUNNELL, R. H. 1968. Enrichment of fruit products and fruit juices. J. Agr. Food Chem. *16*, 177–183.
42. BROOKE, C. L. and CORT, W. M. 1972. Vitamin A fortification of tea. Food Technol. *26*(6), 50–52.
43. PADEN, C. A., WOLINSKY, I., HOSPIN, J. C., LEWIS, K. C., LINEBACK, D. R. and McCARTHY, R. D. 1979. Fortification of accessory food items with vitamin A. Lebensm. Wiss. Technol. *12*, 183–188.
44. WILLS, R. B. H. and DWYER, M. A. 1978. Fortification of tea with thiamin. Nutr. Rep. Int. *18*, 197–202.
45. LINDESAY CLARK, A. 1990. Thiamin in our bread and wine? Med. J. Austr. *153*, 115.
46. PRICE, J. and THEODOROS, M. T. 1979. The supplementation of alcoholic beverages with thiamin: a necessary preventive measure in Queensland. AUS-AUST. N.Z.J. Psychiatry *13*(4), 315–320.
47. WOOD, B. and BREEN, K. J. 1980. Clinical thiamine deficiency in Australia; the size of the problem and approaches to prevention. Med. J. Austr. *1*, 461–464.
48. MEILGAARD, M. C. 1982. Technical aspects of the enrichment of beer with thiamin. J. Stud. Alcohol *43*(5), 427–433.
49. CRANE, S. and PRICE, J. 1983. The attempted enrichment of beer with thiamin alkyl disulphides. J. Nutr. Sci. Vitaminol. (Japan) *29*, 381–387.
50. BUDGE, M. and PRICE, J. 1983. Public reaction to a proposal to fortify beer with thiamin. J. Food Nutr. *39*, 147–151.
51. YELLOWLEES, P. M. 1986. Thiamin deficiency and prevention of the Wernicke-Korsakoff syndrome. Med. J. Austr. *145*, 216–218.
52. WOOD, B. 1987. Thiamin in beer. Med. J. Austr. *146*, 170.
53. ROUSE, I. L. and ARMSTRONG, B. K. 1988. Thiamin and alcoholic beverages: to add or not to add? Med. J. Austr. *148*, 605–607.
54. WODAK, A., RICHMOND, R. and WILSON, A. 1990. Thiamin fortification and alcohol. Med. J. Austr. *152*(2), 97–99.
55. VAN DER WESTHUYZEN, J., DAVIS, R. E., ICKE, G. C. and METZ, J. 1985. Fortification of sorghum beer with thiamin. Int. J. Vit. Nutr. *55*(2), 173–179.
56. BELL, D., ROBERTSON, C. E. and MUIR, A. L. 1987. Carbonated drinks, thiamin deficiency and right ventricular failure. Scott. Med. J. *32*(5), 137–138.
57. RICHARDSON, D. P. 1983. Iron fortification of foods and drinks. Chem. Ind. *13*, 498–501.
58. DUXBURY, D. S. 1987. Nutritional ingredients. Food Proc. *48*(5), 112–114.
59. FENTON-MAY, R. 1975. Fortification of beverages. *In* Technology of Fortification of Foods, Natl. Acad. of Sciences, Washington, DC.
60. BENK, E. 1983. Fruit juices, fruit nectars and fruit beverages with fitness-enhancing additives. Ind. Obst. Gemueseverwert. *68*, 467–469.
61. BENK, E. 1983. Use of minerals in non-alcoholic beverages. Mineralbrunnen *33*, 427–428.
62. BAUERNFEIND, J. C. and DeRITTER, E. 1976. Vitamins. *In* Handbook of Biochemistry and Molecular Biology, 3rd Ed., Physical and Chemical Data, Vol. II, G. D. Fasman (ed.). CRC Press, Cleveland.
63. BAUERNFEIND, J. C. and CORT, W. M. 1974. Nutrification of foods with added vitamin A. Crit. Rev. Food Technol. 4, 337–375.

64. BORENSTEIN, B. and BUNNELL, R. H. 1967. Carotenoids: properties, occurrence, and utilization in foods. Adv. Food Res. *15*, 195–276.
65. KLAEUI, H. and BAUERNFEIND, J. C. 1981. Carotenoids as food colors. *In* Carotenoids as Colorants and Vitamin A Precursors, J. C. Bauernfeind (ed.). Academic Press, New York.
66. GORDON, H. T. and BAUERNFEIND, J. C. 1985. Carotenoids as food colorants. Crit. Rev. Food Sci. Nutr. *18*(1), 59–97.
67. COCCODRILLI, G., JR. and SHAH, N. 1985. Beverages. *In* Iron Fortification of Foods, F. M. Clydesdale and K. L. Wiemer (eds.). Academic Press, New York.
68. JOHNSON, P. E. and EVANS, G. W. 1977. Coffee as a low-calorie vehicle for iron fortification. Nutr. Rep. Int. *16*, 89–92.
69. WEINGARTNER, K. E., NELSON, A. I. and ERDMAN, J. W., JR. 1983. Effects of calcium addition on stability and sensory properties of soy beverage. J. Food Sci. *48*, 256–257.
70. ZEMEL, M. B. and SHELEF, L. A. 1986. Calcium fortified soy milk. Eur. Pat. Appl. EPO 195 167 A2.
71. HECKERT, D. C. 1987. Fruit juice beverages and juice concentrates. Nutritionally supplemented with calcium. U.S. Pat. 860607; Eur. Pat. Appl. EPO 244 903 A1.
72. MELACHOURIS, N. and LEE, C. R. 1988. Calcium fortified acid beverages. U.S. Pat. 4740380.
73. SCHOBINGER, U. and DAEPP, H. U. 1978. Fruit and Vegetable Juices: Technology, Chemistry, Microbiology, Analysis, Importance, Law. Ulmer, Stuttgart.
74. GREEN, L. F. 1978. Developments in Soft Drinks Technology. Applied Sciences Publishers Ltd., Essex, England.
75. KOCH, J. 1986. Beverage Evaluation. Ulmer Gmbh & Co., Stuttgart.
76. PILZ, H. 1985. Beverage ABC, 3rd Ed. VEB Fachbuchverlag, Leipzig.
77. KARMAS, E. and HARRIS, R. S. 1987. Nutritional Evaluation of Food Processing, 3rd Ed., Van Nostrand Reinhold Co., New York.
78. RIESE, H. 1987. Fruit juice: a matter of quality. N. Eur. Food Dairy J. *53*(6), 203–209.
79. KOHNSTAMM, L. W. 1986. Fruit juice enhanced soft drinks: how to make them. Beverages *51*(160), 8–12.
80. PRENDERGAST, K. 1985. Whey drinks: Technology, processing and marketing. J. Soc. Dairy Technol. *38*(4), 103–105.
81. HENSHALL, J. D. 1981. Ascorbic acid in fruit juices and beverages. *In* Vitamin C (Ascorbic Acid), J. N. Counsell and D. H. Hornig (eds.). Applied Science Publishers, London.
82. KLAEUI, H. 1974. The technological aspects of the addition of nutrients to foods. Proc. 4th Int. Congr. Food Sci. Technol. *1*, 740–762.
83. AITKEN, H. C. 1956. Vitaminized apple juice. Canada Food Ind. *27*, 34; 1957. Food Eng. *29*(3), 127; 1958. Can. Food Ind. *29*, 63.
84. BAUERNFEIND, J. C. 1958. Role of ascorbic acid in the browning phenomenon of fruit juice. Symp. Frucht-Konzentrate, Bristol, 159–185, Juris Zurich.
85. ESSELEN, W. B. JR., POWERS, J. J. and FELLERS, C. R. 1946. The fortification of fruit juices with ascorbic acid. Fruit Prod. J. and Am. Food Manuf. *26*, 11–14, 29.
86. BUDRENENE, R. V. 1986. Preservation of vitamin C in vitamin enriched apple products. Vopr. Pitan. *5*, 61–62.

87. SCHOBINGER, U. 1979. Investigations on the processing of cloud stable pomaceous fruit juices: A mixture of apple juice and pear juice. Schweiz. Z. Obst. Weinbau *115*, 422–427.
88. BIRCH, G. G., BOINTON, B. M., ROLFE, E. J. and SELMAN, J. D. 1974. Quality changes related to vitamin C in fruit juice and vegetable processing. *In* Vitamin C: Recent Aspects of Its Physiological and Technological Importance, G. G. Birch and K. J. Parker (eds.). John Wiley & Sons, New York.
89. ESPADA, M. A. 1968. Importance of vitamin C in the carbonated beverage industry. Ion *27*, 564–568, 581.
90. MROZEWSKI, S. 1966. Increasing the nutritional value of carbonated beverages. Przem. Ferment. Rolny *10*, 72–73.
91. BRIGHT, R. A. and POTTER, N. N. 1979. Acceptability and properties of carbonated apple juice. Food Prod. Dev. *13*(4), 34–36.
92. BENDER, A. E. 1958. The stability of vitamin C in a commercial fruit squash. J. Sci. Food Agr. *9*(11), 754–760.
93. PELLETIER, O. and MORRISON, A. P. 1965. Content and stability of ascorbic acid in fruit drinks. J. Am. Diet. Assoc. *47*(5), 401–404.
94. DIEMAIR, W. and POSTEL, W. 1965. Ascorbic acid in the preparation of fruit juices and canned vegetables. Wiss. Veroeff. Dsch. Ges. Ernaehr. *14*, 248–259.
95. BAUERNFEIND, J. C. and PINKERT, D. M. 1970. Food processing with added ascorbic acid. Adv. Food Res. *18*, 219–315.
96. EMODI, A. and SCIALPI, L. and ANTOSHKIW, T. 1976. Water-dispersible, optically clear carotenoid colors. Food Technol. *30*(7), 58–60.
97. BUNNELL, R. H., DRISCOLL, W. and BAUERNFEIND, J. C. 1958. Coloring water-base foods with beta-carotene. Food Technol. *12*, 536–544.
98. BAUERNFEIND, J. C. and BUNNELL, R. H. 1962. Beta-apo-8'-carotenal—A new food color. Food Technol. *16*, 76–81.
99. DeRITTER, E. 1976. Stability characteristics of vitamins in processed foods. Food Technol. *30*(1), 48–51, 54.
100. ANON. 1975. Nutritional approach to marketing expands with Vitamin C enriched tomato juice. Food Proc. *36*(11), 31.
101. POPE, G. G. 1973. Effect of time, temperature and fortification level on the retention of ascorbic acid in fortified tomato juice. Diss. Abstr. Int. B, *33*, 5339. Univ. Microfilms, Ann Arbor.
102. SMOOT, J. M. and NAGY, S. 1980. Effects of storage temperature and duration on total vitamin C content of canned single-strength grapefruit juice. J. Agr. Food Chem. *28*, 417–421.
103. BESTON, G. H. and HENDERSON, G. A. 1974. Vitamin C stability in reconstituted beverage products. Can. Inst. Food Sci. Technol. J. *7*, 183–187.
104. DAVIDEK, J., VELISEK, J., and JANICEK, G. 1974. Stability of vitamin C in orange drink. Lebensm. Wiss. Technol. *7*, 285–287.
105. ROBERTSON, J. M. and SIBLEY, J. A. 1974. Ascorbic acid stability in artificial drinks. Food Technol. N.Z. *9*, 13, 15, 17.
106. AMMU, K., RADHKRISHNA, K., SUBRAMANIAN, V., SHARMA, T. R. and NATH, H. 1977. Storage behavior of freeze-dried fruit juice powders. J. Food Technol. *12*, 541–554.
107. GORDON, H. T., JOHNSON, L. E. and WASKO, P. M. 1986. Vitamin fortification

of carbonated beverages. Presentation, Apr. 28-30, Society of Soft Drink Technologists.
108. PREET KAUR I., VANEJA, K. and RAVI, K. 1988. Studies on acceptability and availability of forticants present in certain fortified foodstuffs. Indian Food Packer 42(2), 24-26.
109. UPRETY, M. C. and DAVIS, B. 1964. Elevated temperature studies on the stability of ascorbic acid in certain juice and aqueous vehicles. J. Pharm. Sci. 53, 1248-1251.
110. SAGUY, I., KOPELMAN, I. J. and MIZRAHI, S. 1978. Simulation of ascorbic acid stability during heat processing and concentration of grapefruit juice. J. Food Proc. Eng. 2, 213-225.
111. LEE, Y. C., KIRK, J. R., BEDFORD, C. L. and HELDMAN, D. R. 1977. Kinetics and computer simulation of ascorbic acid stability of tomato juice as functions of temperature, pH, and metal catalyst. J. Food Sci. 42, 640-644, 648.
112. GOULD, W. A. 1978. Quality evaluation of processed tomato juice. J. Agr. Food Chem. 26, 1006-1011.
113. RIEMER, J. and KAREL, M. 1977. Shelf-life studies on vitamin C during food storage: prediction of ascorbic acid retention in dehydrated tomato juice. J. Food Sci. 1, 293-312.
114. RIEMER, J. and KAREL, M. 1978. The anaerobic degradation of ascorbic acid in dehydrated tomato juice. J. Agr. Food Chem. 26, 350-353.
115. GRANZER, R. 1983. Effect of light on ascorbic acid and carotenoid contents and on sensory quality of orange juice in colourless glass bottles. Ind. Obst. Gemuseseverwert. 68, 263-266.
116. ANDREWS, F. E. and DRISCOLL, P. J. 1977. Stability of ascorbic acid in orange juice exposed to light and air during storage. J. Am. Diet. Assoc. 71, 140-142.
117. ROTHER, H. 1958. Injurious effects of light on soft drinks containing orange juice. Naturbrunnen, Sonderdruck 4, 1-3.
118. KITAGAWA, Y. 1968. The effect of ultraviolet rays on vitamin C. III. Changes of the vitamin C in vegetable and fruit juices. Eiyo Shokuryo 20, 461-464.
119. PROCTOR, B. E. and O'MEARA, J. P. 1951. Effect of high-voltage cathode rays on ascorbic acid. Ind. Eng. Chem. 43, 718-721.
120. KEFFORD, J. F., McKENSIE, H. A. and THOMPSON, P. C. O. 1959. Effects of oxygen on quality and ascorbic acid retention in canned and frozen orange juice. J. Sci. Food Agr. 10, 51-63.
121. CHOGOVADZE, S. K. and BAKURADZA, N. S. 1972. Preservation of ascorbic acid by glucose oxidase. Lebensm.-Ind. 19, 284-289.
122. MATHE, I. 1980. Chanes in the composition of orange beverages during storage. II. Szeszipar 28, 51-53.
123. GRESSWELL, D. M. 1974. Vitamin C in soft drinks and fruit juices. In Vitamin C: Recent Aspects of Its Physiological and Technological Importance, Ind.-Univ. Co-op Symp., G. G. Birch and K. J. Parker (eds.). John Wiley & Sons, New York.
124. JOHNSSON, H. and HESSEL, H. 1982. Stability of ascorbic acid in ready-to-drink juices. Var Foeda 34, 267-279.
125. TIMBERLAKE, C. F. 1960. Metallic components of fruit juices: Oxidation and stability of ascorbic acid. III. In model systems resembling black currant juice. IV. In black currant juice. J. Sci. Food Agr. 11, 258-273.
126. SAWTELL, J. W. 1975. Stability of vitamin C in Ribena. J. Assoc. Public Anal. 13 (Dec.), 143-144.
127. SABUROV, N. V. and UL'YANOVA, D. A. 1968. Juices from fruits and berries of the temperate zone of the USSR. Izv. Timiryazevsk. Skh. Akad. 2, 129-139.

128. FERENCZI, S. and KARENYA, A. 1973. Stabilization of ascorbic acid in wines by formation of complexes. Borgazdasag *21*, 65–70.
129. BERSWORTH, F. C. and RUBIN, M. 1958. Preservation of food by complexing trace metals. U.S. Pat. 2,846,317, Aug. 5.
130. LICCIARDELLO, J. J., ESSELEN, W. B., JR. and FELLERS, C. R. 1952. Stability of ascorbic acid during the preparation of cranberry products. Food Res. *17*, 338–342.
131. JOHNSON, R. L. and TOLEDO, R. T. 1975. Storage stability of 55° brix orange juice concentrate aseptically packaged in plastic and glass containers. J. Food Sci. *40*, 433–434.
132. PRIBELA, A. and DANISOVA, C. 1972. Effect of preservatives on vitamin C in juices. Zb. Pr. Chemickotechnol. Fak. SVST (publ. 1974), 363–368.
133. MORSE, L. D. and HAMMES, P. A. 1976. Beverages containing stabilized vitamin C and iron. U.S. Pat. 3,958,017, May 18.
134. HAMMES, P. A. and MORSE, L. D. 1972. Beverages containing stabilized vitamin C. U.S. Pat. 3,652,290, Mar. 28.
135. MORSE, L. D. 1972. Vitamin C-stabilized sweetened beverages. F. Pat. 2,107,77, Jun. 9.
136. NIPPON KAYAKU CO., LTD. 1981. Prevention of deterioration of vitamin C-enriched soft drinks. Jpn. Kokai Tokyo Koho *81*(29), 979, Mar. 25.
137. HIRATA, A. 1968. Polyphosphates as additives for foods: The effects of phosphates as a preservative (stabilizer) for vitamin C. Kaseigaku Zasshi *19*, 162–164.
138. MORSE, L. D. and HAMMES, P. A. 1971. Beverages containing stabilized vitamin C. Fr. Pat. 2,062,249, Jul. 30.
139. MAEDA, E. E. and MUSSA, D. M. D. N. 1986. The stability of vitamin C in bottled and canned orange juice. Food Chem. *22*(1), 51–58.
140. DIGIACOMO, A., CALVARANO, M. and LIVIDE, G. 1973. Vitamin B_1 in the juice of the sweet Biondo Commune oranges of Calabria. Essenze Deriv. Agrum. *43*, 236–244.
141. KLEIN, A., COP, R., CHATRNA, E. and BADALOVA, M. 1970. The stability of vitamin C and tin content in canned fruit juices. Cesk. Hyg. *15*, 49–55.
142. BERRY, R. E., BISSETT, O. W. and VELDHUIS, M. K. 1971. Vitamin C retention in orange juice as related to container type. Citrus Ind. *52*, 12–13.
143. BISSETT, O. W. and BERRY, R. E. 1975. Ascorbic acid retention in orange juice as related to container type. J. Food Sci. *40*, 178–180.
144. MASSAIOLI, D. and HADDAD, P. R. 1981. Stability of the vitamin C content of commercial orange juice. Food Technol. Aust. *33*, 136, 138.
145. CERUTTI, G. 1959. Stability of fruit juices. II. The influence of storing conditions on the keeping quality of tomato juice. Chimica (Milan) *35*, 461–464.
146. JURKOVIC, N., MIHELIC, F. and VRGA, B. 1977. Vitamin C content in tomatoes. Hrana Ishrana *18*, 253–255.
147. SUCKEWER, A., BARTNICK, J. and SECOMSKA, B. 1970. Effect of technological processes on the contents of folic acid in some vegetable products. Rocz. Panstw. Zakl. Hig. *21*, 619–629.

CHAPTER 11

Foods Considered for Nutrient Addition: SNACKS AND CONFECTIONERIES

G. S. RANHOTRA, Ph.D., and J. L. VETTER, Ph.D.

INTRODUCTION

Snacking has become an American pastime, contributing to an increasing percentage of our energy intake; many of us derive up to 20% of our caloric intake from snack foods. These foods also provide nutrients, but most tend to be calorie dense and not nutrient dense. To improve the nutritional profile of snack foods and/or to correct nutrient inadequacies in our food supply, fortification (nutrification) of snack foods may be an appropriate public health measure.

What is Snack and Snacking

Snacking is defined as an eating occasion between the three main meals of the day. Snacks, solids or liquids, have become part of the American lifestyle, with many of us consuming some foods and beverages between meals.[1] Snacks are also an important component of party foods, and they even complement other foods at mealtime.

Snacking is reported as a common behavior among teenagers and students, with many consuming snacks they desired, rather than what someone else suggested they should have.

Snacks accommodate many lifestyles and may substitute for one or more main meals of the day, thus providing a good portion of our caloric intake. They may also provide various nutrients. This, however, may be in conflict with the belief, deeply ingrained in our psyche and often for purely emotional and unscientific reasons, that snacks are generally "empty calories," i.e., provide calories but little or no nutrients.

The nutritional quality of fruits, vegetables and their juices, as well as other snacks known to be high in nutrients (through natural occurrence or nutrification), are rarely under scrutiny.[2] We become uncertain, however, when snack foods tend to be high in fat, sugar and/or sodium. Many of these latter snack foods are now being reformulated to carry a healthful image. It may be emphasized that no single food consumed in moderate portions can determine the quality of an individual's diet in a day; there are good or bad diets, but no good or bad foods.

SNACK AND CONFECTIONERY FOOD MARKET

Around the World

Snack sales around the world continue to rise.[3] In Europe, a trend toward more healthful snacks is spawning a variety of products.[4] For example, in Germany, there has been test marketing of potato chips and corn-based pellet snacks which contain about 20% fat as compared with 30–40% for regular style products. Germany continues to be a unique potato chip market, although nuts represent the largest selling snack category; pretzel-style snacks run neck and neck with potato chips for second place. In England, snacks represent one of the largest segments of the food industry. After potato chips, savory snacks (noncrisp, extruded, reconstituted and otherwise potato or cereal-based products) represent the second leading category. On the strength of a 5-year growth trend, the snack market in Sweden has now reached 4 lb per capita, with potato chips, extruded snacks and nuts representing an impressive increase. Holland and Switzerland also have a robust potato chip market.[4]

Like snacks, the confection market in Europe has also seen a consistent increase in sales and consumption. New products are continually being developed, and some products that have had success in the United States for many years are now being introduced in Europe. Chocolate-coated products account for the most sales.

In Japan, chili-seasoned potato chips and shoestring potatoes now represent 30% of the potato chip market. This is the largest snack category followed closely by corn-based snacks. Third place in total volume goes to fabricated potato chips; snacks based on wheat, rice and corn are also quite popular. In South Africa, the snack market represents primarily different variations of potato chips including American kettle-style chips. Soft drinks, coffee, tea and other beverages constitute a universal snack. Fruits, vegetables and their juices are also popular in many countries.

In the United States

Americans are among the greatest snackers in the world.[5] Based on a survey of 3 nationally representative samples of 5,500 people in 2000 households, Americans consumed 80 billion snacks in 1986.[6] This snack survey also exhibited considerable age-specific behavior. Young children (age 2–5 years) generated 30% more snack occasions than the population average. Young adults (age 18–24 years) reported the lowest snacking level, with 17% fewer snack occasions than the population average. Flavored chips and low-calorie, low-salt products are among the more successful snack items listed in the survey.

As shown in Table 11.1, total snack sales in the United States in 1987 reached and exceeded the $25 billion mark.[7] This represents a 3-fold increase over the 1978 sales. Of the 17 snack categories listed in Table 11.1, 4 (candies, cookies/crackers, potato chips, and snack cakes/pies) alone account for over ⅔ of the total sales. Many products under these major categories are found in almost all American households, and several of the newly developed ones are targeted for the entire family.

The overall confectionery category (hard candies, chocolate bars, caramels, toffees, etc.) in the United States seems quite healthy, although sales of super-premium chocolates is declining. This is partly due to the increased availability of regional chocolates at a lower cost.

It is easy to relate to solid foods. In contrast, beverages are less readily perceived as snacks, and many beverage items are not consumed as much for any food value they might have as for their thirst quenching and invigorating effects. This is particularly true for soft drinks, a popular snack item because of their unique carbonation, appealing tastes and flavors.

FOODS CONSUMED AS SNACKS

There exists limited current data concerning the nature of snacks eaten.[1] The information available is often limited to assessments of children's and adolescents' eating patterns. Children, ages 9 through 13 years, are reported[8] most likely to consume desserts between meals followed, in descending order, by fruit and milk. For children 3–5 years old, this order includes bakery products, milk, soft drinks, fruits, milk desserts, candy and bread.[9] For 6–11 years old, the snacks, in order of importance, appear to be bakery products, soft drinks, milk desserts, candy, fruits, salty snacks and bread; a different study lists the same snack items but with a different order of preference by children. Teenagers (boys and girls) most preferred soft drinks, bakery products, milk desserts, salty snacks, fruit, milk, candy, bread and meat.

Consumption of soft drinks has risen sharply during the past 2 decades, from about 20 gallons per person in 1968 to an estimated 40 gallons in mid-1980s[10] (Fig. 11.1). In contrast, coffee consumption dropped from more than 36 gallons to 26 gallons in the same period; consumption of tea remained constant at 7 gallons.

SNACKING OCCASIONS

Snacking has truly become the "fourth meal" in the American diet. According to the 1977–78 Nationwide Food Consumption Survey (NFCS), a 3-times-a-day eating pattern was noted for 39% of the individuals studied while 28% reported four, 14% five and 11% six or more eating occasions (Table 11.2).[11] This survey also established that 59–70% of U.S. children and teenagers had at least one snack during the day.[1,11] Adults tended to snack less frequently and the percentage of adults who snacked

TABLE 11.1
SNACK FOOD MARKET (IN MILLIONS OF DOLLARS) 1978-87

Year	Candy	Cookies/ Crackers	Potato Chips	Corn/ Tortilla Chips	Snack Cakes/ Pies	Snack Nut Meats	Frozen Pizza	Imported & MIsc.	Dried Fruit Snacks
1978	N/A	3060	1489	600	774	842	693	108	N/A
1979	N/A	3335	1653	696	851	948	728	113	N/A
1980	4684	3663	1914	840	885	1089	845	112	70
1981	4939	3960	2130	1029	982	980	896	110	85
1982	5300	4197	2289	1132	1000	1088	878	133	175
1983	5625	4449	2430	1214	1000	1099	896	150	250
1984	6150	4938	2514	1246	1110	1121	923	183	326
1985	6683	5234	2651	1283	1220	1160	1000	279	418
1986	7000	5627	2850	1324	1240	1160	1063	606	508
1987	7300	5820	2890	1401	1364	1098	1079	696	587

Source: Snack Food.[7]

decreased with increasing age. In a 1986 survey,[12] 3 of 4 women reported eating snacks on a given day. This is higher than in 1977 when 3 of 5 women reported eating snacks.

CALORIC AND NUTRIENT CONTRIBUTION OF SNACKS

In the 1977–78 NFCS,[11] snacks accounted for an average of 11% of the total energy intake (Table 11.3) and 7–12% of the intake of vitamins and minerals. For those

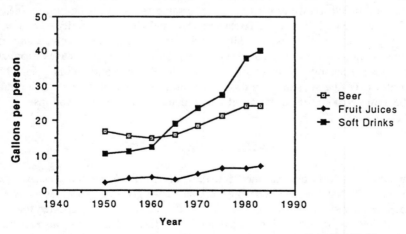

From Pombier[10]

FIG. 11.1. CONSUMPTION OF SOME POPULAR BEVERAGES

Year	Popcorn	Hot Snacks	Extruded Snacks	Meat Snacks	Pretzels	Granola Snacks	Fabricated Chips	Toaster Pastries	TOTALS
1978	99	49	204	197	158	N/A	102	75	8450
1979	111	53	233	214	179	N/A	92	83	9289
1980	135	60	270	233	211	N/A	64	83	15158
1981	153	69	313	254	242	250	85	87	16564
1982	160	72	324	280	248	280	88	94	17738
1983	163	80	334	312	253	350	106	100	18811
1984	176	107	380	345	266	424	121	108	20438
1985	365	456	415	375	271	439	203	168	22620
1986	458	440	467	400	293	359	218	193	24206
1987	554	480	472	424	303	298	262	197	25225

consuming at least one snack in a day, snacks provided 19% of the food energy. They also accounted for 12% of the protein and various percentages of other nutrients. As the number of snacks consumed increased, the amount of energy they contributed also increased. In children, the increased level of snacking made significant contribution to children's intake levels of magnesium and zinc and to adolescents' intake of vitamin B_6, calcium, iron, magnesium and zinc. On days when no snacks were consumed, the meals eaten were not necessarily more nutritious than those meals which included snacks. Based on the data obtained from the *Continuing Survey of Food Intakes by Individuals* in the United States, Weinstock[13] recently compared the percentage of nutrient intake derived from snacks consumed in 1977 and 1985. This comparison, which involved women (19–50 years old) and their children (1–5 years old), showed (Table 11.4) an appreciable increase in 1985 in the intake of both calories and the various nutrients compared.

NUTRIENTS TO ADD OR NOT ADD TO SNACK FOODS

Essential Nutrients

There are 31 nutrients (excluding essential amino acids) that are either known to be essential for man or are presumed to be essential; the essentiality of a few others is being investigated. The Food and Nutrition Board of the National Academy of Sciences[14] has established Recommended Daily Dietary Allowances (RDA) for 19 of these nutrients and indicated approximate and desirable intakes of 12 others. Table 11.5 lists these nutrients. The amounts recommended (not shown) are indicated separately for infants, children, various age groups of men and women, pregnant women, and lactating women.

TABLE 11.2
FREQUENCY OF EATING

Time in a Day	Year	
	1965	1977
One or Two	4	8
Three	32	39
Four	31	28
Five	19	14
Six or More	14	11

Source: Peterkin.[11]

The RDA are the "levels of intake of essential nutrients considered, on the basis of available scientific knowledge, to be adequate to meet the known nutritional needs of practically all healthy Americans."[14] They are not requirements for individuals, but only recommendations. With the exception of allowances for energy, RDAs are estimated to exceed the requirements of most individuals.

Protein, selected amino acids, and minerals and vitamins are the nutrients usually considered for nutrification of foods. Nutritional considerations now also influence the type of fat added to foods. Although not strictly a nutrient, fiber is also being added to a variety of food products, including snacks.

Adding Protein. The RDA for protein for an adult male is set at 63 g;[14] most adults can attain a positive nitrogen balance on 35–40 g dietary protein with protein efficiency ratio (PER) matching or exceeding that of casein. Protein consumption in the United States averages over 100 g/day with about ⅔ originating from animal sources.

From some segment of the population, adding protein to selected snack foods may be justifiable. For example, a breakfast roll was developed in 1972[15] for child nutri-

TABLE 11.3
FOOD ENERGY FROM EATING OCCASIONS[1]
(1977–78 NFCS)

Occasion	All Individuals	Individuals Reporting Occasions
Breakfast	18	21
Lunch	25	32
Dinner	22	45
Supper	22	42
Snack	11	19
Other	2	—

Source: Peterkin.[11]
[1]Values represent percentage of day's intake.

TABLE 11.4
PERCENTAGE OF NUTRIENT INTAKE DERIVED FROM SNACKS

Nutrient	Women 1977	Women 1985	Children 1977	Children 1985
Calories	11	16	13	19
Protein	7	9	8	11
Fat	8	13	11	17
Cholesterol	*	10	*	12
Carbohydrates	15	19	16	22
Dietary Fiber	*	12	*	16
Vitamin A	8	10	9	10
Thiamin	8	11	9	12
Riboflavin	10	13	12	15
Vitamin B_6	7	11	9	12
Vitamin B_{12}	7	10	10	10
Vitamin C	9	12	12	18
Calcium	12	15	13	16
Sodium	*	10	*	11
Iron	8	11	8	11
Zinc	*	11	*	12

Source: Weinstock.[13]
*Data not available.

tion programs. This product was developed to meet precise specifications (PER of 2.5 or more, for example) and contained, besides added vitamins and minerals, soy protein, egg protein and the amino acid lysine. Because disagreement ensued on the merit of recommending a sweet product as a breakfast item, commercial production of this product failed to materialize.

Adding Fats and Oils. According to various estimates, Americans obtain 37–42% of food calories as fat. Excessive fat intake, especially saturated fat, is linked to the development of several important chronic disease conditions, more conclusively coronary heart disease. Americans are advised to limit their calories from fat to no more than 30% and their cholesterol to 300 mg/day.

In an attempt to limit their fat (total and saturated) intake, Americans have been switching to low-fat and reduced-fat foods, and they increasingly choose snacks labeled as made with "100% vegetable shortening or pure vegetable oil."

The term "vegetable oil" may sometimes be misleading.[5] Certain tropical oils—coconut, palm kernel and palm oils—widely used in a variety of snack foods are more highly saturated than even some animal fats (Table 11.6). Saturated fat is strongly linked to elevated blood cholesterol level, a major risk factor in heart disease. It may be added that palm oil, long considered to be hypercholesterolemic in humans, appears less hypercholesterolemic than butter fat and may even inhibit clot formation in animals.[16]

TABLE 11.5
ESSENTIAL NUTRIENTS

| | Nutrients With | |
| | No Established RDA | |
Established RDA	Desirable Intake Proposed	Not Proposed
Protein	Pantothenic Acid	Choline
Calcium	Biotin	Cobalt
Phosphorus	Manganese	
Vitamin A	Fluoride	
Iron	Chromium	
Thiamin	Molybdenum	
Riboflavin	Sodium	
Niacin	Potassium	
Ascorbic Acid	Choride	
Vitamin B_6	Copper	
Vitamin B_{12}		
Vitamin E		
Vitamin K		
Folate		
Iodine		
Magnesium		
Vitamin D		
Zinc		
Selenium		

Source: FNB/NAS.[14]

Tropical oils are used because they function well in food and they are less expensive than unsaturated oils such as soybean, corn, sunflower and peanut oils. The price of all oils does fluctuate, however. This is the reason behind flexi-labeling of foods. This allows a food label to say, for example, "contains one or more of the following oils."

Many food processors have taken note of the health implications of fats/oils used in snacks. A growing number of companies are planning to reduce saturated fat in their food lines by shifting to oils such as canola, cottonseed, soybean and sunflower seed oils. The oil content of some snacks is also being reduced by baking rather than frying the products. Some snack producers are, in fact, launching national campaigns promoting low-fat, cholesterol-free products.

Carbohydrates (Utilizable). According to the 1977 "Dietary Goals" report,[17] Americans obtain 46% of their food calories from carbohydrates, about equally distributed between complex carbohydrates (primarily starches) and simple sugars (naturally occurring and those added to foods). This report recommends that we increase calories from carbohydrates to 58% with ¾ of these originating from complex carbohydrates; several other guideline reports make a similar recommenda-

TABLE 11.6
PERCENTAGE OF FATTY ACIDS IN FATS AND OILS

Type Of Oil in Snacks	Saturated	Mono-unsaturated	Poly-unsaturated
Coconut	86	6	2
Palm Kernel	81	11	2
Beef Tallow	50	42	4
Palm	49	37	9
Cottonseed	26	19	51
Peanut	19	46	30
Sesame Seed	15	40	40
Soybean	15	23	58
Olive	14	72	9
Corn	13	24	59
Safflower	9	12	74
Canola (Low Erucic acid rapeseed)	7	55	33

Source: Anon.[5]
Note: The total percentage of the three types of fats in oil and shortenings does not add up to 100 because these items also contain small amounts of other substances.

tion.[18] Many snack foods are a good source of complex carbohydrates and they are low in simple sugars.

Adding Fiber. As we discover the various health benefits of fiber, and as health conscious Americans strive to include fiber-rich foods in their diet, it affords the snack food processors an opportunity to position their products as sources of fiber. Fruits and vegetable snacks and snacks made with whole grains would be a good source of fiber. Fiber can also be added to such products as cookies, crackers, tortilla chips, fruit snacks, extruded snacks, pretzels, granola bars and several other formulated products.

Fiber is no longer considered a nonessential in our diet. Americans consume 10–15 g of total dietary fiber a day; a doubling of this amount is now recommended by the National Cancer Institute[19] and the Federation of the American Societies for Experimental Biology.[20]

Fiber represents a diverse group of components: cellulose, hemicellulose, pectin, gums, mucilages, lignin and others. These fractions, except lignin, are also complex carbohydrates. In the 1985 report titled "Dietary Guidelines for Americans,"[21] the following advice has been offered about fiber:

> Eating foods high in fiber has been found to reduce symptoms of constipation, diverticulosis, and some types of irritable bowel syndrome; it has been suggested that habitual intake of diets low in fiber may increase the risk of colon cancer.

As outlined in Fig. 11.2,[22] while water-soluble fiber may help normalize elevated blood cholesterol and glucose levels, insoluble fiber may be more useful in the prevention and management of intestinal disorders. Processing may affect the content and the ratio of insoluble and soluble fiber in a food; resistant starch, often formed during processing, is now considered a fiber component.

Adding Vitamins and Minerals. Nutrification of snack foods primarily focuses on vitamins and minerals identified to be deficient in our food supply but may also include other nutrients. Sodium, an essential nutrient, presents a different picture.

Many of us consume sodium well in excess of our need. For hypertensive (having high blood pressure) individuals who are also sensitive to sodium, a reduction in

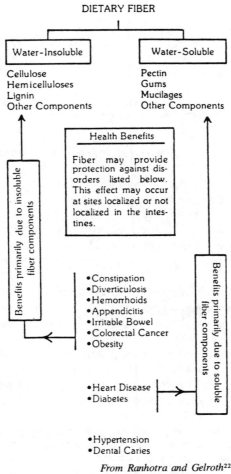

From Ranhotra and Gelroth[22]
FIG. 11.2. CLASSIFICATION AND HEALTH BENEFITS OF FIBER

TABLE 11.7
SODIUM IN FROZEN PIZZA
(Weight = 100 g)

Pizza Type	Sodium in Pizza (mg)			
	Crust	Cheese and Sauce	Topping	Total
Cheese	302 ± 25	222 ± 53	—	524 ± 72
Hamburger	293 ± 37	204 ± 55	114 ± 21	611 ± 70
Bacon	308 ± 24	262 ± 50	110 ± 34	679 ± 104
Pepperoni	357 ± 32	221 ± 18	164 ± 39	742 ± 52
Combination	290 ± 27	187 ± 75	132 ± 35	609 ± 47

Source: Ranhotra et al.[23]

sodium intake is now widely recommended as an effective approach to control hypertension.

About 3 g of sodium (expressed as salt) is usually adequate for most Americans. We consume 2–3 times more, with ⅓ (or more) of this intake originating from processed foods alone; processed foods use some 70 different sodium-containing ingredients.

Many snack foods tend to be high in sodium. Table 11.7 shows the sodium content of a few popular types of commercially produced frozen pizzas.[23] It is obvious that this snack food is high in sodium. However, several low-sodium and reduced sodium (salt) snacks are now being added to the numerous choices of low-salt snacks available from major snack processors. There is an eager market waiting for sodium-reduced snacks. It is well to remember that saltiness is an acquired taste and given sufficient exposure to low-salt and reduced salt snacks the consumer is likely to develop a liking for them. Spices are also a natural for flavor enhancement when salt is reduced and the sodium content of added spices is often negligible. Table 11.8 lists the various spices the snack producers can use.

Several snack food items carry a nutrition label (discussed later); listing of sodium information, as part of the nutrition label, is now mandatory. Foods can also be labeled to just provide sodium information. Table 11.9 lists the terminologies the manufacturer can use to convey sodium information.

In contrast to the health implications of excessive sodium, potassium may help lower blood pressure.[24] Thus, adding potassium to selected snack foods may add to consumer appeal.

High Intensity Sweeteners and Fat Substitutes. For individuals on restricted diets and those wishing to limit their caloric intake, snack foods are being reformulated to be low in calories, fat, saturated fat, cholesterol and high in noncaloric bulk. For this purpose, a variety of high intensity sweeteners (including heat stable ones), fat substitutes and bulking agents are either currently being marketed or in-

TABLE 11.8
THE SALT-REDUCED SNACK FOODS SPICE CHART

Crackers & Wafers
  Sesame seed
  Poppy seed
  Caraway seed
  Freeze-dried chives
  Onion powder
  Garlic powder
  Thyme
  Mixed vegetable flakes
  Chili powder (salt-free)
  (Individually or mixtures
     of above)

Graham Crackers
  Cinnamon
  Nutmeg and allspice
  Ginger and cinnamon

Rusks and Toasts
  Anise
  Cinnamon
  Clove and ginger

Cookies
  Cinnamon
  Cloves
  Nutmeg
  Allspice
  (Individually or mixtures
     or above)
  Anise seed
  Ginger and mustard
  Poppy seed
  Sesame seed

Snack Pies
  Apple-cinnamon, nutmeg
  Peach-cinnamon, allspice
  Cherry, nutmeg
  Berry, nutmeg, cinnamon

Snack Cakes
(including doughnuts)
  Cinnamon
  Cloves
  Nutmeg
  Allspice
  (Individually or a
     mixture of above)

Candy
  Cinnamon
  Nutmeg
  Cloves
  Allspice
  Sesame seed
  Poppy seed
  Ginger

Potato Chips
  Chili powder
  Ground black pepper
  Onion powder
  Garlic powder
  Herb blend (oregano,
     basil and garlic powder)
  Ginger

Pretzels
  Black pepper
  Onion powder
  Garlic powder
  Sesame seed
  Caraway seed
  Chili powder

Cheese Curls
  Chili powder
  Curry powder
  Onion powder
  Caraway seed
  Sesame seed
  Freeze-dried chives

Popcorn
  Oregano and garlic powder
  Chili powder and cumin
  Thyme and basil
  Caraway and mustard
  Black and red peppers

Granola-type Bars
  Cinnamon
  Ginger and sesame seed
  Nutmeg and cloves

Pizzas
  Oregano
  Basil
  Crushed red pepper
  Cumin
  Thyme
  Onion powder
  Garlic powder

Nuts
  Cinnamon
  Chili powder
  Curry powder
  Apple pie spice

Onion Rings
  Onion powder
  Garlic powder
  White pepper

Corn Chips
  Onion powder
  Garlic Powder
  Chili powder
  Curry powder
  Black pepper

TABLE 11.9
SODIUM LABELING OF FOODS

Label	Sodium Content
Sodium Free	Less than 5 mg per serving
Very Low Sodium	35 mg or less per serving
Low Sodium	140 mg or less per serving
Reduced Sodium	Reduction of the usual level by 75%
Unsalted, No Salt Added, Without Added Salt	Processed without the normally used salt

tensely being developed. It is estimated that close to 100 million Americans regularly buy low-calorie foods and beverages, twice as many as in the 1970s.

Caffeine. Because of its widespread use, concern is frequently expressed over undesirable health effects of long-term use of caffeine. Caffeine is found in many snack food items containing cocoa and chocolate, but beverages (Table 11.10) are the main source of caffeine in the American diet.[25] Like sodium, restricted use of ingredients containing caffeine is likely to appeal to many who enjoy snacks but wish to limit caffeine intake.

ADDING NUTRIENTS TO SNACKS

Food consumption and health survey studies have shown that fortifying widely consumed foods with synthetic (pure) nutrients is one of the most effective means of correcting nutritional inadequacies in the population.[26] For example, cereal enrichment with niacin was followed by a continued decline in deaths from pellagra;[27] the addition of two other vitamins (thiamin and riboflavin) in the cereal enrichment action in the 1940s was equally effective in correcting dietary inadequacies of these nutrients. The addition of iron to grain products also helped markedly reduce the incidence of iron-deficiency anemia. Goiter in the U.S. population was practically eliminated by iodizing common salt in the 1930s. Vitamin D was added to milk about the same time to help prevent rickets. Vitamin A is now routinely added to vegetable-fat spreads to guard against the deficiency of this critical nutrient.

Vitamin/mineral supplements can also correct nutritional deficiencies. Supplement usage is usually not recommended, however, except under well-defined need situations such as excessive menstrual bleeding, pregnancy, breastfeeding, inadequate energy intakes (e.g., weight reducing diets) and a food intake pattern which excludes animal-derived products.

Nutrition education can also ensure nutritional adequacy of the diet. Although educational efforts often prove to be a slow process, some[28] feel that an educational approach offers more potential at less cost than does fortification or any other form of food modification.

TABLE 11.10
CAFFEINE CONTENT OF SOME BEVERAGES

Beverage	Caffeine (mg)
Coffee (5 oz. cup)	
Drip	110–150
Percolated	64–124
Instant	40–108
Decaffeinated	2–5
Tea (5 oz. cup)	
1-Minute brew	9–33
2-Minute brew	20–46
5-Minute brew	20–50
Instant	12–28
Chocolate Drinks	
Hot Cocoa (6 oz.)	2–8
Chocolate Milk (8 oz.	2–7
Soft Drinks (12 oz.)	
Jolt	72.0
Mountain Dew	54.0
TAB	46.8
Coca-Cola	45.6
Diet Coke	45.6
Mr. PIBB	40.8
Dr. Pepper	39.6
Sugar-Free Dr. Pepper	39.6
Pepsi-Cola	38.4
Diet Pepsi	36.0
Pepsi Light	36.0
RC Cola	36.0
Canada Dry Jamaica Cola	30.0
Canada Dry Diet Cola	1.2

Source: IFT-EPFSN.[25]

In the 1960s, the Food and Drug Administration (FDA) prohibited adding nutrients to most snack foods, since they do not have, unlike foods such as bread and pasta, established standards of identity, and they also fail to meet certain other criteria. Even in the current FDA recommendations on fortification,[29] snack foods are not included; FDA policy continues to favor fortification of dietary staples rather than snacks.

This concern, on FDA's part, may be misplaced. Many snacks, no doubt, have low nutrient density, but the potential problem of nutrient inadequacies arises only when snack foods are predominantly included in one's diet at the exclusion of foods high in nutrient density. It is well to recognize, also, that snacks provide a sizable portion of energy in the diets of the individuals consuming one or more snacks in a day.

Not all snacks need be fully fortified. First, where the need exists primarily for extra energy (as for physically active individuals), foods with low nutrient density may be the right choice and they may not be unduly fortified. Second, the food industry needs to look at not only the effect of their own products on the health of the American people, but to collectively consider the entire pattern of the nutrients in the food supply before making decisions to fortify foods.[30]

Thus, deemphasizing overfortification and reflecting upon the role of snacks which may be primarily a source of energy, most snack foods can be fortified to ensure good nutrition for all segments of the U.S. population. Fortification benefits the consumer.

The following criteria should be reviewed before deciding on nutrification; when most, if not all, of these can be satisfied, nutrification of snack foods may be considered seriously.

(1) The intake of nutrients in the absence of fortification, is below a desirable intake (usually 70% of the RDA) of a significant number of people.
(2) The food from which the nutrient is to be derived is likely to be consumed in quantities that will make a significant contribution to the diet of the population in need. More than one food carrier can be chosen.
(3) The addition of nutrient is unlikely to create an imbalance of essential nutrients.
(4) There is reasonable assurance that the intake of a nutrient will not be excessive enough to become toxic.
(5) The nutrient which may justifiably be added to snack foods is stable under most storage and usage conditions.
(6) The nutrient added is physiologically available for the food.
(7) The cost of nutrification is reasonable.

Nutrient Intakes and Deficiencies

Mean nutrient intake somewhat below the RDA does not mean existence of malnutrition. The risk of some individuals having inadequate intakes increases as the mean intake of a nutrient falls well below 70% of the RDA. Table 11.11 lists the percentage distribution of 37,785 individuals with nutrient intakes at specified levels of 1980 RDA;[31] it is obvious that several nutrients can be identified as problem nutrients in the United States. The continued deficiency of these (and other) nutrients in our food supply was reaffirmed in women and children in a NFCS reported in 1986.[12] Table 11.12 shows the magnitude of these inadequacies.

Choice of Foods to Nutrify

According to the NFCS,[11,12] a majority of the Americans consume one or more snacks in a day (Table 11.2). These eating occasions may provide about 1/5 of our

TABLE 11.11
PERCENTAGE DISTRIBUTION OF INDIVIDUALS WITH NUTRIENT INTAKES AT SPECIFIED LEVELS OF RDA

	% of Individuals Receiving		
Nutrient	100% and Over of RDA	70–99% of RDA	Less than 70% of RDA
Energy	24	44	32
Protein	88	9	3
Calcium	32	26	42
Iron	43	25	32
Magnesium	25	36	39
Phosphorus	73	19	8
Vitamin A	50	19	31
Thiamin	55	28	17
Riboflavin	66	22	12
Niacin	67	24	9
Vitamin B_6	20	29	51
Vitamin B_{12}	66	19	15
Vitamin C	59	15	26

Source: Pao and Mickle. Based on 1977–78 NFCS.

caloric need. Snacks are not staple foods such as bread, rice, tortillas, pastas, but their caloric contribution is sizable. By exercising prudent judgment to not indiscriminately fortify all snacks, many snack foods can be nutrified to correct nutritional inadequacies.

Nutrient Toxicity

Vitamin and mineral toxicity is a distinct possibility where nutrient intakes well exceeds the RDA. Undesirable effects, trivial to major, have been reported with the use of excessively high doses of vitamin and mineral supplements. However, the mineral/vitamin safety index shown in Table 11.13 underscores a high margin of safety for most minerals and vitamins.[32] Selective fortification of snack foods is, thus, unlikely to lead to a situation of toxicity where proper nutrification practices are followed.

Nutrient Stability

The virtual elimination of deficiency diseases among the U.S. population is a remarkable testimonial to the effectiveness of adding nutrients to foods. Most of

TABLE 11.12
MEAN INTAKES OF NUTRIENTS BELOW THE RDA
(19–50 Years Women)

	Vitamins			Minerals			
	B_6	Folacin	E	Calcium	Magnesium	Zinc	Iron
19–34 years old	63	52	90	82	71	62	61
35–50 years old	61	52	92	75	73	59	58
All Women	62	52	91	79	72	60	60

Source: NMD-HNIS.[12]

these nutrients are reasonably stable under conditions of processing and food usage. Mineral elements are relatively more stable than vitamins. Water-soluble vitamins, e.g., vitamin C, thiamin and riboflavin, may be subject to loss during processing, as are several essential amino acids. Table 11.14 summarizes the stability characteristics of a number of nutrients.[33] Where loss occurred during processing, its magnitude often varies. In a study where cookies were made with enriched flour, ¾ of the thiamin was found to be lost during processing;[34] thiamin is quite unstable in neutral or alkaline pH media. For most nutrients, losses, when occuring, are usually of a lesser magnitude, however (Table 11.14). Furthermore, some stabilized and coated nutrients have extended usage under unfavorable or stressful situations.

Physiological Availability of Nutrients

The mere addition of a nutrient, which is poorly available or unavailable physiologically, to a food may meet label requirement but would defeat the very purpose of nutrification. Fortunately, nutrients that have traditionally been added to foods are well absorbed and utilized. Depending on the processing conditions and the presence of promoters and inhibitors (of nutrient absorption) in a food or a meal, biological availability of a nutrient added to a food may change somewhat, but a drastic change usually does not occur. For example, the addition of soy protein to zinc-fortified cookies resulted in only a small, less than ¼, reduction in the biological value of zinc.[35]

Cost of Nutrification

The ingredient cost to fortify foods at appropriate levels typically adds only a fraction of a cent to the cost of the food. As shown in Table 11.15, 12 vitamins added to a food to provide 100% of the USRDA cost about ½ cent; if a few selected minerals are also included, the cost may still be below 1 cent.

TABLE 11.13
MINERAL AND VITAMIN SAFETY INDEX

Mineral	Recommended Adult Intake[1]	Minimum Toxic Dose	Safety Index
Calcium	1,200 mg	12,000 mg	10
Phosphorus	1,200 mg	12,000 mg	10
Magnesium	400 mg	6,000 mg	15
Iron	18 mg	100 mg	5.5
Zinc	15 mg	500 mg	33
Copper	3 mg	100 mg	33
		<3 mg[2]	<1
Fluoride	4 mg	20 mg	5
		4 mg[3]	1
Iodine	0.15 mcg	2 mg	13
Selenium	0.2 mcg	1 mg	5
Vitamin A	5,000 IU	25,000 to 50,000 IU	5 to 10
Vitamin D	400 IU	50,000 IU	125
		1,000 to 2,000 IU[4]	2.5 to 5
Vitamin E	30 IU	1,200 IU	40
Vitamin C	60 mg	2,000 to 5,000 mg	33 to 83
		1,000 mg[5]	17
Thiamin (B_1)	1.5 mg	300 mg	200
Riboflavin	1.7 mg	1,000 mg	588
Niacin	20 mg	1,000 mg	50
Pyridoxine (B_6)	2.2 mg	2,000 mg	900
		200 mg[6]	90
Folacin	0.4 mg	400 mg	1,000
		15 mg[7]	37
Biotin	0.3 mg	50 mg	167
Pantothenic acid	10 mg	10,000 mg	1,000

Source: Hathcock.[32]
[1]The highest of RDA (except those for pregnancy and lactation) or the USRDA, whichever is higher.
[2]For those with Wilson's disease.
[3]Level producing slight fluorosis of dental enamel.
[4]For infants and also for certain adults with certain infections or metabolic diseases.
[5]To produce slightly altered mineral excretion patterns.
[6]For antagonism of certain drugs; 2000 mg for most adults.
[7]For antagonism of anticonvulsants in epileptics; 400 mg for most adults.

ADDING NUTRIENTS TO CONFECTIONERIES

Candies and other confections are popular snack foods for young and old alike. They are eaten primarily for enjoyment rather than for nutrition. While hard candies chiefly consist of carbohydrates and, thus, contain very few nutrients, soft confections contain a variety of ingredients (milk solids, chocolate, nuts, enriched flour, fruits, etc.), which do provide nutrients.

TABLE 11.14
STABILITY OF NUTRIENTS

Nutrient	Effect of pH			Air or Oxygen	Light	Heat	Maximum Cooking Losses (%)
	Neutral pH 7	Acid < pH 7	Alkaline > pH 7				
Vitamins							
Vitamin A	S	U	S	U	U	U	40
Ascorbic acid (C)	U	S	U	U	U	U	100
Biotin	S	S	S	S	S	U	60
Carotene (pro-A)	S	U	S	U	U	U	30
Choline	S	S	S	U	S	S	5
Cobalamin (B_{12})	S	S	S	U	U	S	10
Vitamin D	S			U	U	U	U	40
Folic acid	U	U	S	U	U	U	100
Inositol	S	S	S	S	S	U	95
Vitamin K	S	U	U	S	U	S	5
Niacin	S	S	S	S	S	S	75
Pantothenic acid	S	U	U	S	S	U	50
p-Aminobenzoic acid	S	S	S	U	S	S	5
Pyridoxine (B_6)	S	S	S	S	U	U	40
Riboflavin (B_2)	S	S	U	S	U	U	75
Thiamin (B_1)	U	S	U	U	S	U	80
Tocopherol (E)	S	S	S	U	U	U	55
Essential amino acids							
Isoleucine	S	S	S	S	S	S	10
Leucine	S	S	S	S	S	S	10
Lysine	S	S	S	S	S	U	40
Methionine	S	S	S	S	S	S	10
Phenylalanine	S	S	S	S	S	S	5
Threonine	S	U	U	S	S	U	20
Tryptophan	S	U	S	S	U	S	15
Valine	S	S	S	S	S	S	10
Essential fatty acids	S	S	U	U	U	S	10
Mineral salts	S	S	S	S	S	S	3

Source: Harris.[33]
S: Stable (no important destruction).
U: Unstable (significant destruction).

In the not too distant past, specialty candies such as "high-protein bars" were produced utilizing a variety of protein sources, such as nonfat dry milk, casein mixtures, soy protein isolates and cottonseed. The protein source is added last to avoid the detrimental effect on the biological quality of protein that occurs when protein is cooked (Maillard reaction) with sugar. Vitamins and minerals were also added to a variety of confections. The goal of these various projects was to develop candies that would be nutritionally balanced.[36] The nutrification step was also aimed

TABLE 11.15
COST OF VITAMIN FORTIFICATION
(100% U.S. RDA)

Nutrient	USRDA	Approximate Cost (dollar)[1]
Vitamin A	5000 IU	0.00071
Vitamin D	400 IU	0.00009
Vitamin E	30 IU	0.00099
Vitamin C	60 mg	0.00080
Thiamin	1.5 mg	0.00006
Riboflavin	1.7 mg	0.00010
Vitamin B_6	2.0 mg	0.00010
Vitamin B_{12}	6.0 mcg	0.00010
Niacin	20 mg	0.00016
Folic acid	0.4 mg	0.00005
Pantothenic acid (as calcium salt)	10 mg	0.00018
Biotin	0.3 mg	0.00180
		0.0051

[1]Approximate cost of bulk ingredients as of 10/90; total food nutrification costs includes charges in premix preparation, for nutrient losses in the food during manufacturing and projected shelf storage, quality control and laboratory assays.

to increase the options available to the consumers, particularly those in the vulnerable group, for improving their diet nutritionally.

Although some confectionery products are still being fortified with protein and pure vitamins and minerals, the intensity of purpose for the confectionery industry to develop such products has greatly diminished, influenced in part by the debate on the merit of nutrifying confections.

NUTRITIONAL PROFILE AND CONTRIBUTION OF SNACK FOODS

Individuals reporting snacking occasions in 1977–78 NFCS[11] obtained about 1/5 of their energy from snacks (Table 11.3). Although one cannot always base consumption trends on data obtained from surveys conducted several years ago, indications are that caloric intake from snacking occasions may even be higher today than it was in the 1970s.

With the exception of some beverages and confectionery items, such as candies and sugar wafers, snack foods also contribute some nutrients to our diet. This contribution is best assessed comparing nutritional profiles of snacks against our nutrient needs. RDA[14] provides a meaningful measure of this need, but USRDA (Table 11.16), now widely used for nutrition labeling of foods, may be an even better standard of reference.

TABLE 11.16
U.S. RECOMMENDED DAILY ALLOWANCE (USRDA)

Nutrient	Adults and Children Over 4 Years
Protein	65 g[1]
Vitamin A	5,000 IU
Vitamin C	60 mg
Thiamin	1.5 mg
Riboflavin	1.7 mg
Niacin	20 mg
Calcium	1.0 g
Iron	18 mg
Vitamin D	400 IU
Vitamin E	30 IU
Vitamin B_6	2.0 mg
Folate	0.4 mg
Vitamin B_{12}	6 mcg
Phosphorus	1.0 g
Iodine	150 mcg
Magnesium	400 mg
Zinc	15 mg
Copper	2 mg
Biotin	0.3 mg
Pantothenic acid	10 mg

Source: NNC.[37]

[1]If protein efficiency ratio of protein is equal to or better than that of casein, USRDA is 45 g for adults and pregnant or lactating women, 20 g for children under 4 years of age and 18 g for infants.

Nutrition Labeling

Started in 1973, nutrition labeling of foods is aimed to "devise a set of standards upon which the individual could base the choice of what to eat." Nutrition labeling of foods is essentially voluntary, except when adding a nutrient to fortify a food or when making nutritional claims (on the label or in advertising) about a food. The FDA suggests that manufacturers conduct numerous tests on their products in order to list the correct nutrition information. The nutritional values of labeled foods, including snacks, are required to fall within a 20% range of what is stated on the package. The snack food industry enjoys a good reputation with the FDA for providing accurate information on nutrition labels.

Over 50% of the packaged foods commercially produced in the United States now carry a nutrition label; this percentage is likely to increase. To provide information in a clear and concise manner, the form, language and position of the label must meet rigid standards. To base claims of nutritional contribution made by a food, a new set of standards labeled USRDA evolved.[37] These standards, developed by the FDA, can be used for labeling both the general food supply and dietary supplement and special dietary foods. They are based on the RDA.[14] Although USRDA are listed separately for adults and children, children under 4 years, infants, and pregnant and lactating women, only the first mentioned set (Table 11.16) is widely used. In this set, the USRDA for protein is 45 g if the PER of protein in the product evaluated is equal to or greater than that of casein, and 65 g if the PER is less than that of casein. Protein with a PER less than 20% of that of the casein may not be stated on the label in terms of a percentage of the USRDA. All labels must list the first eight nutrients shown in Table 11.15 even if some of these are quite low or missing in a food.

Every nutrition label must show certain information. This includes (1) serving size (portion) and the number of servings per package, (2) the amounts of energy, protein, fat, carbohydrates (in grams), and sodium (in mg) furnished by a serving, and (3) the percentage of the USRDA for the first eight nutrients listed in Table 11.1 furnished in a serving. Additional information may include (1) the percentage of the USRDA for one or more of the other 12 nutrients (Table 11.15), (2) the percentage of calories that comes from fat and the amounts of polyunsaturated fat and saturated fat, (3) the amounts of dietary fiber, and (4) information for a serving of the food cooked or prepared in combination with other foods according to the directions given on the label.[38] New FDA regulations require that when manufacturers choose to include information on cholesterol, then they must provide complete nutrition label and state the amount of cholesterol (mg/serving) as well as of fatty acids (polyunsaturated and saturated).

Nutritional Contribution

All foods we enjoy, including snack foods, belong in diet when consumed in moderation. Snack foods, however, do not in all instances measure up to dietary staples in their nutritional profile. Many do provide several nutrients. Table 11.17 underscores this point. Such a table can be expanded to include many more snack foods to focus on their present nutritional contribution to our daily diet and where nutrients may be added to make them better foods.

Nutritional Contribution Through Nutrification

Snacking is a common practice with most Americans. Some snacks contribute nutrients because those nutrients occur naturally; others provide a good portion because nutrients are added. For example, most grain-based snacks use enriched flour; Table 11.18 shows the contribution of this enrichment toward nutrient intake in the U.S. diet.[39] As for other nutrients, vitamin D added to foods, with or without standards of identity, was found to be virtually the exclusive source in the diet of 162 women who were generally at low risk for nutrient deficiency,[40] and margarines now contribute a major portion of vitamin A in our diet.

TABLE 11.17
NUTRITIONAL CONTRIBUTION OF SELECTED SNACK FOODS
(% USRDA)

	Danish	Chocolate Chip Cookie	Cake Donut	Saltines	Cheese Crackers	Plain Yogurt (Skim Milk)	Carrots (raw)	Potato Chips	Apple (raw)	Banana	Beverage (Cola)	Orange Juice	Chocolate Candy
Serving Size (g)	65	40	42	14	14	245	110	20	150	175	247	248	28
Calories (Kcal)	270	210	160	60	80	120	45	110	80	100	90	110	150
Protein	8	4	2	2	2	20	2	2	*	2	*	2	4
Vitamin A	4	*	*	*	*	4	240	*	2	4	*	10	2
Vitamin C	*	*	*	*	*	4	15	4	10	20	*	180	*
Thiamin	4	4	6	6	6	6	4	2	2	4	*	15	2
Riboflavin	6	4	6	4	4	25	2	*	2	4	*	4	6
Niacin	2	4	4	4	4	*	4	4	*	4	*	4	*
Calcium	4	2	2	2	2	30	4	*	*	*	*	2	6
Iron	4	4	4	4	2	*	4	2	2	4	*	2	2

Source: Peterkin et al.[38]
Asterisk indicates none or less than 2% of the USRDA. Some grain produced used enriched flour.

TABLE 11.18
CONTRIBUTION OF CEREAL FORTIFICATION TOWARDS NUTRIENT INTAKE

Nutrient	Total Contribution From Cereal Foods (%)	Contribution Through Fortification (% of Total)
Thiamin	42	71
Riboflavin	28	64
Niacin	30	63
Iron	33	55

Source: Cook and Welsh.[39]

In contrast to most solid foods, carbonated beverages are primarily a source of energy. The use of soft drinks has increased greatly during the past 15 years with a parallel decrease occurring in milk consumption.[41,42] Based on the 1977–78 NFCS,[11] it was found that soft drinks and milk intakes were negatively correlated ($r = -0.22$). In examining the correlation of soft drinks intake with intake of energy and 14 nutrients, a negative correlation was found with calcium (-0.11), magnesium (-0.06), riboflavin (-0.09), vitamin A (-0.08) and ascorbic acid (-0.06). This indicates that soft drinks would contribute to a low intake of these nutrients, especially for the teenagers who seem to have substituted soft drinks for milk at meals.

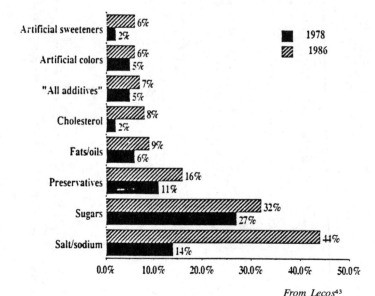

From Lecos[43]

FIG. 11.3. FOOD INGREDIENTS WHICH WERE "AVOIDED" OR LIMITED BY CONSUMERS MORE IN 1986 THAN IN 1978 WITH THE AID OF NUTRITION INFORMATION ON PACKAGING

Some soft drinks are now fortified with fruit juices. At the level used, sometimes as little as 10%, added juices do not make these beverages a nutritious product, but they do add some nutrients. Some thirst quenchers are heavily fortified with minerals as a replacement for losses during physical activity. The nutritional significance of this is, however, debated. Calcium, a critical nutrient in the U.S. diet, is being added to juices, soft drinks, and even milk. With many health professionals, this also remains a controversial issue as the evidence that a high-calcium diet can prevent osteoporosis is far from conclusive. Some soft drinks have been fortified with protein sources such as isolated soy protein but have not gained popularity. Protein is not limiting in the U.S. diet, but it can be a consideration for some technologically developing countries.

FUTURE TRENDS

Americans have been the target of a growing amount of information during the past 10 years about how the foods they eat, or do not eat, may reduce the risk of major killer diseases especially heart disease, cancer and high blood pressure. This educational outpouring is partly a result of the efforts of various government agencies and health organizations[15] and the wide coverage they have received in the mass media.[43] Food industry messages on such dietary links as fiber and cancer, calcium and osteoporosis, and sodium and hypertension have also heightened public awareness of healthy eating. This awareness may become further enhanced if FDA's proposed regulations allowing health messages take a firm hold.

In view of these rapid developments, public perception of formulated snack foods may require some dramatic changes by the industry for snack foods to achieve a realistic health perception by the consumer. Figure 11.3 provides a guideline snack food processors can use when reformulating or developing snack foods—being mindful, of course, that consumers often ignore nutrition information on the food package and pay more attention to unit pricing and product dating and to the eating characteristics ingrained in their psyches.

REFERENCES

1. MORGAN, K. J. 1982. The role of snacking in the American diet. Cont. Nutr. 7(9), 1–2.
2. EZELL, J. M., SKINNER, J. D. and PENFIELD, M. P. 1985. Appalachian adolescents' snack patterns: Morning, afternoon and evening snacks. J. Am. Diet. Assoc. 85(11), 1450–1454.
3. CRAFT, C. B. 1986. Snack sales grow around the world. Chipper/Snacker (Snack World Now) 43(9), 24–26.
4. LEVY, B. 1987. Snack markets around the world. Snack World 44(11), 30–32.

5. ANON. 1987. Beware of snacks made with pure vegetable oil. Tufts Univ. Diet Nutr. Let. 5(3), 1–2.
6. MRCA's Consumer Information Service. 1988. Age determines snack consumption. Food Eng. 60(2), 23.
7. EDITORS. 1988. $25.2 billion snack market ripe for future challenges. Snack Food. Jun, M2–M40.
8. VANBUREN, J. B. 1981. Food intake assessment of elementary children. Thesis, Iowa State University, Ames.
9. PAO, E. M. 1981. Eating patterns and food frequencies in children in the United States. In Food, Nutrition and Dental Health, J. J. Hefferen, W. A. Ayer and H. M. Koehler (eds.). Fourth Annual Conference, Am. Dental Assoc. Health Found. (Vol. 3), Chicago.
10. POMBIER, J. 1988. Beverages—the thirst for knowledge. Hazelton Food Sci. Newslet. 25 (Mar./Apr.), 1–5.
11. PETERKIN, B. B. 1980. Nationwide Food Consumption Survey, 1977–78. Presented at the West. Hemisphere Nutr. Congr. VI, Aug. 11, Los Angeles.
12. NMD-HNIS. 1987. Nationwide Food Consumption Survey. Continuing survey of food intake by individuals—1986. Nutrition Monitoring Division, Human Nutrition Information Service (USDA). Nutr. Today 22(5), 36–39.
13. WEINSTOCK, C. P. 1989. The grazing of America: a guide to healthy snacking. FDA Consumer 23(2), 8–13.
14. FNB/NAS. 1989. Recommended Dietary Allowances, 10th Ed. Food and Nutrition Board, National Academy of Sciences, Washington, DC.
15. AIB. 1972. Breakfast rolls. Am. Inst. Baking, Bull. 160.
16. ANON. 1987. New findings on palm oil. Nutr. Rev. 45(7), 205–207.
17. UNITED STATES SENATE. 1977. Select Committee on Nutritionand Human Needs—Dietary Goals for the United States. Washington, DC.
18. RANHOTRA, G. 1985. Dietary Recommendations: 1977–1985. Tech. Bull., Am. Inst. Baking 7(8), 1–4.
19. NCI. 1984. Cancer Prevention. U.S. Department of Health and Human Services, National Institutes of Health-National Cancer Institute, Bethesda, MD.
20. PILCH, S. M. 1987. Physiological effects and health consequences of dietary fiber. LSRO-Federation of American Societies for Experimental Biology, Bethesda, MD.
21. USDA/USDHHS. 1985. Guidelines for Americans, 2nd Ed. Home and Garden Bull. 232, USDA and U.S. Dept. Health and Human Services, Washington, DC.
22. RANHOTRA, G. and GELROTH, J. 1985. Dietary fiber. Tech. Bull., Am. Inst. Baking 7(10), 1–4.
23. RANHOTRA, G. S., VETTER, J. L., GELROTH, J. A. and NOVAK, F. A. 1983. Sodium in commercially produced frozen pizza. Cereal Chem. 60(4), 325–326.
24. TOBIAN, L. 1988. Potassium and hypertension. Nutr. Rev. 46(8), 273–276.
25. IFT-EPFSN. 1987. Evaluation of caffeine safety. Inst. Food Technol., Expert Panel on Food Safety and Nutr. Food Technol. 41(6), 105–113.
26. LACHANCE, P. A. 1986. The cereal-grain fortification gap. Roche Public Iss. Repts., Hoffmann-La Roche, Nutley, NJ.
27. MILLER, D. F. 1977. Cereal enrichment/pellagra—USA. . . . In perspective. Cereal Foods World 22(9), 458.
28. DYMSZA, H. A. 1974. Nutrition improvement debate: Supplementation of foods vs. nutrition education. Food Technol. 28(7), 55–56.

29. ANON. 1980. Guidelines for addition of nutrients to foods: Addition of nutrients. Fed. Reg. *45*(18), Jan. 25.
30. MILLER, S. A. 1987. Food fortification "horse race" seen as potential public health risk. Food Chem. News *28*(48), 52–53.
31. PAO, E. M. and MICKLE, S. J. 1981. Problem nutrients in the United States. Food Technol. *36*(9), 58–69, 79.
32. HATHCOCK, J. N. 1985. Quantitative evaluation of vitamin safety. Pharm. Times *52*(5), 104–113.
33. HARRIS, R. S. 1988. General discussion on the stability of nutrients. *In* Nutritional Evaluation of Food Processing, 3rd Ed., E. Karmes and R. S. Harris (eds.). AVI/Van Nostrand Reinhold, New York.
34. RANHOTRA, G. S. and GELROTH, J. A. 1986. Stability of enrichment vitamins in bread and cookies. Cereal Chem. *63*(5), 401–403.
35. RANHOTRA, G. S., LEE, C. and GELROTH, J. A. 1979. Bioavailability of zinc in cookies fortified with soy and zinc. Cereal Chem. *56*(6), 552–554.
36. FRANKE, I. 1988. Confectionery manufacture: New technologies using starch as gelling agent, aerated compounds, cracknel and new confectioneries using vitamins and proteins. Food Mark. Technol., Sept., 30–34.
37. NNC. 1975. Nutrition Labeling: How It Can Work For You. Natl. Nutr. Consortium, Bethesda, MD.
38. PETERKIN, B., NICHOLS, J. and CROMWELL, C. 1975. Nutrition Labeling: Tools For Its Use. Agr. Inf. Bull. 382, USDA, Washington, DC.
39. COOK, D. A. and WELSH, S. O. 1987. The effect of enriched and fortified grain products on nutrient intake. Cereal Foods World *32*(2), 191–196.
40. SUBER, A. M. and BOWERING, J. 1988. The contribution of enrichment and fortification to nutrient intake of women. J. Am. Diet. Assoc. *88*(10), 1237–1242, 1245.
41. MORGAN, K. J., STUTTS, V. J. and STAMPLEY, G. L. 1985. Consumption patterns of the U.S. population. J. Am. Diet. Assoc. *85*(3), 352–354.
42. GUENTHER, T. M. 1986. Beverages in the diets of American teenagers. J. Am. Diet. Assoc. *86*(4), 493–499.
43. LECOS, C. 1988. We are getting the message about diet-disease link. FDA Consumer *22*(4), 6–9.

CHAPTER 12

Foods Considered for Nutrient Addition: CONDIMENTS

J. CHRISTOPHER BAUERNFEIND, Ph.D.

INTRODUCTION

In order to carry out a successful food nutrification program for a population in a given geographical area, one or more centrally processed food ingredients regularly and widely consumed must be part of the diet of the respective targeted population. There are many parts of the world where no centralized food processing exists or, if it does exist, the resulting processed food is not universally consumed by the population under study. However, a household survey of the region might reveal regularly purchased and consumed items, or a dietary accessory ingredient[1] such as a seasoning, flavoring or sweetening agent which conceivably could serve as a carrier or vehicle to which nutrients could be added at the point of origin of the item or at some distribution stage before consumption.[1]

MSG

One condiment receiving favorable attention in several countries as a potential nutrient carrier is the water-soluble substance, monosodium-L-glutamate hydrate (MSG). MSG[2] as a flavor or taste enhancer has had a long history of use in foods, first in the form of seaweed extractive and, later, with the 1908 discovery of its enhancing properties, as a pure salt. Some investigators have even concluded on the basis of physiological data that the taste of MSG and related chemical structures is independent of the four basic tastes (bitter, salty, sour and sweet) and have labeled the new basic taste, "umani."[2,3] MSG is used in a variety of meat, poultry and vegetable dishes, in pure form or in a seasoning blend; it has ⅓ the sodium content of table salt. In the United States it is marketed under the name Accent®; in some Asian countries it is known as vetsin.

The acid form of MSG, L-glutamic acid, is an amino acid and exists in the human body in free and protein-bound form. Glutamate is widely distributed in natural foods. It is more plentiful in protein-rich foods and less in low protein foods, such as vegetables. When added to food as an enhancer there is an optimal concentration (up to 0.8% of a food, by weight) beyond which the palatability of the food decreases, thus its usage is self limiting. Consumption of glutamates as a natural component of food greatly exceeds added MSG use levels.[2]

Because of its wide usage, MSG has been one of the most studied substances in the world's food supply. Extensive acute and chronic animal toxicity studies and feeding trials on human infants and adults form the basis on which MSG has been declared to be safe and efficacious. MSG addition to food is accepted in the United States by the Food & Drug Administration (FDA) but its presence must be disclosed on the label. It is listed in the Generally Recognized As Safe (GRAS) substance list. MSG is also approved by the World Health Organization (WHO) and the Food & Agricultural Organization (FAO) and is listed in the *Codex Alimentarius*, supporting its continued consumption.[2-4]

Vitamin A: Philippine Studies

In the past decade research was undertaken as a pioneering venture[4,5] to evaluate the feasibility and efficacy of nutrifying MSG with added vitamin A. Rationale for its selection in a Philippine study resulted from dietary surveys of food frequency use. Of 4 foods consumed frequently, MSG was chosen because surveys revealed 77–94% of the children consumed it at least once a week and often several times a week. Furthermore, in the Philippines, MSG had the following benefits; (1) it was produced at two locations, thereby easing monitoring problems for a nutrified product; (2) it was a pure accessory food substance, distributed in sealed packets providing sanitary handling and some environmental protection; and (3) it was a low-price commodity with a fairly rapid turnover from manufacturer to consumer.

In the preparation of a homogeneous MSG/vitamin A blend one must consider the physical and chemical nature of the ingredients. MSG is usually produced in the form of large elongated (needle) crystals. The form of vitamin A for this application must be dry stabilized and water-dispersible. In a *single* province (Cebu) Philippine nutrition study[4-6] the vitamin-MSG blend was prepared by first reducing the MSG crystals to a fine crystal size (100 mesh), adding dry vitamin A (Type 250 SD, 250,000 IU/g, vitamin A palmitate in an acacia-lactose matrix) and a small quantity of a flow-enhancing agent, blending all ingredients in a Nauta mixer and packaging the nutrified MSG in sealed plastic sachets (2.4 g) providing 15,000 IU of vitamin A per sachet. This amount of vitamin A was chosen to provide the daily needs of a family unit of two adults and two children. Stability testing demonstrated a 90% vitamin A retention when stored for 6 months at 23°C; and 76% retention with 6 months storage at 37°C. In the usual MSG manufacturing, packaging, distributing cycle in the Philippines the sachets reach the consumer about 2 months after manufacture, being exposed to a temperature range of 27–34°C and humidity of 57–87%.

Even though the milled crystal approach produced a uniform nutrified MSG and was successful in the first field study, objections arose about future operations on a large scale. The MSG manufacturer took pride in the production of large MSG crystals, objected to milling crystals, and occasionally observed that fine powder released from the nutrified product could cause fouling the sachet seals, leading to a higher percentage of rejects.[4]

Further feasibility studies were initiated utilizing the regular large MSG crystals in the development of a MSG/vitamin A blend. A larger particle size, stabilized vitamin A was required and a subsequent trial with a dry vitamin A beadlet product (Type 325 L, 325,000 IU/g, vitamin A acetate in a gelatin-sugar matrix) was devised. For the subsequent *tri-province* field study[4] the MSG/vitamin A blend (Fig. 12.1) was prepared by weighing out MSG and the vitamin A product into a polyethylene bag, tumbling the bag for uniformity of contents, then gravity feeding the blend through the chute of the packaging machine for sachet filling and sealing. Sachet vitamin content variability by this method was somewhat greater than in the milled crystal approach, but the sachets were judged adequate for the field study.

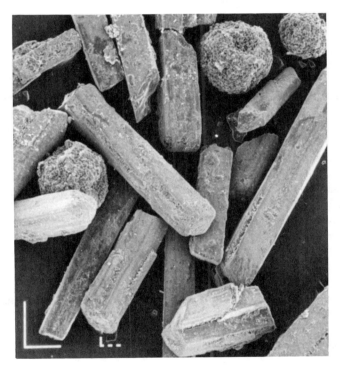

Courtesy of John Gmünder
FIG. 12.1. MAGNIFIED PHOTOGRAPH OF MSG CRYSTALS AND VITAMIN A BEADLETS SHOWING CONTRASTING PHYSICAL SHAPE

However, as the *tri-province* study progressed, some product limitations in the MSG/vitamin A beadlet blend developed over time, including loss of vitamin content due either to variability in mixing, product separation before packaging, environmental stress in the field or a combination of causes.

The earlier *single* province field study occurred in a low economic area of varying ecologic zones on the densely populated island of Cebu. Clinical, biochemical, dietary, demographic and socioeconomic examinations of about 1700 children from 626 families were carried out. The base line survey indicated a high prevalence of xerophthalmia and low serum retinol levels. During the nearly 2 years feasibility trial of the study, 3 intervention modes were identified and compared: (1) a public health and horticultural approach; (2) the provision of periodic massive oral doses of vitamin A (200,00 IU/child); and (3) nutrification of MSG with added vitamin A. In the MSG nutrified group, families were provided with initial sachets and empty ones were replaced with filled ones weekly (15,000 IU/packet). The nutrified MSG intervention[5] was judged the most effective intervention on the basis of clinical observations and biochemical data (Table 12.1). Evidence of clinical xerophthalmia was decreased and the rise in serum retinol was superior in the nutrified MSG intervention.[4-5]

In the later *tri-province* field study two provinces—Nueva Vizcaya and Marinduque—were selected to receive nutrified MSG, with Cebu serving as a control area for a nearly 2 year period. Nutrified MSG was packaged in small sachets (2.4 g), but, rather than delivering the packets weekly to the households, the sachets were made available through the usual marketing channels and had to be purchased by the families in the study. The original design and appearance of the sachet was maintained with a slight labeling modification to indicate the vitamin A addition. No advertising was undertaken to promote the nutrified sachet which was priced the same as the previously unnutrified sachets. To measure the effectiveness of the program, serum retinol levels and prevalence of xerophthalmic signs were observed during the baseline and after the nutrification phase in about 1800 preschool children. More favorable clinical improvements were observed in the nutrified MSG provinces than in the control province and improved serum retinol values occurred.[4-5] The Philippine studies have demonstrated that MSG as marketed in the usual commercial channels can be a useful carrier of added vitamin A and an effective intervention strategy for improving vitamin A status.

There is a growing trend in the Philippines toward marketing MSG in resealable containers of various sizes rather than only in small film sachets. For improved appearance, a whiter colored, dry vitamin A product would be helpful. If only coarse MSG will be marketed in the future, the introduction of a binding agent for greater particle cohesion of MSG crystals and vitamin A particles would mitigate against segregation during manufacturing and distribution of the MSG/vitamin A blend. Bonded, dry vitamin A palmitate (Type 250 CWS) with sucrose crystals proved to be more trouble-free in bulk packaging, as illustrated by the vitamin A nutrified sugar experiences (Chapter 8) in Central America.[7]

TABLE 12.1
XEROPHTHALMIA AND SERUM RETINOL OBSERVATIONS ON CHILDREN
BEFORE AND AFTER A THREE INTERVENTION FIELD STUDY

Intervention	Active Clinical Signs of Xerophthalmia (%)		Levels of Serum Vitamin A (μg/100 mL)	
	Before	After	Before	After
Public health—horticulture	4.9	3.4	19.0	16.4
High-dose capsule	3.1	0.6	19.6	19.6
MSG nutrification	4.2	1.0	21.0	28.5
Total sample[1]	4.1	1.7	19.9	21.5

Source: Latham and Solon.[5]
[1]Sample size: 1407 for clinical signs and 1121 for serum vitamin A levels.

There is also need for a philosophical change in the Philippines, as some believe and may have even promoted the concept that with vitamin A nutrified MSG a "medicine" (vitamin A) has been added to the food product (MSG), while, in actuality, both MSG and vitamin A have nutritive properties and both are food chemical products. All food products are made up of chemicals. Currently, the Philippines are considering a multipreventive approach to vitamin A deficiency control, part of which involves a food nutrification intervention.

Vitamin A: Indonesia Studies

Chronic marginal vitamin A nutriture is a problem for a percentage of children throughout Indonesia. In some areas, clusters of vitamin A deficiency exist. Fifteen provinces out of a total of 27 in Indonesia are considered high risk for xerophthalmia, with the population per province ranging from 5–25 million persons.[8] In its official health plan the Indonesian Ministry of Health has seven goals, one of which is the reduction of xerophthalmia by 70% before the year 2000. MSG, sucrose and wheat flour are known to be consumed by 50–70% of all xerophthalmic children. A decision to nutrify one or all foods has been under evaluation as a national policy.

A one-year field study[9] was undertaken with 10 villages (over 10,000 preschool children) divided into 2 groups. Families in five villages (the experimental group) used vitamin A nutrified MSG in sachets purchased through normal marketing channels; five other villages served as controls. The results of the study revealed that xerophthalmia in the experimental group dropped from 1.24 to 0.15%, and serum retinol values rose from 19.3 to 26.3 μg/dL. Other benefits observed were an increase in hemoglobin levels, improved growth, a lower mortality rate among preschoolers and a rise in the vitamin A level of the breast milk of lactating mothers.

Nutrified MSG for this study was prepared by blending cold water dispersible, dry vitamin A palmitate (Type 250 CWS, 250,000 IU/g) into fine, milled crystals of MSG (100 mesh) with a binding agent (dissolved hydroxypropyl-cellulose) first forming a premix. This was then dried and blended with a larger quantity of regular coarse MSG crystals to produce the final nutrified MSG with a vitamin A potency approximating 3000 IU/g. The objective of the field study was to supply 700 IU of vitamin daily per child from nutrified MSG in the experimental group. This improved, nutrified MSG was developed[10] by the collaborative efforts of the USDA's Office of International Cooperation and Development and Coating Place, Inc. Nutrified MSG retained 84% of its vitamin A potency after 4 months in the marketplace. The cost of the vitamin A nutrification (cost of premix materials) was about 20% over regular MSG production costs before packaging. The study was part of a planned effort toward the adoption of a national policy[9] for Indonesia involving MSG nutrification with vitamin A and increased consumption of dark green, leafy vegetables to eradicate vitamin A deficiency.

The general worldwide (Table 12.2) problem of xerophthalmia (nutritional blindness) resulting from vitamin A deficiency (VAD) is currently estimated to affect millions of children a year. At the 1988 South-East Asian Vitamin A Meeting in Jakarta, VAD was recognized as a systemic disease affecting many millions of children under the age of five in the South-East Asian Region. Many become permanently blind in one or both eyes and others die of increased susceptibility to infectious diseases because VAD unfavorably influences maintenance and function of the immune system. The public health problem of VAD exists in over 70 countries and territories. IVACG, the International Vitamin A Consultative Group is dedicated to the international eradication of vitamin A deficiency.[11]

Iron

Past surveys of nutritional status in countries such as the Philippines have revealed deficiencies of iron and vitamin A, thus raising the question of whether MSG could be nutrified with both nutrients. Laboratory trials support the feasibility, provided the MSG is a milled or is a fine mesh, crystalline product. Two iron sources,[6] micronized ferric orthophosphate (Turners phase II $< 1~\mu$) and zinc stearate coated ferrous sulfate (Durkee) were determined to have favorable color, taste, bioavailability and particle size properties. Each was used with dry, stabilized vitamin A palmitate (Type 250 SD, a fine particle product) in mixing operations with MSG (100 mesh size) to prepare sachets (2.4 g) containing 15,000 IU of vitamin A and 50 mg of iron. Chemical analyses revealed satisfactory product uniformity, and storage trials indicated that the presence of iron did not influence vitamin A retention values. Thus, vitamin A/iron nutrified MSG products also would appear to be satisfactory but would require scaleup production trials and field testing for confirmation.

TABLE 12.2
THE GEOGRAPHICAL DISTRIBUTION OF XEROPHTHALAMIA IN 1987
Countries Classified by Degree of Public Health Significance of Vitamin A Deficiency,
Xerophthalmia and Nutritional Blindness (January 1988)
[Classification of countries according to WHO regions]

	Class 1[1]	Class 2[2]	Class 3[3]
Africa	Benin Burkina Faso Chad Ethiopia Ghana Malawi Mali Mauritania Niger Nigeria U.R. Tanzania Zambia	Angola Kenya Mozambique Uganda Rwanda Burundi	Algeria Botswana Lesotho Madagascar Senegal Zaire Zimbabwe
Americas	Brazil Haiti	El Salvador Guatemala Honduras	Bolivia Ecuador Jamaica Mexico Peru
South-East Asia	Bangladesh India Indonesia Nepal Sri Lanka	Burma Bhutan	Thailand
Eastern Mediterranean	Sudan	Afghanistan Pakistan	Egypt Iran Iraq Jordan Morocco Oman Somalia Syria Yemen
Europe			Turkey
Western Pacific	Philippines Vietnam	Dem. Kampuchea Lao People's Dem. Republic	China Fiji Malaysia

Source: Dr. E.M. DeMaeyer, WHO, Geneva, Jan. 1988.

[1]Class 1: Significant public health problem in part or whole country.

[2]Class 2: Insufficient information but high probability of significant public health problem in part of whole country.

[3]Class 3: Sporadic cases, but prevalence is not such that it constitutes a significant public health problem.

SALT

Salt (sodium chloride, NaCl) is both a condiment and a dietary source of essential nutrients. It is widely consumed on a fairly regular basis. Both sodium and chloride are normal and necessary constituents of body tissues and fluids.

Globally, salt is obtained from different sources by varied operations. Sources include evaporated seawater, inland lake brines, salt wells and salt mines. Salt may be washed, recrystallized, crushed, milled, graded and packaged, all of which increases cost over bulk coarse crystals.[12,13] Evaporated granulated salt of different screen sizes has been purified to a 99.99% grade. Salt around the world varies greatly in quality, in moisture content, in types of impurities, odors, flavors and in particle size. Many populations throughout the world use a type of coarse impure rock or sea salt of large and variable crystal size and high moisture content.[13] As many as 16 trace elements have been identified in 45 indigenous salt samples.[14] Salt exposed to moisture (over 75% humidity) followed by dry periods will cake. The addition of anticaking compounds (tricalcium phosphate, calcium stearate, calcium polysilicate, or magnesium stearate) to salt is a common practice to retard caking tendency.

Advantages claimed for salt as a nutrient carrier include: (1) overconsumption is virtually impossible because of limitation in palatability (2) it is a low cost ingredient; and (3) a developed nutrification technology exists. Potential disadvantages at the local level are: (1) lack of salt uniformity in purity, color and dryness, (2) production by both large and very small or "cottage' industries, the latter raising the issue of monitoring, (3) lack of protective packaging against moisture absorption, and (4) high nutrification costs for more expensive additives (such as some amino acids).

Closely screened, high purity, low-moisture, granular salt nutrified with a combination of nutrients, with an added trace of hydrogenated oil as a bonding agent and an added trace of a flow enhancing agent for nutrifying baked goods and other customized salt mixtures as coatings to nutrify fat-fried manufactured snacks, have been available on the U.S. market for some time.

Vitamin A

In the developing countries there has been an interest in the addition of vitamin A to household salt to increase the vitamin A intake of household members. Issues which need to be addressed in this approach are: (1) Is there a uniform supply of pure, low moisture, screened salt? (2) Can the vitamin A nutrified salt be packaged to avoid high moisture build up in transit and storage? (3) Are the economics favorable to the consumer with or without governmental subsidies to purchase the nutrified product? If the answer is positive to all three questions, it should be possible to nutrify salt using a suitable dry stabilized vitamin A. Vitamin A nutrified salt was rejected by INCAP for Central America on the grounds that daily salt consumption per capita was too low and the cost of vitamin A nutrification potentially too high to make the process feasible on a commercial scale.[15] Favorable vitamin A stability data have been reported on vitamin A nutrified salt prepared from high purity refined salt.[16] Fine crystalline salt nutrified with a premix containing dry stabilized palmitate (Type 250 SD) retained over 90% of the added vitamin A following one year of storage in moisture resistant containers. In a clinical study, vitamin A nutrified salt (440 IU/g) administered to preschool children over a 6 month period was found to be an effective intervention in improving vitamin A status.[17]

α-Tocopherol

Salt is used as a carrier of α-tocopherol in inhibiting carcinogenic N-nitrosamine formation in the processing of bacon.[18] In combination with lecithin, which assists in the aqueous dispersion of tocopherol, the formulation is applied to either brine or dry cured bacon at tocopherol levels of 250–500 mg/kg. Storage of tocopherol coated salt at 70°F for up to three months did not reduce its efficacy. Added tocopherol also compliments the action of added L-ascorbic acid to cured meats in blocking the reaction between nitrite and secondary amine component, thus inhibiting nitrosamine formation (Chapter 15).

L-Ascorbic Acid

The consideration of ascorbic acid addition to salt as a carrier may involve its properties as an essential nutrient but more often the purpose is to act as an enhancer of iron absorbability. Ascorbic acid added to either ferrous sulfate or ferric phosphate containing salt increased iron absorption about threefold in human feeding trials.[19]

Pure L-ascorbic acid, in either granular or powder form, can be kept stable in physical properties and biopotency for years, provided the environment is relatively moisture free initially and kept that way during storage in sealed containers. With moisture pickup ascorbic acid will gradually take on a tan color with very minor loss in potency. In laboratory experiments with analytical grade ingredients, a mixture of NaCl, L-ascorbic acid and $FeSo_4.7H_2O$ developed no discoloration or change in taste, nor change in ascorbic acid content over a 6 month period.[20]

When common Indian salt (usually high moisture type) was nutrified with ferric orthophosphate and ascorbic acid, part of the iron became soluble, but the salt developed a bright pink violet color immediately.[21] With African salt a combination of ferric orthophosphate, ascorbic acid and starch (acting as a discoloration retardant) may be technically feasible and sufficiently bioavailable, but whether local economies would permit such a practical application is in doubt.[20]

Calcium

There has been interest in India for calcium addition[22] to salt, and it can be added to salt relatively inexpensively and at little inconvenience. Public support is needed for such a beneficial intervention for children and child bearing women in calcium deficient areas. When sea water is concentrated, calcium sulfate precipitates out. One suggestion has been to separate, refine, grind and return the calcium product before the final salt concentration stage and produce a standardized 5% calcium nutrified salt. An alternative procedure would be dry mixing calcium sulfate with salt to prepare the same product. Calcium sulfate is bioavailable and in field trials has been shown to improve the growth of children in deficient areas.[23] With iodine deficiency disorders and iron deficiency anemia all as higher priority items, it is likely that progress on calcium nutrified salt will be slow, although no technological or consumer acceptance problems appear troublesome.

Fluorine

Fluorine has been added to salt during the past several decades.[24] In 1967, three quarters of the packeted salt in Switzerland was nutrified with 10 mg of potassium iodide and 200 mg of sodium fluoride per kilogram of salt achieving an ingestion of 1 mg of fluorine per day with a daily salt consumption of 4–5 g. At this rate, urinary excretion of fluorine was about comparable to those obtained from fluoridated water at 1 mg/kg, thus the caries preventing effects should be similar. Hungary, Columbia, Spain, Finland, Sweden and Mexico are other countries in various stages of adopting fluoridation of salt. Data to date indicate fluorine nutrified salt to be a successful alternative to fluoridation of water, especially in areas where water supplies are variable and diverse.

Iodine

Iodine is a necessary component of thyroid hormones. An inadequate dietary intake gradually leads to lowered hormone production and the following consequences: (1) goiter (enlarged thyroid), (2) hypothyroidism, a slowing of physical and mental productivity in adults and irreversible mental retardation in neonates at birth, (3) cretinism, severely affected stature, with deaf mutism and gross neuromuscular symptoms, (4) decreased fertility, (5) increased stillbirths, and (6) decreased child survival. In population surveys, prevalence of goiter can be tabulated in three different stages of development. Iodine urinary excretion values on a per day or per gram of creatinine basis are helpful to judge high, medium and low risk of IDD development. It is estimated that over 600 million persons are at risk of IDD, mostly (Fig. 12.2; Table 12.3) in developing countries.[25] Quantitating the economic consequences of IDD which decreases quantity and quality of the labor force and strains health

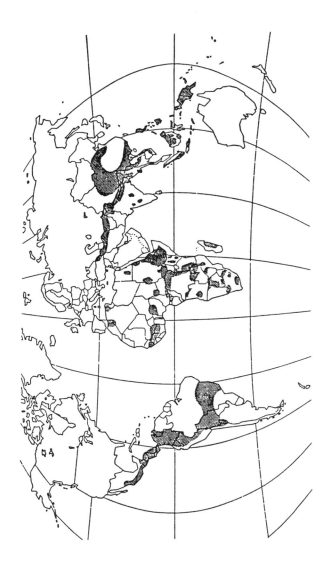

FIG. 12.2. DISTRIBUTION OF IODINE DEFICIENCY DISORDERS IN DEVELOPING COUNTRIES

From ACC/SCN, 1987[6]

TABLE 12.3
IODINE DEFICIENCY DISORDERS IN DEVELOPING COUNTRIES BY WHO REGION

Regions	Total Population (Millions)	Number at Risk (Millions)	Number with Goiter (Millions)	Goiter Prevalence	Number with Overt Cretinism (Millions)
Africa	360	60	30	8%	0.5
South East Asia	1050	280	100	10%	1.5
Asia (other countries)	1070	400	30	3%	0.9
Latin America	360	60	30	8%	0.25
Total	2840	800	190		3.15

Source: ACC/SCN, 1987.[26]

care programs can help to stimulate policy makers to expedite remedial programs. The 39th World Health Assembly in 1986 passed a resolution for the prevention and control of IDD and urged member states to give high priority to IDD and its control by appropriate nutritional programs. The International Council for Control of Iodine Deficiency Disorders works internationally on preventing IDD.[26]

There is an abundance of iodine in the ocean but an uneven scattering over the land. Iodine is an element and was discovered in 1811 and first used as a tincture in successful goiter therapy in 1821. The use of salt as a vehicle for added iodine to control iodine deficiency disorders (IDD) was fist suggested in 1831 by Boussingault in Columbia, South America.[27] In the United States it was Cowie in 1922, recognizing a need for a preventive goiter plan because of the high incidence of goiter, who recommended[28] and developed iodized salt use in Michigan. Marine and Kimball in Ohio were also early leaders.[29] In 1922, Switzerland passed legislation for salt iodization and devised an iodized salt procedure two years later. The virtual disappearance of endemic goiter and cretinism is possible in salt-eating populations if a constant and proper iodated salt program is maintained.[30]

Both iodide and iodate compounds[31] have served as iodine additives to salt. Potassium iodide is cheaper, more soluble and less is needed, but it is more labile under conditions of moisture, high temperature and sunlight, excessive aeration and in the presence of salt impurities. Potassium iodate is a more stable compound and serves better in variable environmental situations. It is regarded as the preferred additive in most applications. With its use there is less need for added stabilizing and drying agents. Calcium and sodium iodized salts also have been employed.

The moisture content of the final nutrified salt should be kept low for better flow properties and to minimize iodine loss in transit and storage. The optimal level of iodine addition[31] must accomodate iodine losses between production and consumption, as well as the average amount of salt consumed per individual in the targeted population. The recommended minimum daily requirement of iodine is 150 mcg. The annual average consumption of salt should be monitored for any population consuming iodine-nutrified salt. The per capita consumption of salt in different countries varies over a range of 2-20 g/day. If consumption decreases per capita as has happened in Finland, Switzerland, the United States and other countries, the iodine content of salt must be increased to maintain recommended iodine daily intake. The cost of iodization includes price of chemicals, processing, protective packaging, and program monitoring. For the iodine range of 40 ppm in salt, the cost approximates $12 per ton[31] including chemicals, iodination procedure, packaging monitoring and administration. Cost per capita is about 7 cents (US) per year as a general guide. Investment and operating costs (Chapter 17) for the basic methods of iodination of salt and the support measures required have been published.[31]

Analyses have been made of reports from Europe, the Americas, Australia, South East Asia and China data before and after a salt prophylactic program (Table 12.4). The reports represent selected populations, not necessarily the whole country, as there are still large areas where IDD prevails due to difficulties encountered in iodized salt distribution.[32]

Success of an iodine nutrified salt program[31] depends on (1) identification and assessment of the IDD program; (2) awareness and support by policy makers and the public for salt iodization; (3) universal iodization by an approved process in all areas (if approved, all salt available to consumers and animals should become iodized); (4) proper packaging and a well-planned distribution to consumers; (5) use of economic and marketing incentives; (6) proper legislation and enforcement to introduce, control and maintain the program, as well as monitoring and periodic evaluation of all phases of the program; and (7) coordination and collaboration among government, industry, health, education and public relation agencies. Spot testing of salt for iodine content is possible with simple field test procedures.[33] Complete eradication of IDD is judged feasible within a 5-10 year period.

Iron

Iron deficiency anemia (IDA) has been and continues to be a major health problem[34-36] in many countries (Table 12.5). IDA is regarded as the most common nutritional disorder influencing as many as an estimated one billion people of all age groups and especially among pregnant women and young children, contributing to maternal morbidity and mortality and low birth weight infants. Severe anemia impairs work capacity, learning ability and immune function, lowering the resistance of the body to infection. Iron deficiency anemia is not defined solely on the basis of low hemoglobin but should include other clinical chemistry parameters, such as serum ferritin, transferrin saturation and protoporphyrin values. Hemoglobin values less than 13 g/dL for men and 12 g/dL for women are indicative of IDA. Body iron balance depends; (1) on iron needed for hemoglobin production; (2) on iron losses from physiological processes and pathological stresses and, (3) on the iron absorbed from the intestines following ingested natural food and supplemental iron sources.

TABLE 12.4
OBSERVATION ON EFFECT OF IODIZED SALT PROPHYLAXIS ON GOITER PREVALENCE

Country Region	Iodine compound in Salt	concentration mg/kg	Duration of observation Years	Prophylaxis Before Goitre %	Prophylaxis After Goitre %	dU-I[1] ug d	Population studied
Guatemala	KIO$_3$	100	13	38	5.2	155	Population
U.S.A. Mich.	KI	100	27	38.6	1.4		Schoolchildren
Colombia							
Candelaria	KI	50	20	83	30	>200	"
Zarzal			20	16	< 9	>200	"
Puerto Tejada			5	98	32		"
Guarcari			5	95	30		
Caldas			15	83	1	>200 ?	"
New Zealand	KI	50	20	15	0.1		"
Equador	KIO$_3$	50	11	24	12		Population
Thailand	KIO$_3$	50	11	84	0	100-150	Schoolchildren
Java	KIO$_3$	40	3	37.2	6.1		Population
Argentina							
Mendoza	KIO$_3$	33	20	46	3.2	155	Schoolchildren
Uruguay	KIO$_3$	33	5	37.8	22.8		Population
Costa Rica	KIO$_3$	33-67	5	?	3.6		Schoolchildren
Finland	KIO$_3$	25	30	>30	2.3	256	"
China							
Chang Ping	KI	20	6	22	2.5		Population
Heba			2	31.5	5.2	105	"
Six Other Communities			12-22	46.8(av) (25-62)	(2,4-10.9)		
India							
Kangra Valley	KI	20	12	38	8.5	204[2]	Schoolchildren
	KIO$_3$	25	12	38	9.1		"
	KIO$_3$	25	6	40.3	17.1		"
Chandigarh	KIO$_3$	25	4	>70	16.4	95	"
Mexico	KI	20	5	93.0	38	50	"
Bulgaria	KI	20	15	56	12		"
Portugal	KI	20	6	51	9.3	145[2]	"
Chechoslovakia							
Bohemia & Moravia	KI	25	14	39.8	9.6	100	6-10 y
				53.1	22.7		11-20 y
				60.3	33.6		21-50 y
				53.7	33.3		51-60 y
Slovakia				27.6	12.6		6-10 y
				42.3	24.7		11-20 y
				52.9	38.5		21-50 y
				41.6	34.2		51-65 y
Brazil	KI, KIO$_3$	10	20	26.5	14.8		
USSR	KI	10	4-5	85	10-15		?
Hungary	KI	10	15	32.5	11.1		Population
Poland	KI	10	9	17.7	1.2		Schoolchildren
Yugoslavia	KI	10	10	71.8	31.7		"
Austria	KI	10	17	45.9	12	65	Schoolchildren
Switzerland							
Berne	KI	5	13[3]	28	16		"
			10[4]	16	1		"
Wallis				71	30		"
Lausanne			14	61.7	0.7		"

Source: Lamberg.[32]
[1] dU-I = Urinary excretion of iodine, μg/d.
[2] I μg/d creatinine.
[3] < 10% iodized salt.
[4] 60–70% iodized salt.

TABLE 12.5
ESTIMATED PREVALENCE OF ANEMIA BY GEOGRAPHIC REGION AND AGE/SEX CATEGORY, AROUND 1980
(POPULATION DATA IN MILLIONS)

Region		Children						Men			Women				
		0–4 Years		5–12 Years				15–59 Years			Pregnant		15–49 Years	All	
		Anemic			Anemic				Anemic			Anemic		Anemic	
	Number	%	Number	Number	%	Number	Number	%	Number	Number	%	Number	Number	%	Number
Africa	85.7	56	48.0	96.6	49	47.3	116.8	20	23.4	17.9	63	11.3	106.4	44	46.8
Northern America	19.6	8	1.6	27.5	13	3.6	76.3	4	3.1	3.4	—	—	64.2	8	5.1
Latin America	52.9	26	13.7	69.8	26	18.1	98.1	13	12.8	9.9	30	3.0	86.5	17	14.7
East Asia*	16.1	20	3.2	25.4	22	5.6	55.8	11	6.1	2.7	20	0.5	46.9	18	8.4
South Asia	212.0	56	118.7	278.4	50	139.2	386.3	32	123.6	41.7	65	27.1	329.4	58	191.0
Europe	33.4	14	4.7	55.0	5	2.7	147.2	2	3.0	5.7	14	0.8	117.5	12	14.1
Oceania	2.3	18	0.4	3.6	15	0.5	6.9	7	0.5	0.4	25	0.1	5.5	19	1.0
USSR	23.1	—	—	3.1	—	—	80.3	—	—	4.0	—	—	68.7	—	—
World*	445.1	43	193.5	587.6	37	217.4	967.7	18	174.2	85.8	51	43.9	825.0	35	288.4
Developing regions	86.1	12	10.3	130.7	7	9.1	346.5	3	12.0	14.8	14	2.0	285.5	11	32.7
Developing regions*	395.0	51	183.2	456.8	46	208.3	621.2	26	162.2	71.0	59	41.9	539.5	47	255.7

Sources: World Health Statist. Quart. 38 (1985); DeMaeyer and Adials.[36]

Notes: *Excluding China. All calculations were made before rounding, figures may thus not add to totals.
Anemia is defined as a hemoglobin concentration below WHO reference values for age, sex and pregnancy status.
Regions are drawn according to United Nations regions; more developed regions include North America, Japan, Europe, Australia, New Zealand and the Union of the Soviet Socialist Republics.
Prevalence rates are estimated from the various studies.

Iron needs are the greatest in instances of rapid expansion of tissue and red cell mass as occurs in infancy, childhood and pregnancy.

The obvious solution to IDA is to increase readily absorbable iron to bolster body tissues and fluids[35-37,38] There are three iron nutrification options, namely the addition of (1) an absorbable form of iron, (2) a facilitator or enhancer of absorption such as ascorbic acid, or (3) both types of compounds to an ingested food carrier. In countries where relative homogeneity of salt consumption is practiced, the addition of a suitable iron compound to salt as part of the refining and packaging process appears readily feasible. However, in practice, nutrification of salt with iron is beset with an array of formidable technological problems.[39-41] Nutrification of salt has been studied in India for over a decade, also in Indonesia and Thailand. An acceptable iron additive for salt is one which will not induce discoloration, nor impart a flavor or odor, and which would be stable and bioavailable when incorporated initially and after storage, and one which would fit into the economy of the country.

Since crystalline salt is a soluble white or nearly white product, a white, water-soluble, nonreactive iron additive would be preferred. Dark, colored, insoluble iron (such as reduced iron, electrolytic iron or carbonyl iron, all bioavailable in fine micronized form) discolor salt and, being dense elemental sources, tend to separate from salt crystals after mixing and shipment. Soluble iron compounds such as ferrous sulfate are absorbed very well but added to salt are chemically reactive, particularly in the presence of impurities and moisture. Oxidation of ferrous iron results in black, green or yellow oxides: reactions with sulfur or phenolic structures likewise produce dark end products. The prooxidant activity of iron, in the presence of oxygen, with or without enzyme assistance, can cause offensive odors and flavors. Light-colored, insoluble iron compounds, such as ferric orthophosphate, have a more favorable density, color, flavor and "cook-up" quality but unless finely micronized are unacceptable because of low iron availability.[37,38]

Over the last decade Indian investigations[40,41] have been directed toward a search for supplementary salt additives which would significantly retard or prevent the troublesome discoloration of iron nutrified salt; and which would also improve the bioavailability of otherwise acceptable iron additives. Orthophosphoric acid (OPA) or sodium hexametaphosphate (SHMP) prevented discoloration but only when these color change preventives were present in excess to the iron source ($FeSO_4$). Furthermore, SHMP, to function as a color preventive, had to be in an acid medium, and so sodium acid sulfate ($NaHSO_4$) was used in conjunction with SHMP. In 18 week storage tests both the $FeSO_4$-SHMP blend and the $FeSO_4$-OPA blend underwent chemical changes, the iron becoming less soluble and less bioavailable. While discoloration was prevented, bioavailability was faulted.

It was observed that $NaHSO_4$ addition to $FePO_4$ increased significantly iron availability. Nutrified salt with $FePO_4$ and $NaHSO_4$ in a 1:2 molar proportion after an 8 month storage test was stable and suffered no loss in iron bioavailability. Nutrified salt of a formulation of 3500 ppm $FePO_4$ and 5000 ppm $NaHSO_4$ providing 1 mg iron/g salt and a second less expensive formulation of 3200 ppm $FeSO_4$,

2200 ppm OPA and 5000 ppm $NaHSO_4$ were developed. Sodium orthophosphate (SOP) can substitute for OPA which eliminates a liquid additive.

Large scale production of the nutrified salt can be prepared in batch or continuous mixing equipment using 40–50 mesh size crushed salt. Both have been formulated to an iron content of 1 mg/g salt. Estimated cost of production including cost of chemicals and packing in protective bags for the $FePO_4$ formulation is \$25 (US)/ton, and \$16 (US)/ton for the $FeSO_4$ formulation, costs which could be lowered by greater volume production. After field testing, acceptance of nutrified salt was favorable, except initially where crushed salt was unfamiliar. Significant improvement in hemoglobin levels and the reduction of anemia was noted in all nutrified salt test areas with both the $FeSO_4$ and the $FePO_4$ formulations.[40,42] Other encouraging trials have been conducted in South Africa and Thailand.

As of 1990 no noniodized salt is permitted to be produced or sold in India, hence it became necessary to develop a double nutrient nutrified salt, with added iron and iodine. Initial suitability studies of 6 months duration indicate a double nutrient formula of 0.04 g iodine (40 ppm), 3.28 g ferrous sulfate (1000 ppm Fe) and 10 g of stabilizer (a permitted food additive) per kilogram has merit.[43] Progress is continuing in the national practice of salt nutrification in India with critical minerals.[46]

Other Condiments

Other condiments have served as vehicles for iron addition. Fish-sauce, a widely used, high salt condiment in Thailand[44] appears to be of some value as a carrier for iron (III) sodium ethylenediamine-tetra-acetate in reducing IDA in populations regularly consuming fish-sauces. In Bangkok, iodized fish-sauce and iodized soy sauce have been developed. In another study[45] curry powder served as a vehicle for iron (NaFeEDTA) addition in South Africa. The nutrified curry powder was acceptable in terms of color, palatability and stability and produced a significant rise in iron absorption in two of three trials.

INACG, the International Nutritional Anemia Consultative Group, works toward the goal of eliminating anemia.[35]

REFERENCES

1. PADEN, C. A., WOLINSKY, I., HOSKINS, J. C., LEWIS, K. C., LINEBACK, D. R. and McCARTHY, R. D. 1979. Fortification of accessory food items. Lebensm. Wiss. Technol. *21*, 183–188.
2. IFT. 1987. Monosodium glutamate. A Scientific Status Summary by the Institute of Food Technologist's Expert Panel on Food Safety and Nutrition. Food Technol. *41*(5), 143–154.
3. KAWAMULA, Y. and KARE, M. R. 1987. Umani: a Basic Taste Physiology, Biochemistry, Nutrition, Food Science. Marcel Dekker, New York.

4. SOLON, F. S., LATHAM, M. C., GUIRRIEC, R., FLORENTINO, R., WILLIAMSON, D. F. and AGUILAR, J. 1985. Fortification of MSG with vitamin A: The Philippine experience. Food Technol. 39(11), 71–77.
5. LATHAM, M. C. and SOLON, F. S. 1986. Vitamin A deficiency control in the Philippines. In Vitamin A Deficiency and Its Control, J. C. Bauernfeind (ed.). Academic Press, Orlando.
6. BAUERNFEIND, J. C. and TIMRECK, A. 1980. Monosodium glutamate, a carrier for added vitamin A and iron. Philippine J. Sci. 107 (3–4), 203–213.
7. ARROYAVE, G., AGUILAR, J. R., FLORES, M. and GUYMAN, M. A. 1979. Evaluation of sugar fortification with vitamin A at the national levels. Pan. Am. Health Organ. 384.
8. TARWOTJO, I., TILDEN, R., SATIBI, I. and NENDRAWATI, H. 1986. Vitamin A deficiency control in Indonesia. In Vitamin A Deficiency and Its Control, J. C. Bauernfeind (ed.). Academic Press, Orlando.
9. MUHILAL, D. et al. 1986. A Pioneering Project for Combatting Vitamin A Deficiency and Xerophthalmia with MSG Fortified with Vitamin A. Dept. Health. Directorate General of Community Health, Republic of Indonesia, Jakarta, 1988. Am. J. Clin. Nutr. 48, 1265–1276.
10. GREENBURG, K. 1987. USDA technology offers new hope in combating vitamin A deficiency abroad. Nat. Food Rev. NFR-38 (fall), 22–23. USDA Econ. Res. Serv., Washington, DC.
11. BAUERNFEIND, J. C. 1986. Vitamin A Deficiency and Its Control. Academic Press, Orlando.
12. IFT. 1980. Dietary salt. A Scientific Status Summary by the Institute of Food Technologist's Expert Panel on Food Safety and Nutrition on the Committee on Public Information. IFT, Chicago.
13. WOLINSKY, I., LINEBACK, D. R., McCARTHY, R. D. and SEVERSON, G. 1980. Iodination of salt. Baroda J. Nutr. 7, 1–6.
14. KUHNLEIN, H. 1980. The trace element content of indigenous salts compared with commercial refined substitutes. Ecol. Food Nutr. 10, 113–121.
15. ARROYAVE, G. 1971. Distribution of vitamin A to population groups. Proc. III West. Hemisphere Nutr. Congr., 66–79.
16. BAUERNFEIND, J. C. and CORT, W. M. 1974. Nutrification of foods with added vitamin A. CRC Crit. Rev. Food Technol. 4, 337–375.
17. HUSIANI, M. A., BARIZI, D., DJOJOSOEBAGIO, S. and KARYADI, D. 1985. The use of fortified salt to control vitamin A deficiency. Proc. XIII Int. Congr. Nutr., 142.
18. WILKENS, M. F. and GRAY, J. I. 1986. Reduce N-nitrosamines formation in bacon. Food. Eng. 58(5), 68–69.
19. SOLOMONS, N. W. and VITERI, F. E. 1982. Biological interactions of ascorbic acid and mineral nutrients. In Ascorbic Acid, Chemistry, Metabolism and Uses, P. A. Seib and Tolbert, B. M. (eds.). Adv. Chem. Ser. 200. American Chemical Society, Washington, DC.
20. SAYERS, M. H., LYNCH, S. R., CHARLTON, R. W., ROTHWELL, T. H., WALKER, R. B. and MAYET, F. 1974. The fortification of common salt with ascorbic and iron. Brit. J. Haematol. 28, 483–495; Br. J. Nutr. 31, 367–375.
21. RAO, B. S. N. and VYAYASARATHY, C. 1975. Fortification of common salt with iron: Effect of chemical additive on stability and bioavailability. Am. J. Clin. Nutr. 28, 1395–1401.

22. LEVINSON, F. J. and BERG, A. D. 1969. With a grain of fortified salt. Food Technol. *23*(9), 70–72.
23. RAO, G. N. and RAO, B. S. N. 1974. Absorption of calcium from calcium lactate and calcium sulfate by human subjects. Indian J. Med. Res. *64*, 426–429.
24. LOWENSTEIN, F. W. 1983. Present public health aspects of salt fortification. *In* CRC Handbook of Nutritional Supplements: Human Use, M. Rechigl Jr. (ed.). CRC Press, Boca Raton.
25. DUNN, J. T., PRETELL, E. A., DAZA, C. H. and VITERI, F. E. 1986. Toward the Eradication of Endemic Goiter, Cretinism and Iodine Deficiency. Pan American Health Organization, Washington, DC.
26. ANON. 1986; 1987. Organization of the ICCIDD & relation to other international organizations. ICCIDD Newsl. *2*(3), 3–5; *3*(2), 1; 1988. UN Admin. Comm. Cord. Subcommittee on Nutr. ACC-SCN-NPD paper No. 3.
27. BOUSSINGAULT, M. 1833. Memoir sur les salines iodiferes des Andes. Ann. Chem. Phys. *54*, 163–177.
28. MARKEL, H. M. 1987. When it rains it pours: Endemic goiter iodized salt and D. M. Cowie. AJPH *77*(2), 219–228.
29. MARINE, D. and KIMBALL, O. P. 1921. The prevention of simple goiter in man. J. Am. Med. Assoc. *77*, 1068.
30. HETZEL, B. S., DUNN, J. T. and STANBURY, J. B. 1987. The Prevention and Control of Iodine Deficiency Disorders. Elsevier, New York; 1989. Story of Iodine Deficiency, Oxford Univ. Press, London.
31. VENKATESH MANNAR, M. G. 1986. Review of iodine technology: iodinated salt. ICCIDD Newsl. *2*(2), 6–7; 1988. Salt iodination: salt production & processing. ICCIDD Newsl. *4*(3), 9–11; 1988. Salt iodination: iodination technique. ICCIDD Newsl. *4*(4), 11–16.
32. LAMBERG, B. A. 1984. Effectiveness of iodized salt in various parts of the world. *In* Thyroid Disorders Associated with Iodine Deficiency and Excess, R. Hall and J. Köbberling (eds.). Raven Press, New York.
33. TYAHJI, R. 1986. Use of iodated salt in the prevention of iodine deficiency disorders; A handbook of monitoring and quality control. UNICEF/ROSCA, Lodi Estate, New Delhi 110,033, India.
34. WHO. 1975. Control of Nutritional Anemia with Special Reference to Iron Deficiency. Tech. Rep. 580. World Health Organization, Geneva.
35. INACG. 1977. Guidelines for the Eradication of Iron Deficiency Anemia. International Nutritional Anemia Consultative Group, Washington, DC.
36. DeMAEYER, E. and ADIALS—TEGMAN, M. 1985. The prevalence of anemia in the world. Rapp. Trimest. Statist. Sanit. Mond. *38*.
37. COOK, J. D. and REUSSER, M. E. 1983. Iron fortification: an update. Am. J. Clin. Nutr. *38*, 648–659.
38. CLYDESDALE, F. M. and WIEMER, K. L. 1985. Iron Fortification of Foods. Academic Press, Orlando.
39. ZOLLER, J. M. *et al.* 1980. Fortification of non-staple food items with iron. Food Technol. *34*(1), 38–47.
40. ANON. 1982. Working Group on Fortification of Salt with Iron. Use of common salt fortified with iron in the control and prevention of anemia: A collaborative study. Am. J. Clin. Nutr. *2*(35), 1442–1451.
41. RAO, B. S. N. 1985. Salt. *In* Iron Fortification of Foods. F. M. Clydesdale and K. L. Wiemer (eds.) Academic Press, Orlando.

42. ANON. 1983. Use of iron-fortified salt to combat anemia: The Indian experience. Nutr. Rev. *41*(10), 302–304.
43. RAO, B. S. N. 1987. Double fortification of salt with iron and iodine to control anemia and goiter. Nutr. News (NIN, Hyderabad, India) *8*(1), 1–3.
44. GARBY, L. and ARREKUL, S. 1974. Iron supplementation in Thai fish-sauce. Ann. Trop. Med. Parasitol. *68*(4), 467–476.
45. LAMPARELLI, R. D. *et al*. 1987. Curry powder as a vehicle for iron fortification: effects on iron absorption. Am. J. Clin. Nutr. *46*, 335–340.
46. SUBRAMANIAN, P. 1989. Fortification of common salt. *In* Trends in Food Science and Technology. M. R. Raghavendra Rao, *et al*. (eds.). Govt. of India Publ. 139. Jaipur, India.

CHAPTER 13

Foods Considered for Nutrient Addition: DAIRY PRODUCTS

ELMER DeRITTER

INTRODUCTION

Dairy products comprise a wide variety of foods derived from milk, which in the United States is predominantly cow's milk. Other animal species[1] that serve as a source of milk for human nutrition in different parts of the world include the goat, Indian buffalo, sheep, camel, and reindeer. Dairy products may be classified in the following groups: (1) fluid or market milk, which includes homogenized whole milk, vitamin D whole milk, fortified milk, flavored milks, low-fat milks, and skim or nonfat milk; (2) fermented milk and milk products including cultured buttermilk, sour cream, yogurt, acidophilus milk, and kefir; (3) market creams with varying amounts of fat; (4) butter, butter oil, and spreads; (5) concentrated milk products including evaporated whole or skim milk, plain and sweetened condensed whole, low-fat, and skim milks, and condensed buttermilk; (6) dried products, such as nonfat dry milk, dry whole milk, dry buttermilk, dry cream, dry whey and malted milk powders; (7) many varieties of cheese; and (8) frozen desserts including ice cream, frozen yogurt, frozen custard, ice milk, and sherbet. Other groups are ready-made desserts, high fruit puddings, mousses and jellied milk products, whey-base beverages and fabricated or recombined products involving milk ingredients and nondairy items. To indicate the wide product range, a collection of tables has been prepared on milk and milk products covering some 620 items.[2,3]

In 1986 the milk supply in the United States was utilized as follows: 36.4% for fluid milk and cream, 29.3% for cheese, 16.1% for butter; 9.2% for frozen desserts; 1.8% used on farms where produced; 1.5% for evaporated and condensed milk; and 5.7% for other uses.[4] Total 1986 U.S. production of fluid milk products according to the USDA in terms of millions of pounds were: plain whole milk, 25,706; lowfat milk, 21,408; skim milk, 3,329; flavored milk and drinks, 2,634; buttermilk, 1,046; half and half, 0.777; light cream, 0.097; heavy cream, 0.244, eggnog, 0.124, resulting in a total of 56,365.

Utilization of milk and various milk products remains in a dynamic state by the consuming public. Changing life patterns, the appearance of dietary guidelines and the greater consciousness of foods and diet relative to health have influenced changes in the consumption of milk products (Fig. 13.1) by the consumer over the past decade, and continued changes are expected in the near future.[5,6] The industry, however, is in a more flexible and creative stance than in past decades.

NUTRIENT CONTENT OF DAIRY PRODUCTS

Dairy products are a valuable source of many nutrients, especially calcium, phosphorus, iodine, potassium, magnesium, protein and vitamins. They represent an important source, particularly of riboflavin, vitamin B_{12} and, in full fat products, vitamin A.[7,8] Reports on the composition of milk appear regularly in the literature,[9,10] some dealing primarily with the mineral components,[10-13] others with the vitamin distribution[13-17] and some showing comparisons between bovine and human milks. The nutrient content of whole fluid milk, nonfat milk solids and milkfat[8] is given in tabular form (Table 13.1). Reviews on the nutrient content, nutritional value and

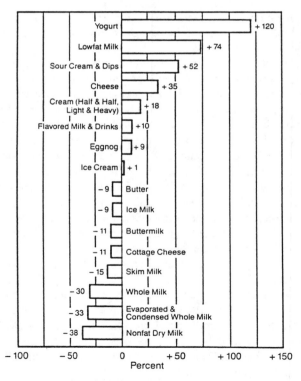

From McBran et al.[6] and Milk Industry Foundation, 1985
FIG. 13.1. PERCENTAGE OF CHANGE
IN PER CAPITA SALES OF DAIRY FOODS 1974-84

TABLE 13.1
NUTRIENT CONTENT OF MILKFAT, MILK SOLIDS-NOT-FAT, AND WHOLE FLUID MILK

The nutrient values are based on whole milk with 3.34 percent fat and 8.67% milk solids-not-fat. The *Handbook 8-1*, includes standard error of the mean.

Nutrient	Per Gram Milkfat	Per Gram Milk Solids-Not-Fat	Per Cup (8 oz, 244 g) Whole Fluid Milk
Energy, kcal[1]	8.79	3.71	150
Energy, kJ	36.78	15.52	627.6
Protein, (N × 6.38), g		0.380	8.03
Fat, g	1.00		8.15
Carbohydrate, total, g		0.536	11.37
Fiber, g		0	0
Ash, g		0.083	1.76
Minerals			
Calcium, mg		13.8	291
Iron, mg		0.006	0.12
Magnesium, mg		1.6	33
Phosphorus, mg		10.8	228
Potassium, mg		17.5	370
Sodium, mg		5.7	120
Zinc, mg		0.044	0.93
Vitamins			
Ascorbic acid, mg		0.108	2.29
Thiamin, mg		0.0044	0.093
Riboflavin, mg		0.0187	0.395
Niacin, mg		0.0097	0.205
Niacin equivalents, mg[2]		0.0987	2.088
Pantothenic acid, mg		0.0362	0.766
Vitamin B_6, mg		0.0048	0.102
Folacin, mcg		0.6	12
Vitamin B_{12}, mcg		0.0412	0.871
Vitamin A, RE[3]	9.3		76
Vitamin A, IU	37.7		307
Cholesterol, mg	4.0		33

Source: National Diary Council.[8]

[1]For rapid estimate of food energy, fat can be assumed to contribute 9 Calories per gram; protein and carbohydrate, 4 Calories per gram.

[2]This value includes niacin equivalents from preformed niacin and from tryptophan. A dietary intake of 60 mg tryptophan is considered equivalent to 1 mg niacin. One niacin equivalent is equal to either of these amounts.

[3]A retinol equivalent (RE) is equal to 3.33 IU of retinol or 10 IU of β-carotene.

trends of particular products include those on cultured dairy foods[18-21] and imitation and substitute dairy products.[22] The levels in milk products of vitamins A, D, E and K, being the fat-soluble vitamins, are directly influenced by the fat level in the milk product. Vitamin A (retinol) in milk is primarily in ester form, but vitamin A activity in milk is also due to provitamin A carotenoids of which beta-carotene is the dominant form. Both preformed vitamin A and the carotenoid content (as well as vitamins D and E) in full-fat fluid milk vary,[22a] being higher during the months when cows are on fresh green pasture (Fig. 13.2) and lower when they are consuming dry forage. Vitamin A values of milk range from 800–1800 IU with an average of approximately 1300 IU per liter or quart.[14] While both principal forms of vitamin D, namely D_2 and D_3, may be present in milk, the total vitamin D content of fluid whole milk varies over the seasons from 5–40 IU/L. The vitamin D content of whole milk was measured by Leerbeck and Soendergaard[23] at 38 IU/L for cow's milk and 15 IU/L for human milk. Hollis *et al.*[24] reported vitamin D levels of 27 and 25 IU/L

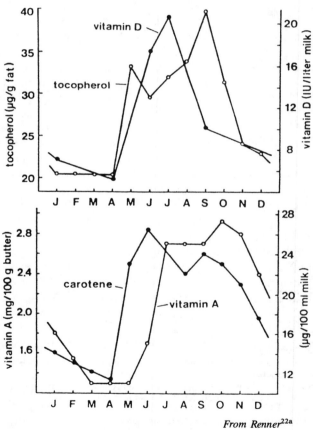

From Renner[22a]

FIG. 13.2. SEASONAL VARIATIONS IN THE CONCENTRATION OF CAROTENE AND VITAMINS A, D, AND E IN COW'S MILK

in cow's and human milk, respectively. Hydroxy analogs of vitamin D, including 25-OH, 24,25-diOH, and 1,25-diOH are present in normal bovine milk.[24,25] Herting and Drury[26] estimated up to 6 times as much alpha-tocopherol in human milk as compared to cow's milk. Human milk contained an average of 1.14 mg of alpha-tocopherol per quart, whereas cow's milk varied from 0.21 mg/quart in early spring to 1.06 mg/quart in mid-fall; evaporated, condensed, and nonfat dry milk contained 0.66, 1.29, and 0.02 mg/reconstituted quart, respectively. Kanno et al.[27] reported mean values of alpha- and gamma-tocopherol in mixed milk for a year at 28.3 (range 17.0–39.3) and 1.5 (range 0.5–2.9) µg/g of fat, respectively. Tsugo and Kanno[28] have reviewed the relation between tocopherols and the oxidized flavor of milk, the antioxidant effect of tocopherols on milk fat, and the synergistic effect of a few compounds on the antioxidant activity of tocopherols. The vitamin K_1 content of cow's milk was found by Allen et al.[29] to be 4.4–17.8; and of human milk; 1.3–2.2 µg/L. More recently Isshiki et al.[30] reported a range of 2–5 µg of phylloquinone and 7–13 µg/L of menaquinone in cow's milk versus 2.1 ± 0.9 µg of phylloquinone and 1.3 ± 1 µg of menaquinone per liter in human milk.

Some nutrients are relatively variable in milk, such as folate,[31] while others such as zinc[32] appear more relatively constant. Still others, like vitamin C, change in nutrient content before the milk reaches the consumer. Freshly drawn cow's milk may contain as much as 20–30 mg of vitamin C per quart or liter compared to human milk at about a 50 mg level. Following extraction from the cow, transportation from farm to the processing plant, pasteurization, packaging, storage and distribution to the consumer, milk contains about half of its original content due to the ease of ascorbic acid oxidation, accelerated by exposure to heat, light and oxygen.[33]

NUTRIFICATION OF DAIRY PRODUCTS

Nutrification of dairy products has a long history and continues to be a widespread practice. One of the major activities in this regard has been the nutrification of both liquid and dry skim milk products with vitamins A and D, since all fat-soluble vitamins are removed with the fat or cream phase in manufacturing skim and low fat milks. The addition of vitamin D to whole milk and evaporated milk has been practiced for many years. Nutrification with vitamins E and K has been considered or carried out primarily in milk-base products intended for infant feeding. Since nonfat dry milk supplies practically no vitamin E, it has been proposed that vitamin E be added to dry nonfat milk offered to developing countries.[26]

Mineral additives have been proposed,[34] those which may be naturally low in milk,[12] such as iron, copper, manganese and zinc, but success in their addition is dependent on prevention of nutrient interactions and/or flavor changes.[35] Research continues on mineral nutrification. Multivitamin and mineral-fortified milk has been produced.[36] Additions per quart were made in the 1950s to adjust the natural levels of these nutrients in milk to levels judged more in nutritional balance when related to human requirements: vitamin A, 4000 IU; vitamin D, 400 IU; thiamin, 1 mg; riboflavin, 2 mg; niacin, 10 mg; iron, 10 mg; and iodine, 0.1 mg. Such fortification of whole fluid milk has been limited today. However in 1959, 34–37 states had approved multivitamin and mineral fortified milks.[37]

At the present time, fluid milks are pasteurized and widely nutrified with vitamins A and D. Despite a slight reduction in the contribution of milk and milk products in the total intake of food energy between 1965 and 1977, the contribution of milk and milk products to total vitamin A intake has increased (Fig. 13.3), while the contribution of nonnutrified nutrients (protein, thiamin, riboflavin, calcium) has remained relatively stable or decreased.[37a] Numerous dairy products have been nutrified or proposed to be nutrified with one or more vitamins and/or minerals to enhance their nutritional value. These include milk products such as milk drinks, yogurt, simulated milk products, desserts, cheese substitutes, etc.

Milk and milk products are closely regulated by federal and state provisions. One type of control is standards of identity for vitamin and mineral fortified milk products as covered in the 1989 Code of Federal Regulations[38] relating to optional and mandatory addition of vitamins A and D (Table 13.2). For those interested in the early development of milk laws and regulations in the United States, the review by Nagano and Wade[39] may be consulted.

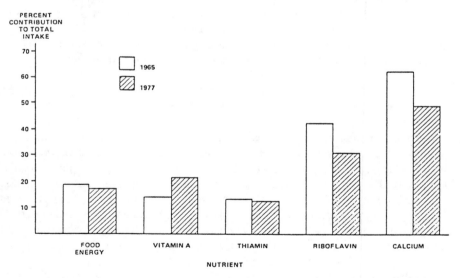

From Heyback et al.[37a]

FIG. 13.3. CONTRIBUTION OF CONSUMPTION OF MILK AND MILK PRODUCTS TO TOTAL INTAKE OF SELECTED NUTRIENTS IN 1965 AND 1977

Source: Data from Nationwide Food Consumption Surveys, 1965–66 and 1977–78.

TABLE 13.2
U.S. CODE OF FEDERAL REGULATIONS ON STANDARDS OF IDENTITY FOR DAIRY PRODUCTS

	Vitamin A		Vitamin D	
Product	Level	Type Requirement	Level	Type Requirement
Milk	not < 2000 IU/qt	optional	400 IU/qt	optional
Acidified milk	not < 2000 IU/qt	optional	400 IU/qt	optional
Cultured milk	not < 2000 IU/qt	optional	400 IU/qt	optional
Concentrated milk	—	—	25 IU/oz	optional
Lowfat dry milk	not < 2000 IU/qt[1]	mandatory	400 IU/qt[1]	optional
Nonfat dry milk	2000 IU/qt[1]	mandatory	400 IU/qt[1]	mandatory
Evaporated milk	125 IU/fl oz	optional	25 IU/oz	mandatory
Evaporated skimmed milk	125 IU/fl oz	mandatory	25 IU/oz	mandatory
Lowfat milk	not < 2000 IU/qt	mandatory	400 IU/qt	optional
Acidified lowfat milk	not < 2000 IU/qt	optional	400 IU/qt	optional
Cultured lowfat milk	not < 2000 IU/qt	optional	400 IU/qt	optional
Skim milk	not < 2000 IU/qt	mandatory	400 IU/qt	optional
Acidified skim milk	not < 2000 IU/qt	optional	400 IU/qt	optional
Cultured skim milk	not < 2000 IU/qt	optional	400 IU/qt	optional
Dry whole milk	not < 2000 IU/qt	optional	400 IU/qt	optional
Yogurt	not < 2000 IU/qt	optional	400 IU/qt	optional
Lowfat yogurt	not < 2000 IU/qt	optional	400 IU/qt	optional
Nonfat yogurt	not < 2000 IU/qt	optional	400 IU/qt	optional
Mellorine	40 IU/g fat	—	—	—

[1]Reconstituted quart.

Rationale

Decades ago the traditional concept in the dairy industry and to some degree the general public was that milk should be consumed as produced by the cow as nature intended and hence should not be manipulated by men. Over time, advances in nutritional knowledge, improved dairy technologies, and economic pressures have altered that position considerably.

With the knowledge of the low natural level of vitamin D in milk and the discernment of nutritional deficiencies, such as rickets in the 1930–40 period, the Food and Nutrition Council of the American Medical Association in 1939, pronounced the addition of not more than 400 units of vitamin D per quart to be in the interest of public health.[40] Irradiation of fluid milk was initiated in the 1928–31 period.[37,41] Since World War II virtually all homogenized fluid whole milk and evaporated milk has been nutrified with the direct addition of vitamin D. The marked decline of rickets in the United States has been attributed, in part, to vitamin D nutrification of milk.[37]

The addition of both vitamin A and D to fluid skim milk used for beverage purposes is widespread today in the United States (Table 13.3). This nutrification prac-

TABLE 13.3
STATE, TERRITORIAL, AND FEDERALLY REGULATED LEVELS
FOR ADDITION OF VITAMINS A AND D TO MILK (USP UNITS/QUART)

Item	Vitamin A in Whole Milk	Vitamin A in Lowfat Milk	Vitamin A in Skim Milk	Vitamin D in Whole Milk	Vitamin D in Lowfat Milk	Vitamin D in Skim Milk
Federal	2,000[1]	2,000	2,000	400[1]	400[1]	400[1]
Alabama	—	2,000	2,000	400	400	400
Alaska	[2]	[2]	[2]	[2]	[2]	[2]
Arizona	[3]	[3]	[4]	400[2]	400[2]	400[2]
Arkansas	[4]	—	[1]	400	—	400
California	[3]	—	[3]	400	—	[3]
Colorado	[3]	—	[5]	400	—	[5]
Connecticut	2,000	[2]	2,000[2]	400	[2]	400[2]
Delaware	[4]	—	[4]	400	—	400
District of Columbia	Illegal	—	2,000	400	—	400
Florida	2,000[2]	2,000[5]	[2]	400[2]	400[5]	[2]
Georgia	2,000	2,000	2,000[2]	400	—	400[2]
Hawaii	—	[2]	[2]	400	[2]	[2]
Idaho	2,000	—	[6]	400	—	[6]
Illinois	[3]	—	2,000	400	—	400
Indiana	[2]	[2]	[2]	[2]	[2]	[2]
Iowa	[3]	[3]	[3]	400	400	400
Kansas	2,000[5]	2,000	2,000	400	400[5]	400[5]
Kentucky	4,000	2,000[1]	2,000	400[1]	400[1]	400[1]
Louisiana	Illegal	2,000	2,000	400	400[1]	—
Maine	2,000[1]	—	2,000[5]	400	—	400[5]
Maryland	2,000	—	2,000	400	—	400
Massachusetts	[2]	[2]	[2]	[2]	[2]	[2]
Michigan	2,000[1]	2,000	2,000	400[1]	400[1]	400
Minnesota	[2]	—	[1]	400	—	400
Mississippi	Illegal	—	2,000	400	—	400
Missouri	2,000[5]	2,000	2,000	400[1]	400[1]	400[1]
Montana	[2]	—	[2]	400	—	400[2]
Nebraska	2,000	—	2,000[2]	400	—	400
Nevada	—	2,000	2,000	400	—	400
New Hampshire	[2]	[2]	2,000	400	[2]	400
New Jersey	2,000	—	[3]	400	—	400
New Mexico	[3,4]	—	[3]	400	—	400
New York	2,000[1]	2,000	2,000[1]	400[1]	400[1]	400[1]
North Carolina	[3]	[5]	2,000	400	[5]	400
North Dakota	2,000	—	2,000	400	—	400
Ohio	[3]	2,000	2,000	400	400[1]	400
Oklahoma	2,000	—	—	400	—	400
Oregon	2,000[2]	2,000[2]	2,000[2]	400[2]	400[2]	400[2]

TABLE 13.3 (*Continued*)

Item	Vitamin A in Whole Milk	Vitamin A in Lowfat Milk	Vitamin A in Skim Milk	Vitamin D in Whole Milk	Vitamin D in Lowfat Milk	Vitamin D in Skim Milk
Pennsylvania	2,000	[1]	2,000	400	[1]	400
Puerto Rico	[3]	[2]	[3]	400	[2]	400
Rhode Island	4,000	—	2,000	400	—	400
South Carolina	[3]	—	2,000	400	—	400
South Dakota	[5]	—	—	400	—	400
Tennessee	[5]	—	2,000	400	400[1]	400
Texas	[4]	—	2,000	400	—	400
Utah	—	—	2,000	400	—	400
Vermont	2,000[1]	2,000[1]	2,000[1]	400[1]	400[1]	400[1]
Virginia	[4]	—	2,000	400	—	400
Washington	[3,4]	5,000	[3]	400	—	400
West Virginia	4,000	—	2,000	400	—	400
Wisconsin	2,000	—	2,000	400	—	400
Wyoming	2,000	—	2,000	400	—	400

Source: Quick and Murphy.[116]
[1]Optional, but when added, not less than quantity shown.
[2]Follows FDA standards.
[3]Quantity not stipulated, but must be declared on the label.
[4]Quantity to be approved by state regulatory authority.
[5]Optional.
[6]Follow U.S. Public Health Service definition.

tice has been justified on the basis that these fat-soluble vitamins are simultaneously removed with the fat in the manufacture of nonfat milk products. Interest in the vitamin A nutrification of sweetened condensed milk was prompted, for example, by such experiences as occurred in Malaya, where it was shown that the vitamin A deficiency diseases of Malayan infants were associated with the consumption of sweetened condensed milk and other modified milk.[42]

In earlier times, nonfat dry milk solids (dry skim milk) produced in developed countries was exported to developing countries as a food supplement primarily for children and pregnant or lactating mothers. Consumption of the high protein supplement accelerated the depletion of the low natural vitamin A reserves, primarily of children, since vitamin A is transported in the body tissues in the form of retinol binding protein complexes. It became obvious that the solution to this vital issue was to export vitamin A nutrified nonfat dry milk.

Since vitamin A deficiency affects mostly young children, UNICEF, with the support of a 1955 joint FAO/WHO Expert Committee Report[43] containing the proposal of vitamin A and D nutrification of surplus world stocks of nonfat dry milk solids for use in underdeveloped countries, began a drive to achieve that goal.[43a] Rickets was also of some concern, and so the vitamin levels were set at 5000 IU of vitamin

A and 500 IU of vitamin D/100 g for export nutrified nonfat dry milk. Time was necessary to develop the technology of producing vitamin A and D nutrified nonfat dry milk solids on a large industrial scale. In 1965, the USDA authorized the vitaminization of nonfat dry milk shipped as food aid under Title II (Food for Peace) of Public Law 480. Further discussions on the nutrification of nonfat dry milk included a tentative list of 74 countries and territories where vitamin A deficiency was a public health problem.[44] Nutrification of foods with vitamin A has not only improved the vitamin A deficiency problems but has also improved iron nutriture of the consuming children, although for total correction of iron deficiency anemia, iron nutrification of food should also be provided.[45]

In general, rationale for vitamin and/or mineral additions to milk products hinges on insufficient nutrient levels in the natural product, on nutrients that are removed or destroyed in some processing procedure, or on a need to supply adequate nutrient levels when for some purpose the milk product serves as the primary or major nutrient source for the nutritional needs of individual or population segments. More recently, calcium nutrified milk products have been introduced,[46] a situation involving a nutrient already naturally in milk. This further amplification appears to have merit from economic considerations and because of great concern about dietary intakes of the mineral in certain age and sex population groups. Iron, another mineral found in dietary surveys to be consumed at inadequate levels, is frequently considered for nutrification in certain milk products. Rees and Monsen[47] contrast iron considerations in the 1970s and 1980s.

Vitamin Forms

The fat-soluble vitamins A, D, E, K and beta-carotene are used for some dairy products in the form of oil solutions or emulsions at desired potency levels for the particular product. For example, vitamin D dispersed in a complete milk carrier is custom packaged for nutrifying fluid milk.[37] Bauernfeind and Parman[48] prepared a liquid concentrate containing vitamin A palmitate and calciferol in hydrogenated coconut oil for use in nonfat dry milk preparation. Conant and Wrenshall[49] used a solution of vitamin A acetate in winterized cottonseed oil at 20,000 IU/g for nutrification of a frozen dessert. Dluzewska et al.[50] fortified sweetened condensed milk using vitamin A palmitate in palm kernel oil homogenized with skim milk and mixed with concentrated full-fat milk. Dry, water-dispersible stabilized beadlet products are manufactured with vitamin A, vitamins A and D, vitamin E, vitamin K, or beta-carotene for blending into dry products or dry products to be reconstituted before consumption.

The water-soluble vitamins (thiamin hydrochloride or mononitrate, riboflavin, niacin, niacinamide, calcium pantothenate, pyridoxine, biotin, folate, and cyanocobalamin) are available in pure, crystalline form for nutrification purposes. For multivitamin nutrification with dry vitamin products, custom-blended premixes are manufactured at desired potency levels and packaged in sizes for batch operations. For example, a mixture of thiamin, riboflavin, and niacin diluted in lactose has been employed and subdivided into packets, each sufficient to enrich 100 gallons of milk.[50a]

Mineral Compounds

Coccodrilli and Shah[51] reviewed the addition of nutrified iron compounds to milk and milk products. For enrichment of pasteurized whole milk, the addition of ferric ammonium citrate prior to heat treatment was recommended.[52,53] Kiran et al.[54] nutrified cow's and buffalo's milk with ferric lactate with or without ascorbic acid. There was no detrimental effect on flavor, color, or rancidity. DeMott[55] determined the effect on milk flavor of nutrifying with iron in the form of various compounds, including ferric pyrophosphate, ferric phosphate, ferrous sulfate, ferric ammonium citrate, ferrous gluconate, and ferrous lactate. Only the two phosphate salts caused minor off-flavors. Tricalcium phosphate with a stabilizer has been employed as one method in the calcium nutrification process.[46]

PROCESSING ASPECTS

Vitamin D fortified milk began with the feeding of vitamin D enriched yeast to the cow which later was replaced by a milk ultraviolet irradiation process and finally by the direct addition of a vitamin concentrate to milk, a process by which greater control could be exercised over vitamin level with less flavor problems. To prepare the concentrate, one type involved dissolution of vitamin D in vegetable oil and in another type vitamin D was dissolved in a water-miscible liquid such as propylene glycol. A third type, a dispersion, was prepared by dissolving vitamin D into butter fat, homogenizing it into a milk product, then canning and sterilizing in size units suitable for nutrifying a given volume of fluid milk or batch of evaporated milk.[37] Either vitamin D_2 or D_3 may be used. This milk base concentrate is most commonly used. The manufacture of the concentrate and its release for milk nutrification is quite a detailed process rigidly monitored, including bioassays for assurance of proper usage and safety. Test procedures involve the basic vitamin, the canned milk concentrate and the final nutrified milk product to satisfy regulations.

When both vitamin A (2000 IU/quart) and D (400 IU/quart) are added to fluid milks, both vitamins can be included in the concentrate so only one addition to milk is required for the resultant vitamin A and D fortified milk. Holland and Winder[56] have discussed the successful manufacture of vitamin A and D nutrified skim milk. Some recent surveys[57-59] of vitamin A and D nutrified fluid milks show wider variations in vitamin content than would be expected; some milk plants have a very small variation from a mean value; others have a wide range. These wider differences are probably a result of operative procedures in the processing plant and warrant a review of (1) the point of addition and type of vitamin concentrate, (2) the uniformity of its addition in continuous operations and (3) subsequent blending operations. Regular review of quality control procedures with periodic vitamin potency testing on any nutrified food product operation is essential, whether in a batch or continous system.

Head and Hansen[60] noted in vitamin A, C, and D nutrified milk no significant changes in vitamin A content on pasteurization and filling operations. Chocolate milk lost a greater amount of ascorbic acid on pasteurization than whole or 1% fat milk. In milk[54] fortified with ascorbic acid (50 mg/100 mL) alone or together with ferric lactate, pasteurization resulted in 10–12% loss of ascorbic acid.

In 1945[61] the feasibility of nutrifying evaporated milk with vitamin C was demonstrated. The effect of preparation, storage conditions and utility of ascorbic acid nutrified evaporated milk has been studied by several investigators.[61–64] It is economically and nutritionally sound to nutrify evaporated milk with 50–100 mg/12 fluid ounces (384.5 mL) for eventual reconstitution to a quart or liter volume, according to Pennsylvania State University researchers.[61,62] Destabilization of milk proteins[61] during sterilization can be avoided by adding sodium ascorbate rather than ascorbic acid. The use of the sodium salt avoids the necessity of adding another buffering agent such as sodium citrate. Conochie[63] also added sodium ascorbate successfully to evaporated milk in a study involving different levels of nutrification. At the 50 mg/L nutrification level of evaporated milk,[61] losses of ascorbic acid due to sterilization were 5.1 and 6.9% when filling and sealing were carried out under nitrogen or vacuum, respectively. A loss of 18.9% was found with normal filling and 23.4% with underfilled cans. At the 100 mg/L nutrification level, percentages of loss were smaller. Bullock et al.,[64] in a report of commercial trials, found the vitamin C content of evaporated milk (fortified by the addition of sodium ascorbate at the rate of 266 g/1000 kg) stored at 21°C for 12 months to remain above the minimum legal standard (Canada Food & Drugs Act) which is equivalent to 14 mg of vitamin C/100 mL of evaporated milk. For optimal stability of vitamin C, it is essential that the cans be sealed under vacuum or nitrogen.[61] Stekel et al.[65] have undertaken detailed field studies on milk products nutrified with vitamin C and iron (ferrous sulfate) for feeding infants and report high iron bioavailability and eradication of anemia in Chile with a program of milk nutrification.

Dluzewska et al.[50] found no significant loss of vitamin A palmitate during nutrification and processing stages of condensed milk. Vitamin D is very stable in milk and is usually not affected by pasteurization, boiling, or sterilization.[14]

Ferric ammonium citrate has been judged to be a suitable additive to milk pasteurized at 81°C by Edmondson et al.,[52] in studies by Kurtz et al.[66] when added to skim milk and skim milk concentrate, and by Wang and King[53] when added to milk. Ranhotra et al.[67] employed a water-soluble citrate phosphate iron complex (16.61% Fe) to fortify milk (38 ppm Fe) with a favorable bioavailability response. Kiran et al.[68] fortified buffalo milk and whey with ferric lactose (25 mg) and ascorbic acid (25 mg/100 mL) and observed that appearance, color, consistency, taste or flavor and keeping quality (3 days, 4 °C) were not affected. Iron availability was good. Fortification of milk with both iron and zinc has been investigated.[69]

Health consciousness, particularly the specter of osteoporosis in older women, has prompted the dairy industry to augment the natural calcium content of milk products by nutrification with added calcium. Within a few years a number of liquid fortified milk products have been marketed, such as Calcimilk (60% more calcium), Bordens' calcium nutrified whole and low-fat milk, Calcium 100, and Vital 15, a low fat, high calcium milk product for women. The interest over calcium nutrification has ushered in a series of reviews dealing with calcification, mineral interactions and calcium bioavailability.[70-72]

Conochie and coworkers[73] contributed greatly to the practical vitamin A nutrification of nonfat dry milk which served as a basis for commercial production of nutrified nonfat dry milk solids in Australia. A batchwise process was proposed in which a synthetic vitamin A acetate oil concentrate was diluted with hydrogenated coconut oil, tocopherol and lecithin as added antioxidants, and homogenized into skim milk concentrate before spray drying. Carr[74] enriched roller-dried nonfat milk using a premix in which vitamin A palmitate was homogenized with hydrogenated coconut oil, soya lecithin, and fluid nonfat milk. This concentrate was mixed with condensed nonfat milk, pasteurized, and roller dried.

Bauernfeind and Allen[75] and Bauernfeind and Parman[48] described both wet-stage and dry-stage procedures for the nutrification of nonfat dry milk with vitamins A and D. In the wet-stage method, antioxidant stabilized vitamin A palmitate (10^6 IU/g) and vitamin D_2 (calciferol) were dissolved and mixed with liquefied hydrogenated coconut fat (melting point 33 °C) to yield a vitamin potency of 10,000 or 25,000 IU of vitamin A and 1000 or 2500 IU of vitamin D/g. The warm vitamin-fat premix is homogenized into warm nonfat milk solids to produce a fine fat emulsion (approximately 1 μ, fat phase) and blended into the appropriate amount of condensed nonfat milk solids and spray dried.

In the dry-stage method, pure stabilized vitamin A palmitate and calciferol in dry beadlet form are introduced uniformly and blended into the constant flow of nonfat dry milk. In either operation, low moisture levels should be attained in the final nutrified dry product. To have a better appreciation of the physical state of the vitamins in the nutrified nonfat dry product, it should be understood that in the wet-stage process the vitamins in the fat carrier are homogenized throughout the condensed milk product, and, hence, are incorporated within each particle of dry milk following spray drying. In the dry-stage process the vitamins remain sealed within the dry beadlet particles uniformly distributed throughout the milk powder and remain so until the nutrified nonfat dry milk is reconstituted with water. The vitamins in nutrified nonfat dry milk manufactured by both processes are fully available biologically.

In a commercial trial (60,000 lb) of the wet-stage manufacturing process of nutrified nonfat dry milk, average recovery of vitamin A in the finished powder, as determined in two different laboratories, was 88 and 90%. Complete recovery of vitamin

D was found by both laboratories. In a large-scale, commercial trial (6,000,000 lb) of the dry-stage process using vitamin A palmitate, Type 250-S beadlets (250,000 IU vitamin A and 50,000 IU vitamin D/g), the vitamin A content found by assay of the finished powder was within 1% of the calculated value.[75] Subsequent studies have appeared by Marquardt[76] on both the wet and dry process, (vitamin A losses favoring the dry process), by Mol et al.[77] on vitamins A and D addition by the wet process, by Slump[78] by the dry process, and also by Killert.[79] A survey[80] of 66 samples of nutrified nonfat dry milk solids from Canadian and U.S. manufacturers showed vitamin A contents of less than 20 to over 30 IU/g of vitamin A, a finding which indicates that processing methods may need to be reviewed and quality control measures intensified.

Freeze-dried cultured milk has been enriched with ascorbic acid (60 mg/kg) and cobalamin (7-10 µg/kg) by adding both vitamins before culturing or drying.[81] A process for enrichment of yogurt with vitamin C was developed[82] in which 20-100 mg of ascorbic acid or its sodium salt were added per 100 g after fermentation. Lowfat yogurt fortified with vitamins A and C made under production conditions and stored for six weeks (3°C) slowly lost vitamin potency, losses being greater for vitamin C than for vitamn A.[83] A process for preparing yogurt with 9 essential vitamins is mentioned by Hannigan.[84] The addition of vitamns to lowfat dairy spreads was investigated in 1987 by Prajapati et al.[85] Mellorine, a vegetable-fat frozen dessert, was nutrified[95] by adding a concentrate of vitamin A in winterized cotton-seed oil (20,000 IU/g) to the dessert mix before pasteurization. The enrichment of milk and milk products with water-soluble vitamins was reviewed by Gregory in 1967.[86] Graham[87] in 1974 reviewed the processing and storage of milk and milk products and the effects of nutrification.

STORAGE ASPECTS

Fluid Milk

Two commercially prepared samples of milk fortified with eight vitamins were tested for stability in the author's laboratory. The first product was stored at 75°F. ($\pm 2°$); and the second, a chocolate-flavored milk, was stored at 86°F ($\pm 2°$). The vitamin stability data for storage periods up to 12 months are summarized (Table 13.4). Riboflavin, niacin, and calcium pantothenate showed good stability. Vitamin A was slightly less stable, while thiamin, ascorbic acid, vitamin B_6, and vitamin B_{12} showed higher losses.

In the United States about a decade ago, production of an ultra-high-temperature (UHT) processed milk began. UHT-processed milk can be stored at room temperature for up to 6 months. Storage stability of vitamin A in fluid milk, either pasteurized or processed by UHT treatment has been reported by LeMaguer and Jackson.[88] In samples stored at 4°C or 20°C, vitamin A losses were minimal in 12 days for

TABLE 13.4
STABILITY OF CANNED, STERILIZED, NUTRIFIED MILK PRODUCTS

Storage Test	Vitamin A (IU)	Thiamin (mg)	Riboflavin (mg)	Ascorbic Acid (mg)	Vitamin B$_6$ (mg)	Vitamin B$_{12}$ (mcg)	Niacin (mg)	Calcium Pantothenate (mg)
Product No. 1								
Initial Content/100 g	392	0.23	0.43	19.9	0.25	0.30	1.28	1.60
% Retention								
6 months at 75°F	94	100	100	82	92	100	98	97
12 months at 75°F	92	74	100	61	66	90	95	95
Product No. 2 (Chocolate-flavored)								
Initial Content/100 g	480	0.25	0.42	3.6	0.30	2.64	2.25	1.72
% Retention								
3 months at 86°F	82	84	100	100	83	76	96	94
6 months at 86°F	90	76	100	100	88	66	96	96
12 months at 86°F	83	48	100	—	88	66	96	100

pasteurized milk and 3 months for UHT-processed milk. Storage for 3 months at 35°C of 2% milk processed by UHT had an adverse effect on vitamin A stability. In low fat (2%) fortified milk[89] sterilized by indirect UHT treatment and stored at 23°C, vitamin A losses appeared to be associated with oxygen content of the containers.

In the author's laboratory homogenized whole milk was fortified with 225 mg/L of sodium ascorbate, pasteurized at 145°F for 30 minutes, and cooled quickly to 50°F. Storage in a refrigerator at 40°F for 5 and 8 days led to losses of vitamin C (reduced and dehydro forms) of 15 and 24%, respectively. Head and Hansen[60] nutrified whole, chocolate, and 1% fat milk with ascorbic acid plus vitamins A and D. Ascorbic acid stability in vitamin A, C and D nutrified milk was studied for up to 36 days at 4°C. The rate of deterioration of ascorbic acid was more rapid initially for chocolate milk, but after 36 days all three types of milk had a retention of about 50%. Addition of the vitamins before or after pasteurization did not significantly influence the stability results. There were no significant changes in vitamin A content during storage.

Evaporated Milk

At the 50 mg/L addition level of ascorbic acid to processed and canned evaporated milk stored for 12 months at room temperature, 47.2% of the ascorbic acid content was lost when the cans were filled normally but only about 32% when filled under nitrogen or vacuum. When underfilled by the normal method, the loss was 83%. At the 100 mg/L fortification level, the corresponding storage losses were lower.[61] Pelletier and Morrison[90] and Bullock et al.[64] also reported stability data on ascorbic acid in evaporated milk. In the latter case, sodium ascorbate was added commercially in two plants to provide 24.8 or 26.2 mg of ascorbic acid/100 mL of evaporated milk. On storage for 12 months at 21°C, the mean losses found were 18 and 21%. When the storage temperature was 36°C, the losses of ascorbic acid in the 2 products were 56 and 55% in 12 months.

Condensed Milk

Sokolov[91] stored sweetened condensed milk nutrified with vitamin A and ascorbic acid for 9 months at 10–15°C. Average loss of vitamin A was 3.8% and of vitamin C, 18.5–21.3%. In a 6-month storage test[92] of sweetened condensed milk nutrified with either a water-miscible vitamin A preparation (100,000 IU/mL) or an oil solution of vitamin A acetate (1,000,000 IU/g), both types were stable at 30 or 40°C. Losses of vitamin A of less than 10% were found[50] on storage of condensed milk nutrified with vitamin A palmitate for 6 months at either 4–6° or 18–20°C. The vitamin A content of nutrified recombined sweetened condensed milk with vitamin A palmitate (200 IU/ounce) added before processing remained fairly constant during storage for up to 12 months as reported by Kieseker and Dunkerley.[93]

Cheese

The stability of added beta-carotene and/or beta-apo-8'-carotenal (vitamin A precursors) in various cheese products, including canned cheese spread, cheddar, primary, and processed cheeses, was shown by Klaeui and Bauernfeind.[94] Addition of the carotenoid was made either to the milk before processing or to the warm cheese. Packaging of the cheese spread was in sealed cans, the cheddar and primary cheeses were waxed wedges, and the processed cheeses were packaged in film. On storage for 12 months at 80–75°F, the retention of carotene was 92–100% and of apo-carotenal, 88–100%.

Frozen Desserts

Bauernfeind et al.[95] observed good retention during processing and storage of synthetic vitamin A added to ice cream. Conant and Wrenshall[49] reported that a solution of vitamin A acetate in winterized cottonseed oil at a potency of 20,000 IU/g could be added to a "Mellorine" mix before pasteurization to provide 10,000 IU/gallon in the finished product. Vitamin A was found to be quite stable: a manufacturing addition overage of 10–15% was suggested to assure label potency claim for the product.

Dry Milk

Storage stability trials of vitamins A and D in nutrified nonfat dry milk have been reported.[48,73,75,77,96–98] Data from laboratory storage trials[75] of such a product made on a commercial scale by the wet-stage process are given in Table 13.5. Losses of vitamin A are relatively low in 12 months at 75° and 86°F, only about 13% in 12 months at 75° and 86°F and only about 30% in 12 months at 98°F. Vitamin D is more stable than vitamin A, particularly at 98°F. Samples of this same milk powder were stored under field conditions in various countries for periods varying from 10–27 months. Stability data on samples returned for assay of vitamins A and D are listed in Table 13.6. Even after 2 years, about ⅔ of the vitamin A was retained from all of the areas in the test. Vitamin D was very stable in all cases. Accelerated storage tests of vitamins A and D_2 in nonfat milk powder prepared by the dry-stage process are shown in Table 13.7. Even at these high temperatures, and in one test at high relative humidity, the stability of vitamin A was good and no significant loss of vitamin D_2 was found. The satisfactory stability of vitamins A and D_2, as shown in Tables 13.5–13.7, as well as the acceptable organoleptic properties and stability on reconstitution,[75] indicate that it is feasible and practical to nutrify nonfat dry milk with vitamins A and D_2 using either the wet- or dry-stage process.

Conochie and Wilkinson[73] found losses of vitamin A to be less than 10% after 6 months storage (40°C) of vitamin A nutrified nonfat dry milk solids. Vitamin A stability during storage of nutrified dry skim milk stored for 3 months (40°C) by

TABLE 13.5
STABILITY OF VITAMINS A AND D_2 IN NUTRIFIED NONFAT DRY MILK

	Wet-stage Process: Laboratory Storage				
	Initial Assay (IU/g)		Storage Temperature	% Retention in 12 Months	
Package	Vitamin A	Vitamin D_2	(°F)	Vitamin A	Vitamin D_2
Box[1]	94.0	11	75	88	91
Can	97.5	11	75	87	91
Box[1]	94.0	11	86	84	83
Can	97.5	11	86	87	91
Box[1]	94.0	11	98	70	100
Can	97.5	11	98	71	91

Source: Bauernfeind and Allen.[75]
[1] 4.5-lb polyethylene-lined chipboard container.

Mol et al.[77] DeBoer et al.[96] reported variable vitamin A levels in nutrified nonfat dry milk solids in a market survey and high storage losses accelerated by heat and light exposure.

In nutrification trials gelatin encapsulated vitamin A beadlets, blended into nonfat dry milk solids, sprayed with hot water (45 mL/400g) for 3 minutes, then dried for 9 minutes with hot air exhibited a 60% vitamin A loss in storage trials. Similar trials without the wetting step showed up to a 10% storage loss.[97] The beadlets are easily dispersed in hot water and once dispersed, the built-in physical stability characteristic is destroyed, hence the above type of results may be expected. Woolard and Edmiston[98] conducted stability tests for two years at ambient temperature of whole milk powders and skim milk powders in bulk packages nutrified with vitamins A, E, and C plus thiamin, riboflavin, niacin, and pyridoxine. All vitamins, except vitamin A, survived storage without loss. The vitamin A loss was rapid in the short term and continued at a reduced rate as time progressed.

Guy and Vettel[99] formulated a chocolate-flavored powder containing milk solids, sugar, eggs, vitamins, and minerals to be reconstituted for beverage use. Adequate storage stability of the product was demonstrated. An instant milk drink with strawberry flavor nutrified with 1400 IU vitamin A and 0.5 mg pyridoxine/25 g was tested for stability in the author's laboratory. Both vitamins showed no significant loss in 6 weeks at 113% for 12 months at 75°F.

Reconstituted Milk

Samples of dry-stage and wet-stage processed, fortified nonfat milk were reconstituted and boiled for either 2 or 30 minutes.[75] The dry-stage milk, which contained 11,700 IU/L of vitamin A after reconstitution, retained 96% of the vitamin A after 2 minutes boiling and 94% after 30 minutes. The wet-stage milk, which

TABLE 13.6
STABILITY OF VITAMINS A AND D_2 IN NUTRIFIED NONFAT DRY MILK

Sample[1] Storage Location	Months of Storage	Wet-stage Process: Field Storage				
		Moisture[2] Content (%)	% Vitamin A Retention		% Vitamin D_2 Retention	
			Lab X	Lab Z	Lab X	Lab Z
Brazil						
Acu	15	6.1	82	81	—	100
Natal	15	6.7	82	87	—	100
Natal	26	7.7	65	52	68	100
Guatemala						
Guatemala City	10	—	96	81	—	100
Puerto San Jose	23	7.3	71	71	75	100
Puerto San Jose	27	7.4	66	64	76	100
Indonesia						
Djakarta	15	6.4	66	88	95	100
Bogor	18	8.9	83	72	80	100
Djakarta	23	7.9	70	64	87	88
Iran						
Tehran	15	5.3	64	95	96	100
Meshed	18	—	105	93	—	—
Tehran	23	5.0	104	102	100+	—
Tehran	27	5.0	87	72	94	100
Kenya						
Nairobi	15	5.7	104	91	—	100
Nairobi	18	—	101	91	—	—
Nairobi	26	6.7	86	65	84	100

Source: Bauernfeind and Allen.[75]
[1]Samples packaged in 4.5-lb polyethylene-lined chipboard containers.
[2]Moisture content of all samples at time of production, approximately 3.5%.

TABLE 13.7
STABILITY OF VITAMINS A AND D₂ IN NUTRIFIED NONFAT DRY MILK

	Dry-stage Process: Laboratory Storage[1]					
	Vitamin A				Vitamin D	
	Laboratory X		Laboratory Z		Laboratory Z	
Sample Storage	(IU/g)	(% Ret.)	(IU/g)	(% Ret.)	(IU/g)	(% Ret.)
Initial	88[2]	—	96.0	—	15	—
500 h/113°F	92	100+	94.3	98	15	100
1000 h/113°F	84	95	86.5	90	15	100
2000 h/113°F	—	—	86.5	90	15	100
3 mos/98°F	85	96	—	—	—	—
3 mos/100°F and 90% Rel. Humidity	—	—	83.8	87	15	100

Source: Bauernfeind and Allen.[75]
[1]Samples packaged in standard 4.5-lb polyethylene-lined chipboard containers.
[2]Claimed value, not assayed.

contained 4700 IU/L of vitamin A, retained 94 and 91% of the vitamin A after 2 and 30 minutes boiling, respectively. Wilkinson and Conochie[100] reconstituted vitamin A nutrified dry skim milk and observed 2 to 22% losses when heating to boiling (10 minutes) and 30% loss after boiling for 30 minutes. Nonfat dry milk solids nutrified with vitamins A and D and stored under different time and heat conditions, reconstituted and held 1 or 3 days at 40°F showed vitamin A retention values of 86–100%.

In the author's laboratory, a milk-base powder was nutrified with the following levels of vitamins per reconstituted quart: vitamin A, 6750 IU; thiamin, 3.38 mg; riboflavin, 5.4 mg; pyridoxine, 2.3 mg; and ascorbic acid, 122 mg. The nutrified liquid was pasteurized and stored for 5 days in a household refrigerator. The percentage of retentions after pasteurization and after storage were as follows: vitamin A, 95 and 95; B_1, 99 and 93; B_2, 100 and 96; B_6, 100 and 100; and vitamin C, 41 and 41.

Infant Products

The stability of a modified liquid milk product fortified with 0.5 or 1.0 mg of vitamin B_6 (pyridoxine) per liter and canned was studied in the author's laboratory. On storage for 12 months at room temperature (72 ±2°F), the losses of vitamin B_6 were 9–10%.

Du[101] nutrified a milk powder for infants with vitamins A, D, E, and C plus thiamin, riboflavin, and niacin and reported the vitamin levels to remain almost unchanged after a 3 month storage period. Samples of a canned, dry infant formula nutrified with vitamin A to provide 2500 IU/quart after reconstitution were tested in the author's laboratory and found to retain the claimed level of vitamin A after storage for 12 months (75 ±2°F).

In reconstituted milk prepared from nonfat dry milk nutrified with vitamin A palmitate or acetate,[102] the vitamin A potency was retained for 48 h at room temperature. However, when the nutrified powder was used to produce khoa by reconstitution and boiling, there was a vitamin A loss of 22% which was preventable by the addition of 5% hydrogenated coconut fat.

Carrier Effect

Skim milk and 2% fat milk were nutrified with vitamin A palmitate in either maize, groundnut, coconut or butter oil as a carrier. The fortified milks, pasteurized and homogenized, were exposed in glass tubes to fluorescent light. Samples with coconut and butter oil showed less light degradation of vitamin A than maize and groundnut oil samples. Furthermore less degradation occurred with increasing level of oil carrier.[103] Degradation rates were increased when homogenization pressures were reduced. Lipid photooxidation did not parallel vitamin degradation during light exposure. Lau et al.[104] also observed improved vitamin A stability in ultra high temperature nutrified liquid milk with higher fat levels.

Light Effect

In addition to vitamin A, riboflavin, and vitamin C loss in nutrified milk upon sufficient exposure of light, a haylike flavor can develop in vitamin A nutrified fluid milk products under certain conditions. The off-flavor is accelerated by high exposure to light and can be retarded by previous antioxidant addition and use of opaque containers. The off-flavor has been attributed to oxidative deterioration of vitamin A.[105] Suyama et al.[106] likened the off-flavor to thermal oxidation products of vitamin A. Beta-ionone and dihydroactinidiolide have a haylike flavor. Addition of ascorbic acid acts as an antioxidant in skim milk and delays vitamin A degradation. Recent studies on the effect of light on vitamin A in milk involve the amount and intensity of light[107] and commercial fluorescent lighting.[108]

Container Effect

Hartman and Dryden[14] mention that the destruction of vitamin A in nutrified skim milk, upon exposure to light, was retarded by the use of amber or brown glass bottles or foil-laminated wax paper cartons. Light at wavelengths 400–500 mμ penetrate deeper into skim milk than whole milk, making the container a critical component of the product. Senyk and Shipe[109] found fiberboard and tinted plastic to give moderate protection against vitamin A loss and riboflavin degradation. Murphy et al.[108] observed paperboard containers to give the best protection against loss of vitamin A potency of fortified skim milk under the stress of retail fluorescent lighting.

Bauernfeind and Allen[75] evaluated various containers for storage of nonfat dry milk enriched with vitamins A and D. Container effectiveness was judged by the retention of vitamin A after a year's storage at 24°C. Retentions of vitamin were 96% for vacuum-packed tin cans, 92% for laminated pouches, 90% for polyethylene bags in cardboard cylinders and for tin cans with air pack, 89% for cardboard cylinders with metal ends, and 81% for polyethylene bags alone.

When milk in clear glass bottles is exposed to sunlight for as little as 2 h, the destruction of riboflavin can be as much as 80%.[14] Singh et al.[110] exposed milk at 4.4°C for 48 h under 300 ft-c light intensity and found 11% loss of riboflavin in both glass and blow-molded polyethylene containers but only 3% loss in paperboard and gold-pigmented, blow-molded polyethylene containers.

Sedlacek et al.[111] studied the effect of packaging on dried milk to which 100–300 mg/L of ascorbic acid, and in some cases also sodium citrate, had been added. In cold storage tests at room temperature and at 37°C, the best ascorbic acid protection was provided by cans filled with nitrogen, followed in decreasing order by cans with air pack, foil-lined paper cartons, and unlined paper cartons.

FUTURE TRENDS

As has been mentioned by Hettinga,[112] this question can be raised: "Why alter milk composition?" Available technology enables milk to be divided into various components.[113–115] When one considers the availability of components resulting from fractionation of other food sources and those nutrients manufactured by chemical or microbial processes, the potential for the creation of new food products becomes greater than in the past. Human nutritional needs, regulatory practices, economic considerations and marketing practices will be the influencing factors in the development of nutrified milk products of the future.

REFERENCES

1. LUQUET, F. M. 1985. Milk and Milk Products Technique et Documentation. Lavoisier, Paris.
2. RENNER, E. and RENZ-SCHAUEN, A. 1986. Nutritional Value Tables for Milk and Milk Products. Velag B. Renner, Giessen, Germany.
3. RENNER, E. and RENZ-SCHAUEN, A. 1987. First Supplement E1/78, Nutrition Value Tables for Milk and Milk Products. Verlag B. Renner, Giessen, Germany.
4. ANON. 1987. Milk Facts. Milk Industry Foundation, Washington, DC.
5. SPECKMANN, E. W. 1986. Present and future health issues and dairy products. Proc. XXII Int. Dairy Congr. The Hague, D. Reidel Publishing Co., Dordrecht.
6. McBRAN, L. D., ALCANTARA, E. N. and SPECKMANN, E. W. 1986. Changing patterns in the dairy industry. In Dietary Fat and Cancer, I. P. Clement, D. F. Birt, A. E. Rogers and C. Mattlin (eds.). Alan R. Liss, New York.

7. SPECKMANN, E. W. 1984. Nutritional characteristics of dairy products. *In* Dairy Products for the Cereal Processing Industry, J. L. Vetter (ed.). Am. Assoc. Cereal Chemists, St. Paul.
8. ANON. 1988. Newer Knowledge of Milks and Other Fluid Dairy Products. National Dairy Council, Rosemont.
9. POSATI, L. P. and ORR, M. L. 1976. Composition of Foods. Dairy and Egg Products, Raw, Processed, Prepared. Agricultural Handbook 8-1, U.S. Dept. of Agriculture, Washington, DC.
10. TISCORNIA, E. 1977. Present knowledge of the chemical composition of food milk. Riv. Soc. Ital. Sci. Aliment. *6*, 423–452.
11. FLYNN, A. and POWER, P. 1985. Nutritional aspects of minerals in bovine and human milks. Dev. Dairy Chem. *3*, 183–215.
12. PENNINGTON, J. A. T., WILSON, D. B., YOUNG, B. E., JOHNSON, R. D. and VANDERVEEN, J. E. 1987. Mineral content of market samples of fluid whole milk. J. Am. Dietet. Assoc. *87*(8), 1036–1047.
13. YAMAUCHI, K. 1979. Chemistry of human milk components. How they differ from cow's milk components. II. Lipids, glucides, minerals, and vitamins. Nippon Nogei Kagaku Kaishi *53*, R49–R60.
14. HARTMAN, A. M. and DRYDEN, L. P. 1974. Vitamins in milk and milk products. *In* Fundamentals of Dairy Chemistry, 2nd Ed., B. H. Webb, A. H. Johnson and J. A. Alford (eds.). AVI/Van Nostrand Reinhold, New York.
15. SCOTT, K. J., BISHOP, D. R., ZECHALKO, A. and EDWARDS-WEBB, J. D. 1984. Nutrient content of liquid milk. J. Dairy Res. *51*(1), 37–57.
16. ANON. 1976. Composition and nutritive value of dairy foods. Dairy Counc. Dig. *47*(5).
17. CREMIN, F. M. and POWER, P. 1985. Vitamins in bovine and human milks. Dev. Dairy Chem. *3*, 337–398.
18. ROGINSKI, H. 1989. Fermented milks. Austr. J. Dairy Technol. *42*(2), 37–46.
19. TAMINE, A. Y. and ROBINSON, R. K. 1988. Fermented milks and their future trends. J. Dairy Res. *55*, 281–307.
20. KLUPSCH, H. J. 1984. Cultured Milk Products, Flavored Milk Drinks and Desserts. Verlag Th. Mann. Gelsenkirchen-Buer.
21. KAMBE, M. 1986. Traditional cultured milks of the world. New Food Ind. *28*(10), 39–50.
22. ANON. 1983. Imitation and substitute dairy products. Dairy Counc. Dig. *54* (1).
22a. RENNER, E. 1988. Effects of agricultural practices on milk and dairy products. *In* Nutritional Evaluation of Food Processing, 3 Ed., E. Karmas and R. S. Harris (eds.). Van Nostrand Reinhold, New York.
23. LEERBECK, E. and SOENDERGAARD, H. 1980. The total content of vitamin D in human milk and cow's milk. Br. J. Nutr. *4*, 7–12.
24. HOLLIS, B. W., ROOS, B. A., DRAPER, H. H. and LAMBERT, P. W. 1981. Vitamin D and its metabolites in human and bovine milk. J. Nutr. *111*, 1240–1248.
25. REEVE, L. E., JORGENSON, N. A. and DeLUCA, H. F. 1982. Vitamin D compounds in cows milk. J. Nutr. *112*(4), 667–672.
26. HERTING, D. C. and DRURY, E. J. E. 1969. Vitamin E content of milk, milk products and simulated milks: Relevance to infant nutrition. Am. J. Clin. Nutr. *22*, 147–155.
27. KANNO, C., YAMAUCHI, K. and TSUGO, T. 1968. Occurrences of gamma-tocopherol and variation of alpha- and gamma-tocopherol in bovine milk fat. J. Dairy Sci. *51*, 1713–1719.

28. TSUGO, T. and KANNO, C. 1969. Distribution of tocopherols in cows' milk and their antioxidant effect. Eiyo To Shokuryo 22, 587–600.
29. ALLAN, V., HARRON, Y. and BARKHAN, P. 1980. Vitamin K metabolism. Vitamin K-dependent proteins. In Proc. Steenbock Symp. 8th, 1979, J. W. Suttie (ed.). University Park Press, Baltimore.
30. ISSHIKI, H., SUZUKI, Y., YONEKUBO, A., HASEGAWA, H. and YAMAMOTO, Y. 1988. Determination of phylloquinone and menaquinone in milk using high performance liquid chromatography. J. Dairy Sci. 71(3), 627–632.
31. HOPPNER, K. and LAMPI, B. 1981. Seasonal variations of folacin levels in market fluid milks. Can. Inst. Food Sci. Technol. J. 14(3), 218–219.
32. JOERIN, M.M. 1978. Zinc levels in bulk bovine milk. N. Z. J. Dairy Sci. Technol. 13(3), 177.
33. BAUERNFEIND, J. C. and PINKERT, D. M. 1970. Food processing with added ascorbic acid. Adv. Food Res. 18, 219–315.
34. SALTMAN, P. and HEGENAUER, J. 1983. Trace elements in milk. Kiel. Milchwirtsch. Forschungsber. 35(3), 381–387.
35. HAZELL, T. 1985. Minerals in foods: dietary sources, chemical forms, interactions, bioavailability. World Rev. Nutr. Dietet. 46, 1–123.
36. CARLSON, W. A. 1960. Multi-vitamin mineral milk. Am. Milk Rev. 22, 60–64.
37. COULTER, S. T. and THOMAS, E. L. 1968. Enrichment and fortification of dairy products and margarine. J. Agr. Food Chem. 16, 158–162.
37a. HEYBACH, J. P., COCCODRILLI, G. D., JR. and LEVEILLE, G. A. 1988. The contribution of consumption of processed foods to nutrient intake status in the United States. In Nutritional Evaluation of Food Processing, 3rd Ed., E. Karmas and R. S. Harris (eds.). Van Nostrand Reinhold, New York.
38. ANON. 1989. Code of Federal Regulations 21, parts 100–169. Off. Fed. Reg. Natl. Archives & Record Admin., Washington, DC.
39. NAGANO, M. and WADA, T. 1978. Studies on milk laws and regulations: Dairy legislation from the 1850s to 1923 in USA. Bull. Coll. Agr. Vet. Med. Nihon Univ. 35, 405–418.
40. ANON. 1939. Fortification of foods with vitamins and minerals. J. Am. Med. Assoc. 113, 681.
41. WECKEL, K. G. 1953. Theory and practice of vitamin D fortification of milk. Quart. Rev. Pediatr. 8, 224–231.
42. LOFTUS HILLS, G. 1953. Vitamin A deficiency in Malaya: Criticism of sweetened condensed milk for infant feeding. Austr. J. Dairy Technol. 8(4), 129–130.
43. ANON. 1955. Joint FAO/WHO Expert Committee on Nutrition. FAO Nutr. Rep. Ser. Q; WHO Tech. Rep. 97.
43a. ANON. 1959. WHO/FAO/UNICEF Protein Advisory group statement. Restricted document, June.
44. ANON. 1976. Vitamin A enrichment of donated foods (with special reference to dry skim milk powder). PAG Bull. 6(4) 1–7; (1973), 3(1), 1–2.
45. MEJIA, L. A. and CHEW, F. 1988. Hematological effect of supplementing anemic children with vitamin A alone and in combination with iron. Am. J. Clin. Nutr. 48(9), 595.

46. ANON. 1986. Calcium milk products satisfy health conscious America. Dairy Field *169*, 21–23.
47. REES, J. M. and MONSEN, E. R. 1985. Iron fortification of infant foods. Clin. Pediatr. *24*(12), 707–710.
48. BAUERNFEIND, J. C. and PARMAN, G. K. 1964. Restoration of nonfat dry milk with vitamins A and D. Food Technol. *18*(2), 52–57.
49. CONANT, H. B. and WRENSHALL, C. L. 1953. Vitamin A fortification of vegetable-fat frozen dessert. Ice Cream Trade J. *49* (9), 24–26.
50. DLUZEWSKA, A., PAWLIK, S., BILINSKA, M. and LOCHOWSKA, H. 1969. Fortification of concentrated and condensed milk with vitamin A. Rocz. Inst. Przem. Mlecz. *11*, 53–69.
50a. JOHNSON, H. J. 1970. Multivitamin food enrichment composition. U.S. Pat. 3,536,494, Oct. 27.
51. COCCODRILLI, G., Jr. and SHAH, N. 1985. Beverages. *In* Iron Fortification of Foods, F. M. Clydesdale and K. L. Wiemer (eds.). Academic Press, New York.
52. EDMONDSON, L. F., DOUGLAS, F. W., Jr. and AVANTS, J. K. 1971. Enrichment of pasteurized whole milk with iron. J. Dairy Sci. *54*, 1422–1426.
53. WANG, C. F. and KING, R. L. 1973. Chemical and sensory evaluation of iron-fortified milk. J. Food Sci. *38*, 938–940.
54. KIRAN, R., AMMA, M. K. P. and SAREEN, K. N. 1977. Milk fortification with a system containing both iron and ascorbic acid. Indian J. Nutr. Diet. *14*, 260–266.
55. DeMOTT, B. J. 1971. Effects on flavors of fortifying milk with iron and absorption of iron from intestinal tracts of rats. J. Dairy Sci. *54*, 1609–1614.
56. HOLLAND, B. K. and WINDER, W. C. 1951. Preparation of modified skim milk. Milk Dealer *40*(11), 43, 92–96.
57. SHIPE, W. F. and SENYK, G. F. 1985. Problems associated with the addition of vitamin A concentrates to fluid milk. J. Dairy Science *68*(Suppl. 1), 94.
58. McGEE, T. S., FRANKE, A. A. and BRUHAN, J. C. 1987. Observations on the availability of vitamin A concentration during processing of fortified milks at plants in California. J. Dairy Sci. *70*(Suppl. 1), 73.
59. TANNER, J. T. *et al.* 1988. Survey of vitamin content of fortified milk. JAOAC *71*(3), 607–610.
60. HEAD, M. K. and HANSEN, A. 1979. Stability of L-ascorbic acid added to whole, chocolate, and low-fat milks. J. Dairy Sci. *62*, 352–354.
61. JOSEPHSON, D. V. and DOAN, F. J. 1945. Ascorbic acid in evaporated milk. Bull. 473, Pa. State Coll., Agr. Exp. Sta., State College.
62. DOAN, F. J. and JOSEPHSON, D. V. 1946. Additional observations on the stability of ascorbic acid and sodium L-ascorbic acid in evaporated milk. J. Dairy Sci. *29*(9), 625–628.
63. CONOCHIE, J. 1958. The stability of sodium ascorbate in evaporated milk. Austr. J. Dairy Technol. *13*(2), 80, 82.
64. BULLOCK, D. H., SINGH, S. and PEARSON, A. M. 1968. Stability of vitamin C in enriched commercial evaporated milk. J. Dairy Sci. *51*, 921–923.
65. STEKEL, A. *et al.* 1985. The role of ascorbic acid in the bioavailability of iron from infant food. Int. J. Vit. Nutr. Res. *27*(Suppl.), 167–175.
66. KURTZ, F. E., TAMSMA, A. and PALLANSCH, M. J. 1973. Effect of fortification

with iron on susceptibility of skim milk and nonfat dry milk to oxidation. J. Dairy Sci. 56, 1139–1143.
67. RANHOTRA, G. S., GELROTH, J. A., TORRENCE, F. A., BOCK, M. A. and WINTERRINGER, G. L. 1981. Bioavailability of iron-fortified fluid milk. J. Food Sci. 46, 1342–1344.
68. KIRAN, R., KAUR, I. P. and VANEJA, K. 1986. Studies on the acceptability and availability of forticants present in milk and whey. J. Food. Sci. Technol. 23(2), 110–111.
69. MOMCILOVIC, B. and KELLO, D. 1979. Fortification of milk with zinc and iron. Nutr. Rep. Int. 20, 429–436.
70. HEANEY, R. P. 1986. Osteoporosis: the need and opportunity for calcium fortification. Cereal Foods World 31(5), 349–351.
71. SMITH, K. T. 1988. Calcium and trace mineral interactions. Cereal Foods World 33(9), 776–781.
72. GREGER, J. L. 1988. Calcium bioavailability. Cereal Foods World 33(8), 796–799; 1987. Nutr. Today, July-August, 4–9.
73. CONOCHIE, J. and WILKINSON, R. A. 1956: The fortification of non-fat milk solids with vitamin A. XIV Int. Dairy Congr. Proc. 1(2), 357–366; 1955. Butter Fat Solids 14, 147.
74. CARR, W. R. 1961. The enrichment of roller-dried nonfat milk with vitamin A. Rhodesia Agr. J. 58(1), 38–41.
75. BAUERNFEIND, J. C. and ALLEN, L. E. 1963. Vitamin A and D enrichment of nonfat dried milk. J. Dairy Sci. 46, 245–254.
76. MARQUARDT, H. G. 1976. Vitaminization of spray dried skim milk. Dtsch. Milchwirtsch. 27(49), 1776; 1979. 30(4), 118–120.
77. MOL, J. J., DAMMAN, A. J. and EISSES, J. 1976. Vitamin enrichment of dried skim milk. Zuivelzicht 68(37), 802–803.
78. SLUMP, H. 1976. Vitaminization of dried skim milk. Zuivelzicht 68(27/28), 637–639.
79. KILLERT, V. 1979. Vitaminization: An example using dried skim milk. Ernaehrung (Vienna) 2, 15–17.
80. NAKAI, S. et al. 1983. Vitamin A and haylike flavor in nonfat dry milk and pasteurized low fat milks. Can. Inst. Food Sci. Technol. J. 16(2), 116–122.
81. RADAEVA, I. A. and PETROVA, ZH.YU. 1973. Enrichment of sour milk products by sublimation drying using vitamins C and B_{12}. Tr. Vseross. Nauchno-Issled. Inst. Molochn. Prom. 32, 35–58.
82. MORIMOTO, K. and KAWAMOTO, K. 1955. Ascorbic acid for the enrichment of yogurt. Mie Diagaku Nogakubu Gakjutsu Hokoku 11, 39–44.
83. ILIC, D. B. and ASHOOR, S. H. 1988. Stability of vitamins A and C in fortified yogurt. J. Dairy Sci. 71, 1492–1498.
84. HANNIGAN, K. J. 1978. Yogurt, the wonder ingredient. Food Eng., May, 118–119.
85. PRAJAPATI, P. S., PATEL, A. A. and GUPTA, S. K. 1987. Ingredients for low fat dairy spreads. Indian Dairyman 39(4), 181–185.
86. GREGORY, M. E. 1967. Review of the progress of dairy science. IV. Nutritive value of milk and milk products. J. Dairy Res. 34, 169–181.
87. GRAHAM, D. M. 1974. Alteration of nutritive value resulting from processing and fortification of milk and milk products. J. Dairy Sci. 57, 738–745.
87a. ARNOLD, S. and ROBERTS, T. 1982. UHT milk: Nutrition, safety and convenience. Nat. Food Rev. NFR-18 (Spring), 2–5.

88. LeMAGUER, I. and JACKSON, H. 1983. Stability of vitamin A in pasteurized and ultra-high temperature processed milk. J. Dairy Sci. 66, 2452-2458.
89. McCARTHY, D. A., KARUDA, Y. and ARNOTT, D. R. 1986. Vitamin A stability in ultra high-temperature processed milk. J. Dairy Sci. 69(8), 2045-2051.
90. PELLETIER, O. and MORRISON, A. B. 1965. Stability of ascorbic acid in evaporated milk. Can. Med. Assoc. J. 92, 1089.
91. SOKOLOV, F. 1954. Fortification of sweetened condensed milk with ascorbic acid and vitamin A. Molochn. Prom. 15(1), 34-35.
92. CONOCHIE, J. and WILKINSON, R. A. 1958. The stability of vitamin A and carotene in sweetened condensed milk. Austr. J. Dairy Technol. 13(1), 27-28.
93. KIESEKER, F. G. and DUNKERLY, J. 1966. Vitamin fortification of recombined sweetened condensed milk. Austr. J. Dairy Technol. 21, 110-111.
94. KLAEUI, H. and BAUERNFEIND, J. C. 1981. Carotenoids as food colors. In Carotenoids as Colorants and Vitamin A Precursors, J. C. Bauernfeind (ed.). Academic Press, New York.
95. BAUERNFEIND, J. C., ROKOSNY, A. D., and SIEMERS, G. F. 1953. Synthetic vitamin A aids food fortification. Food Eng. 25, (6), 81-82, 85, 87.
96. DeBOER, M., DeMAN, L., and DeMAN, J. M. 1984. Effect of time and storage condition on vitamin A in instantized nonfat dry milk. J. Dairy Sci. 67, 2188-2191.
97. DeMAN, J. M., DeMAN, L. and WYGERDE, T. 1986. Stability of vitamin A beadlets in nonfat dry milk. Milchwissenschaft 41(8), 468-469.
98. WOOLARD, D. C. and EDMISTON, A. D. 1983. Stability of vitamins in fortified milk powders during a two-year storage period. N. Z. J. Dairy Sci. Technol. 18, 21-26; 1985, J. Micronutr. Anal. 1, 13-21.
99. GUY, E. J. and VETTEL, H. E. 1975. High quality protein, vitamin, and mineral fortified chocolate-flavored powder for beverage use. J. Dairy Sci. 58, 432-435.
100. WILKINSON, H. A. and CONOCHIE, J. 1958. The stability of vitamin A reconstituted fortified non-fat milk solids: the effect of heat. Austr. J. Dairy Technol. 13(1), 29-31.
101. DU, M. 1983. A research note on multivitamin milk powder for infants. Shipin Kexue (Beijing) 45, 44-47.
102. ANANTAKRISHNAN, C. P. and CONOCHIE, J. 1958. Vitamin A in reconstituted fortified nonfat milk solids. Austr. J. Dairy Technol. 13, 151-154.
103. ZAHAR, M., SMITH, D. E. and WARTHESEN, J. J. 1986. Effect of carrier type and amount on vitamin A light degradation in fortified lowfat and skim milks. J. Dairy Sci. 69, 2038-2044; 1987. 70(1), 13-19.
104. LAU, B. L. T., KAKUDA, Y. and ARNOTT, D. R. 1986. Effect of milk fat on the stability of vitamin A in ultra-high temperature milk. J. Dairy Sci. 69, 2052-2059.
105. WECKEL, K. G. and CHICOYE, E. 1954. Factors responsible for the development of a haylike flavor in vitamin A fortified lowfat milk. J. Dairy Sci. 37(1), 1346-1352.
106. SUYAMA, K., YEOW, T. and NAKAI, S. 1983. Vitamin A oxidation products responsible for haylike flavor production in nonfat dry milk. J. Agr. Food Chem. 31(1), 72-76.
107. GAYLORD, A. M., WARTHESEN, J. J. and SMITH, D. E. 1986. Influence of milk fat, milk solids and light intensity on the light stability of vitamin A and riboflavin in lowfat milk. J. Dairy Sci. 69, 2779-2784.
108. MURPHY, P., ENGELHARDT, R. and SMITH, S. E. 1988. Isomerization of retinyl palmitate in fortified skim milk under retail fluorescent lighting. J. Agr. Food Chem. 36, 592-595.

109. SENYK, G. F. and SHIPE, W. F. 1981. Protecting your milk from nutrient loss. Dairy Field *164*(3), 81–82.
110. SINGH, R. P., HELDMAN, D. R. and KIRK, J. R. 1975. Kinetic analysis of light-induced riboflavin loss in whole milk. J. Food Sci. *40*, 164–167.
111. SEDLACEK, B., RYBIN, R. and TICHA, A. 1957. Storage of dried vitaminized milk with added L-ascorbic acid in different types of packaging: Changes in L-ascorbic acid content in storage. Obaly *3*, 7–10.
112. HETTINGA, D. H. 1988. Why alter milk composition? J. Dairy Sci. *71* (Suppl.), 72.
113. KIRKPATRICK, K. L. and FENWICH, R. M. 1987. Manufacture and general properties of dairy ingredients. Food Technol. *41*(10), 58–65, 85.
114. BYRNE, M. 1989. New potential for dairy ingredients. Food Manufacture *64*(6), 35–38.
115. FLEMING, A. and KENNEY, J. 1989. Will consumers benefit from new dairy technology? Nat. Food Rev. *12*(1), 17–21.
116. QUICK, J. A. and MURPHY, E. W. 1982. The Fortification of Foods: A Review. Agr. Handbook 598. U.S. Dept. of Agriculture, Washington, DC.

CHAPTER 14

Foods Considered for Nutrient Addition: FORMULATED SPECIAL PURPOSE FOODS

R. E. HAGEN, Ph.D., M. R. THOMAS, Ph.D.,R.D.,
and J. J. BUSHNELL

INTRODUCTION

Formulated special purpose foods are among the most sophisticated and technically challenging foods commercially available today. Unlike traditional foods, they are designed for special dietary uses, such as infant feeding, meal substitutes (with normal and restricted calorie content), and foods for the dietary management of patients with medical conditions and chronic diseases. Many formulated special purpose foods constitute a sole source of nutrition for certain patient or consumer groups. Others may provide supplemental enteral nutrition.

"Formulated special purpose foods" usually differ from other general use foods with added nutrients in that

(1) they are designed to supply the particular dietary needs for a defined population of individuals,
(2) ingredient sources including macronutrients (protein, fat, carbohydrate) and micronutrients (vitamins, minerals) are ordinarily selected, processed, and controlled in the formulated special purpose food to meet the requirements of a defined population.

They are, thus, different from basic or traditional foods with added nutrients, e.g., enriched bread, vitamin D fortified milk, calcium supplemented orange juice, and instant breakfasts. With the exception of the added nutrient(s), the nutrients in fortified foods are present at naturally occurring levels rather than at levels designed to fit the nutrient needs of a defined population.

The relationship of these commercial foods to foods that normally constitute a mixed diet has been discussed by Moore.[1] Within each food category, as illustrated in Fig. 14.1, there are wide ranges of scientific and regulatory issues, many of which are discussed elsewhere in this book. Certain technological aspects of formulating foods which serve as sole nutrition sources may not be particularly difficult.[1] This apparent simplicity in their manufacture has attracted a few operators who do not give sufficient attention to details. Understandably, responsible regulatory bodies such as the U.S. Food and Drug Administration continue to face dilemmas on how to police inexperienced, naive, or irresponsible manufacturers without unduly constricting progress and innovation by reputable and capable manufacturers.

A food which purports to be a sole nutrient source is immediately subject to significant constraints in design, manufacture, and control. Some of the more complex products in this class represent an extremely advanced state of the art in the practical and integrated application of nutritional science, food science, food engineering, and quality control systems, including analytical chemistry. Experience has taught that those wishing to succeed in the manufacture of these challenging products need in-depth knowledge of these areas of science and technology.

This chapter, therefore, will focus on the issues raised above with special emphasis on:

(1) Identification of the target population benefitting from a formulated special purpose food.

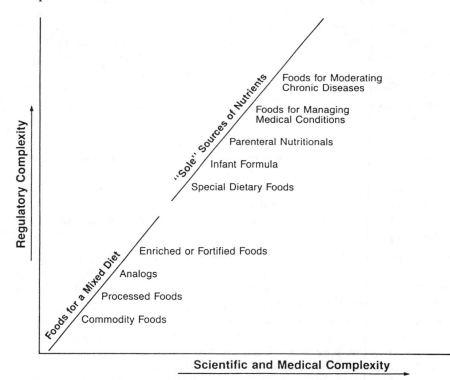

From Moore.[1] Copyright by Institute of Food Technologists
FIG. 14.1. COMPLEXITY OF SCIENTIFIC AND REGULATORY ISSUES FOR VARIOUS TYPES OF FOODS AND NUTRITIONAL PRODUCTS

(2) Medical and nutritional design considerations.
(3) Technologies employed in product and process development.
(4) Manufacture and control systems.
(5) Compliance with applicable laws and regulations.

The goal of these activities is to assure that a formulated special purpose food maintains the desired nutritional and organoleptic qualities throughout shelf-life.

The foods to be discussed are those for normal oral ingestion or for tube feeding. Parenteral nutritional formulas, i.e., those fed intravenously, will not be discussed; however, the reader may consult several reviews.[2,3,4]

INFANT FORMULAS

Evolution of Infant Formulas

Formulated special purpose foods have their heritage in infant formulas, the development of which was spurred by the need to supply proper nutrition for babies when human milk was unavailable. In a major review commissioned by the U.S. Food and Drug Administration (FDA), Anderson *et al.* reported that until the 20th century, there was virtually no safe and reliable alternative to breast-feeding.[5] Few infants not breast fed by mothers or wet nurses survived the first year. At the Paris Foundling Hospital from 1771 to 1777, more than 80% of the 31,000 infants admitted died before their first birthday. Records of the Dublin Foundling Hospital from 1775 to 1799 indicate only 45 of 10,272 infants admitted survived—a mortality rate of 99.6%! In London at that time, for example, it is estimated that among infants that were not breastfed, seven of eight died.[6] The statistics do not distinguish between deaths due to malnutrition and those due to infectious diseases. Undoubtedly, both factors were present.

Use of modified cow's milk for feeding infants dates back to the late 1800s, when sanitary processing of cow's milk first became available. Early infant formulas were made with additions of water and carbohydrate to the heat-treated cow's milk to reduce protein concentration and electrolyte load to levels closer to those of human milk.[7] Wide-scale success with bottle feeding became possible according to Fomon[8] through the application of newer knowledge in three separate areas:

(1) Development of safer water supplies and of sanitary standards for handling and storage of milk;
(2) Development of easily cleansed and sterilized bottles and nipples; and
(3) Alteration of curd tension of milk (through heat treatment).

During the late 19th century, discoveries in chemistry, biology, and medicine began to lay the scientific foundation for the development of human milk substitutes. New methods for protein and fat analyses improved understanding of milk composition.

Causes of infectious diseases and benefits of milk pasteurization became recognized.

The modern era of infant formulas of known composition as complete foods began in 1915 when Gerstenberger and colleagues developed an artificial milk with fat content simulating human milk.[9] As widespread use of carbohydrate modified cow's milk mixtures grew in the United States, it became recognized that they did not provide sufficient vitamins A, D, and C for infants. In the early 1920s, cow's milk formula feedings were supplemented with fish liver oil and orange juice to supply these vitamins. Later, supplements providing vitamins A, D, and C in purified forms were made available.

Since that time, many additional changes have been made in commercial infant formulas so that today, they even more closely simulate human milk, which is generally recognized as the standard for good infant nutrition.[10] Modern infant formulas are formulated to closely mimic the nutritional balance of human milk by combining macronutrients and essential micronutrients. Infant formulas are available as ready-to-use and concentrated liquids, and as dried products (powders).

Design of Infant Formulas, General Considerations

In establishing the nutritional composition of an infant formula, the infant's physiological development and growth are first considered. Research data on nutritional needs of infants, and recommendations by policy groups and expert groups play a key role in this step. Secondly, if certain medical or physical conditions exist, the formula may have to be modified to meet the infant's needs.

Physiology. During the last two months of gestation and the first few months after birth, the human infant physically grows more rapidly than at any other time during its life. Although all organs are maturing and developing, only a few systems that are affected by nutrient intake will be discussed in relation to nutritional needs: the brain, gastrointestinal tract, liver, and kidney as illustrated in Fig. 14.2.

The central nervous system develops rapidly after birth up until about three years of age.[11] Hyperplasia (increase in the number of cells) occurs primarily during gestation and hypertrophy (increase in the size of each cell) postpartum. However, these are not distinct phases. Nutrient deficits of protein, energy, vitamins, and minerals have been shown to affect not only brain size but also brain function. These deficits can have transitional or permanent effects, such as decrease in intelligence quotient (I.Q.).[12]

The stomach, which contains the hydrolytic enzyme pepsin and hydrochloric acid, is the active site for the first part of protein digestion.[13] Secretion of hydrochloric acid and pepsin per unit of body weight is less for the infant than for the adults.[14] In the small intestine, trypsin and chymotrypsin are responsible for further hydrolysis of protein. These enzymes are less active in preterm infants than in full term infants, and both are less active in the infants than in adults.

Enzymes regulating carbohydrate digestion in the infant are fully developed at birth except for pancreatic and duodenal amylase.[15-17] Because of this limitation, starch cannot be fully digested until 3–4 months after birth, when this enzyme begins to function. In the preterm infant, lactase activity may also be limited, resulting in diminished lactose digestion. Thus, preterm infant formulas frequently are designed to use a combination of oligosaccharides and lactose, spreading the digestive burden to take advantage of the mix of available enzymes. These carbohydrate mixtures complement the digestive capacity of the preterm infant.

Fat digestion and absorption is also limited in the preterm and full term infant compared with children and adults.[18,13] Limited secretion of pancreatic lipase limits the rate of triglyceride hydrolysis.[19-22] In addition, bile salt production is low in premature infants, and as a result limits micelle formation, i.e., fat emulsification, in the gastrointestinal tract. Although the infant has lingual lipase which remains active in the stomach, infant formulas designed for premature infants are usually prepared with a combination of medium and long chain triglycerides which are easily digested and absorbed.

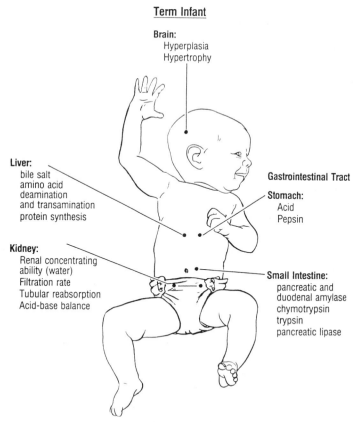

FIG. 14.2. IMMATURE ORGANS SYSTEMS
WHICH AFFECT NUTRIENT NEEDS OF INFANTS

In addition to the incompletely developed capacity to synthesize bile salts, the liver of the newborn infant has a reduced capacity for protein synthesis and protein metabolism.[8] The liver must remove the amine group from amino acids, use it to make nonessential amino acids, or prepare it for excretion via urea or ammonia. Protein intake must be controlled, since the neonatal liver cannot fully adjust to a deficit nor metabolize excesses of amino acids. Proteins must be of high biological value or supplemented with amino acids because the infant's liver cannot compensate for inappropriate amino acid ratios.

One of the primary concerns of developing an infant formula is the renal solute load.[23] The ability of the young infant's kidney to concentrate urine or to dilute the renal solute load by excretion of excess water is less than that of older infants, children, or adults.[24] The filtration rate of blood to form urine is much lower in the newborn and premature infant than in the one-year-old infant. In addition, reabsorption of nutrients such as glucose and phosphate is much lower and appears to develop at a slower rate than formation of urine. The newborn infant can excrete metabolic products from protein metabolism, electrolytes, and water. However, extremes in fluid intake or water losses can cause rapid dehydration. Excessive protein and electrolyte ingestion, as provided by cow's milk, can cause acid/base imbalances. Consequently, the infant needs a controlled protein and electrolyte intake like that provided by human milk or infant formula.

Medical Considerations. Diarrhea and vomiting can become major medical problems in the newborn infant because of its developing kidney and gastrointestinal system. These symptoms can be induced by infection, by inappropriate dietary composition, or by conditions such as heat or stress. Specific medical problems that require specialty formulas will be discussed in later sections on routine infant formulas and exempt formulas.

Preclinical and Clinical Research. Advances in the science of nutrition lagged behind the development of infant formulas and provided little documentation of infant nutrient requirement until the mid-1900s.[25] Technological advances have allowed investigators to approximate the ranges of energy, protein, carbohydrate, and fat needed and tolerated by term and preterm infants. Biochemical measurements and tracer methodology have helped establish recommendations for vitamin and mineral intakes. Although the presence and levels of several ultratrace elements such as selenium, chromium, and molybdenum have been analytically determined in human milk, nutritional requirements for such elements are not well defined.

Until recently, the basis for established nutrient requirements has been the alleviation of clinically defined deficiency disorders. For example, several investigators in the 1950s reported convulsive seizures in infants receiving commercially prepared formula. During the period from 1951–1953, Coursin[25] observed 54 infants from 5 weeks to 2 months of age with hyperirritability and seizures that were attributable to pyridoxine deficiency. All had been fed a commercial liquid cow milk formula from birth and had received no solid foods or supplements of pyridoxine. In 1953, a relatively heat-stable form of pyridoxine was added to commercial formulas, alleviating the problem.

In order to avoid potential problems of this type, infant formula manufacturers conduct preclinical and clinical research on infant formula undergoing significant changes in nutrient level, or manufacturing process.[26] Preclinical research involves the use of animals models to address specific questions about nutrient metabolism. Clinical research involves metabolic balance studies, growth studies, and studies to determine acceptance and tolerance of the formula. These elements of preclinical and clinical research are discussed in more detail later.

Expert Group Recommendations. The Committee on Nutrition (CON) of the American Academy of Pediatrics [10] has published recommendations for nutrient levels in infant formulas. These take into consideration the physiology of the infant, the latest knowledge of infant nutrition, and the Recommended Dietary Allowances [27] developed by the Food and Nutrition Board (FNB) of the National Research Council (NRC). The CON established recommendations on nutrient levels and protein quality for infant formulas.

In addition to the recommendations by the CON and FNB/NRC, recommendations for intakes have been either made or considered by other societies or governing bodies: Codex Alimentarius Commission's Committee on Foods for Special Dietary Use, [28] and the European Society of Pediatric Gastroenterology and Nutrition.[29]

Nutrient Losses. Nutrient losses during manufacturing and processing must be considered when establishing the product formulation and process. This will be discussed in greater detail in the Product and Packaging Development section of the chapter.

Routine Infant Formulas

Milk-based Formulas. Milk-based formulas currently marketed in the Unites States are based on either nonfat milk or a mixture of nonfat milk and demineralized whey. Nutrient profiles in milk-based formulas are patterned after human milk with slight modifications where research shows that higher levels of vitamins and minerals are appropriate. Butterfat is replaced with vegetable oils which provide essential fatty acids. The formula is designed to serve as the sole diet of the infant for at least the first 4–6 months of life and the primary source of nutrients for the first year of life.

Milk-based formulas are designed to provide 67 kcal/dL or 20 kcal/fluid ounce with 1.5 g protein/dL. Protein provides about 9% of total calories, lactose about 40%, and fats approximately 50% of total calories. Iron-fortified formulas in the United States typically provide 1.9 mg iron/100 kcal, or 12 mg/quart although non-fortified formulas providing about 1 mg iron/quart are available as an alternative for those who prefer to provide iron from other sources.

Soy-based Formula. The first soy-based infant formula, Sobee Powder, was introduced in 1929. This contained a full-fat soy flour, provided levels of protein, fat, carbohydrate, and minerals similar to those in infant formulas based on evaporated milk and maltodextrins. This formula powder was used primarily for those infants who had "feeding allergies." In the 1960s protein isolated from soy flour was used to prepare improved soy formulas. Factors in the development of improved soy-based formulas were proper heating of soy protein to reduce trypsin inhibitor activity, the addition of methionine to improve protein quality, and the removal of soluble soy carbohydrates which caused gassy, malodorous stools in infants fed formulas based on soy flour.[30] In contrast to nonfat cow's milk which is a mixture of protein, carbohydrate, vitamins and minerals, the soy protein isolate used in infant formula manufacture contains at least 90% protein on a dry weight basis. Thus, soy formulas require more extensive supplementation with vitamins and minerals than milk-based formulas. Levels of calcium and zinc in soy formulas are adjusted to compensate for binding to the phytate which is present in soy protein isolate. Soy-based formulas are iron-fortified.

Soy-based formulas are commonly used today where cow milk protein and/or lactose should be avoided. These include infants with cow milk allergy, infants with transient or longer term carbohydrate intolerance, and infants with galactosemia. Additionally, soy formulas can be used by infants recovering from diarrhea. They provide appropriate nutrition in a form that is usually well tolerated while the gastrointestinal tract is recovering its full compliment of digestive enzymes.

Specialty Infant Formulas

Specialty or "exempt" infant formulas are also available for infants with feeding problems. (For a definition of "exempt" infant formula, the reader is referred to the Regulatory Considerations section of this chapter). These infant formulas are designed to provide nutritional support for low birth weight infants, as well as those with inborn errors of metabolism such as phenylketonuria, maple syrup urine disease, hereditary tyrosinemia, or other special feeding problems including allergy to milk protein, carbohydrate intolerance, gastrointestinal disease, or chronic diarrhea.

Medical Concerns. The physiological stress of infections, metabolic imbalances, or premature birth increase the infant's nutrient requirements.[31]

Gastrointestinal (GI) infections and feeding problems are each a serious concern. In addition to causing increased requirements, they cause physiological damage and nutrient losses from the GI tract.[32,33] Digestive enzymes, initially reduced by diarrhea, are further depleted by malnutrition during an illness when nutrient intake is compromised. Further, the infection-related damage to the gastrointestinal tract hampers absorption of nutrients, which also contributes to the diarrhea. Thus, a vicious cycle of malnutrition and infection evolves. Infant formulas with casein hydrolysate are targeted to this medical concern.

Protein Hydrolysate Formulas. Commonly, casein, a milk protein, is enzymatically digested to provide the "protein" source for these formulas. The degree of digestion is controlled to yield a mixture of short peptide chains and free amino acids. The hydrolyzed casein is usually supplemented with amino acids so that the protein efficiency ratio (PER) is equal to that of casein. The fat sources for these formulas are medium chain triglyceride and/or vegetable oils which provide essential fatty acids. The carbohydrates provided are usually oligosaccharides, disaccharides other than lactose, or mixtures of these.

The balance of nutrients in these formulas is critical. They must provide adequate amounts of sodium, potassium, chloride, protein, and energy at an acceptably low osmotic load. Such formulas are useful in the management of water and electrolyte losses and accompanying diarrhea, while supporting growth and recuperation.

In addition to dietary management of chronic diarrhea, hydrolysate formulas are used in infants allergic to intact milk protein[34] or food sensitivity,[35] cystic fibrosis,[36] and malabsorption (e.g., short gut).

Formulas for Inborn Errors of Metabolism. The dietary management of some infants with inborn errors of amino acid metabolism is achieved by reducing the level of the offending essential amino acid in order to avoid the accumulation of toxic metabolites of that amino acid. The clinical objective is to provide a sufficient amount of the amino acid for growth and development while limiting the formation and accumulation of toxic byproducts of the altered metabolism.

Hydrolyzed casein is a component of some formulas designed for infants with certain inborn errors of metabolism, since the amino acid content of casein hydrolysate can be modified by further processing. For example, phenylalanine, as essential amino acid, can be markedly reduced by carbon treatment of the hydrolysate. The resulting further modified "protein" is then appropriate for use in formulas for phenylketonuric infants.[37]

Carbohydrate, fat, and energy are supplied at levels comparable to routine formulas. Mineral and vitamin levels are also balanced according to metabolic needs. Preclinical assessment measures, to be described later, are used to assure the necessary protein quality of these specialty formulas.

Formulas for Low Birthweight Infants. The preterm infant offers a significant challenge in the development of infant formula.[38,39] Preterm infants cannot tolerate wide ranges in fluid, electrolytes, protein, lactose, or long chain triglycerides, and, for their size, they require even larger quantities of nutrients (i.e, protein, energy, calcium) for growth and development.[40] For this reason, milk-based premature formulas are prepared with combinations of medium chain and long chain triglycerides, lactose and oligosaccharides (chains of 2–10 glucose units), and added vitamins and minerals. Lactose is included in these formulas to enhance calcium absorption. The protein must be of very high biological value. The studies described in the preclinical and clinical sections are performed as appropriate. These infants are monitored with attention to detailed nutrient assessment techniques.[7]

Other Specialty Infant Formulas. Although only a few exempt formulas can be discussed in this limited space, there are numerous others designed to meet the needs of specific populations. A listing if specialty infant formulas and their composition has been compiled by Moses.[41]

Preclinical Testing of Infant Formulas

New infant formulas and those undergoing substantial changes in formulation may be evaluated preclinically in animal models to verify protein quality, nutritional adequacy, and bioavailability of selected nutrients.[7]

A protein efficiency ratio (PER) assay is performed on infant formulas. In this assay, young rats are fed a diet containing 10% protein from the test sources or products.[8] In the infant formula industry, the PER is conducted using the Association of Official Analytical Chemists (AOAC) assay, "Protein Efficiency Ratio Rat Bioassay."[42]

Clinical Evaluation of Infant Formulas

After assurance of nutritional quality is achieved, infant formulas are carefully evaluated in human infants. Metabolic balance, growth, and acceptance and tolerance studies are frequently used for evaluation of new or modified formulations.[7]

Metabolic balance studies are used to evaluate nitrogen and fat absorption, nitrogen retention, and calcium absorption.[8,43] The experimental formula is compared to control formula containing a reference protein (usually casein), ordinarily for a period of 7-9 days. The metabolic balance study is divided into two separate segments: (1) an equilibration phase (adjustment to the formula) and (2) a 72-h experimental phase where formula intake is measured precisely and all urine and feces are collected. Analyses of collections provide quantitative information on apparent nutrient absorption by the differences between oral intake and fecal excretion. Nutrient retention is calculated as the difference between apparent absorption and losses in urine.

After metabolic studies have documented that the nutrients in question are adequately absorbed and retained, growth studies may be performed. A strict procedure measuring growth of infants for 112 days has been described by Fomon.[44] This unique type of study evaluates the effect of feeding formula over an extended period of time. Upon completion of the study, data on growth parameters and formula tolerance are statistically evaluated.

The acceptance/tolerance and growth study is frequently used as the last in a series of clinical studies to evaluate new or modified formulas.[7] Large-scale studies, some involving 200 or more infants, are used to assess the performance of a formula when fed for several months. The subjects, equally divided into control and test groups, are fed formula from near birth until 3-6 months of age. Each day, parents record the volume of formula consumed, stool characteristics, and instances of any gastrointestinal intolerance. At periodic checkups, the medical staff measures weight, height, and appropriate biochemical and hematological indices.

When formulas designed for premature infants are being evaluated, infants are fed that formula only during the time that they would normally require such a formula. Clinical parameters that may be evaluated include records of illness and medications, biochemical and hematological indices, anthropometric measures, nutrient balances, and formula tolerance.

ENTERAL NUTRITIONAL FOODS

Evaluation, Classification, and General Uses

Enteral nutritional foods constitute another broad category of formulated special purpose foods. Enteral nutritional foods have been defined by the American Society of Parenteral and Enteral Nutrition (A.S.P.E.N.) as "...nutrition provided via the gastrointestinal tract. Oral-enteral nutrition taken by mouth. Tube-enteral nutrition provided through a tube or catheter that delivers nutrients distal to the oral cavity."[45]

A complete formula, Sustagen®, for tube feeding of hospital patients, marketed in 1952 was one of the earliest enteral nutrition foods.[46] This low fat, modified milk formulation provided appropriate levels of all of the then-known nutrients. In broad terms, its concept was that formulations used as the sole diet, or significant parts thereof, should provide the recommended dietary allowances (RDAs) of all micronutrients in a calorie-controlled macronutrient matrix. This remains the foundation of responsibly formulated modern enteral foods designed to be sole sources of nutrition.

Perhaps the best known enteral foods among the lay public are those used to provide complete nutrition and calorie control. In 1960, Metrecal® extended the application of the concept of complete vitamin and mineral nutrition which had previously been developed for infant formulas and tube feeding products for adults.[46] The Metrecal® formulation contained all vitamins and minerals considered by nutritionists to be essential for man, even though RDAs had not been established for many nutrients at that time.[47] Liquid meal substitutes were introduced in 1968 with each serving or "meal" containing about one-third of the daily requirements of all essential vitamins and minerals.

Since that time, a wide range of enteral products have been marketed to meet the nutritional needs of individuals who, due to some disease condition or nutritional problem, may have special dietary needs.[48] Currently, products are available providing varying protein levels and fiber. There are more than 80 nutritionally complete enteral feeds for special dietary (medical) purposes, more than 50 nutritionally incomplete formulas, some 3 dozen formulas for metabolic or genetic disorders, and about 6 oral rehydration products on the market.

Indications for Enteral Nutritionals, General

Enteral foods can be classified by their form (powder or liquid), mode of delivery (tube feeding or normal oral ingestion), and by use.[49] Uses include oral supplements and complete meal replacements.

The feasibility of enteral nutritional support is dependent upon sufficient digestive and absorptive capacity to satisfy the primary nutrient needs of the individual.[3] Intact protein sources can be used for patients with chronic conditions who have normal digestive and absorptive mechanisms for utilization of nutrients. Such patients may include those who are comatose, disoriented, or have head and neck trauma or disease that interferes with normal ingestion. It may also include those which have a chronic disease, such as cancer, that is frequently accompanied by loss of appetite.

In contrast, formulations which provide "protein" in the form of amino acids or short-chain peptides may be suited for those patients with a variety of disorders of the small intestine, pancreas, or liver. Elemental diets based on amino acids or hydrolyzed protein may be used for: diarrhea, infections, radiation therapy, chemotherapy, selective gastrointestinal injury, inflammatory bowel disease such as Crohn's disease, malabsorption syndromes, infection of the pancreas, pancreatic enzyme insufficiency, intestinal or colonic resection (short bowel syndrome), and gastric ulcers.[50-53]

Enteral Nutritional Support in the Management of Chronic Diseases

There are several chronic diseases which may require enteral formula support for long periods of time, such as inflammatory bowel disease or short gut syndrome, chronic kidney failure, cancer, or acquired immunodeficiency syndrome (AIDS). Discussion of nutritional support for these conditions follows.

When gastrointestinal disease is present, the appropriate enteral formula to be used depends upon the length of functional bowel remaining, presence of the ileocecal valve, and various adaptive responses the bowel segment has developed.[3,54] For example, in short gut syndrome, 70-75% of the small intestine has been removed. Such a massive reduction in the length of the intestine may be required as a result of small bowel infarction (blood clot), Crohn's Disease or cancer. If the ileocecal valve and ileum have been removed, there will be reduction in absorption of nutrients including fatty acids, vitamin B_{12}, and fat soluble vitamins.[55] Diarrhea, steatorrhea, bile salt malabsorption, and extensive bacterial colonization frequently occur. Any of these manifestations can result in clinical malnutrition.

Enteral formulas have been used to overcome nutritional deficiencies common in patients with inflammatory bowel disease.[56] Deficits arise from inadequate oral intake, malabsorption, protein-losing enteropathy, and increased metabolic demands. For both short gut and inflammatory bowel disease, either intact protein formula or elemental diets may be used.[57]

Malnutrition usually accompanies cancer, and when malnutrition occurs, prognosis is poor.[58,59] A few of the factors which may contribute to malnutrition in patients with malignancy include: (1) impairment of oral ingestion (oral tumors), (2) aversion to food, (3) taste abnormalities, (4) surgical procedures of the oral pharynx and gastrointestinal tract, (5) chemotherapy and radiation therapy. Available data suggest that enteral nutritional support is effective in reversing immune deficits due to malnutrition and that when reversed, the risk of surgery or further therapies for cancer is reduced.[3]

Individuals with chronic renal failure may need to restrict protein intake to approximately 40 g/day.[3] Conversely, patients undergoing dialysis may require additional protein to replenish losses due to therapy. At least half of the protein intake should be as essential amino acids in dialysis patients. The diet should provide a high energy to nitrogen ratio. In acute renal failure, enteral nutrition may be used to stabilize or reduce the levels of blood urea nitrogen, potassium phosphorus, and magnesium and to enhance recovery.

Infections that accompany acquired immunodeficiency syndrome (AIDS) frequently result in severe diarrhea and malnutrition, requiring nutritional therapy.[60] In AIDS, diarrhea is caused not only by the effect of the virus on mucosal cells [61,62], but also by a secondary infection such as *Campylobacter*.[63] Enteral formulation providing nutrition without contributing to the diarrhea can reduce the risk of infection.[64] If nutritional intervention is not provided early, additional nutrients will be needed to overcome the deficit.

Enteral Nutritional Support in the Management of Acute Diseases

For acute conditions such as trauma and burns, surgery, and acute diarrhea, enteral nutritional formulas are used to provide nutritional support, replenish nutritional stores, and satisfy increased nutrient needs. In several of these circumstances, hormonal changes cause weight loss and depletion of nutrient stores. Until hormone balance is restored, replacement of body protein and stabilization of nutrient losses cannot be achieved, even with aggressive enteral feeding. Without enteral formulations, however, the hypermetabolic state caused by these hormonal changes can be even more debilitating.

In major burns, elevated catecholamine levels cause a hypermetabolic response which accelerates severe depletion of body protein stores.[3,65] Protein is used for energy because of the significant increase in energy demand which accompanies the extensive integumentary damage. Once healing progresses and surface losses are reduced, catecholamine levels return to normal and hypermetabolism subsides. In major burn injuries (>40% of the total body surface area) patients can experience body weight reduction of at least 25% within the first 2 months.[3,66] Death usually occurs when weight loss exceeds 30%. Enteral feeding is the method of choice for feeding burn patients if the gastrointestinal tract is intact and functional. Several investigators have documented that enteral supplementation results in improved nutritional status, improved immune response, and decreased mortality in burn patients.[3] Enteral supplements should provide a high level of energy, protein of high biological quality, and vitamins and minerals.

In the trauma patient, hormonal changes are even greater than in the burn patient.[67] Trauma increases catecholamine levels and also those of other hormones such as insulin. These changes cause increased losses of protein, subcutaneous fat, and carbohydrate stores.[68] These losses can be offset with adequate nutritional support. However, in severe trauma, weight loss in the first 3-5 days is substantial, irrespective of the treatment. For trauma, as in burns, rehabilitation is dependent upon normalized hormone levels, followed by aggressive enteral nutritional support.

Enteral nutritional support is used widely in the management or prevention of perioperative malnutrition.[69] It has been found by several investigators that the risk of postoperative infections is increased in patients with poor nutritional status. Mullen et al. in a prospective study, found that patients identified to be at risk for postoperative complications (a Prognostic Nutrition Index $\geq$ 50%) had a nine-fold higher incidence of major sepsis.[70,71] They also had an eleven-fold greater mortality when compared to those patients thought to be at low nutritional risk.

Acute diarrhea can result from many conditions, i.e., infections, organic causes, drugs. Most diarrheas can be managed through enteral feedings if the osmotic load, the concentration of the nutrients, and electrolyte balance are appropriate. If nutritional needs cannot be met via the gastrointestinal tract or severe diarrhea persists, parenteral nutrition may be required. The gut, however, does not recover as quickly if some form of enteral intake is not provided.[72]

Enteral Nutritionals for Weight Reduction

One of the historical uses of enteral formulations has been in weight reduction.[73,74] Various formulations have been developed to maximize weight reduction and preserve nutritional status. Compared with a typical diet, these formulations have reduced fat and carbohydrate levels, while providing for normal protein intake. Low calorie enteral supplements have been used to complement a weight reduction plan or used in combination with surgery for obesity (gut resection or stomach stapling).

Balance of Nutrient Intake

While nutritional scientists generally agree on the nutritional requirements for healthy infants, children and adults, there are no accepted standards that can be applied to patients with disease or injury. Allowances that apply to healthy individuals still provide the best benchmark for ill or recovering patients.

Several professional societies such as The American Society for Parenteral and Enteral Nutrition, The American Dietetics Association, and the American Medical Association are establishing quality of care guidelines as well as recommendations concerning nutritional therapy. In addition, these societies are publishing recommendations for nutritional assessment of sick patients.[3,75] These nutritional assessment measures help identify individuals in need of enteral nutritional support. They also help document the effectiveness of enteral nutritionals in improving nutritional status.

Much of the knowledge applied to nutritional management of sick patients is derived from a basic understanding of the disease process. Carefully controlled clinical studies are performed to measure the effect of enteral formulations. Clinical trials continue to provide the best means to evaluate alternative nutritional therapy.

PRODUCT AND PROCESS DEVELOPMENT

Development of new formulated special purpose foods involves a number of considerations beyond those encountered in development of other foods. As emphasized in previous sections, the users and their needs must be clearly identified in order to arrive at specific product design parameters, including well-defined nutrient specifications.

Food scientists and engineers must then explore product form, process, and packaging alternatives based on thorough knowledge of their craft. This is best accomplished in a highly integrated process with full consideration given not just to technology, but to the end user (consumer) and the user environment. Marketing issues must be addressed at the design stage, with active participation in critical decisions at each step. Strategies for compliance with all applicable laws and regulations are also made when the clinical and nutritional requirements are being established. Interaction with nutrition scientists and clinical experts is critical at the development stage to assure selected ingredients are compatible with the product design parameters.

Product Development

The discussion that follows keys on infant formula as an example. It is a product with which the authors are intimately acquainted and as one of, if not the most highly controlled foods, presents the most sophisticated example presently available.

Macronutrients. An informative discussion of necessary factors in selection of nutrient sources for infant formulas is given in a paper by Cook.[76] Key elements to be considered in selection of protein, fat, and carbohydrate sources are summarized in Table 14.1.

The source of protein is critical and usually the first decision to be made in designing a formula. Nutritional and medical rationales for use of a selected protein for specific patients were given in the previous section. The most common sources of protein in infant formulas are nonfat cow's or a mixture of cow's milk and reduced minerals whey, soy protein isolate (supplemented with L-methionine), casein, hydrolyzed casein, or crystalline amino acids.

McDermott notes that a major factor dictating finished product characteristics is that infant formulas and enteral formulas are protein-stabilized emulsions with significant quantities of protein in the bulk phase prior to thermal processing.[77] Emulsions stabilized with various combinations of the proteins shown in Table 14.1 will respond differently to a given set of formulation, processing, and storage conditions. Carrageenan, a polysaccharide derived from seaweed, is often used to enhance long-term formula stability. Theuer points out that the functional characteristics needed for whey used in liquid formulas require undenatured whey in the demineralized whey in order to avoid protein precipitation in the final product.[78]

TABLE 14.1
MACRONUTRIENT SELECTION CONSIDERATIONS FOR FORMULATED SPECIAL PURPOSE FOODS

Macronutrient	Common Sources	Factors in Selection	Factors to Monitor in Products
Protein	Nonfat cow's milk Soy isolate w/L-methionine Reduced minerals whey Hydrolyzed casein Crystalline amino acids	Protein equivalency and PER Other nutritional factors Hypoallergenic properties Emulsification/stabilization Organoleptic factors	Amino acid profile Antigenic factors Micronutrients/seasonality Environmental substances Protein gelation/aggregation
Fat (oils)	Corn, soy, coconut Destearinated tallow Medium chain triglycerides (C 8-10)	Essential fatty acids Other nutritional factors Emulsification/stabilization Organoleptic factors	Fatty acids Oxidation susceptibility Environmental substances Fat separation (creaming)
Carbohydrate	Lactose, sucrose Corn syrups, dextrose Maltodextrins Starches	Nutritional value/mineral absorption Digestibility and tolerance Osmolality Organoleptic factors Texture control	Gastrointestinal impact Nonenzymatic browning (Maillard Reaction) Antigenic factors Environmental substances Caramelization reactions

Source: Adapted from Cook[76] and McDermott.[77]

Fat is the next macronutrient building block in most formulas. Fats must provide an adequate level of essential fatty acids and they must be easily absorbed in order to provide needed energy and minimize malabsorption of calcium and other minerals. In addition to the commonly used triglyceride fats listed in Table 14.1, emulsifiers such as lecithin or mono- and diglycerides are normally used to enhance emulsion stability.

Carbohydrate is the third macronutrient to be selected. Lactose, the predominant sugar in human milk, is also the choice for infant formulas designed for normal, healthy infants and for some adult nutritional formulas. The key functional characteristic in selecting a source of lactose is solubility. Lactose is a significant component of common dairy protein sources, such as skim milk and various types of wheys. Disturbances in lactose digestion and absorption are among the most common gastrointestinal problems found in infants and a common problem for many adults. Consequently, some formulas are lactose free and instead contain other carbohydrates such as sucrose, glucose, dextrose, of maltodextrins (see Table 14.1). All listed sugar sources, except sucrose, contain free aldehyde moieties which may participate in nonenzymatic browning reactions in the presence of free amino groups in amino acids and protein. Lactose is generally avoided when designing formulas for infants allergic to cow's milk protein since commercially available lactose may contain small but potentially antigenic amounts of milk protein. Likewise, lactose should be avoided in feedings for infants with the genetic condition, galactosemia.

Nonnutritive dietary fiber is becoming increasingly important in enteral nutritionals designed for adults patients where benefits of bulking agents are desired. Several widely different types of fiber are now in use including various celluloses, brans, and psyllium.

Osmolality. Osmolality is an important characteristic or formulas used as sole nutrition sources.[76] Hyperosmolar infant formulas may have adverse effects in some infants, especially preterm babies, when fed undiluted or too rapidly. Since carbohydrate is a primary determinant of formula osmolality, attention to this factor must be given as part of the formula design. Infant formulas made with monosaccharides (glucose, fructose) have a significantly higher osmolality than those made with glucose polymers or corn syrups. Thus, ingredient selection must balance osmolality and digestibility considerations in arriving at an optimal carbohydrate profile.

Micronutrients. Some important vitamins and minerals are present to a predictable degree in the intact milk proteins used in formulas. Consequently, the naturally occurring levels are supplemented with suitable amounts of essential vitamins and minerals to meet nutrient specifications. Proteins, whose micronutrient contribution is inherently low or reduced by processing (e.g., soy protein isolate), must be supplemented to a greater degree. As with macronutrients, the sources and forms of vitamins and minerals added to infant formulas are chosen with careful attention to purity, solubility, bioavailability, and compatibility with other ingredients.[76] Considerations for selecting nutrient levels have been given earlier.

Finally, the food scientist responsible for developing a product which meets all the stringent nutritional requirements cited above must tailor the formulation to provide the desired palatability, and other organoleptic qualities. Virtually all orally fed products require considerable sophistication both in palatability and eye appeal in order to meet consumer/patient acceptance. In the case of enteral nutritionals designed as food supplements, skillful use of flavorings has earned them wide consumer acceptance.

Process Considerations

Processing options are wide and varied, but generally they begin with consideration of whether the product form should be a canned liquid (ready-to-use or concentrate), powder, or other form. If the product is a liquid, there is a choice of packaging concepts and thermal processing techniques, such as "canning" or the use of aseptic preservation techniques. Conventional canning of low acid foods, the most widely used process involves terminal sterilization, that is, subjecting the product in a filled, hermetically sealed container, i.e., glass or metal, to specified time/temperature cycles according to a predetermined process consistent with Good Manufacturing Practices (GMPs), as required by regulation 21 CFR 113.[79] Aseptic preservation involves achieving commercial sterility of the combined ingredients using an established thermal process *prior* to filling into a sterilized container in an aseptic environment.

In general, packaging technologies used for formulated special purpose foods are selected from those used for other foods. However, packaging technologies employed for this class of foods necessarily need to be compatible with nutrient stability characteristics, as well as other aspects of product integrity, throughout shelf-life. Most liquid formulated special purpose foods can achieve a shelf-life of 12–15 months. Powdered products in properly designed packages may retain essential nutrient, organoleptic, and physical properties for more than three years.

Although publications about formula processing and packaging technology are rare, one such article on thermal processing of liquid formulas recently appeared.[80] (See also the regulatory section of this chapter.) Packard elaborates on other technical considerations in the manufacture of stable formulas which often contain more than 30 ingredients.[81] Tables are presented listing ingredients found in commercial soy-based and milk-based formulas. Milk or milk and whey-based formulas often rely on relatively sophisticated processing technologies wherein cow's milk protein content is lowered with concomitant raising of carbohydrate levels and reduction of minerals. Electrodialysis, ion exchange, ultrafiltration, and gel filtration are processing options.

Extreme care must be taken during process development to assure that the protein/carbohydrate interactions are controlled, that mineral bioavailability is maintained, that potential lipid oxidation is controlled, and that vitamin levels remain acceptable throughout shelf-life. For formulated special purpose foods, the process and formulation must be optimized within the constraints of the required nutritional profile. For this reason, traditional methods for determining protein functionality may not be the most appropriate.[77]

The process must also maintain physical properties that are important to user acceptance. These include color, maintaining viscosity and emulsion properties, and preventing phase separation. The factors which affect heat stability of formulas during sterilization are pH, mineral balance, seasonal variability of the milk, presence of stabilizers, and processing conditions.[77] These parameters properly become the subject of extensive processing studies and as such may influence selection of equipment, sequencing of ingredient additions, mixing and blending techniques, filling and packaging, and finally, precise thermal processing time and temperatures. The Infant Formula Council has published guidelines for the evaluation of physical stability of infant formulas.[82]

In an era of analytical sophistication, responsible manufacturers must also tailor all aspects of ingredient, package, and process selection to minimizing the potential for introduction of undesirable chemical species or microbiological factors. For each product, it is advisable to make a determination on critical control points to assure that essential testing is accomplished. Initial control point determinations and laboratory control strategies are best set in the product design stage when economically sound adjustments can be made in process, package, and ingredients.

Development of Control Systems

Tennyson emphasized the necessity of close coordination of development work with quality control and manufacturing considerations in the early stages of product development.[83] A graphic illustration of the role of various disciplines and their relationship to quality needs is given in Fig. 14.3. Personnel from the various scientific and functional disciplines (nutritional sciences, product development, engineering, quality, control, production, etc.), through close collaboration, are in an excellent position to define those critical material and process factors which can be used to evaluate quality parameters in a final manufacturing process. Also, early laboratory or plant trial batches, if analyzed thoroughly, will provide product composition information and data on the effects of processing on composition and shelf-life.

MANUFACTURING AND QUALITY CONTROL SYSTEMS

Manufacturing Systems

Commercial Processes. Manufacturers of formulated special purpose foods generally utilize combinations of well-known manufacturing systems and equipment. However, specific equipment and processing conditions remain proprietary. Common processing steps for nutritional liquids include ingredient weighing, mixing and homogenizing. Care is taken to standardize the solids level in the liquid product prior to container filling and sealing.

A schematic process flow for liquid formulas is shown in Fig. 14.4. Note that a fat soluble vitamin premix containing vitamins A, D, E, and K is blended with a stream of vegetable oil to assure optimal dispersion prior to intermixing with skim milk and other water soluble ingredients. Minerals are also added in a manner to assure proper dispersion in the final product. A premix of water soluble vitamins is added at a final stage in the process to minimize oxidative degradation of labile vitamins such as vitamin C. The use of vitamin and mineral premixes is discussed more completely in the Nutrient Premix Control section which follows.

Following mixing, liquid product is filled into containers and a closure is applied. Filled containers immediately proceed to pressure heat sterilizers (retorts) where the contents are rendered commercially sterile according to established thermal processing parameters. (For a definition of "commercial sterility," see 21 CFR 113.3.) When the containers are cooled and dry, they are labeled, packed in shipping containers, and held until all quality control testing is completed. If all specifications are met, the batch is released for distribution.

Powdered formulas can be produced in a similar manner up to the point of a liquid bulk product. At that point, however, the liquid is usually spray-dried. The dried bulk powder is then packaged to await release by the quality control unit. A diagram of a flow process for manufacturing powdered infant formulas can be found in Packard's review.[81]

Production Systems. Production can be defined as "a system in which trained people bring together specified materials in a defined, controlled method so as to

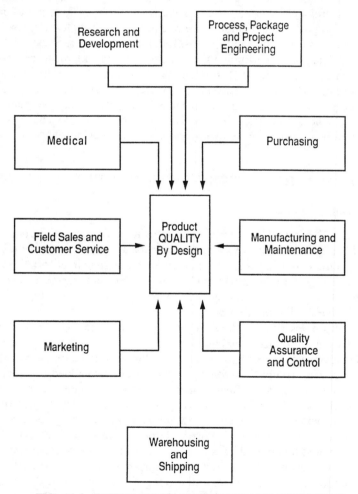

FIG. 14.3. INTERACTION OF CORPORATE FUNCTIONS IN THE DESIGN OF FORMULATED SPECIAL PURPOSE FOODS

SPECIAL PURPOSE FOODS

consistently generate a product of a predetermined quality level."[84] Very important concepts are embodied in this definition. Foremost among them are the selection, qualification, and training of production and maintenance employees, the latter of which are responsible for rigorous preventative maintenance and equipment calibration programs.

Successful manufacture of formulated special purpose foods is built around a strong, integrated set of operating procedures which translate the designed process and good manufacturing principles into specific tasks for production staff. Generally, a batch record (or batch order) containing such instructions is assigned to each batch code of product. Batch records are retained for future reference as may be required by company practice and/or by federal regulations.

It is most important to review operating procedures and systems at each plant to assure that they have been properly designed before use. Particular attention should be given to prevention of contamination, adulteration, or potential misbranding in the final product.

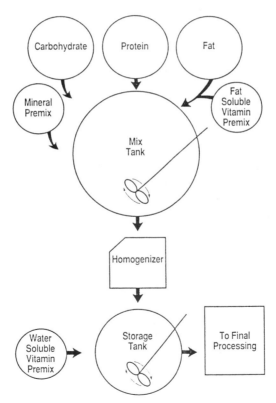

FIG. 14.4. SCHEMATIC PROCESS FLOW
FOR LIQUID FORMULAS

TABLE 14.2
MANUFACTURING CONTROL SYSTEMS

Control System	Features	Benefits
Nutrient systems strategy	Micronutrient blends, other multicomponent nutrient sources or single nutrients are analyzed for each relied-upon nutrient prior to use	Minimize number of separate additions. Direct analytical confirmation of an "indicator nutient" will confirm proper levels in final product
Incoming materials	Nutrient and other critical composition factors are assured prior to use	Avoid products out of specifications
In-process	Testing of indicator nutrients, physical factors, etc., during processing	Allow for adjustments during manufacture
Final product testing	Analyze indicator nutrients, physical, organoleptic, and other parameters prior to distribution release	Assure product specifications/regulatory standards are met
Environmental substances	Employ good manufacturing practices and related critical controls (HACCP)	Assure food safety, prevent adulteration

Quality Control Systems

Although manufacturing controls for formulated special purpose foods are similar to those employed with other foods with added nutrients, several control systems are particularly import, as summarized in Table 14.2.

Nutrient Premix Control System. Manufacture and control of formulated special purpose food products would be subject to many uncontrolled variables were it not for the use of a "nutrient systems" strategy as described in detail by Tennyson.[83] Table 14.3 provides an example of the use of this strategy. By knowing the composition of each of the systems, whether single or multiple ingredient in nature, a manufacturer has the information necessary to assure that each of the nutrients is present in the proper quantity in the finished product. He thus need not analyze for each of them at that stage. Prior to shipment for commercial or charitable distribution, a manufacturer need run only seven assays, as shown in the "indicator nutrient" category in Table 14.3. Thus, for milk solids, the indicator nutrient is protein; vitamin C is the indicator nutrient for the water soluble vitamin premix; and so on. For this nutrient system to achieve the necessary level of control, the composition of each nutrient system or premix must be fully characterized analytically prior to use to assure that each relied-upon nutrient is present at the proper level.

TABLE 14.3
NUTRIENT SYSTEMS FOR AN INFANT FORMULA

	Macro Ingredients			Micro Ingredients			
Nutrients (Indicator Nutrient)	Milk Solids (Protein)	Fat Blend (Fat)	Lactose (Solids)	Water Soluble Vitamin Premix (Vitamin C)	Fat Soluble Vitamin Premix (Vitamin A)	Trace Mineral Premix (Manganese)	Ferrous Sulfate (Iron)
Carbohydrate	X		X				
Protein	X						
Fat		X					
Calcium	X						
Phosphorus	X						
Magnesium	X						
Sodium	X						
Potassium	X						
Chloride	X						
Iodine	X						
Choline	X						
Iron							X
Manganese						X	
Copper						X	
Zinc						X	
Vitamin A					X		
Vitamin D					X		
Vitamin E					X		
Vitamin C				X			
Thiamine				X			
Riboflavin	X			X			
Niacin				X			
Pyridoxine				X			
Pantothenic Acid	X			X			
Vitamin B_{12}				X			
Folic Acid			X				

Responsible manufacturers using the nutrient premix control system have found that it is not possible to predict reliably the nutrient composition of each batch of formulated special purpose foods solely from batch record information. Batch records are of limited value for such purposes, especially when manufacturing "upsets" may occur or for labile nutrients such as vitamin C. Likewise, reliance on "typical" nutrient levels, either in incoming ingredients or in in-process blends, may lead to an unacceptable final product.

Incoming Materials Controls. The above finished product nutrient control system would be cumbersome and potentially economically unmanageable in the absence of sound programs for incoming material control. Specifications which establish realistic limits for essential parameters of raw materials and packaging supplies are the foundation of the integrated control system described in this chapter. Often specifications are derived from the *Food Chemicals Codex*[85] or *U.S. Pharmacopeia/ National Formulary.*[86] If compendial sources do not exist, specifications are crafted from ingredient supplier information, in-house assay information combined with experience gained during the development process.

It is important that ingredient and packaging material supplies are known to meet all critical specifications *before* they are used in manufacture. Strict adherence to this principle not only prevents costly problems in manufacture, but also minimizes the need for agonizing decisions in borderline situations which may arise because of questionable raw material quality.

In-process Control Systems. Many steps are necessarily involved in the manufacture of formulated special purpose foods. Since each step represents an incremental cost addition to the raw materials, manufacturers usually perform certain tests at various intermediate stages. These in-process tests yield information when there is still opportunity to correct any unforeseen deficiencies which could lead to finished products not meeting their specifications. A manufacturer may prudently choose to confirm levels of indicator or labile nutrients (i.e., vitamins A and C) at a bulk formula stage prior to final thermal processing or drying to assure that all necessary nutrient systems are present at the prescribed levels.

Final Product Testing and Product Release. The nutrient premix control strategy for infant formulas described earlier may be useful in designing control systems for other formulated special purpose foods. Key indicator nutrients for each nutrient system, physical properties (color, viscosity, homogeneity, etc.), and flavor are usually tested at the final product stage to assure that all components were properly combined and that no unusual changes occurred during processing and packaging.

The practice of a formal "quality control release" step prior to distribution has served manufacturers well in preventing the release of products into the market place which later prove to be deficient in nutrient content or some other essential property. Recalls due to inadequate nutrient content are not only costly in direct economic terms, but in professional and consumer confidence in the brand as well.

Specifications. Technology for establishing formula product specifications and dealing with analytical data generated during product testing have been reviewed by Schultz.[87] Specifications are designed with the presumption that when they are met, the requirements established for the raw materials, processes or finished formula product will be fulfilled.

At the time of release, a special type of specification sometimes called "Batch Acceptance Limit" may serve as the minimum specification for those nutrients and other quality factors which may change over shelf-life. Examples include vitamins C and A for which decay curves over time can be constructed.

A very useful concept in control of formulated special purpose foods is to consider product specification limits as "laws." That, is, if a product specification is not met, the product will not be released for distribution. Control systems based on case by case exceptions to specifications are very risky especially in the case of formulated special purpose foods designed to be sole sources of nutrition.

Validated Analytical Procedures. Since formulated special purpose foods are generally marketed on the basis of their nutrient properties, it is of utmost importance that measurements of nutrient levels are accurate and precise. Validated chemical or microbiological assays for each product matrix are essential in an analytically based control system.

The 1980 Infant Formula Act, which prescribed levels for 29 nutrients, brought the matter of methods validation for infant formulas to national attention. Industry and government chemists quickly realized they faced an enormous problem, since official analytical methods often did not exist or were otherwise unsuitable for one or more infant formula matrices. Accordingly, scientists affiliated with infant formula manufacturers, the Infant Formula Council, government regulatory agencies, and other interested analytical groups undertook one of the most massive analytical development and validation programs in the history of nutritional chemistry.[88] Collaborative studies are nearing completion for all 29 nutrients in milk-based infant formulas and the final approval is being achieved. However, years of work lie ahead to develop and validate official analytical methods for matrices other than milk.

Environmental Substances Controls. Developing systems to maximize protection from undesirable environmental substances or "contaminants" which could find their way into formulated special purpose foods is a complex matter. Close adherence to Good Manufacturing Practices (GMPs) is clearly the foundation of effective environmental substance control (see the "Regulatory Considerations" section which follows). Additionally, the hazards analysis critical control point (HACCP) approach supplements traditional GMPs to provide an effective and flexible mechanism to afford protection from environmental substances.[89] HACCP is adaptable to the diverse types of products in the general category of formulated special purpose foods. The HACCP approach provides for appropriately trained and experienced individuals within a company to be responsible for identifying and controlling "critical" process points during manufacture to assure that ingredient systems and the final product are protected from contamination or adulteration. Such critical control points are documented in writing subject to review by an appropriate quality control unit of the company.

Water is the predominant ingredient by volume and weight of liquid nutritionals and prepared powdered nutritionals; hence, special care is necessary to assure that water added directly as an "ingredient" meets high standards. Water quality thus becomes a critical control point in the manufacturing cycle.[90]

General purpose water used in processing should minimally meet state, federal, and local regulation for potable water. FDA regulations provide additional guidance on quality attributes for bottled water (21 CFR 103). Testing water supplies on a periodic basis against these standards provides guidance as to any additional water purification which may be necessary. Strategies for further water purification include carbon filtration, defluoridation, and filtration to remove particulates.

Ingredient safety from environmental substances starts at the beginning of the food chain.[91] For dairy ingredients, farm inspections, and regulatory interactions with dairymen subject to the Pasteurized Milk Ordinance[92] all serve as training in good manufacturing practices which help prevent contamination. Criteria for control of pesticides, toxins, and antibiotics are the same under both the PMO for Grade A milk and in USDA regulations which govern manufacturing grade milk. Manufacturers' incoming quality control programs are responsibly designed to monitor incoming milk and dairy products to assure these practices are followed. These same principles apply to other incoming ingredients such as soy proteins, fats, carbohydrates, and minor ingredients.

Finally, an environmental substance control program may involve a testing program to demonstrate on a periodic basis that substances of concern do not present a risk in commercial products. The U.S. Food and Drug Administration has described their Total Diet Studies program [93] which addresses pesticides, selected elements, and other chemicals in a "market basket" of infant and toddler diet samples.[94]

REGULATORY CONSIDERATIONS

The foods discussed in this chapter are generally classified by the U.S. Food and Drug Administration (FDA) as "foods for special dietary use." But before discussing this particular category, it might be well to review the basic legal definition of food as distinguished from drugs. From definitions in Sections 201(f) and 201(g)(1)(C) of the Federal Food, Drug and Cosmetic Act we can conclude that in the eyes of the law, food is intended to affect the structure or function of the body and may consist of food or drink as well as chewing gum or components of these products.

Unlike dictionary definitions of food, the legal definition focuses on what food is not, rather than defining what food is. Fortunately, the Act is more specific in Section 411(c)(3) by referring to foods for "special dietary use" as food intended to be used for the following purposes:

(A) Supplying a special dietary need that exists by reason of a physical, physiological, pathological, or other condition, including but not limited to the condition of disease, convalescence, pregnancy, lactation, infancy, allergic hypersensitivity to food, underweight, overweight, or the need to control the intake of sodium.
(B) Supplying a vitamin, mineral, or other ingredient for use by man to supplement his diet by increasing the total dietary intake.
(C) Supplying a special dietary need by reason of being a food for use as the sole item of the diet.

Foods for special dietary use can be formulated for a wide variety of conditions, but when special dietary foods are labeled with "claims of disease prevention, treat-

TABLE 14.4
LABELING OF FOODS FOR SPECIAL DIETARY USE

Food category	Citation	Requirements[1]
Hypoallergenic foods	21 CFR 105.62	Provide specific information about the quantity or proportion of each ingredient, the specific plant or animal source of each, and information concerning treatment or processing of food or ingredients resulting in a change in allergenic properties
Infant foods	21 CFR 105.65	Provide common or usual name of each ingredient and the specific plant or animal source
Weight control, weight reduction foods	21 CFR 105.66	Provide information on nonnutritive ingredients, including percentage by weight. Regulations define "low calorie" foods and specify where terms such as "sugar-free," "sugarless," etc., may be used
Diabetic foods	21 CFR 105.67	Nutritional labeling requires specific label statement: "Diabetics: This product may be useful in your diet on the advice of a physician. This food is not a reduced calorie food."
Reduced sodium foods	21 CFR 105.69	Provide sodium content in mg/serving

[1]See 21 CFR 105 for complete information.

ment, mitigation, cure, or diagnosis, they must comply with the drug provisions of the act."[95] Thus, labeling is a particularly important factor with foods for special dietary use, since labeling or representation of the product can cause the food to become a drug within the context of the Act.

Specific regulations affecting foods for special dietary use are covered in 21 CFR 105. In this regulation, the definition of "special dietary uses," is further expanded to include "uses for supplying particular dietary needs which exist by reason of age, including but not limited to ages of infancy and childhood" and foods containing artificial sweeteners". . .except when specifically and solely used for achieving physical characteristics in the food which cannot be achieved with sugar or other nutritive sweetener. . ."

The basic focus of regulations of foods for special dietary use (apart from infant formulas which will be considered in depth later) are the labeling requirements for these products (see Table 14.4). The regulations spell out specific requirements for: hypoallergenic foods, infant foods, and products for reducing or maintaining caloric intake or body weight, food for use in the diet of diabetics, and lastly for foods used to regulate sodium intake (21 CFR 105).

Infant Formula Regulations

Infant formula is frequently described as the most highly regulated food product in the United States. This status is appropriate in view of the important role infant formulas play in the diet of infants who receive them. Infant formula serves as the sole source of nutrition for many infants during a critical stage when growth and development are occurring at a rate unequalled at any other time in the life cycle.

The advancing state of knowledge of infant nutrition has been reflected in the evolution of regulations and the recommendations of governmental agencies and various scientific bodies. In 1941, only a few nutrients were specified in the U.S. Food and Drug Administration's (FDA) labeling requirement for infant formulas. These were a part of the general requirement for foods for special dietary purposes.[26,96] The regulations then established minimum requirements for five nutrients.[97] The list of required nutrients expanded to include 17 vitamins and minerals as well as protein, fat, and linoleic acid in 1971. The change in 1971 incorporated the 1967 recommendations of the American Academy of Pediatrics Committee on Nutrition (AAP/CON). The federal government has come to rely increasingly on the expertise of the AAP/CON in establishing nutrient requirements for infants and, more recently, in other areas, including guidelines for clinical testing of infant formula products.

Infant Formula Act of 1980 and Amendments of 1986. The major milestone in infant formula regulation occurred with passage of the Infant Formula Act of 1980 (IFA).[98] This legislation passed virtually unanimously. In it the U.S. Congress provided FDA with specific authority over infant formulas in a manner and to a degree never before encountered with any food product. The enactment was precipitated in large part by a problem involving the marketing of two soy protein infant formula products which contained insufficient chloride to fully meet infants' requirements for this essential nutrient.[99]

The Infant Formula Act of 1980 delegated to FDA in the Department of Health and Human Services (HHS) very broad rule-making authority. Some principal features of the 1980 IFA were to mandate nutrient levels for 29 nutrients, require FDA to establish quality control (QC) procedures, define when an infant formula is adulterated, and to require manufacturers to notify FDA under several specified circumstances. The legal ramifications of the IFA have been discussed by Levin.[100]

In 1986, Congress amended the IFA, providing FDA expanded authority. The combined results are summarized below:

Required Nutrients. Congress built into the Act a table of 29 required nutrients specifying minimum and, in the case of protein, fat, vitamins A and D, iron, iodine, sodium, potassium, and chloride maximum levels, for both milk-based and nonmilk-based formulas (see Table 14.5). At the same time, they granted the Secretary of the Department of Health and Human Services (HHS) the authority to revise the list of required nutrients.[101]

TABLE 14.5
NUTRIENT SPECIFICATIONS FOR INFANT FORMULAS[1]
(21 CFR 107.100)

Nutrients	Minimum Level	Maximum Level
Protein, g	1.8	4.5
Fat, g	3.3	6.0
% calories	30	54
Linoleic acid, mg	300	—
% calories	2.7	—
Vitamin A, IU	250	750
Vitamin D, IU	40	100
Vitamin E, IU	0.7	—
Vitamin K, mcg	4	—
Thiamine (B_1), mcg	40	—
Riboflavin (B_2), mcg	60	—
Vitamin B_6, mcg	35	—
Vitamin B_{12}, mcg	0.15	—
Niacin,[2] mcg	250	—
Folic acid, mcg	4	—
Pantothenic acid, mcg	300	—
Biotin, mcg[3]	1.5	—
Vitamin C (ascorbic acid), mg	8	—
Choline,[3] mg	7	—
Inositol,[3] mg	4	—
Calcium, mg	60	—
Phosphorus, mg	30	—
Magnesium, mg	6	—
Iron, mg	0.15	3.0
Zinc, mg	0.5	—
Manganese, mcg	5	—
Copper, mcg	60	—
Iodine, mcg	5	75
Sodium, mg	20	60
Potassium, mg	80	200
Chloride, mg	55	150

[1]For each 100 kcal of the infant formula prepared for consumption as depicted on the container.
[2]The generic term "niacin" includes niacin (nicotinic acid) and niacinamide (nicotinamide).
[3]Required only for nonmilk-based infant formulas.

Quality Factors. Congress empowered HHS to establish quality factors, including quality factors for required nutrients.

Quality Control Requirements. The Secretary of HHS was required to "establish good manufacturing practices for infant formulas, including quality control procedures that the Secretary determines are necessary to assure that an infant formula provides . . . required nutrients . . . and is manufactured in a manner designed to prevent adulteration of the infant formula."[102]

Infant formula quality control procedure regulations based on the 1980 Act became effective July 19, 1982. Through these regulations, FDA established procedures to assure that infant formulas contain the necessary nutrients at the required levels. Each manufacturer must establish a QC system, but the regulations permit each to adopt the system that is best suited to its needs (21 CFR 106). Other aspects of the mandated QC system are highlighted in Table 14.6.

The 1982 QC procedures also require special testing for infant formulas that have undergone a major change in formulation or processing, including measurements of osmolality, biological value of protein, vitamin D (using the rat bioassay method), and complete nutrient testing.

In addition, the QC procedures require the maintenance of QC records that contain "sufficient information to permit a public health evaluation of any batch of infant formula." These records must be retained for at least one year beyond product shelf-life and be made available to FDA inspectors for review and copying.

Good Manufacturing Practices for Infant Formulas. Congress required HHS to promulgate regulations establishing good manufacturing practices (GMPs) for infant formulas to include the following provisions:

(1) testing each batch for each required nutrient before distribution,
(2) regularly scheduled testing during shelf-life to ensure compliance,
(3) in-process controls to prevent adulteration,
(4) regularly scheduled internal audits by the manufacturer.

Notification. Congress requires manufacturers to register with the Secretary 90 days before introducing a new infant formula into interstate commerce, identifying all establishments at which the formula will be manufactured. Additionally, for new infant formulas and those undergoing a major change, the manufacturer must submit the quantitative formulation and description of the formulation or processing change (where appropriate). The manufacturer must also include assurances that the product meets the quality factors and GMP requirements. Then, after first production and before introduction into interstate commerce, the manufacturer is required to submit written summaries of test results and records demonstrating compliance. Guidelines that reflect FDA policy on notification and testing requirements have been issued by the agency.

Recalls. The amended IFA provides the Secretary with broader authority with respect to recalls than the agency has with other regulated products, including drugs. If the manufacturer has "knowledge" that product in distribution may not provide the required nutrients or is otherwise adulterated or misbranded, he must notify the Secretary. Should the Secretary determine that the infant formula presents a risk to human health, the manufacturer is required to recall the product. The law requires that manufacturers request retailers to post notices of the recall at the retail level and for manufacturers to provide interim reports to FDA on recall progress every 15 days.

TABLE 14.6
ASPECTS OF FDA INFANT QUALITY CONTROL REQUIREMENTS[1]

Ingredient control	Testing for each relied-upon nutrient (individual ingredients and premix)[2]
In-Process control	Master manufacturing control (batch record) system
Finished product evaluation	Sampling and testing to ensure nutrient requirements are met
	Final product analyses for vitamins A, B_1, C, and E[2]
	Periodic analyses on quarterly basis
	Stability testing

[1]The reader should consult 21 CFR 106 for details.
[2]Specifically required by 1986 IFA amendments.

Exemptions. Congress established a category for formulas that would, of necessity, be exempt from one or more provisions of IFA requirement, i.e., level or inclusion of individual nutrients, labeling, quality factors, quality control, or notification requirements. By definition, "exempt formulas" include formulas ". . . represented and labeled for use by infants who have inborn errors of metabolism, or low birthweight, or who otherwise have unusual medical or dietary problems" (21 CFR 107.3). Specific requirements are spelled out in the regulation in two categories based on retail availability. Submissions for exempt status are more extensive than those for "routine" formulas and must include the medical, scientific, nutritional, and technological rationale for the exemption.

Labeling. Detailed labeling regulations for infant formulas describe format and content requirements. These cover nutrient information as well as directions for use, including the use of pictograms and a dilution symbol (21 CFR 107). Background information collected by FDA prior to issuing these regulations was provided by Barnes.[103]

Records. Manufacturers are required to maintain records that demonstrate compliance with GMP and QC procedures, premix nutrient content, microbiological quality and purity of raw materials used in formula powder and finished infant formula, packaging, internal compliance audits, complaints, and product distribution. These records are to be maintained for at least one year beyond the end of the expiration date of the batch and most are required to be available to FDA for inspection purposes.

Other Applicable Regulations

Formulated special purpose foods are subject to all other food regulations as may apply, except where preempted by the specific regulations. For example, many of the formulated special purpose foods discussed in this chapter are produced as ready-to-use liquids or concentrated liquids at or near neutral pH. They must comply with the specific regulations that apply to foods of this type, namely 21 CFR 113, "Thermally Processed Low-Acid Foods Packaged in Hermetically Sealed Containers." All formulated special purpose foods are also subject to the so-called "umbrella' Good Manufacturing Practices regulations in 21 CFR 110.

ACKNOWLEDGMENTS

The authors thank their many friends and colleagues at Mead Johnson Nutritional Group including those whose names may not appear in the Bibliography who developed many of the concepts discussed. We especially wish to thank Drs. G. L. Baker, D. A. Cook, J. L. Moore, P. J. Smith, and T. A. Swinford for their helpful comments and encouragement. Finally, we thank Madonna Yancey for her timely help in typing the manuscript and Marjorie Fuller for her valued assistance in collecting and formatting the authors' references.

REFERENCES

1. MOORE, J. L. 1987. Nutitional equivalency considerations of foods that serve as a sole source of nutrients. Food Technol. *41*(2), 135–140.
2. WRETLAND, A. 1981. Parenteral Nutrition. Nutr. Rev. *39*, 257–265.
3. SILBERMAN, H. and EISENBERG, D. 1982. Parenteral and Enteral Nutrition for the Hospitalized Patient. Appleton & Lange, Norwalk.
4. GILDER, H. 1986. Parenteral nourishment of patients undergoing surgical or traumatic stress. J. Parenter. Enteral Nutr. *10*, 88–99.
5. ANDERSON, S. A., CHINN, H. I. and FISHER, K. D. 1982. History and current status of infant formulas. Am. J. Clin. Nutr. *35*, 381–397.
6. FORSYTH, D. 1911. The history of feeding from Elizabethan times. Proc. Roy. Soc. Med. *4*, 110–141.
7. CORDANO, A. 1984. Pre-clinical and clinical evaluation of new infant formulas. Nutr. Res. *4*, 929–934.
8. FOMAN, S. J. 1974. Infant Nutrition, 2nd Ed. W. B. Saunders Co., Philadelphia.
9. GERSTENBERGER, H. I., HASKINS, H. D., McGREGOR, H. H. and RUH, H. O. 1915. Studies in the adaptation of an artificial food to human milk. Am. J. Dis. Child. *10*, 249–265.
10. American Academy of Pediatrics Committee on Nutrition. 1976. Commentary on breast-feeding and infant formulas, including proposed standards for formulas. Pediatrics *57*, 278–285.
11. PIPES, P. L. 1985. Nutrition in Infancy and Childhood, 3rd Ed. Times Mirror/Mosby College Publishing, St. Louis.
12. WINICK, M., ROSSO, P. and WATERLOW, J. 1970. Cellular growth of cerebrum, cerebellum, and brain stem in normal and marasmin children. Exp. Neurol. *26*, 393.
13. BALISTERI, W. F. 1988. Anatomic and biochemical ontogeny of the gastrointestinal tract and liver. *In* Nutrition During Infancy, R. C. Tsang and B. L. Nichols (eds.). Hanley & Belfus, Philadelphia.

14. AGUNOD, M., YAMAGUCHI, N., LOPEZ, R., LUHBY, A. L. and GLASS, G. B. J. 1969. Correlative study of hydrochloric acid pepsin, and intrinsic factor secretion in newborns and infants. Am. J. Dig. Dis. *14*, 400-414.
15. BORGSTROM, B., LINDQUIST, B. and LUNDH, G. 1960. Enzyme concentration and absorption of protein and glucose in duodenum of premature infants. Am. J. Dis. Child. *99*, 338-343.
16. JAMES, W. P. T. 1970. Sugar absorption and intestinal motility in children when malnourished and after treatment. Clin. Sci. *39*, 305-318.
17. MOBASSALAH, M. and GRAND, R. J. 1987. Physiology of carbohydrate absorption. *In* Pediatric Nutrition: Theory and Practice, R. J. Grand, J. L. Sutphen and W. H. Dietz (eds.). Butterworth's, Boston.
18. KOLDOVSKY, O. 1978. Digestion and absorption. *In* Perinatal Physiology, U. Stane (ed.). Plenum Medical Books, New York.
19. COHEN, M., MORGAN, R. G. H. and HOFFMAN, A. F. 1971. Lypolytic activity of human gastric and duodenal juice against medium- and long-chain triglycerides. Gastroenterology *60*, 1-15.
20. HADORN, B., ZOPPI, G., SHMERLING, D. H., PRADER, A., McINTYRE, I. and ANDERSON, C. M. 1968. Quantitative assessment of exocrine pancreatic function in infants and children. J. Pediatr. *73*, 39-50.
21. NORMAN, A., STANDVIK, B. and OJAMAE, O. 1972. Bile acids and pancreatic enzymes during absorption in the newborn. Acta Paediatr. Scand. *61*, 571-576.
22. HOLT, P. R. 1972. The roles of bile acids during the process of normal fat and cholesterol absorption. Arch. Intern. Med. *130*, 574-583.
23. BERGMANN, K. E., ZIEGLER, E. E. and FOMON, S. J. 1974. Water and renal solute load. *In* Infant Nutrition, 2nd Ed., S. J. Foman (ed.). W. B. Saunders Co., Philadelphia.
24. DRUMMOND, K. N. 1975. The urinary system. *In* Nelson Textbook of Pediatrics, 10th Ed., V. C. Vaughan, III, R. J. McKay and W. E. Nelson (eds.). W. B. Saunders Co., Philadelphia.
25. COURSIN, D. B. 1954. Convulsive seizures in infants with pyridoxine-deficient diet. J. Am. Med. Assoc. *154*, 406-408.
26. COOK, D. A. and SARETT, H. P. 1982. Design of infant formulas for meeting normal and special needs. *In* Pediatric Nutrition: Infant Feedings-Deficiencies-Diseases, F. Lifshitz (ed.). Marcel Dekker, New York.
27. Food and Nutrition Board, National Research Council. 1989. Recommended Dietary Allowances, 10th Rev. Ed., National Academy of Sciences, Washington, D.C.
28. Codex Alimentarius Commission, Joint FAO/WHO Food Standards Program. 1976. Recommended International Standards for Foods for Infants and Children. Food and Agricultural Organization of the United Nations, Rome.
29. ESPGAN Committee on Nutrition. 1977. Guidelines on infant nutrition. I. Recommendations for the composition of an adapted formula. Acta Paediatr. Scand. (Suppl.) *262*, 1-20.
30. FOMON, S. J., THOMAS, L. N., FILER, L. J., ANDERSON, T. A. and BERGMANN, K. E. 1973. Requirements for protein and essential amino acids in early infancy: Studies with a soy-isolate formula. Acta Paediatr. Scand. *62*, 33-45.
31. SOLOMON, N. W. and KEUSCH, G. T. 1982. Nutrition and infection: etiology and mechanism of malabsorption and diarrhea. *In* Pediatric Nutrition: Infant Feedings-Deficiencies-Diseases, F. Lifshitz (ed.). Marcel Dekker, New York.

32. FAGUNDES-NETO, U., LIFSHITZ, F. and CORDANO, A. 1985. Dietary management of postinfectious chronic diarrhea in malnourished infants. *In* Nutrition for Special Needs in Infancy: Protein Hydrolysates, F. Lifshitz (ed.). Marcel Dekker, New York.
33. LIFSHITZ, F. 1985. Nutrition for special needs in infancy. *In* Nutrition for Special Needs in Infancy: Protein Hydrolysates, F. Lifshitz (ed.). Marcel Dekker, New York.
34. ZEIGER, R. S. 1985. Offspring of high-risk allergic families. *In* Nutrition for Special Needs in Infancy: Protein Hydrolysates, F. Lifshitz (ed.). Marcel Dekker, New York.
35. POWELL, G. K. 1985. Use of casein hydrolysate formulas in the diagnosis and management of gastrointestinal food sensitivity in infancy. *In* Nutrition for Special Needs in Infancy: Protein Hydrolysates, F. Lifshitz (ed.). Marcel Dekker, New York.
36. LLOYD-STILL, J. D., SMITH, A. E., SULLIVAN, D. K. AND WESSEL, H. U. 1985. Protein hydrolysates in cystic fibrosis. *In* Nutrition for Special Needs in Infancy: Protein Hydrolysates, F. Lifshitz (ed.). Marcel Dekker, New York.
37. AMPOLA, M. G. 1987. Nutrition in inborn errors of amino acid metabolism. *In* Pediatric Nutrition: Theory and Practice, R. J. Grand, J. L. Sutphen and W. H. Dietz (eds.). Butterworth's, Boston.
38. HEIRD, W. C. 1982. Feeding of low-birth-weight infants. *In* Pediatric Nutrition: Infant Feeding-Deficiencies-Diseases, F. Lifshitz (ed.). Marcel Dekker, New York.
39. BRADY, M. S., RICKARD, K. A., ERNST, J. A., SCHREINER, R. L. and LEMONS, J. A. 1982. Formulas and human milk for premature infants: A review and update. J. Am. Diet. Assoc. *81*, 547–555.
40. PENCHARZ, P. B. 1987. Nutrition of the low-birth-weight infant. *In* Pediatric Nutrition: Theory and Practice, R. J. Grand, J. L. Sutphen and W. H. Dietz (eds.). Butterworth's, Boston.
41. MOSES, N. 1985. Infant formulas and enteral products to meet nutritional needs. *In* Nutrition for Special Needs in Infancy: Protein Hydrolysates, F. Lifshitz (ed.). Marcel Dekker, New York.
42. Association of Official Analytical Chemists. 1984. Protein efficiency ratio rat bioassay. Methods of Analysis, 14th Ed. Assoc. Offic. Anal. Chem., Arlington, VA.
43. CORDANO, A. 1982. Infant formula—clinical evaluation, its uses, and current feeding practices in the United States and developing countries. *In* Advances in Human Clinical Nutrition, J. J. Vitale and Broitman, S. A. (eds.). PSG Publishing Co., Boston.
44. FOMAN, S. J., THOMAS, L. N., FILER, L. J., ZIEGLER, E. E. and LEONARD, M. T. 1971. Food consumption and growth of normal infants fed milk-based formulas. Acta Paediatr. Scand. Suppl. *223*, 1–36.
45. American Society of Parenteral and Enternal Nutrition. Special report: definitions of terms used in A.S.P.E.N. guidelines and standards. J. Parenter. Enter. Nutr. *12*(2), 219.
46. SARETT, H. P. 1967. Contribution of industrial research to human nutrition. Med. Serv. J. Can. *23*, 925–941.
47. SARETT, H. P., LONGNECKER, J. B., BARBORIAK, J. J. and HARKINS, R. W. 1962. Nutritional studies with "900 calorie" diets. J. Assoc. Off. Agric. Chem. *45*, 434–438.
48. BLOCH, A. 1987. Enteral formulas. Nutr. Support Serv. *7*, 23–24.
49. SILK, D. B. A. 1986. Enteral nutrition—the future. Recent Adv. Clin. Nutr. *2*, 203–213.
50. SHILS, M. E. 1977. Enteral nutrition by tube. Cancer Res. *37*, 2432–2439.

51. WILMORE, D. W., McDOUGAL, W. S. and PETERSON, J. P. 1977. Newer products and formulas for alimentation. Am. J. Clin. Nutr. *30*, 1498–1505.
52. THOMPSON, W. R., STEPHENS, R. V., RANDALL, H. T. and BOWEN, J. R. 1969. Use of the "space diet" in the management of a patient with extreme short bowel syndrome. Am. J. Surg. *117*, 449–459.
53. BURY, K. D., STEPHENS, R. V. and RANDALL, H. T. Use of a chemically defined, liquid, elemental diet for nutritional management of fistulas of the alimentary tract. Am. J. Surg. *121*, 174–183.
54. YOUNG, E. A., CIOLETTI, L. A., WINBORN, W. B. and WESER, E. 1980. Comparative study of nutritional adaptation to defined formula diets. Am. J. Clin. Nutr. *33*, 2106–2118.
55. WESER, E., FLETCHER, J. T. and URBAN, E. 1979. Short bowel syndrome. Gastroenterology *77*, 572–579.
56. DRISCOLL, R. H., JR. and ROSENBERG, I. H. 1978. Total parenteral nutrition in inflammatory bowel disease. Med. Clin. North Am. *62*, 185–201.
57. HILL, G. L., BLOCKETT, R. L., PICKFORD, I. R. and BRADLEY, J. A. 1977. A survey of protein nutrition in patients with inflammatory bowel disease: A rational basis for nutritional therapy. Br. J. Surg. *64*, 894–896.
58. COSTA, G. and DONALDSON, S. S. 1979. Effects of cancer and cancer treatment on the nutrition of the host. N. Engl. J. Med. *300*, 1471–1474.
59. DE WYS, W. D. et al. 1980. Prognostic effect of weight loss prior to chemotherapy in cancer patients. Am. J. Med. *69*, 491–497.
60. KOTLER, D. P. 1984. The enteropathy of AIDS. Gastroenterology *86*, 1143 (Abstr.).
61. FOX, C. H., KOTLER, D. P., TIERNEY, A. R., WILSON, C. S. and FAUCI, A. S. 1988. Detection of HIV-L RNA in intestinal lamina propria in AIDS. Gastroenterology *94*, 134 (Abstr.).
62. KOTLER, D. P., TIERNEY, A. R., WANG, J. and PIERSON, R. N. 1987. The magnitude of tissue wasting determines the timing of death in patients with AIDS. Clin. Res. *35*, 368A (Abstr.).
63. CULPEPPERMORGAN, J., KOTLER, D. P., SCHOLES, J. V. and TIERNEY, A. R. 1987. Endoscopic diagnosis of disseminated cytomegalovirus infection in AIDS. Gastrointest. Endosc. *33*, 180 (Abstr.).
64. KOTLER, D. P., BRENNER, S., COUTURE, S., TIERNEY, A. R., WANG, J. and PIERSON, R. N. 1987. Short-term caloric balance in clinically stable patients with AIDS. Clin. Res. *35*, 368 (Abstr.).
65. MOLNAR, J. A., WOLFE, R. R. and BURKE, J. F. 1983. Burns: Metabolism and nutritional therapy in thermal injury. *In* Nutritional Support of Medical Practice, 2nd Ed., H. A. Schneider, C. E. Anderson and D. B. Coursin (eds.). Harper & Row, Hagerstown.
66. GOODWIN, C. W. and WILMORE, D. W. 1983. Surgery and burns. *In* Manual of Clinical Nutrition, D. W. Paige (ed.). Nutrition Publications, Pleasantville, N.J.
67. BLACKBURN, G. L., HOPKINS, B. S. and BISTRAIN, B. R. 1983. Protein-calorie management in the hospitalized patient. *In* Nutritional Support of Medical Practice, 2nd Ed., H. A. Schneider, C. A. Anderson and P. B. Coursin (eds.). Harper & Row, Hagerstown.
68. CLOWES, G. H. A., JR., O'DONNELL, T. F., RYAN, N. T. and BLACKBURN,

G. L. 1974. Energy metabolism in sepsis: Treatment based on different patterns in shock and high output stage. Ann. Surg. *179*, 684–696.
69. McFADYEN, B. V. J., COPELAND, E. M., III and DUDRICK, S. J. 1983. Surgery. *In* Nutritional Support of Medical Practice, 2nd Ed., H. A. Schneider, C. E. Anderson and D. B. Coursin (eds.). Harper & Row, Hagerstown.
70. MULLEN, J. L. 1981. Consequences of malnutrition in the surgical patient. Surg. Clin. North Am. *61*, 465–487.
71. BUZBY, G. P. *et al.* 1980. Prognostic nutritional index in gastrointestinal surgery. Am. J. Surg. *139*, 160–167.
72. TILSON, M. D. 1980. Pathophysiology and treatment of short bowel syndrome. Surg. Clin. North Am. *60*, 1273–1284.
73. BROWN, E. K., SETTLE, E. A. and VAN RIJ, A. M. 1982. Food intake patterns of gastric bypass patients. J. Am. Diet. Assoc. *80*, 437–443.
74. NEWMARK, S. R. and WILLIAMSON, B. 1983. Survey of very-low-calorie weight reduction diets. II. Total fasting, protein-sparing modified fasts, chemically defined diets. Arch. Intern. Med. *143*(7), 1423–1427.
75. BLACKBURN, G. L. *et al.* 1977. Nutritional and metabolic assessment of the hospitalized patient. J. Parenter. Enter. Nutr. *1*, 11–22.
76. COOK, D. A. 1985. The design of infant formulas. *In* Production, Regulation, and Analysis of Infant Formula. Proceedings of a Topical Conference, Association of Official Analytical Chemists, Arlington, VA.
77. McDERMOTT, R. L. 1987. Functionality of dairy ingredients in infant formulas and nutritional specialty products. Food Technol. *43*, 91–103.
78. THEUER, R. C. 1983. Milk protein in infant nutrition: Development and manufacture of infant formula. Kiel Milchwirtsch. Forschungsber. *35*, 423–430.
79. Code of Federal Regulations. 1987. Title 21, Part 113. U.S. Government Printing Office, Washington, D.C.
80. BERRY, M. R. and KOHNHORST, A. L. 1985. Heating characteristics of homogenous milk-based formulas in cans processed in an agitating retort. J. Food Sci. *50*, 209–214, 253.
81. PACKARD, V. S. 1982. Infant formula composition, formulation and processing. *In* Human Milk and Infant Formula. Academic Press, New York.
82. Infant Formula Council. 1982. Methods of Analysis Manual for Infant Formulas. Physical Stability Section AA. Infant Formula Counc., Atlanta.
83. TENNYSON, R. H. 1985. Infant formula quality assurance. *In* Production, Regulation, and Analysis of Infant Formula. Proceedings of a Topical Conference. Association of Official Analytical Chemists, Arlington, VA.
84. KRASAVAGE, K. W. 1987. Personal communication.
85. Food Chemical Codex. 1981. Third Edition. National Academy Press, Washington, D.C.
86. The United States Pharmacopeia/The National Formulary. 1985. United States Pharmacopeial Convention, Rockville, MD.
87. SCHULTZ, R. A. 1985. Quality assurance of analytical data. *In* Production, Regulation, and Analysis of Infant Formula. Proceedings of a Topical Conference. Association of Official Analytical Chemists, Arlington, VA.
88. KUTAK, M. 1985. FDA/IFC collaborative study of infant formula. *In* Production, Regulation, and Analysis of Infant Formula. Proceedings of a Topical Conference. Association of Official Analytical Chemists, Arlington, VA.

89. National Research Council, Food and Nutrition Board, Committee on Food Protection, Subcommittee on Microbiological Criteria. 1985. Expansion of the HACCP system in food protection programs. National Academy Press, Washington, D.C.
90. BARNETT, S. A. and SAUCERMAN, J. R. 1987. Personal communication.
91. DAVIS, J. E. 1987. Personal communication.
92. U.S. Public Health Service, Food and Drug Administration. 1978. Grade A condensed and dry milk products and condensed and dry whey. Suppl. I to the Grade A Pasteurized Milk Ordinance. U.S. Government Printing Office, Washington, D.C.
93. REED, D. V., LOMBARDO, P., WESSEL, J. R., BURKE, J. A. and McMAHON, B. 1987. The FDA pesticides monitoring program. J. Assoc. Off. Anal. Chem. 70, 591–595.
94. GARTRELL, M. J., CRAUN, J. C., PODREBARAC, D. S. and GUNDERSON, E. L. 1986. Pesticides, selected elements, and other chemicals in infant and toddler diet samples October 1980–March 1982. J. Assoc. Off. Anal. Chem. 69, 123–145.
95. U.S. Department of Health and Human Services, Food and Drug Administration. 1984. Requirements of Laws and Regulations Enforced by the U.S. Food and Drug Administration. U.S. Government Printing Office, Washington, D.C.
96. Federal Register. 1941. 6, 5921–5926.
97. FORBES, A. L., MILLER, S. A. and DUY, N. 1985. Food and drug administration's perspectives on infant formula production. In Production, Regulation, and Analysis of Infant Formula. Proceedings of a Topical Conference, Association of Official Analytical Chemists, Arlington, VA.
98. United States Congress. Infant Formula Act of 1980, Public Law 96-359. United States Capitol Health Document Room, Washington, D.C.
99. MILLER, S. A. and CHOPRA, J. G. 1984. Problems with human milk and infant formulas. Pediatrics 74, 639–647.
100. LEVIN, T. M. 1987. Infant Formula Act 1980: A case study of congressional delegation to the Food and Drug Administration. Food, Drug and Cosmetic Law Journal 42, 101–154.
101. Federal Food, Drug, and Cosmetic Act, as amended, Sect. 412(a), (g). 1987. U.S. Government Printing Office, Washington, D.C.
102. Federal Food, Drug, and Cosmetic Act, as amended, Sect. 412(a)(2). 1987. U.S. Government Printing Office, Washington, D.C.
103. BARNES, R. W. 1982. Infant formula label review. J. Assoc. Off. Anal. Chem. 65, 1474–1477.

CHAPTER 15

ADDED ASCORBATES AND TOCOPHEROLS AS ANTIOXIDANTS AND FOOD IMPROVERS

LEONARD E. JOHNSON, Ph.D.
and
WILLIAM J. MERGENS, Ph.D.

INTRODUCTION

It is only natural, when one considers the history of vitamins, to view them primarily as essential dietary factors. This is particularly true today in light of the heightened interest, and numerous studies in progress, pertaining to the possible role of micronutrients and cancer prevention.[1] In a technical sense, however, some of the vitamins have unique chemical properties which make them useful as processing aids in a variety of industries. Two of the more useful families of vitamin compounds in this respect are the ascorbates and tocopherols. These two chemical classes have been used for many years for their technological functions as antioxidants, reducing agents, acidifiers, buffering agents, solvents, etc., providing food manufacturers the opportunity to market many standard and convenience products that might not be possible otherwise.

It is the aim of this chapter to view the chemical properties of these molecules that provide these desirable product attributes to the food manufacturer, as well as to mention many of the recent and/or significant applications that have been reported in the literature.

GENERAL BACKGROUND AND PHYSICAL PROPERTIES

Ascorbic Acid and Derivatives

L-ascorbic acid (a six-carbon, water soluble, white, crystalline compound) is vitamin C (the antiscorbutic vitamin) and has also been called L-xylo-ascorbic acid, hexuronic acid, or cevitanic acid. L-ascorbic acid ($C_6H_8O_6$) resembles the simple sugars in structure and reacts like sugars under some chemical conditions. L-ascorbic acid is one of a pair of enantiomers having the 2-hexenono-1,4-lactone structure.

The other pair is the D- and L-isoascorbic acids, which are also referred to as D- and L-erythorbic acids. The significant U.S. commercial forms of ascorbic acid available to the food industry are L-ascorbic acid, sodium ascorbate, calcium ascorbate, erythorbic acid, sodium erythorbate and the 6-palmitate ester of L-ascorbic acid. The latter, commonly referred to as ascorbyl palmitate, is a unique fat-soluble form of the basic molecule which has found many applications in lipid systems. Outside of the United States, potassium ascorbate and ascorbyl 6-stearate find uses in certain food applications. A summary of the chemical structures of these compounds is presented in Fig. 15.1.

Many other ascorbate derivatives have been reported in the literature and include inorganic esters; alkyl and acyl derivatives at C2, C3, C5 and C6; plus (C5 and C6) esters and acetals.[2] None of these derivatives, except those cited above, are approved for food use. It should be pointed out that derivatization of the C2 and C3 position results in loss of reducing, antioxidant and oxygen scavenging properties in the molecule. C5 and C6 derivatization, on the other hand, does not destroy these properties but rather generally increases the lipid solubility of the parent molecule.

The most important chemical property of the ascorbate moiety is its ease of oxidation through either one- or two-electron transfer reactions. This is possible through the unique enediol grouping ($-COH=COH-$) of these molecules. The chemistry of these reactions as they relate to foods has recently been reviewed.[3] Oxidation proceeds in stages, its rate increasing as the pH is raised, to first form physiologically active (in the case of ascorbic acid) dehydroascorbic acid, a reversible stage. Continuing oxidation results in the irreversible formation of 2, 3-diketo-gulonic acid 3-deoxy-L-pentosone, furfural, reductones and L-threonic acid as the main products of degradation. The physical and chemical properties of ascorbates are summarized in Table 15.1. Both the water-soluble and fat-soluble derivatives are highly stable in the dry state, but are gradually oxidized and become discolored when exposed to humidity and light (salts > acid > C-6 ester derivatives). In solution, all of the compounds listed in Table 15.1 can be oxidized by air with the rate increasing at elevated temperature. Oxidation is also promoted by ions of heavy metals, such as iron and copper. In strongly alkaline solution rapid oxidation will occur, especially in the presence of oxygen. This is true for the fat-soluble derivatives as well, since they become water soluble under such conditions.

Erythorbic acid can be substituted for ascorbic acid in most functional food uses, but this is not always the case. Some comparisons have been made that reveal differences in solubilities and rates of solution between the acids and salts (see Table 15.1); the rate of oxidation of erythorbic acid is greater than ascorbic; the oxygen scavenging ability of erythorbic acid is less efficient than ascorbic acid; and their redox potentials are different.[4] The bread-improving action of L-ascorbic acid is stereo specific; the other three isomers in Fig. 15.1 (II and IV) have negligible action.[5] From a nutritional standpoint, use of erythorbic acid in foods is regulated due to its possible interference with the bioavailability of L-ascorbic acid.[6]

In general the four basic methods for adding water soluble ascorbates to foods are: (1) as the pure crystalline compound(s); (2) premixing with diluent, carrier or other functionally important additives; (3) liquid solution for spray or injection applications; or (4) as wafers or tablets for use in batch-type operations where the pro-

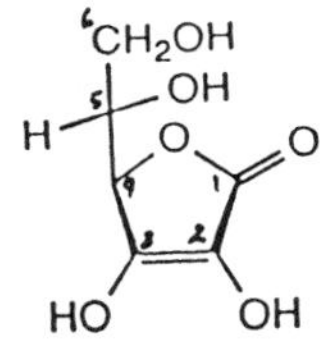

I. ASCORBIC ACID

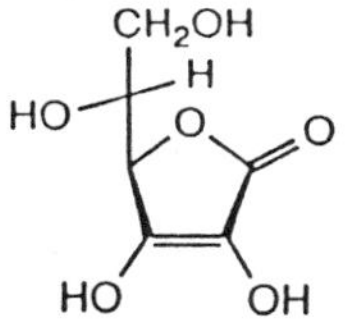

II. ERYTHORBIC ACID

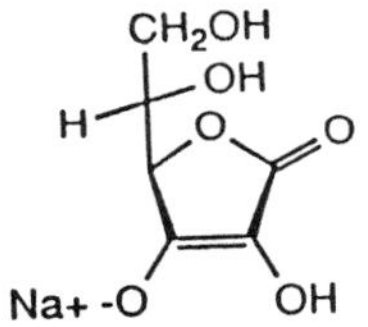

III. SOD. ASCORBATE

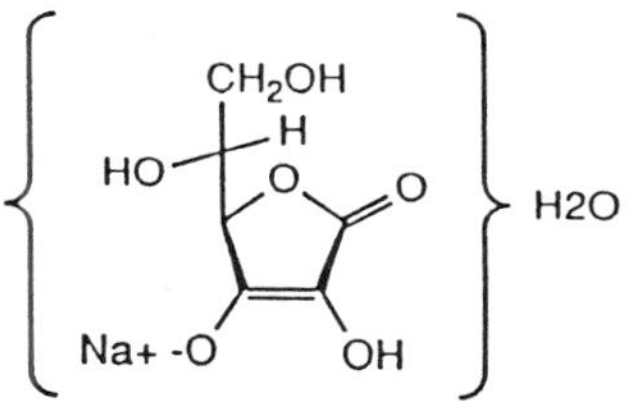

IV. SOD. ERYTHORBATE

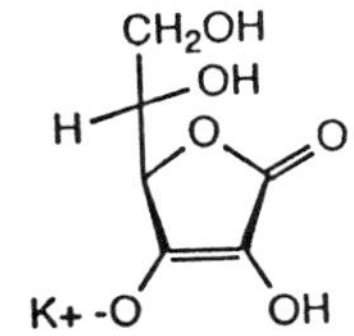

V. POT. ASCORBATE

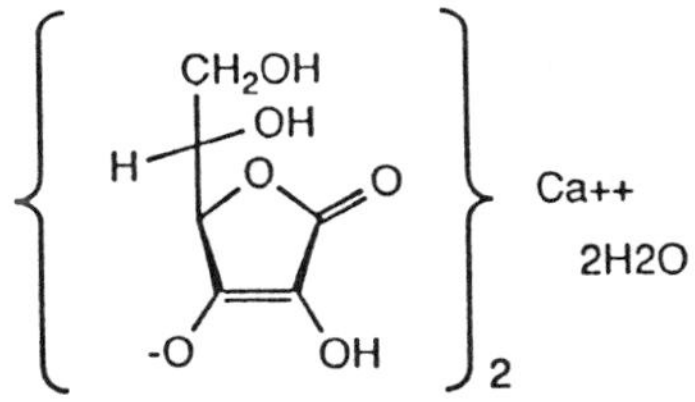

VI. CAL. ASCORBATE

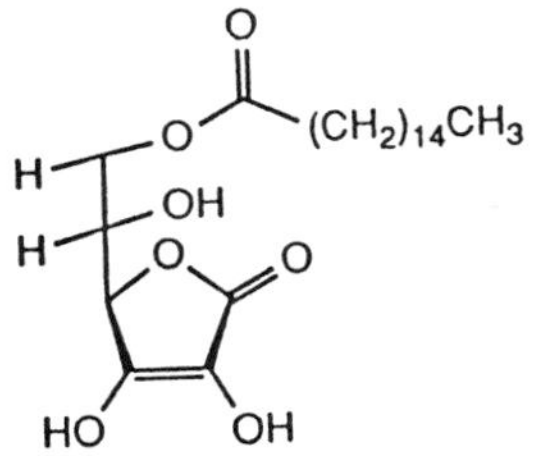

VII. ASCORBYL PALMITATE

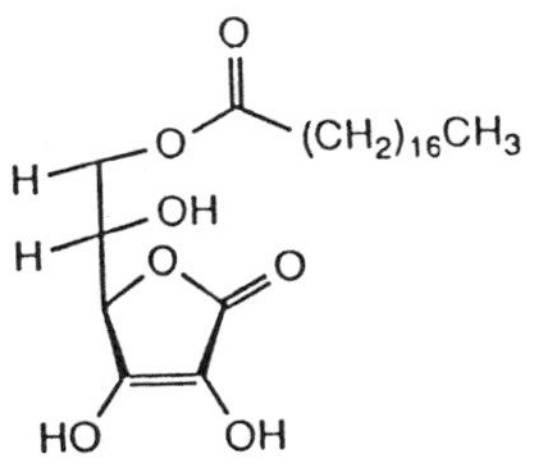

VIII. ASCORBYL STEARATE

FIG. 15.1. CHEMICAL STRUCTURES OF L-ASCORBIC ACID AND DERIVATIVES

TABLE 15.1
PHYSICAL AND CHEMICAL PROPERTIES OF ASCORBIC ACID AND DERIVATIVES

Property	Ascorbic Acid	Sodium Ascorbate	Calcium Ascorbate	Potassium Ascorbate	Erythorbic Acid	Sodium Erythorbate	Ascorbyl Palmitate	Ascorbyl Stearate
Color	white	white	white	white	white	white	white	white
Taste	sour	sl. salty	bitter	sl. bitter	sour	sl. salty	bland	bland
Appearance	crystalline*	crystalline*	crystalline	crystalline	crystalline*	crystalline*	waxy powder	waxy powder
	$C_6H_8O_6$	$C_6H_7NaO_6$	$C_{12}H_{14}Ca_{12} \cdot 2H_2O$	$C_6H_7KO_6$	$C_6H_8O_6$	$C_6H_7NaO_6 \cdot H_2O$	$C_{22}H_{38}O_7$	$C_{24}H_{42}O_7$
Molecular wt.	176.13	198.11	426.35	194.11	176.13	216.12	414.54	442.54
Mp.	190°C	220°C	--	183°C	170°C	--	112°C	114-115°C
Enediol. equiv.	1.0	1.12	1.21	1.10	1.0	1.23	2.35	2.51
$\overset{D}{20}$	+21°	+105°	+96°	+104°	-17°	+96°	+22.5° (NaOH)	+15.8° (EtOH)

pH (10% soln.)	--	7.5	6.8-7.4	7.5	--	5.5-8.0	--
5 mg/mL	3	--	--	--	3	--	--
50 mg/mL	2	--	--	--	2	--	--
Solubility (mg/mL)							
H$_2$O	330	770	500	980	400	160	0.2
95% EtOH	33	<1	<1	<1	--	--	108
EtOH	<1	<1	<1	<1	--	--	120
EtOH 70°C	--	--	--	--	--	--	600
Isopropanol	13	<1	<1	<1	--	--	50
Vegetable oils	<1	<1	<1	<1	--	--	3

*Commercially available in different mesh grades.

cess benefits from the precise addition and one less weighing step for the operator. The fat-soluble ascorbyl palmitate and stearate do not exhibit the facile dissolution properties of their water-soluble counterparts and are usually prepared for application use by prewetting the crystals as a paste for subsequent addition to oils or predissolving the desired quantity in a small portion of oil at elevated temperature prior to batch addition. In order to maximize the stability and efficacy of ascorbate addition to foodstuffs, the following precautions have been recommended:[7] (1) stainless steel, aluminum, or plastic equipment should be used; (2) bronze, brass, copper, monel, cold rolled steel and black iron equipment should be avoided; (3) deaeration (vacuum) procedures and inert gas treatment are recommended where feasible; (4) containers should be filled at a uniform rate to maximum capacity; and (5) when employed, flash heat processing should be used quickly and the containers closed promptly; (6) protect from light and radiant energy; (7) in bottling and canning operations some excess ascorbate should be used to scavenge oxygen from the head space (theoretically, 3.3 mg of ascorbic acid or ascorbic acid equivalent will consume the oxygen in 1 mL of air). These are general guidelines for the proper handling of these compounds in light of the well-known potential instabilities that detract from the desired performance in many applications. More specific processing precautions and chemistries will be addressed under individual applications.

Tocopherols

Tocopherols consist of a group of chemically related compounds that are present naturally in many foodstuffs (fats and oils; nuts and grain products; milk, fish, meats).[8] The tocopherol "family" includes eight members: alpha, beta, gamma and delta tocopherols and the corresponding less saturated tocotrienols. The commercially important antioxidant compounds are alpha, gamma and mixed tocopherols. The latter are usually concentrates occurring as byproducts of oil processing. Usually they contain a maximum of 80% total tocopherols of which 5-20% are nonalpha tocopherols. Other commercially available forms of alpha tocopherol are available in the form of the acetate ester and to a lesser extent the hemisuccinate. These two forms are not active, per se, as antioxidants because the hydroxyl (antioxidant) function has been chemically inerted through esterification. The structures of these compounds are outlined in Fig. 15.2. Each family has three centers of symmetry. Thus, a number of stereoisomers (eight per family) do exist. From a technological point of view, however, when used as food improvers, the stereo chemistry is not important. Rather, the degree and position of methyl substitution on the hydroxy-bearing aromatic ring determines the behavior of these compounds as antioxidants. The four tocopherols differ chemically from each other in the number and position of methyl groups in the aromatic nucleus. Pongracz reported in 1984 that the antioxidant effect of the active hydrogen (hydroxy group) was affected by the degree of ortho methyl substitution.[9] For example, at low tempertaures (20-60°C), alpha tocopherol (ortho,ortho,—CH_3) > gamma tocopherol (ortho, —CH_3) > beta tocopherol (ortho,—CH_3) > delta tocopherol (no ortho substitution). At elevated temperatures (80–120°C), the antioxidant efficiency was delta > gamma > alpha > beta.[10] These investigations were conducted in tocopherol-free lard at 3 concentrations (100, 200 and 1000 ppm). Other studies have shown similar effects with slightly differing relative orders.[11,12,13]

I. TOCOPHEROLS

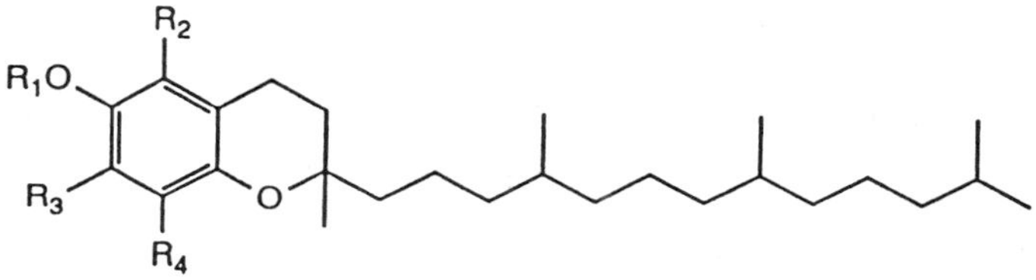

A. Unesterified (antioxidants)

Alpha Tocopherol : $R_2 = R_3 = R_4$ = CH3 R_1 = H
Beta Tocopherol : $R_2 = R_4$ = CH3 ; R_3 = H ; R_1 = H
Gamma Tocopherol : R_2 = H ; $R_3 = R_4$ = CH3 ; R_1 = H
Delta Tocopherol : $R_2 = R_3$ = H ; R_4 = CH3 ; R_1 = H

B. Esterified (not antioxidants)

Alpha Tocopherol Acetate : $R_2 = R_3 = R_4$ = CH3 ; R_1 =

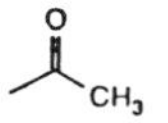

Alpha Tocopherol Succinate : $R_2 = R_3 = R_4$ = CH3 ; R_1 =

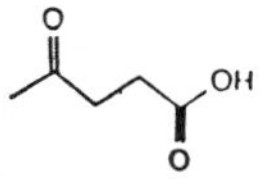

II. TOCOTRIENOLS

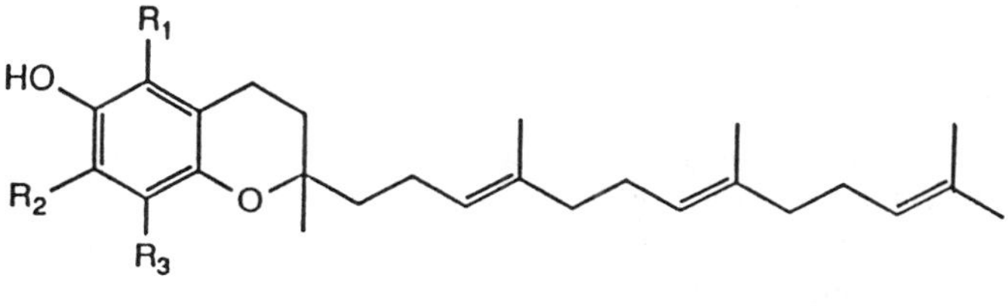

A. Unesterified (antioxidants)

Alpha Tocotrienol : $R_1 = R_2 = R_3$ = CH3
Beta Tocotrienol : $R_1 = R_3$ = CH3 ; R_2 = H
Gamma Tocotrienol : R_1 = H ; $R_2 = R_3$ = CH3
Delta Tocotrienol : $R_1 = R_2$ = H ; R_3 = CH3

FIG. 15.2. CHEMICAL STRUCTURES OF TOCOPHEROLS AND TOCOTRIENOLS

The physical and chemical properties of the most common food-grade tocopherol antioxidants are summarized in Table 15.2. The tocopherols are subject to destruction by oxygen causing the formation of quinones, dimers and trimers. Oxidation is accelerated by exposure to light, heat, alkali, and the presence of certain trace minerals such as iron (Fe^{+3}) and copper (Cu^{+2}). Ferrous and cuprous ions and elemental copper do not react with tocopherol.[14] If ascorbic acid and/or chelating agents are present, they will protect tocopherols from metal-activated oxidation. The tocopherols are more stable to oxidation in acid than in alkali. In the absence of oxygen they are relatively heat and light stable and relatively stable to alkali. Exposure of tocopherol to hydroperoxides and peroxides formed in the development of oxidative rancidity in fats also lowers tocopherol content. During normal handling and processing procedures, foods are usually exposed to one or more of these destructive influences, and the user should select the best alternative available for tocopherol incorporation to minimize tocopherol losses.

Because the tocopherols are freely miscible with oils, they usually present no difficulties in application. The recommended handling procedures include the following: (1) use stainless steel, glass or plastic containers wherever possible; (2) avoid sources of trace iron or copper contamination; (3) minimize air incorporation into tocopherol solutions, especially in an alkaline environment; and (4) protect dilute solutions from exposure to light, especially in the presence of oxygen.

ASCORBATES AND TOCOPHEROLS AS ANTIOXIDANTS

Oxidation is a general term with several specific definitions. It can be thought of as the loss of electrons from a chemical compound or the addition of oxygen to a chemical by enzymatic or nonenzymatic processes. Oxidation can occur in many classes of food components such as proteins, vitamins, minerals, lipids, flavors and colors. Food processors spend a great deal of time and energy in trying to prevent these reactions from occurring, as they quickly deteriorate food quality (appearance, odor) and nutritive value.

Lipid oxidation is probably the best known food oxidation and is often termed autoxidation because it is a free radical reaction that, once started, can sustain itself until some type of termination occurs. A general scheme of autoxidation is shown in Fig. 15.3. The process begins by the abstraction of a hydrogen atom beta to a double bond in an unsaturated triacylglycerol. This process results in a highly reactive free radical that can combine with molecular oxygen to form a peroxy radical which in turn abstracts a hydrogen to form a hydroperoxide. The hydroperoxide can in turn decompose to a peroxy radical and a hydroxyl radical. The latter is one of the most reactive molecular species found in nature. It will react with any available compound in its vicinity.

The lipid hydroperoxides are highly unstable and through a series of reactions form aldehydes, ketones, alcohols and acids that can seriously affect the quality of

TABLE 15.2
PHYSICAL AND CHEMICAL PROPERTIES OF TOCOPHEROLS

	Alpha Tocopherol	Gamma Tocopherol	Mixed Tocopherols
Mol wt	430.17	417.17	—
Mol formula	$C_{29}H_{50}O_2$	$C_{28}H_{48}O_2$	—
Appearance	viscous oil	viscous oil	viscous oil
Sp Gr 25°	0.947–0.958	0.947–0.958	0.920–0.950
Solubility			
H_2O	insoluble	insoluble	insoluble
EtOH	freely soluble	freely soluble	freely soluble
Veg oils	freely soluble	freely soluble	freely soluble
Acetone	freely soluble	freely soluble	freely soluble
Ether	freely soluble	freely soluble	freely soluble
Potency of Commercial Material[2]	97% min.	97% min.	34% total tocopherols[1] or 50% total tocopherols[1]

[1] Not less than 50% of total tocopherols are alpha.
[2] Food Chemical Codex.

```
Initiation*

    RH + initiator  ─────────>  R· + H·


Propagation

    R· + O₂  ─────────>  ROO·

    ROO· + RH  ─────────>  ROOH + R·

    ROOH  ─────────>  RO· + ·OH


Termination

    RH + ·OH  ─────────>  R· + H₂O

    R· + R·  ─────────>  RR

    ROO· + R·  ─────────>  ROOR


*RH = oxidizable molecule
    Initiators:  light (especially UV); heat; trace
    metals; peroxides
```

FIG. 15.3. GENERAL SCHEME OF AUTOXIDATION

a food. These compounds can produce undesirable odors and flavors (rancidity) and react with other food components that affect overall quality. Other types of lipids that can be affected in this way include vitamins (e.g., vitamin A), colors (e.g., beta carotene) and flavor compounds (e.g., orange oil).

Antioxidants can act in two ways to prevent autoxidation. They may act either as chain terminators which break the chain reaction after it has begun, or as oxygen scavengers which prevent the oxidative reactions from starting. The tocopherols act principally by the former, while ascorbates are capable of reacting with a radical as well as scavenging oxygen, as will be discussed below.

Ascorbic acid and its derivatives are effective as antioxidants for several reasons. The unique chemical properties of these compounds allow several functions to occur at the same time. Ascorbic acid, its salts and C-6 ester derivatives are capable of scavenging oxygen. They do so by donating hydrogen to oxygen, making the oxygen unavailable for oxidative reactions. The ascorbates in turn are oxidized to a dehydro form which can regenerate the ascorbic acid. In addition, the ascorbates can chelate metals that catalyse oxidation. Ascorbates are often added to carbonated and noncarbonated beverages and fruit juices because they will scavenge any remaining headspace oxygen that could damage these products. As a rule of thumb, 3 mg of ascorbic acid will scavenge the oxygen in 1 mL of headspce, but in actual practice slightly higher levels of ascorbic acid are used.

Ascorbyl palmitate is a fat-soluble derivative of ascorbic acid formed by combining ascorbic acid at C_6 with palmitic acid (a 16-carbon fatty acid) which is a common food constituent. Ascorbyl palmitate can be added to fat systems directly and has the unique ability to synergise with tocopherols that may be added or occur naturally as in vegetable oils. It is possible that this synergism causes reduced peroxy radical formation resulting from oxygen scavenging by ascorbyl palmitate or the ability of the enediol moeity to regenerate the tocopherol molecule from its radical intermediate. This synergistic effect has received much attention and has been argued extensively in the literature.[15]

USES IN FOODS

Alterations in flavor and appearance brought about by contact and reaction with oxygen, accelerated in certain situations by active oxidases, occupy a prominent position among the causes of deterioration of processed foods.

Ascorbates and tocopherols are truly versatile compounds that possess important functional properties in foods. Apart from their nutritional roles, these molecules can act as useful food antioxidants and food improvers.[16,17] They have been used over the entire range of food products, including: fruits, vegetables, meats and poultry, fish and seafoods, milk, cereal grain flours, snack foods, fats, oils, juices and beverages and even other nutrients such as beta-carotene and vitamin A. They have been used to protect and improve fresh, frozen and heat-treated foods. When used properly, they are safe and very effective. Ascorbates and tocopherols consumed in foods at mealtime continue to have a role in the digestive tract. Ascorbic acid reduces ferric ions to the more easily absorbed ferrous form and both tocopherols and ascorbates reduce mutagens by delaying formation of nitrosamines.[18,19]

The main function of the tocopherols is the prevention of lipid oxidation, and in that role they serve as potent chain breaking antioxidants.[15] Within the tocopherol family, alpha tocopherol has been employed most frequently as an antioxidant. However, there are studies that indicate gamma or delta tocopherol is a better antioxidant than alpha. There are other studies that suggest the efficiency of the various tocopherols (alpha, beta, gamma and delta) vary as a function of storage temperature as well as product type. The particular advantage of using ascorbates and tocopherols in combination is the well-known synergy resulting from the ability for ascorbates to reduce the tocopherol radical back to the ground state tocopherol.

Since its synthesis, L-ascorbic acid has become a widely used food additive.[20] The chemistry of L-ascorbic acid has been reviewed as related to food use[21] as well as its application to food products.[7,22-24] The ascorbates represent a slightly more complex picture than the tocopherols. The unique enediol structure of the C_2-C_3 carbons is common to the ascorbates, erythorbates and C_6 esters. This moiety permits the molecule not only to function as an acidulant, but in multiple functional roles.

The multiple functions of ascorbic acid as an antioxidant in food systems are (1) to scavenge oxygen, (2) to shift the redox potential of the system to a reducing state, (3) to regenerate phenolic fat-soluble antioxidants, (4) to maintain sulfhydryl groups in $-SH$ form and (5) as a weak complexing agent to act synergistically with chelating agents. All of the properties have been put to use in one fashion or another in foods singly or in combination as a food improver. The C_6 esters of ascorbic acid possess these same unique properties plus provide the benefit of limited oil solubility.

When the ascorbates and/or the tocopherols are added to foods to function solely as antioxidants, no nutritional claims are usually made for added nutrient content. This is not only because relatively small amounts are added, but the compounds are undergoing gradual degradation in their role of protecting food components during processing or shelf-life storage prior to consumption. Clearly, when it comes to the evaluation of efficacy of added ascorbates and/or tocopherols to a food product, the complexity of factors often makes it impossible to obtain definitive results from simple model laboratory systems. Pragmatically it is always best to carry out experiments on the foods concerned under practical processing and storage conditions. Many hundred scientific reports exist on adding ascorbates and tocopherols to foods as food improvers. There are reviews[7,22,24] which cover application studies in foods in great detail. Brief mention will only be made here of some food applications.

Fruits and Vegetables

Once fruits and vegetables are excised by a cutting or macerating action, cellular components, formerly in an organized state, are allowed to intermingle and interact.

The end result of some interactions influence unfavorably the appearance, color and flavor of the processed product. Cut plant tissues which discolor readily (apple, banana, peach, etc.) have a relatively low natural ascorbic content and highly reactive phenolases. With the oxidative action of oxygen, enzyme potentiated, on phenolic and flavonoid substrates, reversible, colored orthoquinone compounds form which, unless inhibited, undergo polymerization reactions to irreversible melanin-like structures affecting product appearance and flavor. Added ascorbic acid at the time of excision or very shortly thereafter prevents the above reactions as long as sufficient ascorbic acid remains in a reduced state.

Restaurants, fast food outlets, catering services, institution dining halls, etc., require large volumes of fresh peeled and cut fruit and vegetable products for daily use. In the past, dips and sprays of sulfiting agents were primarily used to delay discolorations. With the recognition of sensitivity reactions of individuals to sulfite, nonsulfite replacement products have been formulated. Dip or spray formulations containing ascorbic acid slow the oxidative discolorations of cut fruits and vegetables.[25-31] Combinations of ascorbic and citric acids for mushrooms, lettuce, carrots and cauliflower,[26,27] ascorbic acid and calcium chloride for sliced apples,[28] ascorbic acid, citric acid and potassium sorbate for peeled potatoes,[29] ascorbic acid, citric acid, calcium chloride and sodium acid phosphate for various fruits and vegetables,[30] and ascorbic acid esters, acidic polyphosphates and cyclodextrins for sliced apples[31] are some of the preparations declared effective for fresh cut fruits and vegetables, treated and held refrigerated for short-time use.

When frozen cut fruits, subject to discolorations, are packed and covered with sugar syrups, and then frozen and subsequently thawed prior to consumption or further food preparatory operations, the oxidative enzymes become active again. Unless adequate ascorbic acid is added to the syrup (0.1–0.25%) covering the fruit prior to freezing, discoloration proceeds quickly during thawing.[22,24,32]

For enzymatic discoloration to occur, the enzyme, the substrate and oxygen must be present at the same moment. When a plant food product is heated sufficiently, the enzyme is destroyed and only the action of oxygen on the substrate remains, a much slower reaction. In heat-treated plant food packaged products, oxygen can be removed by sealing under vacuum or inert gas. Elimination of all oxygen is not always achieved, and added ascorbic acid as an oxygen scavenger has merit as a food improving agent.[32,33]

Juices and Beverages

Juices of fruits, prone to oxidation of their polyphenol composition, likewise undergo color and flavor changes with time, and so ascorbic acid may be added during crushing, pressing and straining of the fruit or to the juice prior to the packaging operation to protect natural color and flavor. Where heat treatment is part of the processing operation and enzyme action is eliminated, added ascorbic acid protects the product from residual oxygen in the container during storage and processing.[33–35]

Soft drinks, either carbonated or heat-sterilized noncarbonated, have flavoring concentrates and colors added.[24,36] Citrus or essential oils containing unsaturated terpenes are highly reactive with oxygen, producing characteristic off-flavors which are slowed in the presence of ascorbates and tocopherols.[37] Added carotenoids, beta-carotene and apocarotenal are color additives which are quite stable in drinks with added ascorbic acid. When essential oils are added, tocopherol may be incorporated in the flavoring oil emulsion for improved resistance to oxidation.

For over 50 years added ascorbic acid has been recognized as a stabilizing agent in beer, reducing oxidation haze and gushing development, also retarding flavor and aroma changes, thereby extending shelf-life of the product significantly. A finished beer of good flavor and clarity ready for packaging should possess a high reducing capacity and a minimum amount of dissolved oxygen and headspace oxygen in the can or bottle for maximum maintenance of product quality. Added ascorbic acid (1–4 g/100 L) serves as an aid toward maintaining the above conditions.[22,38,39]

For over 40 years protection of color, clarity and aroma of wine with added ascorbic acid has been practiced as a replacement for or at reduced levels of sulfurous acid. Additions are made before or after aeration or before bottling. The reducing action of ascorbic acid prevents ferric phosphate precipitation, a development which adds turbidity to wine.[24,40]

Oxidative changes in the cream fraction of cows milk which result in flavors termed "cardboardy, metallic or tallowy" are distasteful in fluid milk and other dairy products. This development, occurring in a minor portion of dairy products, is influenced by oxidation-reduction potential, oxygen content, copper content, light exposure, natural antioxidant content, among the factors involved.[7] Added tocopherol in an aqueous emulsion form with added ascorbic acid inhibits the off-flavor development. If vitamin A has been added previously to the dairy product for improved nutritive value, the introduction of the tocopherol/ascorbic acid combination will also provide improved vitamin A stability during product storage.

Bread and Flour

Since 1935 it has been known that ascorbic acid exerts a marked action on the baking strength of flour.[7] The overall practical advantage of this addition to freshly milled flour (1) enhances loaf texture and volume, (2) gives greater elasticity and gas retention to dough, (3) protects fatty acids, (4) reduces power or minimal time or lowered consistency in continuous dough making and (5) eliminates storage period of unimproved flour. Without ascorbic acid addition, freshly milled flour must be aged for months before use for breadmaking which, requiring storage facilities, is costly. The flour improving properties of ascorbic acid have been widely accepted and practiced in the EEC countries. The oxidized form of ascorbic acid, dehydroascorbic acid formed in bread making and stable in bread dough, is the active compound resulting in the improving action.[24,41,42] Ascorbyl palmitate solubilized in vegetable oil in bread has a shortening-sparing role which results in a softer crumb texture.[43] Ascorbic acid added to semolina dough used in making pasta stabilizes carotenoid color and inhibits lipoxidase action.[44]

Fish and Meat

For many decades it has been observed that frozen fish, particularly of the fatty type, tend to undergo slow enzymic oxidation during storage and become rancid. With this development there is a rusting or yellowing of the frozen flesh, and upon thawing a rancid odor is apparent. This type of product quality loss can be prevented or delayed significantly if an ascorbic acid glaze (a thickened aqueous solution of ascorbic acid) is applied to the fish tissue by a spray or coating procedure in the prepackaging operation prior to freezing.[22,24] The incorporation of tocopherol emulsion in the glaze would appear to be beneficial. Ascorbic acid treatment of frozen shrimp has been useful in delaying black spot development and in stabilization of color.

In the meat curing process, the addition of nitrite salt releases gaseous nitric oxide which reacts with myoglobin to form the nitrosomyoglobin which by subsequent heat denaturation yields nitrosomyochrome, the familiar pink-red color of cured meat products. The addition of ascorbates[7,24,45] (such as sodium ascorbate) to the curing brine in the curing process (1) reduces the amount of nitrite used, (2) reduces the time of curing, (3) contributes to a more uniform color and (4) yields a product with improved flavor (bologna, corned beef, frankfurters, ham, bacon, etc.). There is, however, another role for added ascorbate salts, namely blocking the development of N-nitrosamine formation in cured meats. Added alpha-tocopherol is also a blocking agent for nitrosamine formation.[46] Currently, both compounds are approved by the USDA as additives in the curing of bacon. In another development, literature studies have demonstrated that introducing supplementary levels of alpha-tocopherol in the rations of poultry, cattle, and fish yield edible tissues which are more resistant to oxidative changes.[47,48,48a] Warmed-over flavor is used to describe the rapid development of oxidized flavor in refrigerated cooked meat. Asghar et al.[49] and Bailey[50] reviewed the problem of warmed-over flavor. Membrane-bound alpha-tocopherol stabilized the membranal lipids toward oxidation.[49] More studies on the use of the tocopherols and the ascorbates on this problem may be justified.

Oils and Fats

Fats and oils contain unsaturated fatty acids which with time undergo oxidative and hydrolytic chemical action.[51] As oxidation proceeds, the hydroperoxides break down to give way to aldehydes, ketones, acids, and other cleavage products and polymers. These produce disagreeable odors and flavors, making food products unpalatable to consumers and thereby causing economic loss. Metal chelators deactivating trace metals, antioxidants functioning by reacting with free radicals and singlet oxygen quenching help to delay these deteriorative changes. Antioxidants are used singularly and in combinations to deter changes depending upon the nature and/or source of the fat, oil, or essential oil product.[52,53]

Tocopherols added to beef tallow used to fry potato chips delayed rancidity development.[54] A similar study using lard with added alpha, gamma or delta-tocopherols as a frying oil was effective in stabilizing potato chips.[55] Ascorbyl palmitate (0.02%) reduced peroxide formation in vegetable oil used as frying oil.[56] When ascorbyl palmitate is introduced in a food product, solubilization in oil is a preliminary step.[57] The use of both alpha-tocopherol and ascorbyl palmitate as effective antioxidants in animal fats has been reported repeatedly in the literature.[52,53,58,59] The addition of lecithin to the tocopherol/ascorbyl palmitate formulation increased the stabilizing capacity of the combination[52,53,60,61] for animal fats. Ascorbyl palmitate and lecithin were effective in vegetable oils containing substantial levels of natural tocopherols.[62] Reviews on added tocopherols and ascorbates in fats and oils are available.[63,64]

Beta-carotene, under certain situations, can act as a lipid antioxidant and an efficient quencher of singlet molecular oxygen.[65,66] Flavor deterioration in vegetable salad oils initiated by light can be inhibited effectively without affecting color quality.[67]

REGULATORY ASPECTS

The use of ascorbates and tocopherols as processing aids is subject to government regulations in many countries. Not only do government regulations specify what types of processing aid is permitted, but they also set permitted use levels in the many food applications. Updated, appropriate regulations should always be consulted to determine the permitted use levels for the specific applications of interest.

The uses of tocopherols and ascorbates as antioxidants and food improvers are not only governed by scientific principles but also by regulations, and not all of the tocopherol and ascorbate forms are universally acceptable. For example, erythorbic acid and its salts are permitted in some foods in the United States, but are not allowed in some countries. Similarly, ascorbyl stearate is only widely approved for food use in Japan. Some further comments on the legal aspects of food additives are in order.

The United States

Most ascorbates and tocopherols are "generally recognized as safe," GRAS, for use in foods as processing aids, provided that a standard has not been established by the Food and Drug Administration for the food wherein their use is excluded or permitted within the limitations specified by the standard.

Under GRAS conditions, the quantity added "does not exceed the amount reasonably required to accomplish the intended physical, nutritional or other technical effect on food," and the quantity of processing aid "becomes a component of the food as a result of its use in the manufacturing, processing or packaging of food, and which is not intended to accomplish any physical or other technical effect in the food itself shall be reduced to the extent reasonably possible." And the processing aid "is of appropriate food grade and is prepared and handled as a food ingredient; and the inclusion of processing aids in the list of nutrients does not constitute a finding on the part of the Department that it is useful as a supplement to the diet of humans." (21CFR182.1 [b][1.][2.][3.]).

When a standard for a food product has been established wherein the processing aid is permitted, the standard should be consulted to ensure that the labeling of the food product conforms with the labeling specifications of the standard.

In addition to the regulations established by the Food and Drug Administration, the United States Department of Agriculture has promulgated regulations for the use of ascorbic acid and alpha tocopherol in meat processing. The Alcohol and Tobacco Tax Division of the U.S. Department of Treasury has established a regulation pertaining to the use of ascorbic acid in wine. The standards established by those agencies as they exist are compiled in Tables 15.3, 15.4 and 15.5.

Other Countries

Countries other than the United States have regulations concerning the addition of processing aids to foods, some of which are general and others very specific. For example, considering the use of ascorbic acid as a flour improver, the level of permissible addition ranges from 20–1000 mg/kg of flour (Table 15.6). Some countries permit both ascorbic acid and bromate use, while others only allow L-ascorbic acid.

The Joint FAO/WHO Codex Alimentarius Commission was established to implement the Joint FAO/WHO Food Standards Program. Membership of the commission comprises those member nations of FAO and/or WHO that have notified the organizations of their wish to be considered as members. The purpose of the Joint FAO/WHO Food Standards Program is to elaborate international standards for foods aimed at protecting the health of the consumer, to ensure fair practices in the food trade and to facilitate international trade. Some of these regulations as they relate to ascorbates and tocopherols can be found in Tables 15.6, 15.7, 15.8 and 15.9.

For complete information on specific processing aids and their acceptability for use in given food applications, the full texts of current regulations in the countries of interest must be consulted along with appropriate legal counsel. There are, however, various information sources useful in learning about food regulations, keep-

TABLE 15.3
U.S. REGULATIONS ON ASCORBIC ACID AND
TOCOPHEROL ADDITION TO MEAT

Food	Purpose	Quantity Permitted
Ascorbic acid in: cured pork and beef cuts, cured comminuted meat food product	To accelerate color fixing	70 oz/100 gal pickle at 10% pump level; 0.75 oz/100 lb meat or meat byproduct; 10% solution to surfaces of cured cuts prior to packaging (the use of such solution shall not result in the addition of a significant amount of moisture to the product)
Sodium ascorbate in: cured pork and beef cuts, cured comminuted meat food product	To accelerate color fixing	87.5 oz/100 gal pickle at 10% pump level; 0.88 oz/100 lb meat or meat by product; 10% solution to surfaces of cured cuts prior to packaging (the use of such solution shall not result in the addition of a significant amount of moisture to the product)
d- and dl-alpha-tocopherol in: pump-cured bacon	To inhibit nitrosamine formation	500 ppm; by injection or surface application
Ascorbic acid, erythorbic acid, sodium ascorbate, citric acid, sodium citrate in fresh pork cuts	To maintain color	Maximum: 500 ppm ascorbic acid, erythorbic acid or sodium ascorbate, citric acid, sodium citrate alone or in combination or 1.8 mg/inch^2 of surface area; not to exceed either limit. Total of citric acid and sodium citrate not to exceed 250 ppm.

Source: Bauernfeind,[7] with permission.

TABLE 15.4
U.S. REGULATIONS ON ASCORBIC ACID ADDITION TO ALCOHOLIC BEVERAGES
Alcohol and Tobacco Tax Division
U.S. Department of Treasury Regulations

Food	Purpose of Ascorbic Acid	Quantity Permitted
Wine	To prevent darkening of color and deterioration of flavor, and over-oxidation	Within limitations which do not alter the class or type of the wine (use need not be declared on the label)
Beer	Antioxidant and biological stabilization	To be used only by agreement between U.S. Dept. of Treasury and the brewer

Source: Bauernfeind,[7] with permission.

TABLE 15.5
U.S. STANDARDS OR REGULATIONS OF FOODS
TO WHICH ASCORBIC ACID MAY BE ADDED

Food	Purpose of Ascorbic Acid	Quantity Permitted
Artificially sweetened fruit jelly	Preservative	Not more than 0.1% by weight of finished food
Artificially sweetened fruit preserves and jams	Preservative	Not more than 0.1% by weight of finished food
Canned applesauce	Preservative, nutrient	Not more than 150 ppm, an amount to provide 60 mg/4 oz (113 g)
Canned apricots	Preservative	An amount no greater than necessary to preserve color
Canned artichokes (packed in glass)	Preservative	Not more than 32 mg/100 g of finished food
Canned fruit cocktail	Preservative	Amount no greater than necessary to preserve color
Canned fruit nectars	Preservative, nutrient	Not more than 150 ppm, amounts to provide not less than 30 mg or more than 60 mg/4 fl oz
Canned mushrooms	Preservative	Not more than 37.5 mg/oz of drained weight of mushrooms
Canned peaches	Preservative	Amount not greater than necessary to preserve color
Flour (white, whole wheat, plain)	Dough conditioner	Not to exceed 200 ppm
Frozen raw breaded shrimp	Preservative	Sufficient to retard development of dark spots
Ice cream (the fruit therein)	Acidulant	Such quantity as seasons the finished product and meets the standards for ice cream
Margarine	Preservative	Ascorbyl palmitate and/or ascorbyl stearate 0.02%
Nonfruit water ices	Acidulant	Such quantity as seasons the finished product
Canned asparagus	Preservative	An amount necessary to preserve color
Water ices (the fruit therein)	Acidulant	Such quantity as seasons the finished product

TABLE 15.5 (*Continued*)

Food	Purpose of Ascorbic Acid	Quantity Permitted
Foods for which standards are established and in which nonspecified preservatives may be optional ingredients are:		
Dry whole milk		
Dry cream		
Breads, rolls, buns	Dough conditioners not referred to in standard if the total quantities are not more than 0.5 part for each 100 parts by weight of flour used	
Frozen raw breaded shrimp	Antioxidant preservative—may be used to retard development of rancidity of the fat content	

Source: Compiled by D. M. Pinkert. From Bauernfeind,[7] with permission.

ing abreast of regulatory developments, and determining the current regulatory status of processing aids. Schultz[69] provides a comprehensive review of food law in the United States, and Rothchild's *Food Chemical News Guide* is a weekly, updated compilation of the status of food and color additives, including antioxidants.

The *Food Chemicals Codex* (FCC) is a compilation of specifications provided in the United States by the Food Protection Committee of the National Research Council on the identity and purity of chemicals suitable for use in foods in compliance with

TABLE 15.6
LEGAL STATUS OF L-ASCORBIC ACID AS A FLOUR IMPROVER

Maximum Level Permitted	Country
20 mg/kg	Uruguay
20–50 mg/kg	Chile
50 mg/kg	Holland, Belgium
75 mg/kg	Cypress, Turkey
100 mg/kg	Sudan, Netherlands, Norway, Iceland
200 mg/kg	Italy, Denmark, Canada, Sweden, Iceland, Austria, United States, Indonesia, India, Spain, South Africa, Argentina, Zambia, United Kingdom, Philippines, Gibraltar, Mexico, Japan, France, Kenya, Spain
300 mg/kg	Belgium, Portugal
1000 mg/kg	Finland
GMP[1]	France, Switzerland, Papua-New Guinea, Australia, Malta, New Zealand, Portugal, Malaysia, Bulgaria, Sengapori, Kuwait, Sweden, Norway, Germany

[1]Good manufacturing practice.

TABLE 15.7
STATUS OF TOCOPHEROL AND ASCORBATES AS FOOD ADDITIVES
FROM THE JOINT FAO/WHO EXPERT COMMITTEE ON FOOD ADDITIVES (JECFA)

Additive	ADI[1]	Reference
Ascorbic acid	Not specified[2]	WHO Technical Report Series 669,
Sodium ascorbate	Not specified[2]	25th Report of JECFA, 1981, p. 32
Calcium ascorbate	Not specified[2]	
Potassium ascorbate	Not specified[2]	
Ascorbyl palmitate	1.25 mg/kg b.w.	FAO Nutrition Meeting Report,
Ascorbyl stearate	1.25 mg/kg b.w.	Series No. 53A, 17th Report of JECFA, 1974, p. 146
Alpha-tocopherol	1.5–2 mg/kg b.w.	WHO Food Additives Series 21, 30th Meeting of JECFA, 1986, p. 55
Mixed tocopherols		

[1]ADI: Acceptable daily intake from all sources.
[2]Not specified: indicates that an upper limit has not been specified.

U.S. government regulations. Internationally, the counterpart of the FCC is Codex Alimentarius which is a compilation of standards provided by the Codex Alimentarius Commission under the Joint FAO/WHO Food Standards Program.

CONCLUDING REMARKS

The application of ascorbates and tocopherols to the broad range of food product types discussed in this chapter, attests to the versatility of these compounds in protecting all types of foods from unwanted deterioration.

All of man's foods originate from living organisms which were equipped initially with natural antioxidant systems. The cornerstones of biological antioxidants are the ascorbates and tocopherols. These antioxidants are designed to maintain homeostasis which can be upset by oxidants which may be catalysed by light, temperature, metal ions, cell damage, etc.

As little as 25 years ago in the United States, the number of products on the supermarket shelf were fewer, the markets were smaller and a larger portion of food preparation was done in the home. Today, however, consumer needs continue to shift toward convenience foods, such as, partly or fully cooked frozen products, prepared foods, frozen bakery products, and foods in packages that are ready to "heat and eat." The challenge to deliver these products remains, and so does the need for safe and effective antioxidants, like the tocopherols and ascorbates.

As much as the market and consumer needs have changed, and will continue to change, the goals of the food technologist and the use of antioxidants remain the same, i.e., to produce a product that is safe, nutritious and appealing to the consumer. The use, preferred handling and application techniques have been addressed

TABLE 15.8
FOOD USES OF ALPHA TOCOPHEROL, ASCORBYL PALMITATE
AND ASCORBYL STEARATE FROM CODEX ALIMENTARIUS

Product Oils/Fats	Alpha tocopherol	Ascorbyl Palmitate	Ascorbyl Stearate
Low erucic acid canola, coconut oil, palm oil, palm kernel, grapeseed, babassu, soybean, arachus (peanut), cottonseed, sunflower, rapeseed, maise (corn), sesame, safflower, mustardseed, lard, rendered pork, premier jus, tallow, margarine	GMP	200 mg/kg[1]	200 mg/kg[2]
Refined olive oil	GMP	—	—
Boullions, consommes	50 mg/kg[3]	—	—
Infant formulas (Ready-to-drink)	10 mg/L	—	—
Canned baby foods; processed cereal-based foods for infants and children	300 mg/kg fat	200 mg/kg fat	—

Source: Food and Agricultural Organization of the United Nations.[70]
[1]Singly or in combination with ascorbyl stearate.
[2]Singly or in combination with ascorbyl palmitate.
[3]Alone or in combination with mixed tocopherols.

in the relevant texts. One guide, however, applies to all work with added antioxidants to foods, namely maximum protection from oxidation; the preventive approach is better than the curative. In fact, once oxidation has started, there is no going back. The most important ways to achieve optimal protection of foods from oxidation during the processing and storage have been summarized as follows:[64,68]

(1) Use fresh, unspoiled raw materials.
(2) Observe good manufacturing practices.
(3) Inactivate enzymes to avoid hydrolytic processes.
(4) Eliminate atmospheric oxygen.
(5) Reduce any form of energy by storage at low temperatures and protection from light, particularly UV wavelengths that generate free radicals.
(6) Avoid contact with traces of catalytically active prooxidant metals like copper and iron, heme, and chlorophyll.
(7) Add antioxidants and sequestering agents at the earliest possible stage.

TABLE 15.9
FOOD USES OF ASCORBATES LISTED IN CODEX ALIMENTARIUS

Product	Ascorbic Acid	Calcium Ascorbate	Potassium Ascorbate	Sodium Ascorbate
Vegetable				
Edible fungi; canned mushrooms; canned asparagus	GMP	—	—	—
Table olives	200 mg/kg	—	—	—
Fruits				
Apricot, peach, pear nectars;[1] quick frozen strawberries; concentrated apple juice;[1] apple juice;[1] concentrated pineapple juice;[1] concentrated pineapple juice with preservatives (for mfg. use only);[1] pulpy nectars of small fruits[1]	GMP	—	—	—
Canned fruit cocktail, jams and jellies (Black currant 750 mg/kg)	500 mg kg	—	—	—
Canned tropical fruit salad; quick frozen peaches	750 mg/kg	—	—	—
Canned apple sauce	150 mg/kg	—	—	—
Canned peaches	550 mg/kg	—	—	—
Sweetened (labrusca type) grape juice; concentrated grape juice; grape juice	400 mg/kg	—	—	—
Meats				
Canned corned beef	500 mg/kg	—	—	500 mg/kg ascorbic acid
Luncheon meat; cooked, cured chopped meat; cooked, cured pork shoulder; cooked, cured ham	500 mg/kg[3]	—	—	500 mg/kg ascorbic acid[3]
Fish				
Quick frozen shrimp/prawns	GMP	—	—	—
Quick frozen lobsters; fillets of cod, haddock, hake, flat fish, and ocean perch	—	—	1 g/kg ascorbic acid[3]	1 g/kg ascorbic acid[3]
Miscellaneous				
Minarine	300 mg/kg	—	—	—
Quick frozen french fries	100 mg/kg[2]	—	—	—

TABLE 15.9 (*Continued*)

Product	Ascorbic Acid	Calcium Ascorbate	Potassium Ascorbate	Sodium Ascorbate
Boullions, consommes (ready-to-eat basis)	1 g/kg	1 g/kg ascorbic acid	1 g/kg ascorbic acid[3]	1 g/kg ascorbic acid[3]
Canned baby foods; cereal based foods for infants and children	500 mg/kg	—	500 mg/kg ascorbic acid	500 mg/kg ascorbic acid

[1]Preserved exclusively by physical methods.
[2]Alone or in combination with other sequestrants (e.g., phosphates).
[3]Alone or in combination with erythorbic acid, erythorbate.

REFERENCES

1. MOON, T. and MICOZZI, M. 1989. Investigating the Role of Micronutrients. *In* Nutrition and Cancer Prevention. Marcel Dekker, New York.
2. ANDREWS, G. C. and CRAWFORD, T. 1982. Recent advances in the derivatization of L-ascorbic acid. *In* Ascorbic Acid: Chemistry, Metabolism and Uses, P. A. Seib and B. M. Tolbert (eds.). Advances in Chemistry Series 200, American Chemical Society, Washington, DC.
3. MING-LONG, L. and SEIB, P. A. 1987. Selected reactions of L-ascorbic acid related to foods. Food Technol. *41*(11), 104–107, 111.
4. BORENSTEIN, B. 1965. The comparative properties of ascorbic acid and erythorbic acid. Food Technol. *19*(11), 115–117.
5. LILLARD, JR., D. W., SEIB, P. A. and HOSENEY, R. C. 1982. Isomeric ascorbic acids and derivatives of L-ascorbic acid: Their effect on the flow of dough. Cereal Chem. *59*, 291.
6. HORNIG, D., WEBER, F. and WISS, O. 1974. Influence of erythorbic acid on the vitamin C status of guinea pigs. Experientia *30*, 173.
7. BAUERNFEIND, J. C. 1982. Ascorbic acid technology in agricultural, pharmaceutical, food and industrial applications. *In* Ascorbic Acid: Chemistry, Metabolism, and Uses, P. A. Seib and B. M. Tolbert (eds.). Advances in Chemistry Series 200, American Chemical Society, Washington, DC.
8. BAUERNFEIND, J. C. 1980. Tocopherols in foods. *In* Vitamin E: A Comprehensive Treatise, L. Machlin (ed.). Marcel Dekker, New York.
9. PONGRACZ, G. 1984. Alpha tocopherol as a natural antioxidant. Fette Seifen Anstrichm. *86*(12), 455–460.
10. TELEGDY-KOVATS, L. and BERNDORFER-KRASZNER, E. 1967. The antioxidant mechanism of alpha, beta, gamma, and delta tocopherols in lard. Die Nahrung *11*, 671.
11. JUILLET, M. T. 1975. Comparison of vitamin activity and antioxidant activity of various tocopherols from important vegetable oils. Fette Seifen Anstrichm. *77*, 101.
12. PARKHURST, R. M., SKINNER, W. A. and STURM, P. A. 1970. The effect of various concentrations of tocopherols and tocopherol mixtures on the oxidative stability of a sample of lard. Lipids *5*, 184.

13. LEA, C. H. 1960. Antioxidant activities of the tocopherols (II) influence of substrate, temperature and level of oxidation. J. Sci. Food Agr. *11*, 212–218.
14. CORT, W. M. 1975. Effects of processing by additives on nutrients, Part 3. Effect of treatment by chemical additives. *In* Nutritional Evaluation of Food Processing, R. H. Harris and E. Karmas (eds.). AVI/Van Nostrand Reinhold, New York.
15. NIKI, E. 1987. Antioxidants in relation to lipid peroxidation. Chem. Phys. Lipids *44*, 227–253.
16. KLAEUI, H. 1974. Use of vitamins C and E as antioxidants in food technology. *In* Nat. Synth. Zusatzstoffe Nahr Menschen, 14th Int. Symp., Steinkopff, Darmstadt.
17. JOHNSON, F. C. 1979. The antioxidant vitamins. CRC Crit. Rev. Food Sci. Nutr. *11*, 217–309.
18. MERGENS, W. J. and NEWMARK, H. L. 1980. Antioxidants as blocking agents against nitrosamine synthesis. *In* Autoxidation in Food and Biological Systems, M. G. Simic and M. Karel (eds.). Plenum Publishing Corp., New York.
19. NEWMARK, H. L. and MERGENS, J. W. 1981. Applications of ascorbic acid and tocopherol as inhibitors of nitrosamine formation and oxidation in foods. *In* Criteria of Food Acceptance, J. Solms and R. L. Hall (eds.). Forster Verlag AG/Forster Publishing Ltd., Zurich.
20. REIO, L. 1982. L-ascorbic acid, a widely used additive. Var Foeda *34*(5), 232–266.
21. LIAO, M. L. and SEIB, P. A. 1988. Chemistry of L-ascorbic acid related to foods. Food Chem. *30*(4), 289–312.
22. BAUERNFEIND, J. C. 1953. The use of ascorbic acid in processing foods. Adv. Food Res. *4*, 359–431.
23. BORENSTEIN, B. 1987. The role of ascorbic acid in foods. Food Technol. *41*(11), 98–99.
24. JOHNSON, L. E. and MERGENS, W. J. 1990. Food application studies with added ascorbates and tocopherols as antioxidants. (In preparation).
25. VOIROL, P. 1972. Use of vitamin C on vegetable products. Food Proc. Ind. *41*(490), 27–30.
26. ANON. 1983. Sulfite substitute preserves color in vegetables. Food Eng. *55*(7), 138.
27. RICE, J. 1983. Ascorbic/citric acid: An answer to the sulfite question. Food Proc. *43*(11), 74–75.
28. JOHNSON, L. E. 1984. Unpublished observations.
29. LANGDON, T. T. 1987. Prevention of browning in fresh prepared potatoes without the use of sulfiting agents. Food Technol. *41*(5), 64–67.
30. DUXBURY, D. D. 1988. Stabilizer blend extends shelf-life of fresh fruit and vegetables. Food Proc. *49*(10), 98–99.
31. SAPERS, C. M. and HICKS, K. B. 1988. Inhibition of enzymatic browning in fruits and vegetables. Presentation American Chem. Soc. Meeting, Los Angeles, Sept. 25–30.
32. HENSHALL, J. D. 1974. Vitamin C in canning and freezing. *In* Vitamin C: Recent Aspects of Its Physiological and Technological Importance, G. Birch and K. Parker (eds.). John Wiley & Sons, New York.
33. BAUERNFEIND, J. C. 1985. Antioxidant function of L-ascorbic acid in food technology. Int. J. Vitam. Nutr. Res. (Suppl.) *27*, 307–333.
34. HENSHALL, J. D. 1981. Ascorbic acid in fruit juice and beverages. *In* Vitamin C, J. Counsell and D. Hornig (eds.). Applied Science, London.
35. BIRCH, G. F. *et al.* 1974. Quality changes related to vitamin C in fruit juices and vegetable processing. *In* Vitamin C: Recent Aspects of Its Physiological and Technological Importance, G. Birch and K. Parker (eds.). John Wiley & Sons, New York.

36. GRESSWELL, D. M. 1974. Vitamin C in soft drinks and fruit juice. *In* Vitamin C: Recent Aspects of Its Physiological and Technological Importance, G. Birch and K. Parker (eds.). John Wiley & Sons, New York.
37. JOHNSON, L. E. and CORT, W. M. 1983. Comparison of alternate antioxidants to BHA in citrus oil. Presentation: Soc. Soft Drink Technol. Meeting, Atlanta, Apr. 16-20.
38. RUBACH, K., BREYER, CH. and KRUGER, E. 1980. The behavior of ascorbic acid during the storage of bottled beer. Brauwissenschaft *33*, 162-166.
39. ANDREGG, P. and HUG, H. 1981. Ascorbic acid and antioxidant for beer. Brauerie-Kundschau *92*(10), 241-243.
40. VIDAL-BARRAQUER, J. M. 1979. Problems with stabilization of wines intended for bottling. Bull. O.I.V. *52*(578), 280-308.
41. CHAMBERLAIN, N. 1982. Use of ascorbic acid in breadmaking. *In* Vitamin C, J. Counsell and D. Hornig (eds.). Applied Science, London.
42. KLAEUI, H. 1985. Ascorbic acid as a flour and bread improver. Int. J. Vitam. Nutr. (Suppl.) *27*, 335-343.
43. KOCH, R. L., SEIB, P. A. and HOSENEY, R. C. 1987. Incorporating L-ascorbyl palmitate in bread and its shortening-sparing and anti-firming effects. J. Food Sci. *52*(4), 954-957.
44. MILATOVIC, L. 1985. The use of L-ascorbic acid in improving the quality of pasta. Int. J. Vitamin Nutr. *27*, 345-361.
45. RANKEN, M. D. 1982. The use of ascorbic acid in meat processing. *In* Vitamin C, J. Counsell and D. Hornig (eds.). Applied Science, London.
46. MERGENS, W. J. and NEWMARK, H. L. 1979. The use of alpha tocopherol in bacon processing: An update. Proc. Meat Ind. Res. Conf., Chicago, Mar. 29-30.
47. MARUSICH, W. L. 1980. Vitamin E as an in vivo lipid stabilizer and its effects on flavor and storage properties of milk and meat. *In* Vitamin E: A Comprehensive Treatise, L. Machlin (ed.). Marcel Dekker, New York.
48. POZO, R., LAVETY, J. and LOVE, R. 1988. The role of dietary alpha-tocopherol in stabilizing the canthaxanthin and lipids of rainbow trout muscle. Agriculture *73*, 165-175.
48a. ANON. 1990. Feeding cattle vitamin E promotes fresh beef color. Food Proc. *51*(3), 117.
49. ASGHAR, A., GRAY, J. I., BUCKLEY, D. J., PEARSON, A. M. and BOOREN, A. M. 1988. Perspectives on warmed-over flavor. Food Technol. *42*(6), 102-108.
50. BAILEY, C. 1988. Inhibition of warmed-over flavor with emphasis on maillard reaction products. Food Technol. *42*(6), 123-126.
51. PACQUETTE, G., KUPRANYEZ, D. B., VAN DE VOORT, F. R. 1985. The mechanisms of lipid auto-oxidation. Can. Inst. Food Sci. Technol. J. *18*(2), 112-118.
52. PONGRACZ, G. 1973. Antioxidant mixtures for use in foods. Int. J. Vitam. Nutr. Res. *43*(4), 517-525.
53. CORT, W. M. 1974. Antioxidant activity of tocopherol, ascorbyl palmitate and ascorbic acid and their mode of action. J. Am. Oil Chem. Soc. *51*, 321-325.
54. DOUGHERTY, M. E. 1980. Tocopherols as food antioxidants. Cereal Foods World *33*, 222-223.
55. AOYAMA, M., MARUYAMA, T., NUEYA, I. and AKATSUKA, S. 1986. Effects of addition of tocopherols on oxidative stability of potato chips. J. Japan. Soc. Food Sci. Technol. *33*(6), 407-413.
56. ORY, R. L., St, ANGELO, A. J., GWO, Y. Y., FLICK, Jr., G. J. and MOD, R. R. 1985. Oxidation-induced changes in foods. *In* Chemical Changes in Foods During Processing, T. Richardson and J. Finley (eds.). AVI/Van Nostrand Reinhold, New York.

57. BOURGEOIS, C. F. and CYORNOMAZ, A. M. and PAGES, P. 1982. Solubilization of ascorbyl palmitate in vegetable oils. Rev. Fr. Corps Gras 29(879), 319–324.
58. YANG, J. H., CHANG, Y. S. and SHIN, H. S. 1988. Relative effectiveness of some antioxidants on palm oil and beef tallow. Korean J. Food Sci. Technol. 20(4), 563–568.
59. HA, K. H. and IGARSHI, O. 1988. Disappearance and interrelationship of tocopherol analogues during oxidation of corn oil and synergistic effect of L-ascorbyl palmitate with alpha-tocopherol. J. Japan. Soc. Food Sci. Technol. 35(7), 464–470.
60. HILDEBRAND, D. H., TERAO, J. and KILO, M. 1984. Phospholipids plus tocopherols increase soybean oil stability. J. Am. Oil Chem. Soc. 61(3), 552–555.
61. BOURGEOIS, C. F. and CYORNOMAZ, A. M. 1982. Stabilization of lard by ascorbyl palmitate, alpha tocopherol and phospholipids. Rev. Fr. Corps. Gras 29, 111–116.
62. YANISHLIEVA, N. and MARINOVA, E. 1988. Stability of sunflower oil against autoxidation. Khranit. Prom. 37(6), 17–18.
63. CORT, W. M. 1982. Antioxidant properties of ascorbic acid in foods. In Ascorbic Acid: Chemistry, Metabolism and Uses, P. A. Seib and B. M. Tolbert (eds.). Adv. Chem. Ser. No. 220. Am. Chem. Soc., Washington, DC.
64. KLAEUI, H. and PONGRACZ, G. 1982. Ascorbic acid and derivatives as antioxidants in oils and fats. In Vitamin C, J. Counsell and D. Hornig (eds.). Applied Science, London.
65. BURTON, G. W. and INGOLD, K. W. 1984. Beta-carotene: An unusual type of lipid antioxidant. Science 224 (4649), 569–573.
66. MATSUSHITA, S. and TERAO, J. 1980. Singlet oxygen-initiated photoxidation of unsaturated fatty acid esters and inhibitory effects of tocopherols and beta-carotene. In Autoxidation in Food and Biological Systems, M. G. Simic and M. Karel (eds.). Plenum Publishing Corp., New York.
67. WARNER, K. and FRANKEL, E. N. 1987. Effects of beta-carotene on light stability of soybean oil. JAOCS 64(2), 213–218.
68. JOSSE, R. 1987. Food oxidation and its prevention with the use of natural antioxidants. Presentation: Food Additive Symp., Izmir, Turkey, Nov. 2–8.
69. SCHULTZ, H. W. 1981. Food Law Handbook. AVI/Van Nostrand Reinhold, New York.
70. FAO. 1984. Food and Nutrition Paper No. 30. Food and Agricultural Organization of the United Nations, Rome.

CHAPTER 16

BIOAVAILABILITY OF NUTRIENTS ADDED TO HUMAN FOODS

DAPHNE A. ROE, M.D.

INTRODUCTION

Nutrients added to human foods are used for purposes of enrichment, fortification, formulation of diets of defined composition and to provide functional benefits in processed foods.

Enrichment implies the adding back of nutrients which have been extracted or otherwise lost in the process of food manufacture. Fortification is the process whereby nutrients are added to foods to increase nutrient density above that naturally present, to reduce risk of endemic deficiency. Endemic deficiencies which have been combatted by enrichment include pellagra and ariboflavinosis (vitamin B_2 deficiency). Endemic nutritional deficiencies which have been combatted by fortification include iron and iodine deficiency. Formulation of diets of defined composition is carried out in the preparation of infant foods, as well as special formula foods used in tube feeding and intravenous hyperalimentation regimens for those who cannot consume, digest or absorb normal food. Functional benefits are conferred on processed foods when a nutrient provides flavor or color, when it protects the appearance or quality of the product, or when it confers protection against food toxins[1].

The extent to which nutrients added to food are absorbed and reach the plasma is generally termed bioavailability. The bioavailability of nutrients added to human food is largely related to the form of the nutrient added, as well as to the composition of the food vehicle. However, the bioavailability of added nutrients may be also affected by intestinal function and by concurrent administration of drugs (Table 16.1).

Valid studies of the bioavailability of nutrients added to food intended for human use should utilize human subjects whenever possible. Animal models can yield useful data when they are suitably validated and their limitations understood. Further the subjects who participate in the bioavailability study should be similar in age, sex, physiological status and health status to those for whom the food product is intended. A further criterion of a valid bioavailability study is that the nutrient-enriched food that is given should be processed and prepared in such a way that it is normally consumed.

TABLE 16.1
COMMON DRUG GROUPS AND DRUGS THAT MAY CAUSE
NUTRIENT DEPLETION AND NUTRITIONAL DEFICIENCIES

Drug Group	Drug	Deficiency
Antacids	Sodium bicarbonate	Folate, phosphate, calcium, copper
	Aluminum hydroxide	
Anticonvulsants	Phenytoin, phenobarbital, primidone	Vitamins D and K
	Valproic acid	Carnitine
Antibiotics	Tetracycline	Calcium
	Gentamicin	Potassium, magnesium
	Neomycin	Fat, nitrogen
Antibacterial agents	Boric acid	Riboflavin
	Trimethoprim	Folate
	Isoniazid	Vitamin B_6, niacin, Vitamin D
Anti-inflammatory agents	Sulfasalazine	Folate
	Aspirin	Vitamin C, Folate, iron
	Colchicine	Fat, Vitamin B_{12}
	Prednisone	Calcium
Anticancer drugs	Methotrexate	Folate, calcium
	Cisplatin	Magnesium
Anticoagulants	Warfarin	Vitamin K
Antihypertensive agents	Hydralazine	Vitamin B_6
Antimalarials	Pyrimethamine	Folate
Diuretics	Thiazides	Potassium
	Furosemide	Potassium, calcium, magnesium
	Triamterene	Folate
H² receptor antagonists	Cimetidine	Vitamins B_{12}
	Ranitidine	
Hypocholesterolemic agents	Cholestyramine	Fat
	Colestipol	Vitamin K, Vitamin A, Folate, Vitamin B_{12}
Laxatives	Mineral oil	Carotene, retinol, Vitamins D, K
	Phenolphthalein	Potassium
	Senna	Fat, calcium
Oral contraceptives		Vitamin B_6, folate, Vitamin C
Tranquilizers	Chlorpromazine	Riboflavin

Source: Roe[52] (1989).

Formerly, concerns relative to the bioavailability of added nutrients were that the form of the nutrient was such that absorption was inadequate or, conversely, that the nutrient added imposed the risk of vitamin overload or mineral toxicity. Although these concerns are still of paramount importance, other issues are that the added nutrient could mask a nutrient deficiency or that the added nutrient could reduce the efficacy of a therapeutic drug.

In this review of the bioavailability of nutrients added to conventional foods and formula foods, methods for determining the absorption or the apparent absorption of the added nutrient will be discussed and the findings relative to macro- and micronutrients will be summarized.

METHODS FOR STUDYING BIOAVAILABILITY AND EXAMPLES OF TEST PROCEDURES

Bioavailability of Vitamins Added to Conventional Foods

The bioavailability of vitamins added to foods has been studied in human subjects by three main methods, including change in the serum or plasma level after ingestion of the food, measurement of urinary loss of the vitamin after ingestion of the food with prior tissue saturation, and by use of radiotracer methods for vitamin absorption from the gastrointestinal tract.

Change in plasma level of the vitamin has been used to compare folate absorption from different food products and to examine the effect of drugs on such folate absorption[2,3]. Rat and chick bioassay has also been used to study the bioavailability of folate from different foods[4,5].

Load tests which measure the urinary excretion of a vitamin after body saturation have been used to study the bioavailability (apparent absorption) of riboflavin from food products, and particularly to investigate the effect of food additives on riboflavin absorption[6].

In laboratory animals, intrinsic and extrinsic radiolabelling of foods has been used to examine bioavailability. This was the method selected by Ink et al.[7] to measure the bioavailability of vitamin B_6 from animal-derived foods and the effects of thermal processing on the bioavailability of the vitamin. Intraluminal perfusion of the human intestine has also been used to demonstrate differences in the bioavailability of vitamins from food products. This method was employed by Nelson et al.[8] to compare the bioavailability of vitamin B_6 from orange juice and a synthetic source. When vitamins are added to foods in pharmacological quantities so that active physiological mechanisms for absorption are exceeded and absorption is by passive diffusion, it is valid to study the bioavailability of the added vitamins by pharmacokinetic methods employed to study the bioavailability of drugs which are also absorbed by passive diffusion.

Methods for measuring the bioavailability of specific vitamins are summarized in Table 16.2.

TABLE 16.2
METHODS EMPLOYED IN THE MEASUREMENT OF THE BIOAVAILABILITY OF VITAMINS ADDED TO FOODS

Vitamin	Food	Method	Reference
A	Margarine	Growth of rats	Ames et al.[32]
Folic acid	Breads and other cereals	Folate excretion	Colman et al.[33]
	Frozen foods	Chick bioassay	Graham et al.[34]
Vitamin B_6	Enriched cornmeal; Enriched alfalfa sprouts	Rat bioassay; Intrinsic and extrinsic labelling	Nguyen and Gregory[35] Ink et al.[7]
Riboflavin	Breakfast cereal	Urinary excretion	Jusko and Levy[6]

Bioavailability of Vitamins Added to Formula Foods

Infant Formulas. Bioavailability of vitamins added to infant formulas has commonly been examined by comparing blood levels of the vitamins of concern in breast- and formula-fed infants. Standard references on methods for measuring the bioavailability of vitamins used in infant formulas can be found in Machlin's Handbook of Vitamins[9].

A recent report[9] which explains the rationale and methods employed for a study of the bioavailability of vitamin K in infant formula points up the difficulties which may be encountered relative to interpretation of findings. The need to provide vitamin K in an available form in infant formulas is explained by the risk of vitamin K deficiency in newborn infants. In order to reduce this risk, the Committee on Nutrition of the American Academy of Pediatrics has recommended that prophylactic vitamin K be administered by injection to all newborns. Potential sources of vitamin K to the newborn, other than these injections, include transplacental transfer of the vitamin as phylloquinone and dietary sources of vitamin K including human milk and formulas.

The technical significance of this recent study[9], relative to bioavailability, is the demonstration of a new capability to measure vitamin K in serum and feces and to identify the form of the vitamin present, using the HPLC method[10]. However, because the infants in the study had already received parenteral vitamin K, it was not possible to make a comparison as to the relative bioavailability of the vitamin from the formula as compared to human milk.

Formula Foods Used as Oral Supplements or for Enteral Feeding. The bioavailability of vitamins used in the preparation of formula foods not intended for infants, has been examined by measuring change in vitamin levels following formula intake. Inadvertently, it has also been tested by observation of the extent to which the vitamin in the formula interfered with the therapeutic effect of coumarin anticoagulants which are vitamin K antagonists[11].

TABLE 16.3
METHODS USED IN THE MEASUREMENT OF THE
BIOAVAILABILITY OF MINERALS ADDED TO FOODS

Mineral	Method	Reference
Calcium	Fecal calcium	Sheikh et al.[26]
	Calcium balance	Nicar and Pak[36]
	Radioisotopic methods	Recker[37]
Iron	Intrinsic labelling; Extrinsic labelling	Cook[30]
	In vitro dialysis; Hb repletion	Forbes et al.[14a]
Zinc	Intestinal perfusion; Metabolic balance; Isotropic tracers	Solomons and Cousins[27]

Bioavailability of Minerals and Trace Elements Added to Conventional Foods

In laboratory animals and until recently, in human subjects, radioisotope methods have been considered the most accurate means to study mineral absorption. Because of the risk of radioisotopes, use is now limited. Current methods for studying the bioavailability of iron in human subjects do however include the technique of extrinsic radiolabelling, as well as use of stable isotopes. The method of extrinsic radioiron labelling has made it possible to measure the absorption of iron from composite meals. Effects of enhancers and inhibitors of non-heme iron sources in the food used for fortification can be investigated by this method[12]. The absorption of iron added to conventional foods, as well as from soybean-based and milk-based formulas, has been assessed by measuring utilization of radioactive iron by erythrocytes[13]. Since difference in iron status affects the absorption of nonheme iron, this has to be considered in the selection of an experimental design. An independent measurement of the absorptive capacity of iron should be obtained for each subject included in the study, by determining the absorption of a standard dose of inorganic radioiron or with greater safety by use of a dose of a stable iron isotope. Several alternate techniques employing stable isotopes of iron have been used, and recently these different methods have been compared. Experiments carried out by Fairweather-Tait and Minski[14] indicate that absorption of iron from a meal, labelled with the stable isotope, ^{58}Fe, can be assessed by measuring the ^{58}Fe enrichment of erythrocytes.

Relative bioavailability[14a] of two iron fortification compounds, electrolytic iron and ferric orthophosphate, was related to that of the reference ferrous sulfate with in vitro and rat model depletion-repletion methods in four laboratories to compare values directly with those obtained in a parallel human study. Two depletion-repletion techniques, hemoglobin-regeneration efficiency and an official method of the AOAC were examined. The AOAC method served as the most reliable predictor of iron bioavailability in the human, although in vitro dialysis is a promising technic.

Bioavailability of trace elements is studied by the classical balance method, which has been used for zinc[15], by change of serum level[16], or by extrinsic or intrinsic or stable isotope labelling[17]. Effects of extrusion cooking of high fiber cereal products, using mild conditions, on the apparent absorption of zinc, iron, calcium, magnesium and phosphorus, has been studied by direct measurement of the intake of these minerals from the cereal products, and measurement of the minerals lost via ileostomy bag contents[18]. Methods for measuring the bioavailability of minerals and trace elements added to foods and formulas are summarized in Table 16.3.

OVERVIEW OF CONCERNS RELATIVE TO THE BIOAVAILABILITY OF NUTRIENTS USED IN THE PREPARATION OF FORMULA FOODS

Formula foods include infant formulas, liquid nutrient supplements, enteral formulas used in tube feeding, and parenteral formulas used in intravenous feeding. These products have the common characteristic that they are all prepared from purified or semipurified ingredients and the form of the nutrients present may be unlike that occurring in natural foods. Reasons for use of these ingredients include either commercial availability or better absorption or utilization by individuals with compromised gastrointestinal function for whom they are intended.

The availability of nutrients in formulas which are to be administered by the oral route and/or by other enteral routes, such as via a gastrostomy or a jejunostomy, is tested by measured change in blood levels of nutrients, by balance studies or by functional tests. Bioavailability studies may be carried out in laboratory animals, in normal human subjects, or in patients.

Since bioavailability of nutrients in these products may be decreased by loss of the nutrient from the product due to photodegradation, heat destruction, adsorption of the nutrient onto plastic bags and tubes, or due to loss of stability with storage, testing the stability of nutrients used in the formula foods can be considered an integral part of the procedures for examining the availability of the components.

FACTORS INFLUENCING THE BIOAVAILABILITY OF VITAMINS ADDED TO FOODS OR FORMULAS

Loss of vitamin from formula foods intended for intravenous (parenteral) administration is due to instability of the vitamin and to adsorption of the vitamin onto the plastic tubing of the administration set[19]. Although Gutcher *et al.*[20] suggested that use of retinyl palmitate as a vitamin A source would decrease the instability of the vitamin, in TPN solutions, oxidative losses have been shown to occur unless vitamin E is added to the solution. Instability of vitamin A, added as retinol, is due to photodegradation rather than other oxidative losses[21]. However, photodegrada-

TABLE 16.4
FACTORS INFLUENCING THE BIOAVAILABILITY OF VITAMINS
ADDED TO FOODS AND FORMULAS

Vitamin	Factor	Effect	Reference
β-carotene	Fat	Enhances	Roels et al.[38]
	Lecithin	Enhances	Wolf[39]
	Protein	Increases conversion to vitamin A	Stoecker and Arnrich[40]
	Pectin and methylcellulose	Greater than 10% of diet decreases	Gronowska-Senger[41]
	Tocopherol	Increases	Arnrich and Arthur[42]
Retinyl esters	Fat	Increases	Sivakumar and Reddy[43]
	PUFA	Decreases	Arnrich and Arthur[42]
	Protein	Increases	Arnrich and Arthur[42]
Riboflavin	Glucose polymer	Increases	Levy and Rao[44]
	Sodium alginate	Increases	Levy and Rao[44]
	Hemicellulose	Increases	Roe et al.[45]
Folic acid	Fiber	No effect	Ristow et al.[5]
	Vitamin C	Promotes	Chanarin[46]
Thiamin	Sulfites	Decreases	Gubler[47]
Vitamin B_6	Hemicellulose	Minor reduction	Leklem et al.[48]

tion of vitamins in formulas, as in natural foods such as milk, can be related to the composition of the container. Containers that permit photodegradation of vitamins by fluorescent light sources that emit light in the UV range can decrease the stability of infant formulas kept in storage rooms or cabinets with such lighting. Further, the administration of parenteral formulas to premature neonates who are receiving phototherapy as treatment of hyperbilirubinemia, can be associated with a loss of vitamins in the formula because the light source (which usually has a spectral emission maximum of approximately 420 nanometers) causes loss of riboflavin and also of vitamin A. Another vitamin which may be lost through this type of visible ("blue") light exposure is folic acid.

Effects on vitamin stability of enteral bag composition, as well as freezing and thawing, have been examined with respect to vitamins A, E and riboflavin. When the bag composition was either polyvinyl chloride or polyethylene, and the enteral feeding solution was stored in the frozen state for three months, there was no loss of stability of the vitamins under investigation. However, there were minor losses in vitamin A when the bag was thawed and then held for 12 h in the defrozen state[22].

Other than concerns relative to changes in the bioavailability of vitamins in enteral and parenteral formulas due to instability or degradation outside the body, there are several factors which differentiate the bioavailability of nutrients in these products from the bioavailability of nutrients which are added to conventional foods. These factors include the form in which the nutrient is present, which may vary with the intended route of administration, the concentration of the nutrient, which may influence whether it is absorbed as a physiological substance or as a drug, and the intended route of administration.

Comparisons have been made between the absorption characteristics of vitamins used in the preparation of formulas and those of drugs. Such comparisons indicate that there are factors influencing the bioavailability of the vitamins and the drugs, including both the vehicle and gastrointestinal motility[23]. Other factors which can have a significant effect on bioavailability include the age of the recipient, as well as their health status. Factors linked to age, which can alter bioavailability, include the immaturity of intestinal function in infants and the change in efficiency of nutrient absorption which occurs with aging. The practical importance of these factors is apparent when it is appreciated that formula foods are particularly used in nutritional support of the very young and the very old[24,25]. Factors influencing the bioavailability of vitamins added to foods and formulas are summarized in Table 16.4.

EFFECTS OF ENHANCERS AND INHIBITORS OF MINERAL ABSORPTION, WHICH ARE PRESENT IN FOOD AND FORMULAS, ON BIOAVAILABILITY OF ADDED MINERALS

The bioavailability of calcium added to dairy foods for enrichment purposes is not influenced for human subjects by the anion[26].

The bioavailability of zinc in foods depends on the presence or otherwise of inhibitors such as iron, or soy products and of enhancers such as EDTA[27,28].

The bioavailability of iron in conventional and formula foods is influenced by the iron specie, by the particle size of the iron used in fortification, as well as by other nutrients and non-nutrients in the product. For example, the bioavailability of iron from foods depends on whether the added iron is ferrous sulfate or ferrum reductum, and if the latter, whether the particle size is small enough to permit absorption. Further, there are a number of enhancers and inhibitors of iron absorption in foods. Important enhancers of iron absorption include ascorbic acid and certain amino acids, whereas inhibitors include tannins and phytate[29,29a].

The bioavailability of iron may be facilitated or decreased by chelating agents which are used as intentional food additives. The most widely used chelating agent is EDTA, which is added to food to prevent oxidative damage by free metals. Cook[30] found that EDTA reduced the absorption of non-heme iron when it was present in high concentrations in the food.

Factors influencing the bioavailability of minerals and trace elements are summarized in Table 16.5.

TABLE 16.5
FACTORS INFLUENCING THE BIOAVAILABILITY OF MINERALS
ADDED TO FOOD AND FORMULAS

Mineral	Food	Factor	Effect	Reference
Iron	Infant formula	Vitamin C	Enhances	Derman et al.[13]
Iron	Infant formula	Citric acid	Enhances	Derman et al.[13]
	Bread	Large particle size	Reduces	Pla et al.[49]
	Wheat rolls	Phytate	Reduces	Hallberg et al.[29a]
		Vitamin C	Enhances	
Iron	Infant formula	Soybean	Reduces	Derman et al.[13]
Zinc	Meat substitute	Soybean	Reduces	Sandstrom et al.[28]
Zinc	Bread	Soybean	No effect	Sandstrom et al.[28]

FINDINGS CONCERNING EFFECTS OF DISEASE STATE ON THE BIOAVAILABILITY OF NUTRIENTS FROM FORMULAS

Since the recipients of parenteral- and enteral-feeding solutions are individuals whose nutrition is compromised due to the single or combined effects of gastrointestinal disease, late effects of gastrointestinal surgery and drugs, the bioavailability of the nutrients contained in the feeding solutions may be influenced by these factors. On the other hand, acute folate deficiency which has been reported in patients on parenteral infusions, has been explained by Nichoalds et al.[31] as being due to effects of the high methionine intake on the interconversion of folate metabolites.

Disease-related factors which influence the bioavailability of nutrients from nutrient formulas are listed in Table 16.6.

SUMMARY

Nutrients including vitamins and minerals are added to conventional foods for purposes of enrichment or fortification with the ultimate goal of preventing endemic forms of malnutrition. Nutrients are also added, as intentional additives, for nonnutritional purposes. Further, nutrients are used in the preparation of formula foods intended for infants or for those whose ability to eat or to absorb or utilize nutrients is compromised. The bioavailability of an added nutrient depends on the form in which that nutrient is used, and on the composition of the food to which the nutrient is added. The bioavailability of added nutrients is also influenced by whether they are absorbed as physiological or pharmacological substances. Immaturity of the gut, presence of disease, or the use of drugs may reduce the absorption of nutrients used

TABLE 16.6
DISEASE-RELATED FACTORS WHICH INFLUENCE THE BIOAVAILABILITY
OF AND REQUIREMENT FOR NUTRIENTS FROM NUTRIENT FORMULAS

Disease	Factor	Nutrient	Reference
Inflammatory bowel disease	Decrease in absorptive function	Folic acid	Roe[50]
	Gut resection	Vitamin B_{12}	Roe[50]
	Antibiotic used	Biotin and vitamin K	Roe[50]
	Use of sulfasalazine	Folic acid	Roe[50]
Cystic fibrosis	Maldigestion due to loss of pancreatic function	Vitamins A and D	Floch[51]
	Antibiotics	Vitamin K	Floch[51]

in formula foods. Methods used to assess the bioavailability of added nutrients include in vitro tests of nutrient stability, animal bioassays, and human studies. Extrapolation of animal bioassay findings to the human being may be misleading.

REFERENCES

1. NEWSOME, R. L. 1987. Use of vitamins as additives in processed foods. A scientific status summary by the Institute of Food Technologists' Expert Panel on Food Safety and Nutrition. Inst. Food Technologists, Chicago, IL.
2. RHODE, B. M., COOPER, B. A. and FARMER, F. A. 1983. Effect of orange juice, folic acid and oral contraceptives on serum folate in women taking a folate-restricted diet. J. Am. Coll. Physicians 2, 221–230.
3. ROE, D. A. 1981. Intergroup and intragroup variables affecting interpretation of studies of drug effects on nutritional status. In Nutrition in Health and Disease and International Development, XII Intern. Congr. Nutr. Alan R. Liss, New York.
4. ABAD, A. R. and GREGORY, J. F. 1987. Determination of folate bioavailability with a rat bioassay. J. Nutr. 117, 866–873.
5. RISTOW, K. A., GREGORY, J. F. and DAMRON, B. L. 1982. Thermal processing effects on folacin bioavailability in liquid model food systems, liver and cabbage. J. Agric. Food Chem. 30, 801–806.
6. JUSKO, W. J. and LEVY, G. 1975. Absorption, protein binding and elimination of riboflavin. In Riboflavin, R. S. Rivlin (ed.). Plenum Press, New York.
7. INK, S. L., GREGORY, J. F. and SARTAIN, D. B. 1986. Determination of pyridoxine beta-glucoside bioavailability using intrinsic and extrinsic labeling in the rat. J. Agr. Food Chem. 34, 857–861.
8. NELSON, E. W., LANE, H. and CERDA, J. J. 1976. Comparative human intestinal bioavailability of vitamin B_6 from a synthetic and from a natural source. J. Nutr. 106, 1433–1437.
9. MACHLIN, L. J. 1984. Handbook of Vitamins: Nutritional, Biochemical and Clinical Aspects. Marcel Dekker, New York.

10. GREER, F. R., MUMMAH-SCHENDEL, L. L., MARSHALL, S. and SUTTIE, J. W. 1988. Vitamin K_1 (phylloquinone) and vitamin K_2 (menaquionone) status in newborns during the first week of life. Pediatrics 81, 137-140.
11. LEE, M., SCHWARTZ, R. N. and SHARIFI, R. 1981. Warfarin resistance and vitamin K. Ann. Intern. Med. 94, 140-141.
12. HALLBERG, L. 1981. Bioavailability of iron from different meals. In Nutrition in Health and Disease and International Development, XII Intern. Congr. Nutr. Alan R. Liss, New York.
13. DERMAN, D. P. et al. 1987. Factors influencing the absorption of iron from soya-bean protein products. Brit. J. Nutr. 57, 345-353.
14. FAIRWEATHER-TAIT, S. J. and MINSKI, M. J. 1986. Studies on iron availability in man, using stable isotope techniques. Brit. J. Nutr. 55, 279-285.
14a. FORBES, A. L. et al. 1989. Comparison of in vitro, animal, and clinical determinations of iron bioavailability: International Nutritional Anemia Consultative Group Task Force Report on Iron bioavailability. Am. J. Clin. Nutr. 49, 225-238.
15. CREWS, M. G., TAPER, L. J. and RITCHEY, S. J. 1980. Effect of oral contraceptive agents on copper and zinc balance in young women. Am. J. Clin. Nutr. 33, 1940.
16. KIVISTO, B., ANDERSSON, H., CEDERBLAD, G., SANDBERG, A-S. and SANDSTROM, B. 1986. Extrusion cooking of a high-fibre cereal product. 2. Effects on apparent absorption of zinc, iron, calcium, magnesium and phosphorus in humans. Brit. J. Nutr. 55, 255-260.
17. PECOUD, A., DONZEL, P. and SCHELLING, J. L. 1975. The effect of foodstuffs on the absorption of zinc sulfate. Clin. Pharmacol. Ther. 17, 469.
18. ARVIDSSON, B., CEDERBLAD, A., BJORN-RASMUSSEN, E. and SANDSTROM, B. 1978. A radionuclide technique for studies of zinc absorption in man. Int. J. Nucl. Med. Bio. 5, 104-109.
19. CHIOU, W. L. and MOORHATCH, P. 1973. Interaction between vitamin A and plastic intravenous infusion bags. JAMA 223, 328.
20. GUTCHER, G. R., LAX, A. A. and FARRELL, P. M. 1984. Vitamin losses to plastic intravenous infusion devices and an improved method of delivery. Am. J. Clin. Nutr. 40, 8-13.
21. RIGGLE, M. A. and BRANDT, R. B. 1986. Decrease of available vitamin A in parenteral nutrition solutions. JPEN 10, 388-392.
22. DAVIS, A. T., FAGERMAN, K. E., DOWNER, F. D. and DEAN, R. E. 1986. Effect of enteral bag composition and freezing and thawing upon vitamin stability in an enteral feeding solution. JPEN 10, 245-246.
23. ROE, D. A. 1984. Food, formula and drug effects on the disposition of nutrients. World Rev. Nutr. Dietet. Karger (Basel) 43, 80-94.
24. ZEMAN, F. J. and NEY, D. M. 1988. Applications of Clinical Nutrition. Prentice Hall, Englewood Cliffs, New Jersey.
25. FLOCH, M. H. 1981. Nutrition and Diet Therapy in Gastrointestinal Disease. Plenum Medical Book Co., New York, pp. 327-344.
26. SHEIKH, M. S., SANTA ANA, C. A., NICAR, M. J., SCHILLER, L. R. and FORDTRAN, J. S. 1987. Gastrointestinal absorption of calcium from milk and calcium salts. New Engl. J. Med. 317, 532-536.
27. SOLOMONS, N. W. and COUSINS, R. J. 1984. Zinc. In Absorption and Malabsorption of Mineral Nutrients. Alan R. Liss, New York.

28. SANDSTROM, B., KIVISTO, B. and CEDERBLAD, A. 1987. Absorption of zinc from soy protein meals in humans. J. Nutr. *117*, 321–327.
29. COOK, J. D., MORCK, T. A., SKIKNE, B. S. and LYNCH, S. R. 1981. Biochemical determinants of iron absorption. Nutrition in Health and Disease and International Development, XII Intern. Congr. Nutr. Alan R. Liss, New York.
29a. HALLBERG, L., BRUNE, M. and ROSSANDER, L. 1989. Iron absorption in man: Ascorbic acid and dose-dependent inhibition by phytate. Am. J. Clin. Nutr. *49*, 140–144.
30. COOK, J. D. 1977. Absorption of food iron. Fed. Proc. *36*, 2028–2032.
31. NICHOALDS, G. E., MENG, H. C. and CALDWELL, M. D. 1977. Vitamin requirements of patients receiving total parenteral nutrition. Arch. Surg. *112*, 1061.
32. AMES, S. R., LUDWIG, M. I., SWANSON, W. J. and HARRIS, P. L. 1952. Biochemical studies on vitamin A. X. A nutritional investigation of synthetic vitamin A in margarine. J. Am. Oil Chemists Soc. *29*, 151–153.
33. COLMAN, N., GREEN, R. and METZ, J. 1975. Prevention of folate deficiency by food fortification. II. Absorption of folic acid from fortified staple foods. Am. J. Clin. Nutr. *28*, 459–464.
34. GRAHAM, D. C., ROE, D. A. and OSTERTAG, S. G. 1980. Radiometric determination and chick bioassay of folacin in fortified and unfortified frozen foods. J. Food Sci. *45*, 47–51.
35. NGUYEN, L. B. and GREGORY, J. F. III. 1983. Effects of food composition on the bioavailability of vitamin B_6 in the rat. J. Nutr. *113*, 1550–1560.
36. NICAR, M. J. and PAK, C. Y. C. 1985. Calcium bioavailability from calcium carbonate and calcium citrate. J. Clin. Endocrinol. Metab. *51*, 391–393.
37. RECKER, R. R. 1985. Calcium absorption and achlorhydria. New Engl. J. Med. *313*, 70–73.
38. ROELS, O. A., TROUT, M. and DUJACQUIER, R. 1958. Carotene balances in boys in Ruanda where vitamin A deficiency is prevalent. J. Nutr. *65*, 115–127.
39. WOLF, G. 1980. Vitamin A. *In* Human Nutrition: A Comprehensive Treatise. R. Alfin Slater and D. Kritchevsky (eds.). Plenum Press, New York.
40. STOECKER, B. and ARNRICH, L. 1973. Patterns of protein feeding and the biosynthesis of vitamin A from carotene in rats. J. Nutr. *103*, 1112–1118.
41. GRONOWSKA-SENGER, A., SMACZYNY, E. and DOBKOWICZ, B. 1980. The effect of fiber on the utilization of carotene in laboratory rats. Bromatol. Chemia. Toksykol. *13*, 129–134.
42. ARNRICH, L. and ARTHUR, V. A. 1980. Interactions of fat soluble vitamins in hypervitaminoses. Ann. N.Y. Acad. Sci. *355*, 109–118.
43. SIVAKUMAR, B. and REDDY, V. 1972. Absorption of labelled vitamin A in children during infection. Brit. J. Nutr. *27*, 229–304.
44. LEVY, G. and RAO, B. K. 1972. Enhanced intestinal absorption of riboflavin from sodium alginate solution in man. J. Pharm. Sci. *61*, 279–280.
45. ROE, D. A., WRICK, K., McLAIN, D. and VAN SOEST, P. 1978. Effects of dietary fiber sources on riboflavin absorption. Fed. Proc. *37*, 756.
46. CHANARIN, I. 1969. The Megaloblastic Anaemias. Blackwell Publishing Co., Oxford.
47. GUBLER, C. J. 1984. Thiamin. *In* Handbook of Vitamins. L. J. Machlin, (ed.). Marcel Dekker, New York.
48. LEKLEM, J. E. 1977. Vitamin B_6 enrichment of wheat flour: Stability and bioavailability.

Report to the Food & Nutrition Board, Committee on Food Protection of the National Academy of Science. Technology of Fortification of Cereal-Grain Products, May 16–17.
49. PLA, G. W., HARRISON, B. N. and FRITZ, J. C. 1973. Comparison of chicks and rats as test animals for studying bioavailability of iron, with special reference to use of reduced iron in enriched bread. JAOAC 56, 1369–1373.
50. ROE, D. A. 1985. Nutrition and diet in relation to chronic disease and disability. *In* Nutrition for Family and Primary Care Practitioners, A. B. Lasswell, D. A. Roe and L. Hochheiser (eds.). George Stickley Co., Philadelphia.
51. FLOCH, M. H. 1981. Nutrition and diet therapy in gastrointestinal disease. Plenum Medical Book Co., New York, pp. 210–212.
52. ROE, D. A. 1989. Diet and Drug Interactions. Van Nostrand Reinhold, New York.

CHAPTER 17

ENGINEERING ASPECTS OF NUTRIFYING FOODS

DARYL B. LUND, Ph.D.

INTRODUCTION

The addition of vitamins, minerals, amino acids, and other nutrients to foods for the purpose of improving the health and well-being of people has been widely practiced since the 1940s. The technological aspects are straightforward once the nutrient has been selected and a suitable vehicle in the diet has been determined. In this chapter, the engineering considerations for adding a nutrient(s) to a food will be covered omitting detailed engineering design (e.g., sizing various pieces of equipment within a total plant process). In addition, information on nutrient bioavailability (e.g., iron in cereals), stability (e.g., vitamin A in fats and oils), nutrient-product interaction (e.g., yellowing of rice by riboflavin), and cost of the nutrient will not be presented here but can be found in nutrient-specific chapters in this book.

This chapter will present a discussion on factors affecting the point in the process for addition of the nutrient and methods of nutrient addition using numerous examples from current practice.

FACTORS AFFECTING POINT-OF-ADDITION

One of the most important factors affecting point-of-addition of a nutrient or mixture of nutrients is stability of the nutrients. Vitamins are subject to a variety of reactions which diminish or eliminate their biological function. For example, vitamin A is subject to oxidation, hydrolysis, and biomolecular reactions, and the importance of any one of these deteriorative mechanisms is dependent on time, temperature and composition of the milieu. Consequently, it is generally advisable that nutrients, especially vitamins, be added to the food after operations which involve heating, aeration and washing.[1]

In considering the point-of-addition, the unit operations downstream from addition must be reviewed from the standpoint of effect on nutrient stability. For example, minerals can be added to doughs which are going to be extruded, whereas vitamins generally are not because of their susceptibility to degradation during ex-

NUTRIENT ADDITIONS TO FOOD

TABLE 17.1
METHOD OF NUTRIFICATION AND PREFERABLE POINT OF ADDITION OF MICRONUTRIENT TO FOOD

Food	Pure or Direct	Solution, Emulsion or Dispersion			Dry Premix			Preferable Point of Addition	Comments
		Measured Volume	Coating or Spray	Tablet or Wafer	Nutrients in Dry Carrier	With Processed Micronutrients			
Baked items	—	—	x	x	x	x		In water-flour mix	Enriched flour as alternative may be used
Beverages	x	x	—	—	—	x		Before pasteurization	Ascorbic acid[1]
Bread	—	—	—	x	x	x		In water-flour mix or yeast slurry	Enriched flour as alternative may be used
Breakfast cereals, dry	—	—	x	—	—	—		After toasting	Mix for uniformity
Cake mixes	—	—	—	—	x	x		During mixing stage	Watch out for segregation
Candy, hard	x	—	—	—	—	x		On slab or during mixing	Heat-labile nutrients on slab, others during mixing
Candy, soft	—	—	—	—	x	x		To chocolate or filling	Sometimes with flavoring
Cereals, cooked	—	—	—	—	x	x		Last mixing stage	Cooking water[2]
Cheese, processed	—	x	—	—	x	—		During blending	—
Cheese, primary	—	x	—	—	—	x		To milk before curding	—
Chowders, processed	x	—	—	—	x	x		During blending	—
Corn grits	—	—	—	—	x	x		End of milling	Must not segregate. Coated particle premix may be used[2]
Corn meal	—	—	—	—	x	x		During milling	Must not segregate
Dessert mixes	—	—	—	—	x	x		During mixing	Watch out for segregation
Farina, wheat	—	—	—	—	x	x		During milling	Must not segregate. Cooking water[2] Coated particle premix may be used
Flour, wheat	—	—	—	—	x	x		During milling	Additives must be 100 mesh or more. Stable to 13.5% moisture content.

ENGINEERING ASPECTS

Product						Point of addition	Ascorbic acid[1]
Fruit juices	x	—	—	—	—	Before pasteurization	—
Gelatin, dry	x	—	—	x	x	During mixing	Must not segregate
Infant food, dry	x	—	—	x	x	During mixing	Or homogenized in condensed product and spray dried
Infant food, liquid	x	—	—	—	x	Prior to homogenization or blending	—
Margarine	x	—	—	x	—	To tank before churning	—
Mellorine, parevine	x	—	—	x	x	To mix before homogenizing	—
Milk, dry	x	—	—	—	x	Dry blending before instantizing	Or homogenized in condensed product and spray dried
Milk, liquid, semi-solid	x	—	—	x	—	Prior to homogenization	—
Pasta products	—	—	x	—	x	In water-dough mix	Enriched semolina as alternative may be used
Peanut butter	x	—	—	—	x	With salt addition	—
Potato chips	—	—	—	—	x	Coat after toasting	Or with salt addition
Potato granule	—	—	x	—	x	Solution before drying	Watch out for segregation if dry mixed
Protein beverages	x	—	x	—	x	Prior to homogenization	Should not settle out
Rice	—	—	—	—	x	After milling	Cooking water[2] Protective coating[3] Riboflavin addition[4]
Salt	x	—	—	—	x	To be dry mixed	Must not segregate. Coated particle premix may be used.
Semolina, durum wheat	—	—	—	—	x	During milling	Must not segregate. Coated particle premix may be used.
Snack foods	—	—	x	—	x	After heat processing for liable nutrients; before extruding for others	—

TABLE 17.1. (*Continued*)

Food							When added	Remarks
Soups, dry	x	—	—	—	x	x	During mixing	Watch out for segregation
Soups, processed	—	x	—	—	x	x	Before pasteurization	—
Soy flour or grits	—	—	—	—	x	—	During mixing	Must not segregate. Coated particle premix may be used.
Sugar	x	—	—	—	x	—	To be dry blended	Must not segregate. Coated particle premix may be used.
Tea leaves	—	—	x	—	—	—	After drying and then blended	—
Vegetable juice	x	—	—	—	—	x	Before pasteurization	Ascorbic acid¹
Vegetable or salad oil	x	—	—	—	—	—	Followed by blending	Use dark glass or opaque container for light sensitive nutrients
Vegetable dressings (emulsified)	x	—	—	—	—	x	Before emulsifying	Use dark glass or opaque container for light sensitive nutrients

Source: Bauernfeind and Brooke.[2]
[1] If ascorbic acid is added, avoid iron, copper and brass equipment and unnecessary exposure to oxygen.
[2] Cooking water should not be discarded.
[3] If product is washed before cooking, a water-resistant protective coating must be applied to the kernel premix.
[4] If riboflavin is added, a yellow color will be imparted to the white-rice.

trusion cooking. Vitamin premixes are usually added to products just prior to packaging in order to maximize retention of the vitamin. The most severe downstream processing unit operations in terms of vitamin degradation are those involving heat (including mechanical energy in homogenizers) and aeration (due to oxidative losses). Table 17.1 summarizes the method of nutrification and preferable point-of-addition for a number of foods.[2] It can be seen that most foods are preferably fortified using a dry premix.

As a general guideline, addition is preferred at that point in the process which will: (1) provide sufficient agitation to ensure that the nutrients are uniformly distributed, (2) present the food at some fixed, known volume or weight (either total or rate basis) to provide proper ratio between nutrients and food, (3) provide for ease of addition and (4) eliminate as many adverse processing conditions as possible.[3]

METHODS OF NUTRIENT ADDITION

The most common methods of adding nutrients to dry foods are dry mixing and spray coating.

Mixing

For liquid or semimoist foods, the nutrient is dissolved or dispersed in a liquid carrier (water or oil) and subsequently blended or homogenized into the product. In both cases, for continuous systems it is common to use a precision feeder (for either solid or liquid) to introduce the desired amount of nutrient into the product. For batch systems, the liquid or solid is added to the product per the requirements for the batch, and the batch is subsequently mixed in a mixing vessel. In order to avoid incorrect addition to the batch, preweighed tablets or packets of nutrient premix can be obtained from nutrient suppliers for fast, easy addition to the batch.

Feeders. For continuous processes, such as flour production, it is necessary to add the nutrient(s) at a rate compatible with the flow rate of the product in order to have the correct dilution of the nutrient in the product. Since the nutrient must be blended with the product in a precision blender, it is essential to design the system based on the specifications of the precision blender. Precision blenders will be discussed in the next section and, therefore, suffice it to say that blenders can blend ratios from 1/1 up to 1/100,000 and the continuous feeder will be sized depending on the blender requirements.

The feeder can either consist of a volumetric or mass feeder or can be a part of a pneumatic system if the product is pneumatically conveyed. For flour, for example, a pneumatic system of conveying flour allows the volumetric feeder to be placed anywhere in the system convenient to the pneumatic equipment, since the nutrient premix can be pneumatically conveyed to point-of-addition.[4] This system requires an air blower, an ejector unit and pneumatic lines to carry the nutrients to point-of-addition. It is important that the point-of-addition be followed by some type of mixing, since the dilution rate in flour is usually 0.1–0.3 g premix/kg flour. Roll-type and variable speed screw-type feeders are shown in Fig. 17.1 and 17.2, respectively. The choice of one over the other is largely personal, since both types come in a variety of adjustable sizes.

Frequent monitoring and preventive maintenance are required for proper functioning of the feeder. It is also essential to check adjustment on the feeder periodically to ensure proper feed rate. If the flow rate of the product varies significantly throughout the production day, then it is desirable to have an adjustable feeder which is controlled through a feed forward control system by the flow rate of the product. In this case, the product flow rate could be determined by a weighing belt and the feeder rate could be adjusted based on the product flow rate. The flow rate of the premix or nutrient can be determined from the formula:

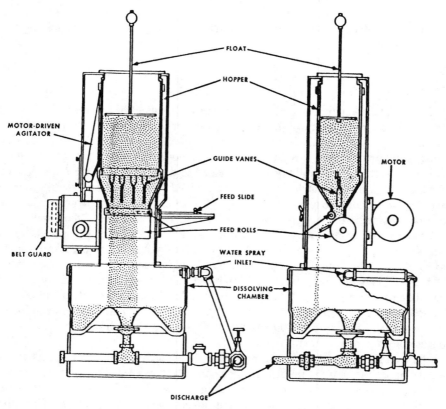

FIG. 17.1. ROLL-TYPE VOLUMETRIC FEEDER WITH SLIDE BAR FEED-RATE ADJUSTMENT

Flow rate of nutrient = (Dilution rate of nutrient)(Flow rate of product)

For example, it is desired to add a premix at a rate of 0.5 oz/cwt of product and the product flow rate is 100 cwt/h, then the flow rate of premix is:

$$\frac{0.5 \text{ oz}}{\text{cwt}} \frac{100 \text{ cwt}}{\text{h}} = 50 \frac{\text{oz}}{\text{h}} = 0.83 \frac{\text{oz}}{\text{min}} = 23.6 \frac{\text{g}}{\text{min}}$$

In order to ensure proper overall operation, it is advisable to monitor daily the disappearance of premix and verify that it coincides with the desired amount corresponding to the production rate. This will also be useful to verify to regulatory agencies that the nutrient or premix is being added to the product in accordance with regulations.

Mixers. Mixing is one of the most widely utilized unit operations in the food industry, and, therefore, equipment manufacturers are generally well-prepared to correctly size the mixer and provide information on characteristics such as power, mix time, temperature rise and operating parameters (e.g., rpm). Fortunately, it is a relatively simple operation and equipment costs are usually modest in comparison to other operations such as heating, grinding and packaging.

Although there are numerous factors which affect mixing effectiveness, they can be broadly categorized as either (1) ingredient attributes or (2) equipment attributes. Ingredient attributes which can greatly affect mixer effectiveness include: (1) parti-

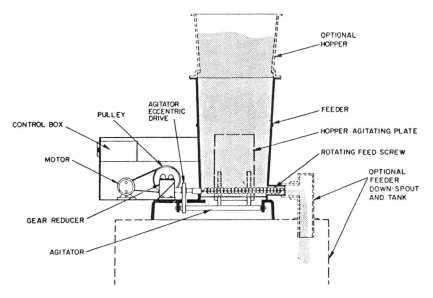

FIG. 17.2. VARIABLE SPEED-DRIVE SCREW-TYPE FEEDER

cle shape, (2) particle size, (3) density, (4) hygroscopicity, (5) electrostatic properties and (6) adhesive characteristics. In order to properly check out equipment, preliminary mixing trials should be conducted. Most supply houses of premixes and individual nutrients can make recommendations on their appropriate product when you specify your product. Two of the most important properties of the nutrient or premix are particle size and particle density. For best efficiency of mixing and maintenance of mix uniformity during storage and distribution it is best to have a particle size and density approximating that of the product. Since most dry biological material will have close to the same density, it is only necessary to determine the bulk density. If, for example, the product has been previously agglomerated for ease of solubilizing or wetting, then it may be desirable to have the premix supplied as an agglomerate with or without a carrier.

Mixer attributes which are most important include mechanical energy input, particle attrition, ease of loading and unloading, cleanability and mixing time. Again, most mixer manufacturers can recommend appropriate mixer equipment given the requirements of the mixing operation. Information which must be supplied includes nature of materials to mixed (density, particle size, etc.), batch or continuous operation, temperature limits, and moisture content.

One of the most commonly used horizontal batch or continuous mixer is the ribbon mixer (Fig. 17.3). The trough-like unit has a rotating shaft extending through

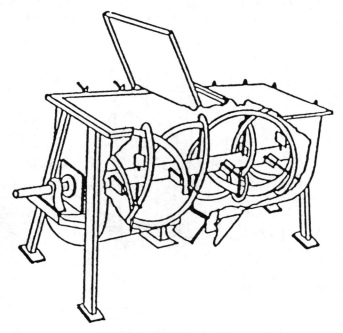

FIG. 17.3. RIBBON MIXER

ENGINEERING ASPECTS 481

the trough onto which are attached two helical ribbons that rotate in opposite directions. As a result, the material moves back and forth from one end of the vessel to another while at the same time being lifted. A popular vertical batch mixer is the inverted cone-type with circulating screw agitators (Fig. 17.4). Both the ribbon and vertical cone mixers can be used for mixing liquids into solids by mounting spray nozzles carrying the liquid above the trough or into the cone, respectively.

Spray Application

If the nutrient or premix is in liquid form or if the nutrient is added after the product has been manufactured (e.g., ready-to-eat cereal), then it is desirable to apply the premix to the product by spraying. This is an excellent technique for applying minute quantities of premix to an unusually shaped product. As with blending, this process technology has been well established so equipment manufacturers are confident in sizing equipment and assuring uniform coverage.

The most popular method is to position spray nozzles over a belt conveyer or blender or spraying into a rotating drum. The drum blending method is generally used with ready-to-eat (RTE) cereals after cooking because the cereals are subjected to high temperatures for relatively long times during cooking. Figure 17.5 is a schematic diagram for producing a flaked and a puffed cereal.[12] The vitamin spray is applied immediately after cooking the cereal to minimize exposure to oxygen and

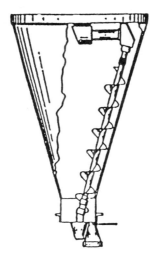

FIG. 17.4. VERTICAL
CONICAL MIXER WITH
CIRCULATING
SCREW AGITATOR

high temperature and provide residual heat for evaporation of the water in the spray solution.

For nutrients which are sensitive to oxidative deterioration, it is necessary to build in an adequate protection system, such as an antioxidant and an oxygen barrier. BHA and BHT have been incorporated into vitamin premixes to protect against oxidation.[5] An effective oxygen barrier for vitamin A is sucrose, as shown in a recent study by Johnson et al.[5] Sucrose was mixed with a vitamin premix containing vitamins A, C and B_1 (thiamin) and sprayed onto two RTE cereals. The stability of the vitamins was measured over a 12 month period. From Table 17.2, it can be seen that the vitamin premix containing 15–20% sucrose applied to Raisin Bran resulted in no loss of vitamin A compared to nearly 30% loss in Corn Flakes after 12 months. The authors attributed the increased stability to the protective oxygen barrier effect of sucrose. On the other hand, vitamin C loss in Raisin Bran was nearly 60% after 12 months compared to approximately 30% in Corn Flakes. Johnson et al.[5] attributed the more rapid vitamin C loss in Raisin Bran to the fact that Raisin Bran had 6% moisture (in order to minimize hardening of the raisins) compared to 2–3% moisture in the Corn Flakes. From this example, it can be seen that there are numerous interacting variables that effect vitamin stability including method of addition, presence of protective chemicals, moisture content, and temperature.

Infusion

Infusion of nutrients, especially those that are heat stable, is also used in RTE cereals. Minerals are added to water along with flavoring and coloring agents which is then admixed to cereal grains. The cereal kernels soak up the aqueous solution, resulting in an infusion of nutrients into the kernels. Since all of the water is taken

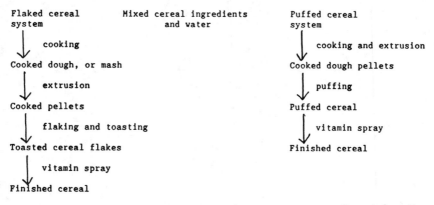

From Anderson[12]

FIG. 17.5. PRODUCING FLAKED AND PUFFED CEREAL

TABLE 17.2
VITAMIN STABILITY IN CEREALS AS AFFECTED BY SUGAR
IN THE VITAMIN SPRAY SOLUTION

Cereal Types and Spray Solution Used	Time in Storage	Vitamin Assays of Cereal Stored at Ambient Room Temperature					
		Vitamin A		Vitamin C		Thiamin	
		IU/Oz	% Loss	Mg/Oz	% Loss	Mg/Oz	% Loss
Raisin bran							
Sprayed with	Initial	2180	—	27.6	—	0.81	—
vitamins in 15–20%	6 Months	2230	0	18.9	22	0.73	10
sugar solution	12 Months	2230	0	11.2	59	0.72	11
Corn flakes							
Sprayed with	Initial	1430	—	18.8	—	0.49	—
vitamins in < 1%	6 Months	1170	18	17.1	9	0.50	0
sugar solution	12 Months	1040	27	13.4	29	0.46	6

Source: Johnson et al.[5]
[1]Cereal type not intended to denote any particular brand.
[2]Both spray solutions contained BHT as an antioxidant.
[3]Vitamin A palmitate.
[4]Sodium ascorbate.
[5]Thiamin mononitrate.

up by the kernels there is no loss of nutrient, and the infused grain can now be cooked and subsequently processed. The main advantage of infusion is that the nutrient, color and flavor are distributed into the kernel resulting in a uniform concentration. Thus, upon soaking the product in liquid such as milk, the nutrient, color and flavor stay in the grain and are not totally released until mastication.

Ingredient Carrier

A popular method of fortifying formulated foods with fat-soluble vitamins is to add the vitamin directly to the lipid or fat constituent prior to formulation of the product. Successful examples include vitamins A, D and E addition to oil used for margarine, fortification of vitamin A in peanut butter, and adding vitamin A and D to milk.[6]

The process is relatively simple and requires a system for accurately dispersing the vitamin into the oil. A liquid-liquid mixer is required or a stirred batch tank. Usually the vitamin is delivered to the plant site in small quantity packages suitable for adding directly to the batch tank. This avoids any mistakes which can be made at the plant, especially for nutrients which can be toxic at sufficiently high concentrations.

CASE STUDIES

Three case studies will be briefly reviewed in order to illustrate the principles of the technology of fortification with minerals and vitamins.

Cereal Fortification

Wheat flour has been routinely fortified since the enrichment program was instituted in 1941. A typical process flow chart is presented in Fig. 17.6. Enriching is accomplished just prior to bagging or bulk delivery usually by dry mixing a nutrient premix with the flour. Although this method works effectively for adding nutrients to a milled cereal, it can not be applied to whole grains. For whole grains the nutrient must either be infused into the grain or coated onto the kernel surface.

One of the most important applications of enrichment is with polished white rice. In the United States, the Standard of Identity for Enriched Rice was established in 1958. In the initial process, rice was infused with an aqueous solution containing thiamin, niacin, and iron; the impregnated kernels were then coated with a rinse-resistant coating. A schematic of the process which was invented by Hoffmann-LaRoche[8] is given in Fig. 17.7. The rice is spray coated with a vitamin premix of thiamin hydrochloride and nicotinamide dissolved in sulphuric acid, allowed to dry in hot air and then followed by application of two coats of protective mixture. The protective mixture, an alcoholic solution of gums and resins, is applied, followed immediately by an application of talc and ferric pyrophosphate. After drying, the process is repeated to increased the iron to the desired level. The purpose of the coating is to prevent dissolution of the water-soluble vitamins when the rice is rinsed or soaked prior to cooking. The fortified rice is then mixed with white milled rice at a ratio of 114 g premix to 50 lb of white milled rice (blending ratio of 1:200).

This process, or others substantially similar to it, were used successfully with little modification until Bramall[9] reported a new four step manufacturing technique (Fig. 17.8). The RCL (Rice Growers Cooperative Limited) process consisted or spraying a liquid mixture of ferric pyrophosphate suspended in an acid solution of the vitamins onto rice, allowing the rice to dry, and finally bagging the premix for subsequent distribution to blending plants where it was diluted 1:200 with white milled rice. The uniqueness of the process was the elimination of gums and resins to facilitate sticking the ferric pyrophosphate onto the kernels by choosing acidic conditions such that starch hydrolysis at the kernel surface generated a thin sticky sugar layer. Sulfuric acid could not be used because ferric pyrophosphate with sulfuric acid produced brown basic ferric sulfates. It was claimed that this process is vastly superior to the Hoffmann-LaRoche process because (1) production rate was doubled, (2) production costs were reduced, since only 4 stages were used rather than 13 with the older process, and (3) safety was improved, since there was no need to handle solvents, hot melt gums and strong oxidizing acids. The process has been a commercial success and is used extensively to produce the RCL fortified rice premix.

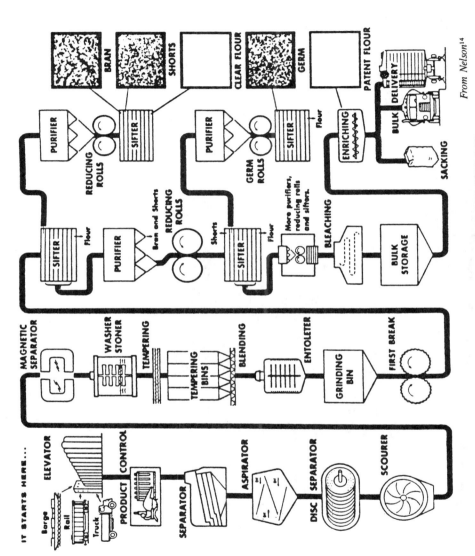

FIG. 17.6. SIMPLIFIED FLOW CHART FOR FLOUR MILLING

From Nelson[14]

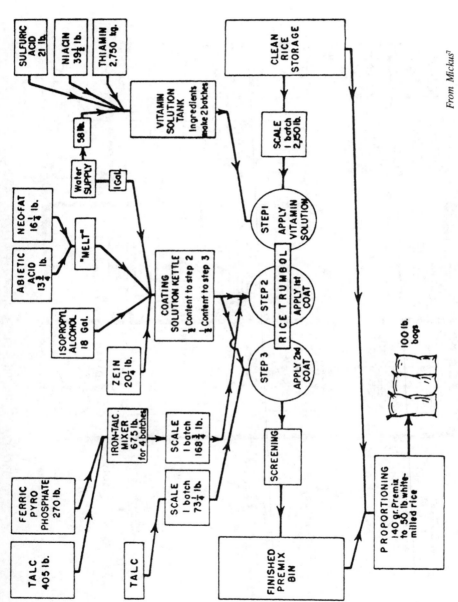

FIG. 17.7. SCHEMATIC OF THE RICE ENRICHMENT PROCESS

From Mickus[7]

Another technique to produce enriched rice is to manufacture an artificial rice kernel for blending with milled rice.[10] The concept is to produce an enriched artificial kernel from wheat flour (75%), waxy (glutinous) rice flour (20%) and non-waxy (nonglutinous) rice flour (5%). After addition of thiamin, these ingredients are blended with water, kneaded into a dough and shaped like rice grains using a granulator, a device commonly used to make macaroni or noodles. After steaming to gelatinize the surface layer, the artificial kernels are dried. The primary disadvantage of this technique is that the artificial rice kernels lose integrity upon cooking and, therefore, can only be used in countries that eat "sticky" rice, a rice gruel for which the rice is cooked until it is soft and "sticky."

Fortification of Tea

In 1974, Crowley et al.[11] described an AID project to develop a procedure to fortify tea with Vitamin A for Pakistan. The solution to the problem was to spray a 50% sucrose solution/Vitamin A emulsion onto tea (Fig. 17.9). The Vitamin A emulsion was palmitate ester of Vitamin A in an acacia and water-based solution with BHT and dl-alpha tocopherol as antioxidants and sodium benzoate as preservative. The cost of fortifying tea using this technique at an annual production of

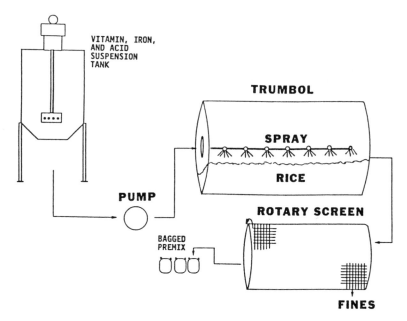

From Brammal[9]

FIG. 17.8. PRODUCTION OF VITAMIN-ENRICHED RICE PREMIX

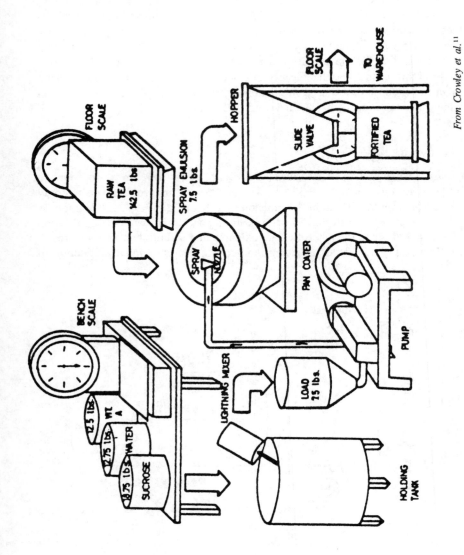

FIG. 17.9. DIAGRAMMATIC FLOW SHEET FOR FORTIFICATION OF TEA WITH VITAMIN A

From Crowley et al.[11]

TABLE 17.3
ESTIMATED COST OF FORTIFYING TEA, WITH 500,000 LB/YEAR CONCENTRATE PLANT (1974)

Item	Cost/Lb ($)
Total ingredients	0.698
Quality control costs	0.011
Labor costs	0.009
Maintenance (@ 15% equipment cost/year)	0.006
Depreciation (buildings 20 years, equipment 10 years)	0.012
Utilities	0.001
Total manufacturing costs	0.737
Incremental cost (Replacing tea with concentrate @ $0.60/lb)	0.137
Costs of fortifying @ 250 IU/g	0.0068

Source: Crowley et al.[11]

500,000 lb/year are shown in Table 17.3. Although the costs represent 1974 dollars, it is relevant to note that ingredient costs are 94.7% of the total manufacturing costs and maintenance and depreciation are only 2.4% of total costs. This is an important point to consider in fortification process design, since the nutrient cost can be considerable forcing the adoption of relatively low cost technology for the process.

Iodination of Salt

One of the most important technological developments has been the iodination of table salt for the control and elimination of goiter. Iodine as the iodide or iodate of potassium, calcium or sodium is added at a rate sufficient to meet the recommended minumum daily requirement of 150 μg. If the per capital salt consumption is assumed to be 5 kg/year and there are 50% losses in transit and storage, then the additional level of potassium iodate is 37 ppm.

There are 4 methods commonly used for salt iodination:[13] (1) dry mixing, (2) drip feed addition of iodine, (3) spray mixing, and (4) submersion. In the dry mixing process a mixture of potassium iodate and an anticaking agent is prepared in a ratio of 1:9. One part of this stock mixture is then added to 10 parts of salt and the premix is introduced onto a screw conveyor at a fixed rate. This process is suitable for powdered salt only and has been applied in several countries in South and Central America.

In drip feed addition, potassium iodate solution is continuously dripped onto salt which has been discharged onto a belt conveyor at a fixed rate. The drop rate is adjusted to the speed of the conveyor. This gives a uniform coating to the salt crystals. Experience has shown that a capacity of 5 tons per hour is ideal for a drip feed concentration which requires only a low pressure head to maintain the required flow rate. This method has been adopted in several Asian countries, including Indonesia.

TABLE 17.4
COMPARISON OF SALT IODINATION METHOD

	Drip	Spray	Dry Mix	Submersion
Type of salt				
Refined powder, dry	++	+++	+++	NA
Unrefined powder, dry	++	+++	+++	NA
Unrefined powder, moist	++	+++	+++	NA
Unrefined crystal, dry	++	++	+	+
Unrefined crystal, moist	+	+	+	++
Cost				
Capital	Medium	High	High	Low
Operating	Medium	High	High	High
Cost to consumer	Medium	High	High	Medium

Source: Mannar.[13]
+++ = good, ++ = satisfactory, + = poor, NA = not applicable.

In spray mixing, crystallized salt is crushed to a coarse powder and ultimately potassium iodate solution is sprayed onto either a bed of salt on a conveyor or a falling stream of salt in a spray chamber. The concentration of solution and the spray rates are adjusted to yield the required dose of iodate. A batch-type system has been developed in India for small manufacturers who do not have continuous spray mixing plants. The batch system consists of a ribbon blender fitted with an overhead drip or spray arrangement. The continuous and batch systems are being used in India, Bangladesh and Vietnam.

In the submersion process, the salt is spread in a shallow tank either manually or mechanically to a thickness of 25–30 cm. A saturated solution of sodium chloride containing a predetermined quantity of potassium iodate is prepared and then admitted into the tank until the salt is completely submerged. After approximately 10–15 minutes, the solution is drained from the salt crystals and the salt is allowed to dry. This method is being adopted in several areas in India.

A comparison of the methods for salt iodination is given in Table 17.4 and the economics for capital investment and operating costs for a continuous batch iodination plant are shown in Tables 17.5 and 17.6, respectively.

SUMMARY

Nutrifying foods is a relatively simple concept but in practice may be difficult to achieve. The ingredients and nutrients are chemically reactive species subjected to time, temperature and environment which may promote or allow chemical alteration resulting in loss of quality and/or functionality. The engineering design of processes which are economically viable must take this reactivity into account. Con-

TABLE 17.5
INVESTMENT AND OPERATING COST FOR A CONTINUOUS SALT IODINATION PLANT

TYPE: Continuous spray mixing			
CAPACITY: 5 tons/h (20,000 tons/year assuming 2 shifts/day and 250 working days in a year)			
A. Capital Cost			US $
1. Plant consisting of feed hopper, belt conveyor, spray chamber, screw conveyor platforms, SS drums, air compressor, piping and spares for 2 years working			35,000
2. Hand trolleys and weighing machine			2,000
3. Laboratory equipment and chemicals			1,000
4. Transport, clearing and forwarding, installation and commissioning			10,000
Subtotal			48,000
5. Building 1200 sq. m. including fencing, lighting, piping and drainage			360,000
6. Office and workshop equipment			5,000
Total capital investment for setting up a 20,000 TPY salt iodination plant at a new location			$413,000

B. Cost of iodination

Basis: Production of 20,000 tons/year of iodinated salt using spray mixing plant (2 shifts, 250 days/year)

1. Cost of chemical 50 ppm KIO			
1000 kg US $30/kg			30,000
2. Processing cost			
a. Labor supervision			
Manager	1	US $500/month	
Shift chemist	2	US $300/month	
Shift foreman	2	US $300/month	
Operator	8	US $150/month	
Workers	30	US $100/month	
Watch and ward	6	US $150/month	81,600
b. Maintenance, spares and lubricants			
i. 2% on buildings and civic works			3,600
ii. 5% on plant, equipment and lab accessories			2,150
c. Power			
Cost of power for salt crushing and iodination			
10 KWH/h: 40,000 KWH US $0.10			4,000
3. Administration overheads, ⅓ of 2 (a)			27,200
4. Depreciation			
3% on buildings and civil works	10,800		
10% on plant and equipment	4,300		15,100
Total cost of iodination of 20,000 tons			$163,650
Cost of iodination of 1 ton of salt = US $8.18.			

Source: Mannar.[13]

TABLE 17.6
INVESTMENT AND OPERATING COST FOR A BATCH IODINATION PLANT

TYPE: Batch spray mixer
CAPACITY: 1 ton/h (250 kg batch capacity, 4 batches/h): 4000 tons/year assuming 2 shifts/day and 250 days in a year.

A. Capital cost US $

1. Plant comprising of ribbon blender with overhead spray arrangement, SS drum, hand pump, piping and spares — 10,000
2. Hand trolley and weighing machine — 1,500
3. Laboratory equipment and chemicals — 750
4. Transport, clearing and forwarding, installation and commissioning — 2,500

Subtotal — 14,750

5. Building 20m × 12m: 240 sq. m. US $300/sq. m. Brick walls with AC sheet roofing including fencing, lighting, piping and drainage — 72,000
6. Office and workshop equipment — 2,000

Total capital investment for setting up a 4000 tons/year batch iodination plant at a new location. — $88,750

B. Cost of iodination

Basis: Production of 4000 tons/year of iodinated salt using a batch spray mixing plant for two shifts, 250 days/year.

1. Cost of chemical 50 ppm KIO_3
   200 kg US $30/kg — 6,000
2. Processing cost
   a. Labor and supervision

Manager/chemist	1	US $400/month
Foreman	1	US $300/month
Operator	4	US $150/month
Worker	10	US $100/month
Watch and ward	3	US $150/month

   Subtotal — 33,000

   b. Maintenance, spares and lubricants
      i. 1% on building and civil works — 720
      ii. 5% on plant and equipment and laboratory accessories — 710
   c. Power/fuel
      Cost of power for crushing and iodination of salt 5 KWH/h: 20,000 KWH US $0.10 — 2,000
3. Administrative overheads, ⅓ of labor — 750
4. Depreciation
   3% on building and civil works   2,160
   10% on plant and equipment   1,420 — 3,580

Total cost of iodination of 4000 tons of salt — 46,760
Cost of iodination of 1 ton of salt = US $11.69

Source: Mannar.[13]

sequently, selection of mixers, feeders, spray systems, extruders, dryers and packaging systems are paramount in assuring a successful nutrification application.

These selections must be made within economic boundaries dictated by a consumer who is increasingly cost conscious. Furthermore, the cost of the micro- or macronutrient may be sufficiently large so that equipment and operating costs are, of necessity, a relatively small fraction of total cost.

In 1973, Bauernfeind and Brooke[2] published Table 17.1 giving guidelines for nutrifying 41 processed foods. This is an excellent summary of methods of addition and preferable point-of-addition and can serve still today as a practical guide to nutrification.

ACKNOWLEDGMENT

This is contribution No. D10209-9-89 from the Department of Food Science, New Jersey Agricultural Experiment Station, Cook College, Rutgers, The State University of New Jersey.

REFERENCES

1. BORENSTEIN, B. 1975. Vitamin fortification technology. *In* Technology of Fortification of Foods. National Academy of Sciences, Washington, DC.
2. BAUERNFEIND, J. C. and BROOKE, C. L. 1973. Guidelines for nutrifying 41 processed foods. Food Eng. *45*(6), 91–97, 100.
3. PARMAN, G. K. and SALINARD, G. J. 1963. Vitamins as ingredients in food processing. *In* Food Processing Operations, Vol. II, M. A. Joslyn and J. L. Heid (eds.). AVI/Van Nostrand Reinhold, New York.
4. BARRETT, F. and RANUM, P. 1985. Wheat and blended cereal foods. *In* Iron Fortification of Foods, F. M. Clydesdale and K. L. Wiemer (eds.). Academic Press, New York.
5. JOHNSON, L., GORDON, H. T. and BORENSTEIN, B. 1988. Vitamin and mineral fortification of breakfast cereals. Cereal Foods World *33*(3), 278, 281, 283.
6. BAUERNFEIND, J. C. and CORT, W. M. 1974. Nutrification of foods with added vitamin A. Crit. Rev. Food Technol., 337–375.
7. MICKUS, R. R. 1955. Seals enriching additives on white rice. Food Engr. *27*(1), 91–93, 160.
8. FURTER, M. R. and LAUTER, W.M. 1949. Fortifying grain products. U.S. Pat. 2,475,133.
9. BRAMALL, L. D. 1986. A novel process for the fortification of rice. Food Technol. Aust. *38*(7), 281–284.
10. ARIYAMA, H., TATAZAWA, S. and NAGASAWA, S. 1952. Method of thiamine enriched rice. Vitamin *5*, 408.
11. CROWLEY, P. R., FULLER, C. E., NELSON, J. H., SMITH, D. E., SWANSON, J. L. and WELLS, F. B. 1974. A technology for the fortification of tea with vitamin A. Proc. IV Int. Congr. Food Sci. Technol. *5*, 180–189.

12. ANDERSON, R. H. 1985. Breakfast cereals and dry milled corn product. *In* Iron Fortification of Foods, F. M. Clydesdale and K. L. Wiemer (eds.). Academic Press, New York.
13. MANNAR, M. G. V. 1988. Salt Iodinization. Part 2: Iodination Technique. IDD News. *4*(4), 11–16.
14. NELSON, J. H. 1985. Wheat: Its processing and utilization. Am. J. Clinical Nutr. *41*, 1070–1076.

CHAPTER 18

NUTRIENT INFLUENCE ON OPTIMAL HEALTH

GEORGE CHRISTAKIS, M.D., M.P.H.*

> *When health is absent,*
> *Wisdom cannot reveal itself,*
> *Art cannot become manifest,*
> *Strength cannot fight,*
> *Wealth becomes useless,*
> *and intelligence cannot be applied.*
>
> Herophilus, 300 BC

INTRODUCTION

The purpose of this chapter is to provide examples of the remarkable interrelationships existing between micronutrients, health and disease. The previous chapters have clearly indicated that the technological aspects of manipulating food composition have advanced significantly in the past decade. It is apparent that the 1990s will witness further advances, and that much applied research utilizing epidemiological, metabolic ward and clinical trial methodologies will be required to study the effect of the nutrient and nonnutrient components of foods in decreasing the risk of disease and maintaining and improving health.[1]

NUTRITION-HEALTH INTERRELATIONSHIP

Health can be defined as a continuous state of soundness and vigor of body and psyche. A discussion of the influence that nutrients and nonnutrients might have on "optimal" health requires a definition of this optimal condition. It may be defined as that state of physiological well-being that is most effective in maintaining health and preventing disease. It is a state of physiological well-being that supports a relatively disease-free, long, useful and happy life.

---

*The author thanks Dr. Paul Lachance for his editorial review and Tables 18.3 and 18.4.

The next issue is: What are some of the interrelationships between the intake of food components, especially nutrients and health and disease? Figure 18.1 presents a paradigm and conceptualization of an optimal nutrition/optimal health interrelationship which can be derived from optimal eating patterns. The latter are, in turn, conditioned by host and environmental factors such as age, sex, race, ethnic, cultural, genetic, physical activity and other variables. Figure 18.1 depicts how insufficient, as well as excessive, nutrients and other dietary component intakes, such as fiber, carotenoids, cholesterol, etc., can impact on disease pathogenesis based on the current data from ongoing studies of disease-diet relationships. Some nutrients which appear to exert carcinogenic effects such as calories, fat and protein or anticarcinogenic effects such as fiber, some minerals, beta-carotene, and certain vitamins, as well as possible mechanisms of their action, were reviewed[2] in 1989. Disproportionate or "unbalanced" intakes of specific classes of compounds, such as vitamins, minerals and amino acids, comprise the second category of influences on health which have specific vitamin-vitamin and vitamin-mineral and other internutrient interrelationships. Conversely, how disease affects micronutrient intake is a third mechanism of the nutrition-health axis. How nutrient and food factors contribute to the risk of chronic disease is the fourth mechanism. We now recognize that a number of nonnutrient components of food (e.g., phenolics, sterols, naturally occurring toxicants and protective factors) also interplay with nutrients in determining optimal health.

In order to maintain health, the effect of nutrient adequacy, insufficiency or excess on the immune system is key to both combating and preventing disease and

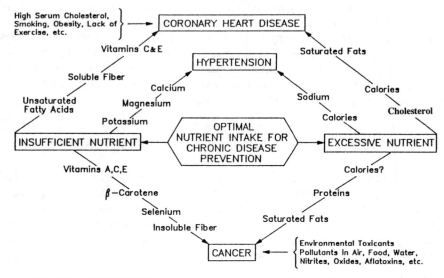

FIG. 18.1. EMERGING DEFINITION OF OPTIMAL NUTRIENT INTAKE CONSIDERING NUTRITIONAL DETERMINANTS OF CHRONIC DISEASE

maintaining health.[3] Scientific papers on the role of minerals and vitamins in insufficient or adequate intakes in relation to immune functions and disease resistance, first presented at a 1989 symposium, were published[4] in 1990. Another significant issue is the effect of nutrient intake on the integrity of mental and psychological functioning.[5–8] The influence of dietary carbohydrate and specific amino acids on neurotransmitter synthesis, cognitive functions and on appetite[9] further exemplifies the critical manner in which nutritional status influences "optimal health."

In 1981, Pao and Mickle reported that from 9–15% of participants in the USDA Nationwide Food Consumption Survey met less than 79% of the Recommended Dietary Allowance for 1 or more of 7 vitamins.[10] Such persons may become patients of physicians who do not consider nutritional status as part of their history and physical examination profiles. Clinicians must also consider contributing factors to both primary and secondary micronutrient deficiencies. These include poverty, ignorance, persons on low-calorie weight reducing diets, fad dieting, abnormal eating patterns, persons who smoke or consume alcohol excessively, those who take medications, such as oral contraceptives and many other categories of illicit, nonprescription and prescription medications. Much more research is surely needed, but this does not preclude clinicians from recognizing and applying the extensive knowledge we now have in nutrition in order to foster optimal health.

Subclinical Nutrient Deficiencies

Subclinical nutrient deficiencies, or the "marginal" vitamin deficiencies cited in Chapter 1, may represent a substantial subgroup of persons who do not have signs or symptoms of deficiency disease, but whose micronutrient plasma or tissue levels may be in the "low" or "deficient" range. Since micronutrients are cofactors or precursors of compounds involved in a myriad of metabolic pathways, it is indeed possible that suboptimal micronutrient intake may induce or be associated with dysfunctional metabolic or immunologic effects. For example, recent studies suggest that while serum vitamin A levels did not reflect depleted liver stores of vitamin A, conjunctival cell evidence of vitamin A deficiency could be assessed even when the clinical examination of the eyes and serum vitamin A levels were normal. Supplementation of these subjects improved their visual abnormalities.[11] Further examples of clinical, and thus preventive medicine, roles for micronutrients are discussed in this chapter.

Secondary Nutrient Deficiencies

Secondary nutrient deficiencies may be defined as resulting from a specific disease which interferes with the ingestion, digestion, absorption, storage, transport, utilization, metabolism and excretion of micronutrients. Many categories of diseases cause secondary nutrient deficiencies through a wide array of mechanisms. Central nervous system disorders can affect appetite, smell, taste, and swallowing. Tumors in the mouth, esophagus, stomach and colon may affect digestion, or partially or completely block food passage through the gastrointestinal tract.

Individuals with secondary micronutrient deficiencies comprise a largely unrecognized source of patients. In order to appreciate how pathologic changes in the gastrointestinal tract can induce nutrient losses through a "secondary" or disease-based cause, Table 18.1 indicates the specific site or absorption of selected vitamins. Only some of the biochemical mechanisms are cited — either postulated or already elucidated — as examples of metabolic rationales for carefully evaluating the patient for clinical and laboratory evidence of one or more micronutrient deficiencies, and their molecular pathogenetic basis. Table 18.2 illustrates this relationship of nutrition to clinical medicine for selected vitamins. Unraveling the dietary pattern-disease interrelationship will likely be the direction that nutrition will take in the near future,[12] which could open new therapeutic horizons.

Treatment of Disease With Nutrients

The third area in which micronutrients contribute to health is the treatment by vitamins and minerals of nonnutrition-based diseases as illustrated in later sections.

Prevention of Disease With Nutrients

The fourth and most recent and exciting prospect for both clinical medicine and public health is the prevention of chronic disease through manipulation of the nutritional and environmental determinants or "risk factors" of chronic diseases, such as coronary heart disease, hypertension, stroke, diabetes and cancer. This is exemplified in the resemblance in the composition of the dietary patterns recommended for decreasing the risk of atherosclerosis on the one hand and cancers on the other hand. Moreover, if the carbohydrate intake is predominantly complex carbohydrates with approximately a 1:1 ratio of insoluble and soluble fiber sources, and if the sodium, potassium and calcium intake as recommended is adhered to, the eating pattern can also be that of the prevention of hypertension and diabetes as well, especially if obesity is prevented, or if present, treated. Diet as a part of lifestyle changes can reverse coronary heart disease.[13] Thus, health providers, from physicians to public health workers, have the challenge and responsibility of including nutrition education and health counseling as an integral part of services offered to their patients.

CLINICAL AND PREVENTIVE MEDICINE ROLE OF SELECTED MICRONUTRIENTS

An emerging, fascinating, and controversial area which merits consideration for food fortification and/or micronutrient supplementation has been referred to as the

TABLE 18.1
SITES AND MECHANISMS OF ABSORPTION OF VITAMINS
BY THE GASTROINTESTINAL TRACT

Vitamin	Absorption Site	Absorption Mechanism	Comments
B_1	Proximal small intestine	Probably active transport via phosphorylation; possible passive diffusion	(1) Rate-limited at dosage over 10 mg (2) Absorption $<$ by ⅓ in alcoholics due to $<$ receptor sites, not in phosphorylation
B_2	Proximal small intestine	Probable passive diffusion $B_2 \rightarrow$ FMN in intestine	$<$ Absorption with age
B_6	Jejunum + proximal ileum	Passive maximum in 60–90 seconds; can alter membrane permeability and $>$ absorption of amino acids	
Folate	Proximal small intestine	Enzymatic deconjugation of polyglutamates $\rightarrow$ monoglutamates; rate of absorption is inversely proportional to glutamyl side chain	Present as polyglutamates in food
B_{12}	B_{12} + intrinsic factor (IF) in ileum	Needs IF in parietal (acid) gastric cells; methylated in liver; transcorrin (an alpha-globulin) transports it	Pancreatic extract protects IF-B_{12} complex in stomach; gastric protease releases B_{12}
C	Proximal small intestine	Sodium-dependent, gradient coupled carrier in jejunum, absorptive capacity 20–40g/day	
A, Beta-carotene	Duodenum, jejunum	Beta-carotene $\rightarrow$ vitamin A (retinol) $\rightarrow$ retinal (intestinal wall) $\rightarrow$ retinyl ester; beta-carotene dioxygenase, aldehyde reductase requires NADH or NADPH; retinoic acid also found in tissues; pre-albumin transport mechanism	Bile-lipid mixture required pancreatic enzyme release retinyl esters in food; vitamin E deficiency impairs vitamin A absorption; low fat diets impair vitamin A absorption
D	Jejunum, probably also ileum	Hormone-like; transported as hydroxycholecalciferol 1,25(OH)D_3 complexed with a globulin; 1,25(OH)$_2D_3$ in kidney as active form	
E	Intestine	Probably stored in liver; transportd with lipoproteins	Present in food as vitamin E esters
K_1	Small intestine	Probably transported with chylomicrons	GI flora can produce it

Note: $>$ = increase; $<$ = decrease.

TABLE 18.2
PATHOGENETIC BASIS OF SECONDARY VITAMIN DEFICIENCIES

Pathogenetic Basis	Disease/Condition
Vitamin A	
Inadequate lipolysis	pancreatitis, pancreatic insufficiency
Inadequate micelle formation	biliary cirrhosis, bile acid insufficiency
Mucosal cell injury	sprue, chronic diarrhea, acute protein calorie malnutrition
Mucosal cell injury and hypoalbuminemia-reduced vitamin A storage	hepatitis, cirrhosis, hepatocellular carcinoma, liver toxins (ex. CCL_4)
Tubular reabsorption of apo-retinol binding protein	tubular or glomerular renal dysfunction
Decreased transport or utilization of vitamin A	hepatitis, measles, upper respiratory tract infections
Decreased plasma retinol	intestinal flukes, liver flukes, hookworm
Decreased vitamin A absorption	ascariasis, giardiasis, chronic salmonellosis
Decreased vitamin A storage	liver flukes, schistosomiasis
Decreased vitamin A storage or RBP synthesis	alcoholic cirrhosis
Cadmium, copper toxicity	Decreased reabsorption of RBP or vitamin A
Vitamin D	
Decreased vitamin D absorption	tropical sprue, regional enteritis, jejunal diverticulosis, gastric resection, jejunal-ileal bypass, patients receiving TPN
Increased intestinal sensitivity of $1,25(OH)_2D$ results in increased intestinal absorption of Ca^{++}	idiopathic hypercalcinuria
Liver is primary site of $25(OH)D$; synthesis of bile salts required for vitamin D absorption, liver is also site of $25(OH)D$ via transcalciferin, which $\rightarrow$ malabsorption of vitamin D	primary biliary cirrhosis obstructive jaundice $<$ in $25(OH)D \rightarrow$ bone disease
Kidney synthesizes $1,25(OH)_2D$, the Ca^{++} homeostatic hormone	renal failure, uremia, anephric patients; results in: renal osteo-dystrophy, growth retardation, osteitis fibrosa, osteo-malacia, osteoporosis, osteosclerosis
Parathyroid hormone affects synthesis of $1,25(OH)_2D \rightarrow >$ intestinal Ca^{++} transport	primary hyperparathyroidism; $\rightarrow$ osteomalacia
$<$ Serum $1,25(OH)_2D$	Hypoparathyroidism; $\rightarrow <$ serum Ca^{++}

TABLE 18.2 (*Continued*)

Pathogenetic Basis	Disease/Condition
Parathyroid X-linked dominant genetic disorder	vitamin D-resistant rickets
Drugs which affect vitamin D	diphenylhydantoin, phenobarbital, oral contraceptives → < serum A, E & $1,25(OD)_2D$; can cause osteomalacia
Vitamin K	
Newborn has < PT levels	hemorrhagic disease of the newborn
Gut of newborn is sterile; breast milk & formulas low in vitamin K	
< Absorption of vitamin K	protracted antibiotic therapy, long-term TPN, obstructive jaundice, biliary fistula, pancreatic insufficiency, steatorrhea, diarrhea
Vitamin C	
Support collagen synthesis and fiber cross-linking to form new tissue of high tensile strength	postsurgical wound healing, burns, pressure sores, periodontal disease
Support of immune competence > mobility of WBC's, inhibition of autooxidation; > serum immunoglobulin and antibody formation	infections
> Metabolism of vitamin C	smoking
Thiamin	
Decreased absorption	diarrhea, sprue, ulcerative colitis, achlorhydria, biliary disease, alcoholism
< Utilization	hepatitis, cirrhosis, diabetes ?
> Requirement	fever, infections, high carbohydrate diets
Inadequate intake associated with > alcohol intake, which → anorexia, < absorption, utilization of B_1, and transketolase levels; < transketolase and B_1 levels	alcoholism Wernicke and Korsakoff's syndromes
Niacin	
Malabsorption syndromes with intraluminal dysfunction	cystic fibrosis, diverticulosis, gastric-ileal resection, hepatobiliary disease, pancreatic insufficiency, surgical blind loop, Zollinger-Ellison syndrome
Mucosal transport defects	amyloidosis, celiac disease, drugs, gut ischemia, lymphoma, parasites, radiation injury, tropical sprue, Whipple's disease

TABLE 18.2 (*Continued*)

Pathogenetic Basis	Disease/Condition
Lymphatic origin	congestive heart failure constrictive pericarditis intestinal lymphangiectasia
Digestive malfunction	Hartnup disease, tryptophan malabsorption, amino acid imbalances (leucine overload) niacin malabsorption, iron overload
Defective coenzyme/apoenzyme relationships	B_6, B_2 as well as B_1 deficiencies anti-vitamin drug effects: cycloserine, deoxypyridine, hydralazine, INH, penicillamine; protein deficiency: burns, fever, fistulas, hepatic cirrhosis, PCM, protein-losing enteropathy, thyrotoxicosis
Metabolic blocks, shunts	antimetabolites, amino acid imbalances tryptophan conversion: carcinoid syndrome, diabetes, acute intermittent porphyria
> Requirement	carcinomatosis large benign or malignant tumors > metabolic activity: convalescence, prolonged fevers, scurvy, stress
Vitamin B_6	
Tryptophan metabolic dysfunction	oral contraceptives, marijuana B_6 antagonists
Unknown mechanisms	uremia, liver disease, breast cancer celiac disease alcoholism (with or without liver distress) stress
Niacin and riboflavin deficiencies	B_3 and B_2 required for interconversions of B_6; B_6 required for tryptophan → niacin B_6 < → > vitamin C excretion
Folic acid	
> DNA synthesis by hyperactive bone marrow	hemolytic anemias
Malabsorption	tropical, nontropical sprue Crohn's disease (jejunitis) zinc deficiency (folate polyglutamate hydrolysis impairment) thyrotoxicosis, tissue repair
> Excretion	> biosynthesis: cold stress, oral contraceptives, lactation, pregnancy, salicylates, tryptophan overload

TABLE 18.2 (*Continued*)

Pathogenetic Basis	Disease/Condition
	systemic disease: Hodgkin's leukemia, multiple myeloma, polyuropathies, TBC, typhoid, bladder, cancer, renal disease
Malignancies	solid tumors, hematopoietic cancers cancer patients in general
Inborn errors of folate metabolism	defective absorption < folate-dependent enzymes homocystinuria Tesch-Nyhan syndrome (defective purine salvage pathway)
$B_{12} <$, > pteglu required both for B_{12} and folate deficiency patients	B_{12} deficiency, ? iron <, ? scurvy
Vitamin B_{12}	
Inability to secrete intrinsic factor, failure to absorb cobalamins; autosomal dominant trait	pernicious anemia, gastrectomy destruction of gastric mucosa (by strong acids or alkalies)
Competitive utilization of cobalamins by bacterial overgrowth	surgical blind loop, strictures, anastomoses diverticula, tapeworm infestation small bowel diverticula
Small bowel defects (generally, causes unknown)	celiac sprue, tropical sprue Gasbeck-Imerslud syndrome, ileal resection
Inborn errors of cobalamin malabsorption; failure to synthesize one coenzyme	deficiency of trans-cobalamin II methylmalonic aciduria
Impaired absorption	Zollinger-Ellison syndrome drugs: PASA, colchicine neomycin, metformin, phenformin

"protector effect" of certain micronutrients. Following are brief examples of some of the vitamins and minerals which appear to have these attributes and their possible mechanisms of action.

Beta-carotene and Vitamin A

Significant dietary intake of beta-carotene, apparently distinct from its function as a vitamin A precursor, appears to decrease the risk of lung,[14–21] gastric,[22] esophageal[23] and cervical cancer.[24] This effect apparently is not shared by vitamin A itself. However, both beta-carotene and vitamin A may decrease oral cancer,[25] and breast cancer[26,27] risk.

Beta-carotene can "quench" singlet oxygen and block its ability to induce free-radical formation. Free-radical formation can injure and destroy subcellular components such as lysosomes and mitochondria, with resultant cell injury. Free-radicals may also injure DNA molecules and repeated injury is believed to initiate the neoplastic process. Beta-carotene further acts as a potent antioxidant, especially as a lipid antioxidant, and thus reduces the formation of superoxides and peroxides through this mechanism.[28,29]

The potential use of vitamin A to prevent the cancers cited above must also be tempered by findings that excess intakes of vitamin A, but not carotenoids, may be associated with increased risk of cancer of the prostate in elderly men[30] and recurrence of bladder cancer.[31] Nevertheless, the development of prostate cancer has been associated with low serum vitamin A.[32]

Beta-carotene and vitamin A may also be involved in the maintenance of immunocompetence.[4] Retinol stimulates tumor-cell killing properties in the in-vitro model[33] and enhances immune function in animal models.[34,35] In a human trial of the effect of vitamins on immunity, 180 mg/beta-carotene daily increased T_4 helper lymphocytes but not the T_8 suppressor lymphocytes.[36] While it has been recognized that smoking reduces vitamin C serum levels, it also appears to reduce beta-carotene levels as well.[37] There is limited evidence that cataract development may be also related to deficient intake of beta-carotene, as well as riboflavin, vitamin C and E.[38] A rationale for further research with beta-carotene and other antioxidant "protector" compounds lie in their ability to prevent oxidative and free-radical damage resulting from extensive exposure of the eye to oxygen and light.[28]

Vitamin B_6

Clinical states in which vitamin B_6 may be indicated are diabetic neuropathy, premenstrual syndrome, carpal tunnel syndrome, reduced bladder cancer risk and homocystinuria. Vitamin B_6 is required for the synthesis of serotonin and dopamine, and the decreased synthesis of these vital brain neurotransmitters may induce water retention, mood changes, sleep disturbances and increased appetite for carbohydrates.[39] Influence of vitamin B_6 intake relative to health categories such as asthma, cardiovascular disease, carpal tunnel syndrome, diabetic neuropathy, immune function and premenstrual syndrome was reviewed[40] in 1990.

Folic Acid

Folic acid deficiency has been suggested as a cause of neural tube defect (NTD) for over 25 years or more.[41] The work of several different investigators now lends strong support to this hypothesis. Milunsky et al.[42] prospectively examined a group of 23,491 women at approximately the 16th week of gestation for the relation of multivitamins and folic acid intake to NTD. Use of folic acid containing multivitamins during the first six weeks of pregnancy had a statistically protective effect. These results when considered in the light of two other recent studies[43,44] provide evidence for the reduction of NTD occurrence of more than 50% when multivitamins containing folic acid (400 µg) are taken during the first 6 weeks of pregnancy. Only optimal dietaries provide levels of folic acid approaching 400 µg; therefore, women contemplating pregnancy whose long-term dietary histories are suboptimal should be encouraged by physicians to consume foods nutrified with folic acid or consider use of supplements containing folic acid.

Low maternal folate serum levels associated with greater incidence of infant birth defects and the effect of folic acid intake on cardiovascular disease were reviewed[45] in 1990.

Vitamin C

In addition to its many other metabolic functions (such as its key role in iron absorption, histamine metabolism, and immunocompetence), vitamin C is required for the conversion of tyrosine to dopamine and other neurotransmitters, and for the biosynthesis of carnitine.[46] Ascorbic acid also scavenges peroxyl and superoxide radicals and cycloperoxidase-derived hypochlorous acid.[47] Ascorbic acid may conceivably reduce the toxic effects of pesticides and pollutants, which is of particular significance to certain categories of industrial workers.[46,55]

Nitrosamine formation is decreased in the presence of vitamin C, which also reduces the mutagenicity of gastric juice.[48] It has therefore been postulated that the progression of atrophic gastritis to gastric cancer may be reduced by consuming one gram of vitamin C daily. Consumption of about 230 mg of vitamin C or more daily has been also associated with a 40% decrease in the risk of developing colorectal cancer.[49]

The possible role of vitamin C in the prevention of atherosclerosis and myocardial infarction remains mystifying. The enzyme 7-alpha-hydroxylase regulates the conversion of cholesterol to bile acids which are excreted into the stool. Since it is well known that increased fecal sterol excretion is one mechanism of reducing serum cholesterol, the association between serum cholesterol and vitamin C has merited study.[50] Other studies fail to support a consistent hypocholesterolemic effect of vitamin C, although several studies suggest that HDL may be increased.[51]

Ascorbic acid also increases fibrinolytic activity and decreases platelet aggregation and adhesion, both important factors in thrombosis, a direct cause of myocardial infarction, especially in the presence of atherosclerotic arteries. Decreased stroke incidence in the United States had been associated with increased vitamin C-rich fruit and vegetable intake, as well as new generations of antihypertensive agents. Steinberg has recently reported that oxidized LDL-cholesterol in the arterial wall may be important in the metabolic pathogenesis of atherosclerosis.[52] Vitamin C protects human LDL from oxidation induced in vitro by copper choloride.[53]

Human plasma lipid peroxidation induced by exposure to a water-soluble radical initiator or to the oxidants generated by polymorphonuclear leucocytes does not occur when ascorbate is present.[54] Ascorbate is apparently the only plasma oxidant that completely protects plasma lipids against detectable peroxidative damage induced in vitro by aqueous peroxyl radicals.[55] On the basis of the latter research, an increase in the RDA for ascorbate from 60–150 mg has been suggested.

An inverse relationship between hypertension and vitamin C intake was demonstrated in NHANES I subjects.[56] In Finland[57] and in Japan,[58] plasma ascorbic acid levels confirmed this association. One gram of vitamin C daily given to women with hypertension was found to reduce systolic and diastolic levels and to decrease serum cholesterol.[57]

Another disease in which vitamin C may prove useful is cataract formation. Oxidation of proteins in the lens of the eyes, followed by protein polymerization and crystal formation appears to be a basic pathogenetic process.[59] The human lens also contains a relatively high concentration of ascorbic acid and antioxidant enzymes to protect the eye against light and oxygen, and its resultant lipid photoperoxidation. Vitamin C also inhibits lipoxygenase enzymes. Protective compounds in the lens, such as ascorbic acid, decrease with age, which may help explain the natural history of cataracts. Cataractous lenses were found to contain less than half the concentration of vitamin C compared to normal lenses. In an epidemiological trial of 300–600 mg of vitamin C per day, control subjects had a 4-fold higher relative risk of developing a cataract compared to the subjects receiving vitamin C.[59]

Vitamin E

Relatively high serum levels of vitamin E and selenium have been implicated in decreasing the risk of several cancers compared to a relative risk of 1.0 for subjects with low serum levels.[60] When serum levels in vitamin E, C and beta-carotene were studied, subjects in the higher ranges of vitamin E, C and beta-carotene had a risk rate of 0.27, 0.38, and 0.47 respectively, compared to 1.0 for the control subjects.[19,61]

Provocative research has focused on the study of the peripheral vascular effects of alpha-tocopherol in improving lower extremity circulation. Vitamin E appears to improve walking ability and intermittent claudication.[62] Women on oral contraceptives have increased platelet aggregation which returns to normal ranges with 200 mg of vitamin E per day.[63] It is well recognized that vitamin E inhibits the oxidation of arachidonic acid which increases prostaglandin synthesis, resulting in thromboxane formation and increased platelet aggregation. Vitamin E also inhibits the cycloxygenase and lipoxygenase required for prostaglandin synthesis.

Vitamin E intake relative to health benefits in the case of cancer, cardiovascular disease, cataracts, physical activity, immunity and infection, fibrocystic breast disease, hemolytic anemia, neurological disorders and sickle cell anemia was reviewed[64] in 1990.

Minerals

There are remarkable interrelationships existing between micronutrients, and thus their relationship to optimal health. Table 18.3 excerpted from the *Handbook of Vitamins, Minerals and Hormones*,[65] provides a substantial documentation of mineral-mineral and mineral-vitamin interrelationships. The details of the table are not tabulated in other reviews, and such a treatise is much needed. This chapter cannot cite all the references, nor expand on the detailed inferences of the table. The documentation of the interrelationships serves to demonstrate the complexity of the issues, but also the critical importance of food systems in the delivery of a balanced array of nutrients that are vital to realizing optimal nutrition and thus disease prevention.

The influence of copper, iron, selenium and zinc on immune response and disease resistance was reviewed[4] in 1990.

OPTIMAL EATING PATTERNS

From the above discussion, improved health may be gained by: (1) minimizing environmental insults to health such as exposure to pollutants, be it from tobacco smoke or industrial sources, and (2) fostering an optimal intake of nutrients and other protective factors. Decreasing the risk of chronic disease and even reversing the pathology of certain disease conditions requires adopting eating patterns consistent with those promulgated by the USDA/DHHS dietary guidelines[66] and by the NCI to thwart the incidence of cancer.[67] The nutrient delivery[68] of these recommendations (Table 18.4) is substantially greater than that evolved by the RDA Committee of the Food and Nutrition Board of the National Academy of Sciences. Evidently, the philosophy for the evolution of the RDA versus the other two Dietary Guidelines is substantially different. The RDA emanates from a philosophy of assessing the minimal needs to prevent nutritional deficiencies and the addition of a statistical augmentation to arrive at recommended intakes sufficient to cover 97.5% of the population. In contrast, the dietary recommendations of USDA/DHHS/NCI emanate from a philosophy directed to reducing susceptibility to major public health diseases. An ever-increasing number of basic and clinical studies, few of which have been cited in this chapter, emphasizes the need of an "optimal" level of nutrient intake to realize "optimal" health.

CONCLUSION

Truly, it would be a great "step forward for mankind" if our more recent knowledge concerning "optimal nutrition" were applied by clinicians and public

TABLE 18.3
MINERAL-MINERAL RELATIONSHIPS AND VITAMIN-MINERAL RELATIONSHIPS

Calcium
    Relationship of Calcium to Other Minerals
        Mg—absorption antagonist, synergist in bone and metabolism
        Na—antagonist or synergist to Ca, depending on organ and concentration
        K—antagonist or synergist to Ca, depending on organ and concentration
        PO_4—absorption synergist (antagonist in excess Ca), synergist in bone
        F—absorption antagonist
        Fe—utilization stimulated by Ca (hematopoiesis)
    Relationship of Calcium to Vitamins
        Vitamin D—synergist in absorption
        Vitamin A—synergist in absorption
        Vitamin C—synergist in bone growth

Phosphorus
    Relationship of Phosphorus to Other Minerals
        Ca^{2+}—absorption and metabolic synergist to PO_4; antagonist in excess
        Mg^{2+}—synergist to PO_4 in metabolism
        Na^+, K^+—synergists in PO_4 absorption
        Sr^{2+}, Be^{2+}, Ba^{2+}, Al^{3+}—sequester PO_4 in the gut
        Fe^{2+}—segregates PO_4 in the gut
    Relationship of Phosphorus to Vitamins
        Inositol—hexaphosphate ester (phytate) segregates divalent ions in gut
        B-complex—most B-complex vitamins require PO_4 for biological activity
        Vitamin D—increased absorption of PO_4 in gut and in kidney

Potassium
    Relationship of Potassium to Other Minerals
        Na-Synergistic in Na-K pump, antagonistic in intracellular reactions
        Ca—Antagonist in absorption, synergist in effects on smooth muscle
        Mg—Antagonist in absorption, synergist in anesthetic actions
        PO_4—Synergist in pH maintenance (intracellular)
        HCO_3—Synergist in CO_2 transport in RBCs
    Relationship of Potassium to Vitamins
        B_6—Involved in electrolyte balance
        D—Involved in Ca-K antagonisms in absorption (?)

Sodium
    Relationship of Sodium to Other Minerals
        K-Synergist in Na-K pump, antagonist in intracellular reactions
        Ca—Antagonist in absorption, synergist in bone metabolism
        Mg—Antagonist in absorption, synergist in bone metabolism
        PO_4—Synergist in pH maintenance
        HCO_3—Synergist in CO_2 transport (as $NaHCO_3$)
    Relationship of Sodium to Vitamins
        B_6—Involved in electrolyte balance
        D—Possible synergist in bone metabolism with Na

TABLE 18.3 (*Continued*)

Magnesium
  Relationship of Magnesium to Other Minerals
    Ca—Antagonist or synergist to Mg, depending on system
    Na—Antagonist or synergist to Mg, depending on system
    K—Antagonist or synergist to Mg, depending on system
    F—Absorption antagonist
    PO_4—Absorption antagonist
  Relationship of Magnesium to Vitamins
    B_1—Cofactor in glucose metabolism
    D—Absorption synergist
    B_6—Mg acts as binding agent in enzyme reactions
    C—Synergist in collagen synthesis

Zinc
  Relationship of Zinc to Other Minerals
    Cu—Absorption and metabolic antagonist to Zn
    Cd—Absorption and metabolic antagonist to Zn; major toxin
    Fe—Absorption and metabolic antagonist to Zn
    Cr—Absorption antagonist (competitive)
    Ca—Absorption antagonist (competitive)
    Mn—Absorption antagonist (competitive)
    P—Absorption antagonist (competitive)
  Relationship of Zinc to Vitamins
    A—Mobilized from liver by Zn
    D—Affects Zn intestinal absorption in some animals
    E—Synergist with Zn
    B_6—Synergist with Zn
    Niacin—NAD a cofactor with many Zn metalloenzymes

Iron
  Relationship of Iron to Other Minerals
    Co, Zn, Cd, Cu, Ni, Mn—Competitive absorption inhibitors
    Mo—With Fe in xanthine oxidase
    Cu-As ceruloplasmin acts as ferroxidase
    Cu—With Fe in cytochrome oxidase
    Pb—Inhibits heme synthesis
    Zn—Deficiency mimics Fe deficiency anemia
    Se—With Fe in glutathione peroxidase
    Co—As B_{12} synergizes hemoglobin production
  Relationship of Iron to Vitamins
    B_2—Cofactor with iron for succinc and NAD dehydrogenase (FAD)
    B_6—Deficiency increased Fe absorption
    B_{12}, folic acid—Synergize Fe, control pernicious anemia

Copper
  Relationship of Copper to Other Minerals
    Fe, Cd, Hg, Ag, Zn—Competitive absorption inhibitors for Cu

TABLE 18.3 (*Continued*)

    SO_4, Mo—Intestinal sequestrants for Cu
    Fe—Synergistic with Cu in heme synthesis
    Zn, Cd—Present with Cu in metallothionin
  Relationship of Copper to Vitamins
    B_6—Cofactor for various Cu metalloenzymes
    B_2—FAD a cofactor for diamine oxidase (Cu enzyme)
    C—Inhibits absorption of Cu
    C, folic acid, B_{12}—Partially compensate for Cu-deficiency anemia

Iodine
  Relationship of Iodine to Other Minerals
    Mg—Cofactor for T4-activated enzymes
    Br, NO_3, ClO_4—Iodide transport inhibitors
    Co^{2+}—Metabolic antagonist
  Relationship of Iodine to Vitamins
    A—T4 needed for liver synthesis of vitamin A
    C—Synergist in cold survival
    B_{12}—Absorption aided by T4
    Niacin—Synergist in mitochondrial metabolism
    B-complex—Deficiency develops in hyperthyroidism

Fluorine
  Relationship of Fluorine to Other Minerals
    Mg—Metabolic and absorption antagonist; metabolic synergist
    Ca—Metabolic and absorption antagonist
    Fe—Absorption antagonist; metabolic synergist
    Al—Absorption antagonist
    Cl—Absorption and metabolic antagonist
    HCO_3—Replaced by F in bone
    Mo—Synergistic in tooth development
  Relationship of Fluorine to Vitamins
    Vitamin D—Antagonist in Ca absorption (intestinal)

Cobalt
  Relationship of Cobalt to Other Minerals
    I—Co^{2+}-antagonized thyroid absorption of I
    Mo—Synergist with Co^{2+}-antagonized thyroid absorption of I
    Cu—Synergist with Co^{2+} in RBC production (as B_{12})
    Zn—Synergist with Co^{2+} in RBC production (as B_{12})
    Fe—Antagonist in absorption of Co^{2+}; synergist in RBC production (as B_{12})
    Mn—Antagonist in absorption of Co^{2+}
  Relationship of Cobalt to Vitamins (see also vitamin B_{12})
    B_{12}—Co is central atom
    C—Increases Co^{2+} absorption in gut (chicks)
    Folic acid—Cofactor with B_{12} in prevention of anemia

TABLE 18.3 (*Continued*)

Chromium
  Relationship of Chromium to Other Minerals
    Zn, V, Mn, Fe—Absorption inhibitors or competitors
    Mg—Synergist in Cr in enzyme action
    Zn—Synergist with insulin and Cr
  Relationship of Chromium to Vitamins
    Niacin—Part of GTF
    B_6—Synergist with Zn and Cr
    Pantothenic acid—Synergist in stress response

Manganese
  Relationship of Manganese to Other Minerals
    Mg—Can substitute for Mn as cofactor, certain enzymes
    Cr—Improves glucose tolerance (similar to Mn)
    Cu, Zn, Fe—Co-metals in superoxide dismutases
    Fe, Cu, V, Mg—Metabolic antagonists
    Zn—Metabolic synergist
    Ca, PO_4, Fe, Co—Absorption antagonists
  Relationship of Manganese to Vitamins
    K, C—Synergist in blood clotting
    B_1—Synergists in acetylcholine synthesis
    Biotin—Cofactor for pyruvate carboxylase
    Choline—Synergist in lipotropic action

Molybdenum
  Relationship of Molybdenum to Other Minerals
    F^-—Synergist in tooth development
    Fe^{2+}—Cofactor in various heme enzymes
    SO_4, Zn—Nutritional antagonists
  Relationship of Molybdenum to Vitamins
    FAD (B_1)—Cofactor for xanthine and aldehyde oxidase
    NAD (B_3)—Cofactor for xanthine dehydrogenase

Selenium
  Relationship of Selenium to Other Minerals
    Hg, Cu, Ag, Cd, Tl, SO_4—Antagonists to Se (absorption)
    Hg, Tl, Cd, Ag, As—Metabolic antagonists to Se
    As—Causes biliary excretion of Se
    SO_4—Increases urinary output of Se
    Hg—Potentiates toxicity of trimethyl selenomium
    Fe—Found in glutathione peroxidase (Se)
  Relationship of Selenium to Vitamins
    E—Synergist as antioxidant
    C—Synergist as antioxidant
    Niacin—Glutathatione functions require it (NAD)
    CoQ—Se involved in synthesis of CoQ

Source: Excerpted from Kutsky.[65]

TABLE 18.4
RECOMMENDED DIET:
HEALTH FACTORS OF USDA/NCI RECOMMENDED DIETARIES

Dietary Health Factor	USDA[1]	HHS (NCI)[2]	RDA (1989) Adult
Calories	1695	1604	> 1520
Protein (g)	84 ± 8	84 ± 5	50–63
Total fat (g)	59 ± 6	52 ± 6	Not specified
% Calories from fat	31%	30%	30%
Polyunsaturated fat (g)	15 ± 4	12 ± 4	Not specified
% Calories from PUFA	8%	6.7%	Not specified
Saturated fat (g)	19 ± 4	17 ± 4	Not specified
% Calories from saturated fat	10%	9.5%	< 10% of calories
P/S ratio	0.8	0.8	Not specified
Cholesterol (mg)	238 ± 97	188 ± 33	< 300 mg
Total carbohydrate (g)	216 ± 15	212 ± 12	> 200 g
Dietary fiber	28 ±	30 ±	Not specified
Total vitamin A activity	9689	11183	800–1000 RE (μg)
Preformed vitamin A (IU)	919	1018	Not specified
Provitamin A (carotene) (mg)	5.2	6.0	Not specified
% Provitamin A (carotene)	90.5	90.9	Not specified
Vitamin E (total)	27	23	8–10
Vitamin C (mg)	225	217	60
Thiamin (B_1) (mg)	1.7	1.6	1.1–1.5
Riboflavin (B_2) (mg)	1.9	1.8	1.3–1.7
Niacin (B_3) (mg)	24	24	15–19
Vitain B_6 (mg)	1.4	1.3	1.6–2.0
Vitamin B_{12} (mg)	3.2	2.9	2.0
Folic acid (mg)	353	381	180–200
Calcium (mg)	1004	1017	800
Phosphorus (mg)	1371	1420	800
Sodium (mg)	1887	1955	> 500
Potassium (mg)	3464	3480	> 2000
Magnesium (mg)	362	388	280–350
Iron (mg)	14	14	10–15
Zinc (mg)	13	13	12–15

[1] U.S. Dept. of Agriculture.[66]
[2] U.S. Dept. of Health and Human Services, Natl. Cancer Inst., National Inst. of Health.[67]

health practitioners so that these major illnesses could be reduced in the general population. Given the aforementioned relationships among nutrient intake, nutritional status and disease, and vice versa, it is important that medical students, residents in all specialties of medicine, and practicing physicians receive a basic grounding in nutritional principles, therapy and the role of nutrition in preventive medicine. They will then be more prepared to practice 21st century clinical and preventive medicine and help reduce the morbidity and mortality caused by the major clinical and public health problems discussed above.

Reduction of the burgeoning costs of health care can be accomplished through the simple and effective means of nutrition education, nutrient manipulation through dietary and supplemental means, and through food product fortification as discussed in the previous chapters. Fortunately, the data base supporting the relationship between diet and health is extensively documented in two U.S. government publications. These landmark reviews indicate that preventive and clinical nutritional approaches are available to combat the problems of chronic diseases.[1,69]

The Recommended Dietary Allowances have been extremely valuable in defining nutrient intakes required for populations to avoid outright nutritional deficiencies. We now seem to be on the threshold of an expanded definition of micro- and macronutrients which will help to reduce the epidemics of chronic disease, such as coronary heart disease, diabetes, hypertension, and cancer, which are, by far, the major causes of morbidity and mortality in developed countries.

REFERENCES

1. Committee on Diet and Health, Food and Nutrition Board, National Research Council. 1989. Diet and Health: Implications for Reducing Chronic Disease Risk. National Academy Press, Washington, DC.
2. MOON, T. E. and MICOZZI, M. S. 1989. Nutrition and Cancer Prevention. Marcel Dekker, New York.
3. BENDICH, A. et al. 1990. Antioxidant vitamins and their function in immune responses. Adv. Exp. Med. Biol. 262, 35–55.
4. BENDICH, A. 1990. Micronutrients and Immune Functions. Ann. N. Y. Acad. Sci., Vol. 587. N.Y. Acad. Sci., New York.
5. HAAS, R. H. 1988. Thiamin and the brain. Am. Rev. Nutr. 8, 483–515.
6. FINE, E. J. et al. 1990. The neurophysiological profile of vitamin B_{12} deficiency. Muscle Nerve 13(2), 158–164.
7. GRAY, G. E. 1989. Nutrition and dementia. J. Am. Dietet. Assoc. 89(12), 1795–1802.
8. JACOBS, L. G. et al. 1990. Mania and gait disorder due to cobalamin deficiency. J. Am. Geriatr. Soc. 38(4), 473–474.
9. FERNSTROM, J. D. 1990. Aromatic amino acids and monoamine synthesis in the central nervous system: Influence of diet. J. Nutr. Biochem. 1, 508–517.
10. PAO, E. M. and MICKLE, S. T. 1981. Problem nutrients in the United States. Food Technol. 35(9), 58–62, 64, 66–69 and 79.
11. FLORES, H., CAMPOS, F., ARAUJO, C. R. C. and UNDERWOOD, B. A. 1984. Assessment of marginal vitamin A deficiency in Brazilian children using the relative dose response procedure. Am. J. Clin. Nutr. 40, 1281–1289.
12. FELDMAN, E. B. 1989. The future direction of nutrition research: Unraveling the diet-disease connection. J. Nutr. 119(2), 323–324.
13. ORNISH, D. et al. 1983. Effects of stress management training and dietary changes in treating heart disease. JAMA 249(1), 54–59; 1990. Can life style change reverse coronary heart disease? Lancet 336(8708), 129–133.

14. MacLENNAN, R., DaCOSTA, J., DAY, N. E., LAW, C. H., NG, Y. K. and SHANMUGARATNAM, K. 1977. Risk factors for lung cancer in Singapore Chinese, a population with high female incidence rates. Int. J. Cancer 20, 854–860.
15. SAMET, J. M., SKIPPER, B. J., HUMBLE, C. G. and PATHAK, D. R. 1985. Lung cancer risk and vitamin A consumption in New Mexico. Am. Rev. Respir. Dis. 131, 198–202.
16. PAGANINI-HILL, A., CHAO, A., ROSS, R. K. and HENDERSON, B. E. 1987. Vitamin A, beta-carotene, and the risk of cancer; a prospective study. J. Natl. Cancer Inst. 79, 443–448.
17. FONTHAN, E. T. H., PICKLE, L. W., HAENSZEL, W., CORREA, P., LIN, Y. and FALK, R. T. 1988. Dietary vitamins A and C and lung cancer risk in Louisiana. Cancer 62, 2267–2273.
18. NORMURA, A. M., STEMMERMANN, G., HEIBRUN, L. K., SALKELD, R. M. and VUILLEUMIER, J. P. 1985. Serum vitamin levels and the risk of cancer of specific sites in Hawaiian males of Japanese ancestry. Cancer Res. 45, 1–4.
19. MENKES, M. S., COMSTOCK, G. W., VUILLEUMIER, J. P., HELSING, K. J., RIDER, A. A. and BROOKMEYER, R. 1986. Serum beta-carotene, vitamins A and E, selenium, and the risk of lung cancer. N. Engl. J. Med. 315, 1250–1254.
20. GEY, K. F., BRUBACHER, G. B. and STÄHELIN, H. B. 1987. Plasma levels of antioxidant vitamins in relation to ischemic heart disease and cancer. Am. J. Clin. Nutr. 45, 1368–1377.
21. WALD, N. J., THOMPSON, S. G., DENSEM, J. W., BOREHAM, J. and BAILEY, A. 1988. Serum beta-carotene and subsequent risk of cancer: Results from the BUPA study. Br. J. Cancer 57, 428–433.
22. YOU, W. C. et al. 1988. Diet and high risk of stomach cancer in Shandong, China. Cancer Res. 48, 3518–3523.
23. TUYNS, A. J., RIBOLI, E., DOORNBOS, G. and PEQUIGNOT, G. 1987. Diet and esophageal cancer in Calvados (France). Nutr. Cancer 9, 81–92.
24. BROCK, K., BERRY, G., MOCK, P. A., MacLENNAN, R., TRUSWELL, A. S. and BRINTON, L. A. 1988. Nutrients in diet and plasma and risk of in situ cervical cancer. J. Natl. Cancer Inst. 80, 580–585.
25. STICH, H. F., ROSIN, M. P., HORNBY, A. P., MATHEW, B., SANKARANARAYANAN, R. and NAIR, M. K. 1988. Remission of oral leukoplakias and micronuclei in tobacco/betel quid chewers treated with beta-carotene and with beta-carotene plus vitamin A. Int. J. Cancer 42, 195–199.
26. WALD, N. J., BOREHAM, J., HAYWARD, J. L. and BULBROOK, R. D. 1984. Plasma retinol, beta-carotene, and vitamin E levels in relation to the future risk of breast cancer. Br. J. Cancer 49, 321–324.
27. KATSOUYANNI, K. et al. 1988. Risk of breast cancer among Greek women in relation to nutrient intake. Cancer 61, 181–185.
28. KRINSKY, N. I. 1990. Carotenoids in medicine. In Carotenoids: Chemistry and Biology, N. I. Krinsky et al. (eds.). Plenum Press, New York.
29. STÄHELIN, H. B., GEY, F. and BRUBACHER, G. 1989. Preventive potential of antioxidative vitamins and carotenoids on cancer. Int. J. Vit. Nutr. Res. 30 (Suppl), 232–241.
30. KOLONEL, L. N., HANKIN, J. H. and YOSHIZAWA, C. N. 1987. Vitamin A and prostate cancer in elderly men: enhancement of risk. Cancer Res. 47, 2982–2985.

31. MICHALEK, A. M., CUMMINGS, K. M. and PHELAN, J. 1987. Vitamin A and tumor recurrence in bladder cancer. Nutr. Cancer 9, 143-146.
32. REICHMAN, M. E. et al. 1990. Serum vitamin A and subsequent development of prostate cancer in the first National Health and Nutrition Examination Survey Epidemiologic Follow-up Study. Cancer Res. 50, 2311-2315.
33. MORIGUCHI, S., KOHGE, M., KISHINO, Y. and WATSON, R. R. 1988. In vitro effect of retinol and 13-cis retinoic acid on cytotoxicity of human monocytes. Nutr. Res. 8, 255-264.
34. SCHWARTZ, J. and SHKLAR, G. 1988. Regression of experimental oral carcinomas by local injection of beta-carotene and canthaxanthin. Nutr. Cancer 11, 35-40.
35. SCHWARTZ, J., SUDA, D. and LIGHT, G. 1986. Beta-carotene is associated with the regression of hamster buccal pouch carcinoma and the induction of tumor necrosis factor in macrophages. Biochem. Biophys. Res. Comm. 136, 1130-1135.
36. ALEXANDER, M., NEWMARK, H., and MILLER, R. G. 1985. Oral beta-carotene can increase the number of $OKT4^+$ cells in human blood. Immunol. Lett. 9 221-224.
37. STRYKER, W. S., KAPLAN, L. A., STEIN, E. A., STAMPFER, M. J., SOBER, A. and WILLETT, W. C. 1988. The relation of diet, cigarette smoking, and alcohol consumption to plasma beta-carotene and alpha-tocopherol levels. Am. J. Epidemiol. 127, 283-296.
38. BUNCE, E. B., KINOSHITA, J., HORWITZ, J. 1990. Nutritional factors in cataract. Ann. Rev. Nutr. 10, 233-254.
39. MERRILL, JR., A. H. and HENDERSON, J. M. 1987. Diseases associated with defects in vitamin B_6 metabolism or utilization. Ann. Rev. Nutr. 7, 137-156.
40. GABY, S. K. 1990. Vitamin B_6: Health benefits. In Vitamin Intake and Health: A Scientific Review, S. K. Gaby et al. (eds.). Marcel Dekker, New York.
41. SCOTT, J. M., KIRKE, P. N. and WEIR, D. G. 1990. The role of nutrition in neural tube defects. Am. Rev. Nutr. 10, 277-295.
42. MILUNSKY, A. et al. 1989. Multivitamin/folic acid supplementation in early pregnancy reduces the prevalence of neural tube defects. JAMA 262, 2847-2852.
43. MULINASE, J., CORDERO, J. F., ERICKSON, J. D. and BERRY, R. J. 1988. Periconceptual use of multivitamins and the occurrence of neural tube defect. JAMA 260, 3141-3145.
44. SMITHELLS, R. W. et al. 1983. Further experiences of vitamin supplementation for prevention of neural tube defect recurrences. Lancet 1, 1027-1031.
45. GABY, S. K. and BENDICH, A. 1990. Folic acid: Health benefits. In Vitamin Intake and Health: A Scientific Review, S. K. Gaby et al. (eds.). Marcel Dekker, New York.
46. CLEMENTSON, C. A. B. 1989. Vitamin C, Vol. I, II, and III. CRC Press, Boca Raton, Fla.
47 GABY, S.K. and SINGH, V. N. 1990. Vitamin C. In Vitamin Intake and Health: A Scientific Review, S. K. Gaby et al. (eds.). Marcel Dekker, New York.
48. TANNENBAUM, S. R. and MERGENS, W. 1980. Reaction of nitrite with vitamins C and E. Ann. N.Y. Acad. Sci. 35, 267-277.
49. KUNE, S., KUNE, G. A. and WATSON, L. F. 1987. Case-control study of dietary etiological factors: The Melbourne colorectal cancer study. Nutr. Cancer 9, 21-42.
50. GINTER, E., CERNA, O., BUDLOVSKY, J., BALAZ HRUBA, R., ROCH, V. and LASKO, E. 1977. Effect of ascorbic acid on plasma cholesterol in humans in a long-term experiment. Int. J. Vit. Nutr. Res. 47, 123-124.

51. JACQUES, P. F., HARTZ, S. C., McGANDY, R. B., JACOBS, R. A. and RUSSELL, R. M. 1987. Ascorbic acid, HDL, and total plasma cholesterol in the elderly. J. Am. Coll. Nutr. *6*, 169–174.
52. STEINBERG, D., PARTHASARATHY, S., CAREW, T. E., KHOO, J. C. and WITZTUM, J. L. 1989. Beyond cholesterol. Modifications of low-density lipoprotein, N. Engl. J. Med. *320*(14), 915–924.
53. ESTERBAUER, H. et al. 1989. The role of vitamin E and carotenoids in preventing oxidation of low-density lipo-proteins. Ann. N.Y. Acad. Sci. *570*, 254–267.
54. FREI, B., STOCKER, R. and AMES, B. N. 1988. Antioxidant defenses and lipid peroxidation in human blood plasma. Proc. Natl. Acad. Sci. (USA) *85*, 9748–9752.
55. FREI, B., ENGLAND, L. and AMES, B. N. 1989. Ascorbate is an outstanding antioxidant in human blood plasma. Proc. Natl. Acad. Sci. (USA) *86*, 6377–6381.
56. McCARRON, D. A., MORRIS, C. D., HENRY, H. J. and STANTON, J. L. 1984. Blood pressure and nutrient intake in the United States. Science *224*, 1392–1398.
57. SALONEN, J. T. et al. 1988. Blood pressure, dietary fats, and antioxidants. Am. J. Clin. Nutr. *48*, 1226–1232.
58. YOSHIOKA, M., MATSUSHITA, T. and CHUMAN, Y. 1984. Inverse association of serum ascorbic acid level and blood pressure or rate of hypertension in male adults aged 30–39 years. Int. J. Vit. Nutr. Res. *54*, 343–347.
59. ROBERTSON, J. M., DONNER, A. P., and TRAVITHICK, J. R. 1988. Supplementary vitamin E: a cataract preventive in man? Presented at the 7th Congress of Intl. Soc. for Eye Res., Nagoya, Japan.
60. SALONEN, J. T., SALONEN, R., LAPPETELAINEN, R., MAENPAA, P. H., ALFTHAN, G. and PUSKA, P. 1985. Risk of cancer in relation to serum concentrations of selenium and vitamins A and E: Matched case-control analysis of prospective data. Br. Med. J. *290*, 417–420.
61. TUYNS, A. J., RIBOLI, E. and DOORNBOS, G. 1985. Nutrition cancer of the esophagus. *In* Diet and Human Carcinogenesis, J. V. Joossens et al. (eds.). Elsevier Science Publishers, New York.
62. HAEGER, K. 1982. Long-term study of alpha-tocopherol in intermittent claudication. Ann. N.Y. Acad. Sci. *393*, 369–375.
63. RENAUD, A., CIAVATTI, M., PERROT, L., BERTHEZENE, T., DARGENT, D. and CONDAMIN, P. 1987. Influence of vitamin E administration on platelet functions in hormonal contraceptive users. Contraception *36*, 347–358.
64. GABY, S. K. and MACHLIN, L. J. 1990. Vitamin E. *In* Vitamin Intake and Health: A Scientific Review. S. K. Gaby et al. (eds.). Marcel Dekker, New York.
65. KUTSKY, ROMAN. 1981. J. Handbook of Vitamins, Minerals and Hormones, 2nd Ed. Van Nostrand Reinhold Co., New York.
66. U.S. Dept. of Agriculture. 1981. Ideas of better eating—Menus and recipes to make use of dietary guidelines. U.S. Government Printing Office, Washington, DC.
67. U.S. Dept. of Health and Human Services, Natl. Cancer Inst., Natl. Inst. of Health. 1984. Diet, nutrition and cancer prevention: A guide to food choices (NIH Publ. No. 85-2711). U.S. Government Printing Office, Washington, DC.
68. LACHANCE, PAUL A. 1991. Diet-Health Relationship. Proceedings of the Am. Chem. Soc. Symposium "Food Safety Evaluation." Aug. 27, 1990. ACS, Books, Washington, DC. (In press).
69. The Surgeon General's Report. 1988. U.S. Department of Health and Human Services, Public Health Service, DHHS (PHS) Publ. No. 88-50210.

General Reading References

ABDULLA, M., NAIR, B. M. and CHANDRA, R. K. 1985. Health Effects and Interactions of Essential and Toxic Elements. Nutr. Res. Suppl. *1*. Univ. Hospital, Lund, Sweden.
BENDICH, A. *et al*. 1990. Micronutrients and the Immune Functions. Ann. N.Y. Acad. Sci., Vol. 587. N.Y. Acad. Sci., New York.
BERGER, H. 1988. Vitamins and Minerals in Pregnancy and Lactation. Raven Press, New York.
BLACKBURN, G. L. 1989. Nutritional Medicine: A Case Management Approach. Saunders, Philadelphia.
BODWELL, C. E. and ERDMAN, J. W. 1988. Nutrient Interactions. Marcel Dekker, New York.
BOURNE, G. H. 1988. Sociological and Medical Aspects of Nutrition. World Review of Nutrition and Dietetics Series, Vol. 55. S. Karger, Basel.
BOURNE, G. H. 1990. Aspects of Some Vitamins, Minerals and Enzymes in Health and Disease. World Review of Nutrition and Dietetics Series, Vol. 62. S. Karger, Basel.
BURNS, J., RIVERS, J. M. and MACHLIN, L. J. 1987. Third Conference on Vitamin C. Ann. N.Y. Acad. Sci., Vol. 498. N.Y. Acad. Sci., New York.
CORNATZER, W. E. 1989. Role of Nutrition in Health and Disease. Thomas, Springfield, Ill.
DAKSHINAMURTI, K. 1990. Vitamin B_6. Ann. N.Y. Acad. Sci., Vol. 585. N.Y. Acad. Sci., New York.
DIPLOCK, A. T., MACHLIN, L. J., PACKER, L. and PRYOR, W. A. 1989. Vitamin E: Biochemistry and Health. Ann. N.Y. Acad. Sci., Vol. 570. N.Y. Acad. Sci., New York.
FINBERG, L. and LAUER, R. M. 1988. Prevention of Adult Atherosclerosis During Childhood. Ross Laboratories, Columbus, OH 43216.
GABY, S. K., BENDICH, A., SINGH, V. N. and MACHLIN, L. J. 1990. Vitamin Intake and Health: A Scientific Review. Marcel Dekker, New York.
HAYAISHI, D. and MINO, M. 1987. Clinical and Nutrition Aspects of Vitamin E. Elsevier, New York.
HENRYK, D., ERDMAN, J., KRINSKY, N. I., BENDICH, A. and LACHANCE, P. 1988. Symposium on carotenes in food and in health. Clin. Nutr. *7*(3), 97–125.
KRINSKY, N. I. *et al*. 1989. Carotenoids: Chemistry and Biology. Plenum Press, New York.
LEKLEM, J. E. and REYNOLDS, R. D. 1988. Clinical and Physiological Applications of Vitamin B_6. John Wiley & Sons, New York.
MACHLIN, L. J. 1991. Handbook on Vitamins, 2nd Ed. Marcel Dekker, New York.
McLAREN, D. S. and McQUID, M. M. 1988. Nutrition and Its Disorders, 4th Ed. Churchill Livingston, London.
MOON, T. E. and MICOZZI, M. S. 1989. Nutrition and Cancer Prevention: Investigating the Role of Micronutrients. Marcel Dekker, New York.
National Research Council, Food and Nutrition Board. 1989. Diet and Health: Implications for Reducing Chronic Disease Risk. National Academy Press, Washington, DC.
NORMAN, A. W., SCHAEFER, H. G. and v. HERRATH, D. 1988. Vitamin D: Cellular and Clinical Endocrinology. DeGruyter, Berlin.
ORNISH, D. 1990. Reversing Heart Disease. Random House, New York.
ROE, D. A. 1989. Diet and Drug Interactions. Van Nostrand Reinhold, New York.
SHILS, M. and YOUNG, V. 1988. Modern Nutrition in Health and Disease, 7th Ed. Lea & Febiger, Philadelphia.
SIDRANSKY, H. 1985. Nutritional Pathology: The Role of Nutrition in the Disease Process. Marcel Dekker, New York.

SOMOGYI, J. C. and HEJDA, S. 1989. Nutrition in the Prevention of Disease. Bibl. Nutr. Dieta, Vol. 44. S. Karger, Basel.

TVER, D. F. 1989. Nutrition and Health Encyclopedia. Van Nostrand, Reinhold, New York.

WALTER, P., BRUBACHER, G. and STÄHELIN, H. B. 1989. Elevated Dosages of Vitamins. Hogrefe & Huber, Lewiston, N.Y.

WHO Expert Committee. 1990. Prevention in Childhood and Youth of Adult Cardiovascular Diseases: Time for Action. Tech. Rep. Ser. 792. World Health Organization, Geneva.

WHO Study Group. 1990. Diet, Nutrition and the Prevention of Chronic Disease. Tech. Rep. Ser. 797. World Health Organization, Geneva.

WINICK, M. 1987. Nutrition in Health and Disease, 2nd Ed. John Wiley & Sons, N.Y.

CHAPTER 19

CONSUMER NUTRIENT LABELING ISSUES

JESSE F. GREGORY, III, Ph.D.

INTRODUCTION

Nutrition labeling regulations and practices are in a major state of flux. Current labeling policies in the United States, which have changed little since their time of implementation in 1973, have been the target of considerable criticism and intense scrutiny, especially over the past two years. Nutrition labeling in this country is mainly voluntary, although labeling becomes mandatory when a food is fortified or a nutrition claim is made (see Chapter 20 for further discussion). Currently, only about 60% of packaged foods presently display nutrition labeling.

Considerable criticism has been directed toward the current system of nutrition labeling mainly on the basis of the following issues: (1) as stated above, nutrition labeling of packaged foods is incomplete; (2) there is also little or no nutrition information provided for fresh foods, (i.e., meats, poultry, seafoods, fruits and vegetables); (3) current nutrition labeling is incomplete concerning certain food components of potential health significance (e.g., dietary fiber, saturated fat, calories from fat, and cholesterol); (4) current emphasis in labeling is on required micronutrients; and, (5) many aspects of current labeling practice (e.g., non-standardized serving size and potentially ambiguous ingredient listings) contribute to confusion of consumers.

In the fall of 1989, the FDA and USDA commissioned a one-year study by the National Academy of Sciences/Institute of Medicine to make recommendations concerning improvement of the coverage, content, format, and regulatory aspects of nutrition labeling. Prior to the release of the study, in July of 1990 the FDA published proposed new nutrition labeling regulations for foods under their jurisdiction (i.e., all foods except meat and poultry products). During September of 1990, the NAS/IOM report was released to the sponsoring agencies as originally contracted, which was within the period of public comment for the proposed regulations. The NAS/IOM report was far reaching and contained the following major recommendations: (1) nutrition labeling should be required for nearly all packaged foods, under both FDA and USDA jurisdiction; (2) nutrition information concerning fresh foods, including meats, poultry, seafoods, fruits and vegetables, should be provided to consumers; (3) the content of nutrition labels should be modified to provide more complete listing of food components of public health concern in the context of chronic disease; and (4) nutrition information should be available to consumers for major items purchased in restaurants and other food service establishments.

During the same time period, legislative momentum developed in the U.S. Congress with respect to nutrition labeling. In 1989, 11 bills were introduced which had bearing on nutrition labeling.[1] These proceedings culminated with the passage of the Nutrition Labeling and Education Act of 1990, signed by the President on Nov. 7. This act, which applied only to foods under FDA jurisdiction, included some, but not all, of the recommendations of the NAS/IOM Committee, and it paralleled much of the regulatory proposal published by the FDA in July 1990. Many of the details of implementation were assigned to the FDA to be developed within a two-year period. The major elements of the new law include: (1) mandatory nutrition labeling of most packaged foods; (2) labeling of the top 20 items in each class of fresh foods under FDA jurisdiction (fruits, vegetables, and seafoods); and (3) modification of nutrition label content to emphasize nutrients of concern in chronic disease.

It should be emphasized that nutrition labeling is not a practice unique to the United States. Many other countries have employed at least partial nutrition labeling, often on a voluntary basis, during the 1970s and 1980s. Changes in labeling requirements similar to those of the U.S. legislation are in progress in the European Economic Community.[2] Because many of the changes have not yet been implemented, and the details remain to be finalized, the precise nature and impact of the various programs is unclear (Table 19.1).[3]

The remainder of this chapter will focus on issues of nutrition labeling with emphasis on those of direct bearing on consumers. In view of the coming changes in nutrition labeling, along with the uncertainties of their ultimate specific form, this chapter will deal mainly with (1) consumer expectations and the role of nutrition labeling as a tool in the nutrition education of the consumer, (2) the impact of new nutrition labeling policies on the food industry, especially with respect to consumer perceptions in food development and marketing, and (3) labeling issues with respect to micronutrients.

CONSUMER ISSUES IN NUTRITION LABELING

Nutrition labeling in expanded and modified form is a costly undertaking for the public, both as consumers and taxpayers. In its July 1990 proposal,[4] the FDA estimated that implementation of a new labeling system costs would initially include: $215 million for analytical costs, $77 million in relabeling, and $25 million for point-of-purchase displays, with a total one-time cost of approximately $315 million. The agency also estimated $60 million annual continuing costs for recurring relabeling, analytical, and administrative costs. Even if these figures are not fully accurate, their magnitude indicates the substantial expense of such a program. The cost of the labeling program mandated by the Nutrition Labeling and Education Act of 1990 (H.R. 3562), which will be technically similar to that of the July 1990 FDA proposal, will probably be of similar order.

These costs of improved nutrition labeling must be weighed against its benefits. Among these benefits, improved nutrition labeling should aid consumers in making dietary choices. Expanded nutrition labeling should have the effect of giving consumers greater access to food composition data and, thus, should serve as a vehicle in nutrition education toward the selection of healthy diets. It should also provide more specific information for individuals on medically required diets. Another potential effect is less tangible; that is, greater disclosure of nutrient content may be an added incentive to manufacturers to formulate foods of reduced fat, sodium, etc.

Another aspect of the cost-benefit analysis is the question of how effectively consumers will use improved nutrition labeling. It should be noted that the new legislation mandates educational efforts by the Department of Health and Human Services to educate consumers about "(1) the availability of nutrition information in the label or labeling of food, and (2) the importance of that information in maintaining healthy dietary practices" (H.R. 3562). Shortly prior to passage of this legislation, a coalition designated the Food Label Education Coalition was formed by the National Food Processors Association, government agencies, industry, consumer and health organizations with the mission of developing guidelines on how to formulate messages to explain how to use nutrition labeling. These and similar educational efforts are vital to the success of nutrition labeling in improving dietary habits.

Many consumers are clearly aware and concerned about the influence of diet on health. Consumer interest in nutrition and nutrition information provided through food labeling has been shown to be high, but the level of understanding of nutrition by many consumers has frequently been found to be inadequate. This has been thoroughly reviewed in the NAS/IOM nutrition labeling report, to which the reader is referred for a more detailed discussion and analysis.[5]

Several recent studies have provided insight into the nutrition knowledge of consumers, their interest in and use of nutrition labeling, and its role in food selection. The International Food Information Council and American Dietetic Association jointly sponsored a Gallup survey of 772 randomly selected adult subjects concerning their attitudes, perceptions, and knowledge concerning diet and health.[6] Over 80% of subjects were either "fairly concerned" or "very concerned" about diet affecting future health. The results demonstrated a general knowledge of nutrition principles, as indicated by the following results: (1) 95% believed that balance, variety and moderation are keys to healthy eating, (2) 77% were familiar with basic food groups, and (3) 60% could name at least 3 different food groups. The response of these subjects to questions concerning fat and cholesterol indicated a high awareness of these diet components. For example, 87% believed that changing dietary habits can lower blood cholesterol levels, and 67–74% reported eliminating either fats, saturated fats, or cholesterol from their diet due to health concerns. In spite of this evidence of

TABLE 19.1
COMPARISON OF NUTRITION LABELING PROGRAMS OF THE UNITED STATES FDA, CANADA, EUROPEAN COMMUNITIES, AND CODEX ALIMENTARIUS COMMISSION

	United States (FDA)	Canada	Commission of the European Communities	Codex Alimentarius Commission
Background	NL regs were promulgated in 1973. Purpose was to establish system for identifying nutr qualities of food. Regs changed little in the 70s and 80s. In July 1990, major revisions were proposed to require NL on most foods, revise list of required nutrients, and establish standard serving sizes	Guidelines on NL published in 1988. Purpose was to set out a uniform system of NL to be used in Canada	Council of the EC adopted common position on NL in Feb 1990. Purpose was to benefit consumer and avoid possible technical trade barriers. Final adoption as Council directive subject to review by European Parliament	Codex guidelines on NL promulgated in 1985. Purpose was to ensure that NL is effective, is not false or misleading, and that no nutr claims are made without NL
Scope	PRA to require NL on most foods, applies to foods regulated by FDA, thus excludes meat/poultry products and alcoholic beverages. PRA applies only to foods that are meaningful sources of nutrients and exempts or makes subject to special labeling requirements certain other foods (e.g., foods provided by restaurants/restaurant-type services; foods provided by grocery store, self-service or deli/bakery counters; foods sold by small businesses; infant formulas; foods for special dietary use)	Guidelines do not apply to formulated liquid diets and infant formulas, which have specific regulatory requirements *Authority*: CG, CR	PD concerns NL of foodstuffs to be delivered to the consumer. Also applies to foodstuffs for restaurants, hospitals, canteens and similar mass caterers, and to foodstuffs intended for particular nutr uses. PD does not apply to diet integrators/food supplements and to natural waters or other waters intended for human consumption. *Authority*: ECPD	Guidelines apply to labeling of all prepackaged foods to be offered to the consumer or for catering purposes. Foods for special dietary uses may have additional provisions *Authority*: CODEXG

LABELING

When required	*Authority:* USPRA Mandatory on most foods (exceptions cited above) *Authority:* USPRA	Voluntary except specific nutr info required by regs when claims are made, vit or min are added, or in the case of foods for special dietary use: *Authority:* CG, CR —Addition of vit or min or claim about vit or min content triggers declaration of that nutrient(s) content in the food. EXCEPT: A claim about sodium or potassium content triggers declaration of sodium and potassium content (CR) —A claim about energy or other nutrient(s) content triggers declaration of energy or that nutrient(s) content in the food. EXCEPT: A claim about fatty acid or cholesterol content triggers declaration of total fat, *cis*-polyunsaturates, *cis*-monounsaturates, saturates, and cholesterol (CR)	Voluntary except when a nutr claim is made *Authority:* ECPD —A claim about sugars, saturates, fiber or sodium content triggers declaration of energy, value and the content of pro, carb, sugars, fat, saturates, fiber and sodium. —A claim about energy or other nutrient(s) content triggers declaration of energy or that nutrient(s) content in the food, plus declaration of energy, pro, carb and fat Also declaration of polyunsaturates and/or monounsaturates and/or cholesterol triggers declaration of saturates	Nutrient declaration should be voluntary except when nutr claims are made *Authority:* CODEXG —including but not limited to claims about energy value and the content of pro, fat, carb and vit/min; —not including quantitative or qualitative declaration of nutrient(s) on label if required by national legislation A claim about energy or a nutrient(s) content should trigger declaration of energy or that nutrient(s) content in the food plus declaration of energy, pro, available carb and fat A claim about fatty acids should trigger declaration of saturates and polyunsaturates A claim about carb should trigger declaration of total sugars content
Basis for declaring amounts	Must declare nutr info on per serving basis: May also declare nutr info per 100 g (ml)	Must declare nutr info on per serving basis: May also declare nutr info per 100 g (ml) (cr)	Must declare nutr info on per serving basis: May also declare nutr info per portion if no. portions in package is stated	Should declare nutr info on per 100 g (ml) basis, or per single portion package: May also declare nutr info per serving or per portion if no. portions in package is stated.

TABLE 19.1 (Continued)
Nutrition Labeling Comparisons: Overview

	United States (FDA)	Canada	Commission of the European Communities	Codex Alimentarius Commission
Basis for declaring amounts (cont.)	Must list no. servings/container Must declare amounts as sold May also declare amounts as prepared for consumption Must declare serving size in both US and metric measures May also declare serving size in familiar household measures Serving (portion) size is defined Single serving container is defined Standard serving sizes are established for food product categories	Must declare amounts as sold (CR) Recommend also declaring amounts as prepared for consumption (CG) Must declare serving size in metric units using same unit as net quantity declaration (CR) Recommend also declaring serving size in household measure or common unit (CG) Typical serving sizes are recommended for food product categories (CG)	Must declare amounts as sold May declare amounts as prepared for consumption where appropriate if preparation instructions are given Must declare amounts in metric units	Should declare amounts in metric units

*Abbreviations used: NL, nutrition labelling; USPRA, U.S. proposed regulatory amendment (*Federal Register* (55)139:29487–29517 and 29517–29533, July 19, 1990 proposed rule) (Note: Information may change with publication of final rule); CG, Canadian Guidelines on Nutrition Labelling (Department of Health and Welfare, Canada, 1988); CR, Canadian Regulation (Food and Drug Regulations, with amendments to December 6, 1989); ECPD, European Community Proposed Directive (Common Position Adopted by the Council on February 22, 1990, with a view to the Adoption of a Directive on Nutrition Labelling for Foodstuffs; CODEXG = Codex Guidelines on Nutrition Labelling (Codex Alimentarius Commission/Guideline 2-1985); nutr, nutrition; info, information; vit, vitamins; min, mineral; carb, carbohydrate; pro, protein.

Source: Crane *et al.*[3] © Williams & Wilkins 1990.

nutrition knowledge, misconceptions were clearly apparent. For example, the concept of "good foods" versus "bad foods" was prevalent. This was indicated by findings such as (1) 65% of subjects reported that all foods should contain less than 30% calories from fat, and (2) 33% of subjects reported that high-fat foods cannot be part of a healthy diet when balanced with low-fat foods. Of interest was the observation that 68% of subjects reported that magazines, newspapers, and television were sources of nutrition information, while doctors and dietitians only accounted for 13% and 3%, respectively, and food packages/labeling accounted for only 2% (Table 19.2). The results of this study indicate a need for effective nutrition education to enable consumers to make effective use of the information provided in nutrition labeling.

The Food Marketing Institute (FMI) has sponsored a series of annual studies of consumers' views and shopping patterns (conducted by Opinion Research Corporation), which evaluates current behavior and attitudes of consumers. The results of the 1990 study,[7] indicated that consumer concern about nutrition is high; 96% of subjects indicated that nutrition is a factor in food selection, of nearly equal importance as taste, safety and price (Table 19.3). Approximately 90% of subjects reported that they paid attention to the nutritional content of food either somewhat or a great deal, and 65% of all subjects reported that their diet "could be at least somewhat healthier." Low fat, cholesterol, salt (sodium), calories, and sugar were the food components of greatest concern, followed by attention to vitamin/mineral content (Table 19.4), which may be associated with the emphasis on these nutrients in the news media and popular press. These findings are consistent with the philosophy of recent considerations in nutrition labeling, i.e., focus on macronutrients associated with overconsumption and chronic disease rather than intake of essential micronutrients. Over 80% of all subjects indicated that they read labels either always or sometimes in purchases of packaged foods with respect to expiration date, ingredients, and nutrition. An even higher percentage of subjects reported that they always read ingredient and nutrition label panels when making a first-time purchase (Table 19.5).

The 1990 FMI study also indicated that the consumers were split on their perceived adequacy of information on current nutrition labels. Fifty percent of subjects reported that current labels provided all or most of the information needed for meal planning, dietary and health concerns in purchasing, while 50% were generally negative. The FMI study did not evaluate the ability of subjects to interpret and utilize the nutrition label information, although previous studies have indicated difficulty in this regard.[5,6]

The FMI study provided significant information concerning another important aspect of labeling, that of health claims. Although only 8% of subjects indicated that health claims were "very believable," over half (52%) reported that claims were "somewhat believable," and 39% stated that claims were either "not very" or "not at all believable." Thus, these consumers exhibited a substantial degree of skepticism; however, 73% of subjects reported that health claims influenced food

TABLE 19.2
SOURCES AND USEFULNESS OF NUTRITION INFORMATION FOR CONSUMERS[6]

	Source of Information (%)	Advice "Very Useful" (%)
Magazine/newspaper	46	23
Television	22	23
Doctor	13	55
Books	10	51
Family	4	44
Dietitian	3	61
Food/labels packages	2	—
Friends	2	46
Government	1	26

Source: IFIC.[6]

purchases either "somewhat" or "a great deal." The subjects who doubted health claims did so for a variety of reasons. The influence of health claims on food purchases, as reported in the FMI study,[7] is shown in Table 19.6.

The use of health claims in food labeling is controversial. Valid health benefits may be a legitimate element in food marketing, although the potential for misleading claims is high. One component of the Nutrition Labeling and Education Act of 1990 should increase the accuracy of health claims. This specifies that such claims will be authorized "only if the Secretary determines, based on the totality of publicly available scientific evidence (including evidence from well-designed studies conducted in a manner which is consistent with generally recognized scientific procedures and principles), that there is a significant scientific agreement, among experts qualified by scientific training and experience to evaluate such claims, that the claim is supported by such evidence" (H.R. 3562).

The National Food Processors Association (NFPA) sponsored a study which examined consumer knowledge and opinions concerning food labeling and nutrition

TABLE 19.3
IMPORTANCE OF VARIOUS FACTORS IN FOOD SELECTION[7]

	Percentage of Respondents				
Attribute	Very Important	Somewhat Important	Not too Important	Not at all Important	Not Sure
Taste	88	9	2	*	*
Nutrition	75	21	3	*	*
Product safety	71	20	1	1	1
Price	66	28	1	*	*

Source: Adapted from FMI.[7]
* = Less than 0.5%. May not add to 100% due to rounding.

TABLE 19.4
NATURE OF SHOPPERS' ATTENTION TO NUTRITIONAL CONTENT OF FOOD[7]

Attribute or Component	Percentage of Respondents Indicating Attention[1]
Fat content, low fat	40
Cholesterol levels	39
Salt content, less salt	28
Calories, low calories	21
Sugar content, less sugar	18
Vitamin/mineral content	13
Preservatives	6
Fiber content	6
Food/nutritional value	5
Protein value	5
Making sure we get a balanced diet	4
Chemical additives	4
Freshness, purity, no spoilage	4
Ingredients/contents	4
Less red meat	4
Carbohydrate content	4

Source: FMI.[7]
[1]Responses less than 4% not shown.

(conducted by Opinion Research Corp.)[8] The results of this survey indicated that consumers frequently read both nutrition labeling and ingredient listings, especially on first-time purchases (Table 19.7), in agreement with the FMI findings. Consumers reported that they most often read label information concerning the content of sodium, fat, calories, cholesterol, and sugar, and they also reported having the greatest interest in these constituents. The subjects reported that their attention to nutrition label-

TABLE 19.5
FREQUENCY OF READING FOOD LABELS

Label Component	Always	Sometimes	Rarely	Never	Not Sure
All Purchases					
Expiration Date	72	20	1	*	*
Ingredients	36	48	12	4	*
Nutrition	36	45	14	5	*
First-time purchases only					
Ingredients	53	35	8	5	*
Nutrition	49	38	7	5	1

Source: FMI.[7]
* = Less than 0.5%.

TABLE 19.6
INFLUENCE OF FOOD MANUFACTURERS' HEALTH CLAIMS
ON FOOD PURCHASES

Degree of influence	Percentage of Respondents
A greal deal	25
Somewhat	48
Not very much	17
Not at all	10
Not sure	1

Source: FMI.[7]

ing and ingredient listings was primarily due to general interest and next to avoid a specific component or ingredient.

The NFPA study did not directly examine the nutrition knowledge of consumers, although the subjects were indirectly asked about their understanding of food labeling information. A lack of attention to food labeling was more frequently due to a lack of interest rather than a lack of understanding. In contrast to this observation, many previous studies have indicated a widespread lack of practical knowledge of nutrition among consumers.[5] For example, a recent evaluation by the Consumer Federation of America[9] indicated that consumers' understanding of nutrition was "inadequate." Particularly noteworthy was the observation that only 30% of subjects understood the concept of the RDA. Since the USRDAs, which originated from the RDAs, are the current means of presentation of micronutrient contents in current nutrition labeling, these results indicate the potential for major problems in the understanding of nutrition labeling by many consumers.

Additional evidence concerning inadequate working knowledge of nutrition was provided by a 1988 Health and Diet Survey conducted jointly by the FDA and National Heart Lung and Blood Institute. This study indicated that 55% of the subjects believed that high fat foods cause heart disease, while 25% believed that high-fat foods cause cancer.[10] Only 34% of the subjects knew that cholesterol and fat were not identical. These findings indicate common sources of confusion and misinterpretations, and provide further evidence of the need for better nutrition education.

In view of the many studies of the nutritional awareness of consumers, it is interesting to consider the changes that have occurred since the period shortly after the advent of nutrition labeling. Among the many aspects of the 1973-74 FDA Consumer Nutrition Knowledge Survey,[11] 47% of subjects indicated that they understood everything provided in nutrition labeling, while 51% reported that they did not understand some or all of the label contents. The study also indicated that 75% of subjects believed that all members of their households were getting a balanced diet. On the basis of a series of questions to test knowledge of nutrition and food components, the existence of misconceptions was clear. For example, nearly half of consumers reported that natural vitamins were nutritionally better than added ones chemically

TABLE 19.7
FREQUENCY OF FOOD LABELING READING[8]

Label Component	Always	Sometimes	Rarely/Never
First-time purchases			
General labeling	40	39	20
Ingredients	44	36	20
Nutrition	44	37	19
All subsequent purchases			
General labeling	18	45	45
Ingredients	15	44	40
Nutrition	16	46	37

Source: NFPA.[8]

synthesized. With respect to food labels, 70% of subjects indicated that they paid attention to price, but only 26% paid attention to nutritional value (defined as calories, vitamins, and minerals) and only 17% were attentive to ingredient listings. Slightly better results were obtained in the results of a similar FDA survey two years later.[12] These data and those of the 1990 FMI and NFPA studies indicate that contemporary consumers' awareness of the nutritional quality and food composition has increased markedly in the past 16–17 years. In the 1973–74 FDA survey, nearly half of the subjects reported that the content of vitamins and minerals was "very important" when listed on the nutrition label. This again contrasts with the 1990 FMI data in which only 13% of subjects indicated that they paid most attention to vitamin/mineral content, with fat and cholesterol content much more prominent (40%) in the 1990 survey. In summary, although the 1973–74 results indicated limitations in the nutrition knowledge of consumers, optimism was high concerning the perceived benefits of nutrition labeling. Of the consumers surveyed, 75% reported that they would use nutrition labeling in food choices, and 52% believed that "they would derive quite a bit of benefit from nutrition labels." The current overhaul of the nutrition labeling system is in progress because these anticipated benefits were never fully realized.

CONSUMERS, FORTIFICATION, AND REVISION OF NUTRITION LABELING

The Nutrition Labeling and Education Act of 1990 does not specify a format of revised labeling, and the FDA is conducting consumer evaluations to study the most suitable format. Various graphical or pictorial approaches have been proposed to aid in interpretation of nutrition label information.[8,13] However, the NFPA study indicated a preference of consumers, *among the choices given*, for clearly presented labeling data in numerical form (Fig. 19.1).[8] The NAS/IOM Committee on Nutrition Components of Food Labeling recommended further systematic testing of for-

What Consumers Want On Food Labels

Four hundred consumers were asked to rank various label formats according to helpfulness. The label on this page (Format #5) was found to be "very helpful" by 80 percent of the respondents.

Consumers want more information on fiber, fats and cholesterol to help them link diet and health.

Consumers said they wanted a clear numerical comparison between the amount of a nutrient and its recommended daily allowance.

BREAKFAST CEREAL

Nutrition Information Per Serving

Serving size: 1 oz. (28 g)
Servings per container: 16

	Cereal	Cereal With ½ Cup Vit. A & D Fortified 2% Milk
Calories	100	170
Protein	4 g	8 g
Carbohydrates	21 g	27 g
Complex carbohydrates	14 g	14 g
Simple sugars	5 g	11 g
Fiber	2 g	2 g
Total Fat	2 g	4 g
Saturated	.	2
Unsaturated	2 g	2 g
Cholesterol	0 mg	10 mg
Sodium	160 mg	220 mg
Potassium	100 mg	290 mg

Percentage of U.S. Recommended Daily Allowances (% U.S. RDA)

Protein	6	15
Vitamin A	30	35
Vitamin C	**	2
Thiamine	25	30
Riboflavin	20	30
Niacin	35	35
Calcium	2	15
Iron	35	35

**Contains less than 2% of the U.S. RDA for this ingredient.

Nutritional Profile — Cereal with 2% Milk

	Amount	Recommended Daily Allowance
Calories	170	2000 calories daily average recommended by U.S. RDA
Total fat	4 g	67 g daily maximum as part of a 2000 calorie diet
Saturated fat	2 g	.22 g daily maximum as part of a 2000 calorie diet
Cholesterol	10 mg	300 mg maximum for adults with high blood cholesterol (Heart, Lung, Blood Institute)
Sodium	220 mg	2200 mg as mid-range of safe and acceptable level for adults (National Academy of Sciences)

Ingredients

Whole Oat Flour (with Oat Bran), Whole Wheat Flour, Brown Sugar, Maltodextrin, Malted Barley Extract, Baking Soda, Salt, Vitamin A Palmitate, Niacinamide, Reduced Iron, Zinc Oxide (A Source of Zinc), Calcium Pantothenate, Pyridoxine Hydrochloride, Vitamin D, Thiamine Mononitrate, Riboflavin, Folic Acid, Vitamin B$_{12}$, BHT, BHA.

Courtesy of The National Food Processors Assoc.[8]

FIG. 19.1. PROPOSED LABEL REPORTED BY 80% OF RESPONDENTS IN NFPA STUDY TO BE "VERY HELPFUL" FOR EVALUATING BREAKFAST CEREAL

mats, and did not include sample graphical formats but also did not specifically recommend against them.[5] It should be noted that the NFPA study only involved *format* of labeling, not the *content* of the label.

Label format issues may strongly affect the presentation of vitamin and mineral contents, and may indirectly affect nutrification practices. The FDA has proposed that micronutrients be expressed in food labeling using a new reference system termed the Recommended Dietary Intake (RDI) in lieu of the USRDA system.[4] The USRDAs are based on the 1968 RDA values and represent the highest RDA within the various age ranges. In contrast, the proposed RDI is a population-based weighted average of the RDAs of the various age ranges above age 4 years. Because it is a weighted average, the proposed RDI by definition is lower than the USRDA for each nutrient. If the conversion to the proposed RDI system is implemented under the new labeling law, this will be another aspect requiring attention in consumer education.

Another implication of conversion to the proposed RDI system is the level of nutrification/fortification used in common foods. For example, would ready-to-eat breakfast cereal products currently fortified to 25% of the USRDA for selected nutrients be fortified to 25% of the proposed RDI or would current levels be maintained? If current fortification levels were maintained, labeling expressed as a percentage of the proposed RDI would indicate values greater than the current 25%, which may be a source of confusion for consumers. In contrast, if fortification was performed at 25% of the proposed RDI, then a reduction in the levels of added nutrients in the diet would result.

Another question of format of micronutrient data involves the use of a numeric system (as percentage of USRDA or proposed RDI) or based on a system of semiquantitative descriptors or ranges. The NAS/IOM report recommended adoption of the semiquantitative system in which micronutrient content would be expressed as one of three categories (per serving):

A very good source (over 20% of [standard]) of:
A good source (11–20% of [standard]) of:
Contains (2–10% of [standard]) of:

As a marked deviation from currently used labeling practice for micronutrients, the semiquantitative system has both advantages and disadvantages. The current numeric system (as percentage of USRDA) implies that the nutrient content is known with a high degree of accuracy and precision. While that is usually true in the case of formulated, fortified foods, many foods exhibit a higher degree of natural variability. In addition to natural variability, the uncertainty is compounded by the imprecision inherent in many methods of food analysis. The semiquantitative system would not relieve the manufacturer of the need for suitable analysis, this proposed system would better represent the actual micronutrient content of many foods. This system may have the added benefit to manufacturers of not requiring relabeling when minor changes in composition occur (e.g., due to reformulation). Another argument supporting a semiquantitative system is that it may be more easily interpreted by consumers who have difficulty with quantitative data (i.e., percentages). The selection of the 20% limit was based on the fact that relatively few foods naturally provide substantially more than this amount of a given nutrient in a typical serving. For example, milk is considered a good source of calcium, and it provides 35% of the 1989 RDA for this nutrient per serving. Similarly, chicken breast, a typical muscle-based food, contains 29% of RDA for vitamin B_6 per serving.[5] A major potential disadvantage of a semiquantitative system is that it may be more difficult for a consumer to evaluate his/her total intake of various nutrients in a meal or over a day's time.

Another effect of the semiquantitative approach to micronutrient labeling is that it could affect standard levels of fortification. For example, there would be little incentive for manufacturers to fortify products at levels greater than the minimum needed for the highest category (e.g., 20% of USRDA or proposed RDI per serving). This could have direct impact on the formulation and marketing of products now fortified at higher levels. There are a few foods that naturally have very high levels of a certain nutrient (e.g., orange juice, 100% of RDA for vitamin C per serving; carrots, 300% of RDA for vitamin A per serving). Changes to a semiquantitative method of labeling may affect the marketing of such products naturally rich in certain nutrients.

SUMMARY AND CONCLUSIONS

The expansion and revision of nutrition labeling is expected to have a significant impact on the nutritional awareness and food selection of consumers. While studies have shown that interest and awareness is already reasonably high, misconceptions and misunderstanding of basic principles of nutrition are widespread. Therefore, an effective education program is an essential adjunct to improved nutrition labeling.

Although revisions in nutrition labeling may initially appear to have little direct impact on the practice of food fortification, as discussed here, the format of future labeling may have highly significant effects. The resolution of these issues will be interesting and highly important to stated goals of optimal health through improvement of nutrition.

REFERENCES

1. PORTER, D. V. 1989. Food Labeling. Congressional Res. Serv., The Library of Congress, Washington, DC.
2. EEC (European Economic Community). 1990. Council Directive of 24 September 1990 on Nutrition Labelling for Foodstuffs. Offic. J. Eur. Commun., No. L 276/40–44.
3. CRANE, N. T., BEHLEN, P. M., YETLEY, E. A. and VANDERVEEN, J. E. 1990. Nutrition labeling of foods: A global perspective. Nutr. Today 25, 28–35.

4. FDA (Food and Drug Admin.). 1990. Food labeling; Reference Daily Intakes and Daily Reference Values; Mandatory Status of Nutrition Labeling and Nutrient Content Revision; Serving Sizes; Proposed Rules. *In* Federal Register 55 (139), 29476-29533, July 19.
5. NAS/IOM (Natl. Acad. of Sci., Inst. of Med.). 1990. Nutrition Labeling. Issues and Directions for the 1990s. D. V. Porter and R. O. Earl (eds.). National Academy Press, Washington, DC.
6. IFIC (Int. Food Inform. Counc.). 1990. How are Americans Making Food Choices. Results of a Gallup Survey. Int. Food Inform. Counc., Washington, DC.
7. FMI (Food Marketing Inst.). 1990. Trends. Consumer Attitudes & the Supermarket 1990. Food Marketing Inst., Washington, DC.
8. NFPA (Natl. Food Proc. Assoc.). 1990. Food Labeling and Nutrition: What Americans Want. Natl. Food Proc. Assoc., Washington, DC.
9. Food Chemical News. 1990. CFA Test Finds Consumer Knowledge on Nutrition Lacking. Oct. 1, p. 28. Washington, DC.
10. SLAVIN. J. L. 1990. Communicating nutrition information. Whose job is it? Food Technol. *44*, 70-74.
11. FDA (Food and Drug Admin.). Div. of Consumer Studies. Office of Nutr. and Consumer Sci., Bur. of Foods. U.S. Dept. of Health, Educ., and Welfare. 1976. Consumer Nutrition Knowledge Survey. Rept. I, 1973-74. DHEW Publ. No. (FDA) 76-2058.
12. FDA (Food and Drug Admin.). Div. of Consumer Studies. Office of Nutr. and Consumer Sci., Bur. of Foods. U.S. Dept. of Health, Educ., and Welfare. 1976. Consumer Nutrition Knowledge Survey. Rept. II, 1975. DHEW Publ. No. (FDA) 76-2079.
13. CSPI (Center for Sci. in the Publ. Interest). 1989. Food Labeling Chaos: The Case for Reform. Center for Sci. in the Pub. Interest, Washington, DC.
14. NAS/NRC (Natl. Acad. of Sci., Natl. Res. Counc.). 1989. Recommended Dietary Allowances, 10th Ed. National Academy Press, Washington, DC.

CHAPTER 20

REGULATION OF FOOD FORTIFICATION: UNITED STATES

ANTHONY J. IANNARONE, LL.M.

Regulation of food fortification in the United States involves a number of separate regulatory mechanisms, which taken together form a comprehensible pattern, albeit with some fuzziness along the fringes. While our focus is on the present-day situation, it is perhaps helpful to observe that for the greater part of its existence the Food and Drug Administration (FDA), the most important U.S. federal governmental agency involved in this area, had little by way of specific regulations to govern fortification. (For those interested in some further background see Hutt,[1] Vetter[2] and Frattali.[3]) Basically, control of food fortification was exercised through the more general elements of FDA's statutory authority, together with whatever standards of identity were in force. The one specific statutory provision which strengthened its authority was Section 403(j) of the *Federal Food, Drug, and Cosmetic Act* (*FD& C Act*), [21 USC Sect. 343(j)] which provides as follows:

> Section 403. A food shall be deemed to be misbranded —
>
> (j) If it purports to be or is represented for special dietary uses, unless its label bears such information concerning its vitamin, mineral, or other dietary properties as the Secretary ["Secretary" refers to the Secretary of Health and Human Services; the Commissioner of FDA acts through delegated authority from the Secretary] determines to be, and by regulations prescribes as, necessary in order to fully inform purchasers as to its value for such uses.

Such regulations as were adopted in 1941 pursuant to this authority remained with little substantive change or controversy until Jun. 20, 1962. On that day began a historic battle over the regulation of nutrients in dietary supplements and as additives to food, which in many ways is still continuing.

On Jun. 20, 1962, FDA published in the *Federal Register* (27 Fed. Reg. 5815) a notice of its intention to revise its earlier regulations. These revisions would have provided that a food or dietary supplement represented for special dietary use as a result of its providing a particular nutrient or nutrients, would be restricted to label declarations of only those nutrients recognized by competent authorities as essential and of significant value in human nutrition. A change in the nutritional reference standard from Minimum Daily Requirements (MDR) to Recommended Dietary Allowances (RDA) was also proposed. There were also other elements, which, taken together, set off an unprecedented number of critical comments and communications to the FDA. In the face of this, the proposal was withdrawn, but the FDA's desire to increase its control of dietary supplements and fortified foods was still very much alive.

At about this time FDA also suffered a legal setback. Acting to stem what it considered to be irrational fortification, FDA sought to set an example by instituting suit against New Dextra Brand Fortified Cane Sugar, a product with some 19 added nutrients. FDA contended the labeling was misleading in various respects involving the product's role in the American diet. The federal district court ruled against FDA on all counts, its botton-line conclusion being that, despite FDA's negative view, it had no authority to prohibit the sale of the food in the marketplace, because FDA had no power under the *FD& C* Act to determine what foods should be included in the diet. The lower court decision was affirmed on appeal.[4]

Furthering its intent, FDA published new regulations in the *Federal Register* on Jun. 18, 1966 (31 Fed. Reg. 8521). Those regulations were to take effect on Dec. 14, 1966 (180 days from the publication date) unless stayed. Among the many provisions were the establishment of eight classes of foods that could be fortified with vitamins and minerals, including iodized salt and breakfast cereals, and restrictions as to which nutrients could be added and in what amounts. The 1962 idea of substituting the RDA for the MDR — probably the most progressive element — was retained. It is interesting to note that vitamin B_6, vitamin E, biotin and pantothenic acid, 4 of the 13 essential vitamins for man, would not have been allowed. A new storm of protest erupted, the regulations were stayed one day before they were to become effective, and the process was begun for conducting the so-called vitamin-mineral hearings.

These administrative hearings, once begun, consumed a nearly 2-year period from May 21, 1968 to May 14, 1970, during which time hundreds of witnesses testified, thousands of documents were presented for consideration, and a transcript of more than 30,000 pages was produced.

These hearings and the political clout stemming from the recommendations of the 1969 White House Conference on Food, Nutrition and Health led to a major regulatory publication on "Food Labeling" in 1973 [Fed. Reg. *38* (13), 2123 et seq., Friday, Jan. 19, 1973]. This included final rules or policy statements on "Food Label Information Panel," (original proposal Fed. Reg. *37*, 6493, Mar. 30, 1972) "Labeling of Foods with Information on Cholesterol and Fat and Fatty Acid Composition," (original proposal Fed. Reg. *36*, 11521, Jun. 15, 1971) and "Label Designation of Ingredients for Standardized Foods" (clarifying original publication in Fed. Reg. *37*, 5120, Mar. 10, 1972).

Also included in the 1973 publication (for some of the history leading to the 1973 *Federal Reg.* see publication "Vitamin, Mineral and Diet Supplements."[5]) were proposed rules on "Imitation Foods;" "Proposed Labeling of Flavor, Spices, and Food Containing Added Flavor;" "Exemptions from Food Labeling Requirements;" "Special Dietary Foods;" "Frozen Desserts;" "Nutrition Labeling of Certain Standardized Foods;" "Dietary Supplements of Vitamins and Minerals;" and "Food Labeling."

Many of these were incorporated in one form or another into the current regulations; others did not survive. The history here is detailed, arduous, and generally unnecessary for our purpose. However, for those who may have an interest it may be helpful to list some of the intervening publications spanning this period of regulatory turmoil (Table 20.1) which saw thousands of comments pouring into the FDA, several appeals to the federal courts, and congressional intervention in 1976 through the Rogers-Proxmire bill which amended the *Food Drug and Cosmetic Act* (21 U.S.C. Sect. 343).

Without dwelling further on history, one important concept which emerged from all this is the "U.S. Government Recommended Daily Allowances" (USRDA). These are based on the Recommended Dietary Allowances (RDA) established by a committee report of the National Research Council (NRC), published by the National Academy of Sciences (NAS) in 1968 (7th Ed.).[6] The RDA, however, contain a number of different categories including males and females, different age groups, pregnant women and lactating women.

For regulatory and labeling purposes, the FDA combined the RDA, generally on the basis of the highest level in any particular category, into four categories of USRDA: (1) infants, (2) children under 4 years of age, (3) adults and including children 4 or more years of age, and (4) pregnant and lactating women. Although the 8th edition (1974)[7] and 9th edition (1980)[8] of the National Academy of Sciences publication on the RDA included some changes from the 7th edition (1968), the FDA has not changed the USRDA, which basically remain the same as originally published on January 19, 1973. The 10th edition of the National Academy of Sciences publication originally scheduled for 1985 was delayed because of certain controversial recommendations. It was ultimately published in late 1989 with recommendations for lowered levels of a number of nutrients.[9]

The FDA, of course, retains the power to change the USRDA in line with changes in the RDA, and in 1990 has proposed to do so based on the 10th edition of *Recommended Dietary Allowances.* (See Addendum at the end of this chapter.) Changes in the USRDA would have a substantial impact on food processors in terms of making formulation and labeling changes. This would also be the case with manufacturers of dietary supplements, since the dietary supplement regulations published on October 19, 1976, continue to be widely used as guidelines despite their revocation in 1979. While there are increasing scientific indications that certain nutrients are beneficial at levels higher than the USRDA, there is virtually no evidence that

TABLE 20.1
FEDERAL REGISTER FOOD LABELING PUBLICATIONS

Date		Title
Mar. 14, 1973	Vol. 38, No. 39, p. 6949	Food labeling
Aug. 2, 1973	Vol. 38, No. 148, p. 20701	Food and drug products; definitions, identity, and label statements
Jun. 14, 1974	Vol. 39, No. 116, p. 20877	Food labeling
May 28, 1975	Vol. 40, No. 103, p. 23243	Food for special dietary uses
Jan. 6, 1976	Vol. 41, No. 3, p. 1115	Food labeling; label declaration of ingredients requirements
Oct. 19, 1976	Vol. 41, No. 203, p. 46155	Food for special dietary uses
Jul. 19, 1977	Vol. 42, No. 138, p. 37165	Special dietary foods label statements
Aug. 24, 1979	Vol. 44, No. 106, p. 49665	Foods for special dietary uses; vitamin and mineral products; revocation of regulations

intakes at or about USRDA levels cause any untoward effects, and, in general, the USRDA provide wide margins of safety. In these circumstances, the advantages of consistency in the USRDA stand in opposition to adjustments for compatibility with the RDA, in the absence of compelling scientific reasons.

Before returning more specifically to the main subject of this chapter, one must observe a word of caution. There is reference in what follows to regulatory particulars and requirements as of the time of this writing. Over a course of time there are changes (e.g., see Addendum); therefore, anyone subject to the regulations should always check the most up-to-date sources. This can be done with the latest version of the *Code of Federal Regulations*, in conjunction with the *Federal Register* or more easily through a looseleaf service such as the *Food Drug and Cosmetic Law Reporter* published by Commerce Clearing House, Inc., Chicago, Illinois.

DEFINITION OF FORTIFICATION

There are generally four types of nutrient additions to foods:

(1) Additions to increase the amounts of nutrients already present to higher levels.
(2) Additions to add nutrients which are not already present.
(3) Additions to "restore" to natural levels nutrients lost or reduced at one or more stages during the chain of events leading to the final product.
(4) Additions of "nutrients" for technical rather than nutritional purposes.

When reference is made herein to fortification in a general way, the intent is to encompass the first three types of additions briefly described above. As used more specifically for regulatory purposes, however, "fortification" encompasses the first two types of additions described above and "restoration" is used for the third type. These distinctions are discussed in the preamble to FDA's policy "Nutritional Quality of Foods; Addition of Nutrients" (Guidelines for Addition of Nutrients to Foods) [Fed. Reg. 45 (18), 6314–6315, Jan. 25, 1980]. As originally proposed, however, FDA designated type 1 above as "enrichment" and type 2 as "fortification" [Proposed rule "General Principles Governing the Addition of Nutrients to Foods," Fed. Register 39, (116), 20900, June 14, 1974]. In general, the terms are interchangeable, but enrichment is used in the case of foods such as enriched bread and enriched flour, where "enriched" is part of the name of the foods by virtue of specific regulatory provisions [See for example 21 *Code of Federal Regulations* (CFR) Sect. 137.165].

In the case of restoration, while in common parlance this would include any degree of restoration, such as adding vitamin C to potato flakes, FDA's definition includes only complete restoration as defined in their Guidelines for Addition of Nutrients to Foods. This will be the subject of later discussion.

Regarding the fourth type of nutrient addition described above, namely, for technical nonnutrient purposes, this is of considerable significance for the food industry, but is excluded from the present discussion, because it does not fall within the general description of fortification set forth above. Examples of such uses are beta carotene (provitamin A) and riboflavin, which are both approved color additives (21 CFR Sect. 73.95 and 21 CFR Sect. 73.450), and ascorbic acid (vitamin C) and tocopherols (vitamin E), which are GRAS preservatives (antioxidants) (21 CFR Sect. 182.3013 and 21 CFR Sect. 182.3890).

GUIDELINES FOR ADDITION OF NUTRIENTS TO FOODS

Under general principles of legal interpretation, that which is more specific takes precedence over the more general. In discussing the regulation of food fortification by FDA, however, it is perhaps more logical to begin with the more general and leave the more specific to later discussion. As will be seen, FDA has a number of regulatory vehicles for control of food fortification, but to develop specific regulations for each fortified food would be difficult and time consuming. It would also tend to be inflexible and create significant gaps between advances in food technology and nutritional knowledge, on the one hand, and changes in fortification practices on the other. In an attempt to fill the gaps and exercise some control in the interest of rational fortification, in 1974 FDA proposed to establish general principles governing the addition of nutrients to foods (39 Fed. Reg. 20900, Jun. 14, 1974). A final policy statement, "Nutritional Quality of Foods; Addition of Nutrients" was published in 1980 [45 Fed. Reg. 6314, Jan. 25, 1980].

As stated at the outset of the final publication:

> This statement establishes a . . . policy concerning the nutrient fortification of foods and is expressed as a series of guidelines which manufacturers are urged to follow if they elect to add nutrients to a manufactured or processed food. This final policy statement is to promote the rational addition of nutrients to foods in order to preserve a balance of nutrients in the diet of American consumers. It is not intended to encourage widespread nutrient fortification of foods but rather to provide a consistent set of guidelines to be followed when foods are nutritionally improved by the addition of discrete nutrients (vitamins, minerals, or protein).

Thus, while this fortification policy has been incorporated into the *Code of Federal Regulations* [21 CFR Sect. 104.20], it is still important to note that it is not a regulation as such, but "guidelines." Nevertheless, persons fortifying outside of these guidelines (or other specific regulations controlling fortification), may be subject to close scrutiny under FDA's general powers. As clearly stated at the outset of the 1980 *Federal Register* publication:

> FDA will continue to determine in specific situations whether labeling claims about nutrient additions may be false or misleading in the case of foods fortified in ways not provided for in these guidelines. . . . Before making a claim relating to fortification, a manufacturer should have the types of specific data identified in the guideline to document the appropriateness of the claim [Ibid at p. 6317].

These principles or guidelines provide several bases for addition of nutrients to foods, and FDA has indicated that foods fortified in accordance with these guidelines will be regulated as general purpose foods and not as special dietary foods (45 Fed. Reg. 6315).

1. Correction of Dietary Insufficiency

The first basis for addition of a nutrient(s) to a food is "to correct a dietary insufficiency recognized by the scientific community to exist and known to result in nutritional deficiency disease . . ." [21 CFR Sect. 104.20(b)]. There must be "sufficient information . . . available to identify the nutritional problem and the affected population groups," and the food must be "suitable to act as a vehicle for the added nutrients." The food, of course, must not be covered by a specific regulation, and in this case FDA urges manufacturers contemplating such a course to contact them beforehand. Also, the allowable nutrients are those specified in Table 20.2 in connection with fortification based on calories.

This first concept is theoretically sound, but not too likely to be used more than rarely, if at all. There is little overt deficiency disease in the United States (food fortification based on standards of identity having eliminated most of that which did

TABLE 20.2
REQUIRED NUTRIENTS FOR CALORIC DENSITY FORTIFICATION UNDER 21 CFR SECT. 104.2(d)(3)

Nutrient and Unit of Measurement	USRDA[1]	Amount per 100 Kcal
Protein (optional), gram (g)	65[2]	3.25
	45	2.25
Vitamin A, international unit (IU)	5000	250
Vitamin C, milligram (mg)	60	3
Thiamin, milligram (mg)	1.5	0.075
Riboflavin, milligram (mg)	1.7	0.085
Niacin, milligram (mg)	20	1.0
Calcium, gram (g)	1	0.05
Iron, milligram (mg)	18	0.9
Vitamin D (optional), international unit (IU)	400	20
Vitamin E, international unit (IU)	30	1.5
Vitamin B_6, milligram (mg)	2	0.1
Folic acid, milligram (mg)	0.4	0.02
Vitamin B_{12}, microgram (mcg)	6	0.3
Phosphorus, gram (g)	1	0.05
Iodine (optional), microgram (mcg)	150	7.5
Magnesium, milligram (mg)	400	20
Zinc, milligram (mg)	15	0.75
Copper, milligram (mg)	2	0.1
Biotin, milligram (mg)	0.3	0.015
Pantothenic acid, milligram (mg)	10	0.5
Potassium, gram (g)	([3])	0.125
Manganese, milligram (mg)	([3])	0.2

[1]U.S. Recommended Daily Allowance (USRDA) for adults and children 4 or more years of age.
[2]If the protein efficiency ratio of protein is equal to or better than that of casein, the USRDA is 45 g.
[3]No USRDA has been established for either potassium or manganese, daily dietary intakes of 2.5 g and 4.0 mg, respectively, are based on the 1979 Recommended Dietary Allowances of the Food and Nutrition Board, National Academy of Sciences–National Research Council.

exist some decades ago) and insufficiency short of that continues to be resisted as a concept by nutritional conservatives. Wider use of the latter concept basically depends on 3 elements: (1) generally accepted criteria for nutritional adequacy, (2) continuing survey data showing that those criteria are not being met by significant numbers of people, and (3) recognition that insufficiency, as opposed to overt deficiency, has negative health implications. As to the latter, there is much accumulating evidence that this is so, but the entrenched proponents of educating people to eat balanced diets continue to resist fortification and supplementation as appropriate means to provide at least partial nutritional solutions.

2. Restoration

This concept should be accepted as one which is eminently sound, namely, addition of a nutrient(s) (i.e., one or more of those specified in Table 20.2 in connection with fortification based on calories) "to a food to restore such nutrient(s) to a level representative of the food prior to storage, handling, and processing . . ." [21 CFR Sect. 104.20(c)]. The restoration guideline involves 4 conditions: (1) adequate scientific documentation that the loss or losses are equivalent to at least 2% of the USRDA in a normal serving, or 2% of 2.5 g of potassium and 4 mg of manganese, which have no USRDA; (2) the losses cannot be prevented with good manufacturing practices and normal storage and handling procedures; (3) all specified nutrients lost in a measurable amount of 2% or more (considering all ingredients of the food product that contribute nutrients) must be restored; and (4) the food products must not be subject to fortification by more specific regulations (e.g., a standard of identity).

Significant changes in food distribution and processing practices over the years, along with changes in eating styles and habits, combine to make nutrient restoration a desirable public health measure. The disappearance of local farms, increases in the number of working wives and mothers, use of more preprepared foods, more meals eaten away from home, and increased use of fast foods are some of a number of factors that may be mentioned in this connection. Nevertheless, food processors have not availed themselves of this FDA-endorsed concept, possibly because of the testing requirements, technological problems of dealing with a number of nutrients, and increased costs with no perceived competitive advantage. With regard to the latter, however, a processor using restoration is entitled to include a labeling claim such as "fully restored with vitamins and minerals" or "fully restored with vitamins and minerals to the level of unprocessed _____" (common or usual name of the food to be filled in) [21 CFR Sect. 104.20(h)(1)]. Thus, with increased scientific knowledge and interest in nutrition, the practice of restoration may still emerge as an important fortification modality.

3. Fortification in Proportion to Total Caloric Content

This is another fortification concept which has not been adopted by the food fortification industry. Under this concept a nutrient(s) listed in Table 20.2 "may be added to a food in proportion to the total caloric content of the food, to balance the vitamin, mineral and protein content . . ." [21 CFR Sect. 104.20(d)]. The conditions are that (1) a "normal serving of the food contains at least 40 kilocalories," (2) the food is not subject to more specific regulations controlling nutrient additions, and (3) the final food product contains all of the nutrients listed in Table 20.2 (except for protein, vitamin D and iodine, which are optional) in the amounts listed "per 100 kilocalories based on a 2,000 kilocalorie total intake as a daily standard . . . ." If this type of fortification is practiced, a label claim is allowed stating "vitamins and minerals (and 'protein' when appropriate) added are in proportion to caloric content" [21 CFR Sect. 104.20(h)(2)].

This concept is much more controversial than those discussed above. The main opposing arguments were directed to the daily caloric standard (originally proposed as 2,800 Kcal, 2,000 Kcal being favored by many), the technical difficulties inherent in dealing with so many nutrients (including flavor problems), and arguments in favor of protein content as a standard rather than kilocalories. In any case, while this concept as enunciated in the guidelines may be sound from the standpoint of nutritional science, at least at this point, there are practical reasons why it is unlikely to be put into widespread use.

4. Miscellaneous

The guidelines go on to provide that nutrients may be added to foods as provided by applicable regulations. Such specific regulations will be discussed below, but there are other important provisions of the guidelines which should be mentioned.

In addition to describing nutrient additions FDA considers to be appropriate, the guidelines also include a brief statement relating to FDA's view of the inappropriate:

> The Food and Drug Administration does not encourage indiscriminate addition of nutrients to foods, nor does it consider it appropriate to fortify fresh produce; meat, poultry, or fish products; sugars; or snack foods such as candies and carbonated beverages [21 CFR Sect. 104.20(a)].

One can certainly appreciate this viewpoint, while still asking the question whether it is good nutritional practice to ignore the realities of everyday eating practices. If large numbers of people, for whatever reasons, choose to obtain a significant percentage of their caloric requirements from snack foods, why not allow micronutrient additions within the framework of the concepts outlined above? Again one is faced with the established view of the nutritional conservatives that the answer lies in educating people to eat sound, well-balanced diets, regardless of the overwhelming evidence that for a whole host of reasons people simply do not.

Returning to what is appropriate, the guidelines also provide that a nutrient added to food should (1) be "stable in the food under customary conditions of storage, distribution, and use;" (2) be "physiologically available from the food;" (3) be present at a level where there is assurance that there will not be "excessive intake . . . considering cumulative amounts from other sources in the diet;" and (4) be "suitable for its intended purpose and . . . in compliance with provisions . . . governing . . . safety . . ." [21 CFR Sect. 104.20(g)].

Provisions as to labeling, other than those listed above, include the traditional provision that any claims or statements about nutrient addition should not be false or misleading [21 CFR Sect. 101.4(h)]; that when labeling claims are permitted the terms" 'enriched,' 'fortified,' 'added,' or similar terms may be used interchangeably

... unless an applicable federal regulation requires use of specific words or statements" [21 CFR Sect. 101.4(h)(3)]; and, in the case of foods which replace traditional foods and have nutrients added to avoid inferiority (i.e., ones with common or usual names to be discussed later) [21 CFR Sect. 101.3(e)(2)], no claim of nutrient addition is appropriate, except a listing of the nutrient ingredients as part of the ingredient statement.

As noted a number of times in these guidelines, there are more specific regulations controlling food fortification, which are applicable to the particular foods or types of foods which they cover, and the discussion will now proceed with a review of those regulations.

STANDARDS OF IDENTITY

The authority of the FDA to establish food standards derives from Sect. 401 [21 USC Sect. 341] of the *FD& C Act*. In relevant part, Sect. 401 provides:

> Whenever in the judgment of the Secretary such action will promote honesty and fair dealing in the interest of consumers, he shall promulgate regulations fixing and establishing for any food, under its common or usual name so far as practicable, a reasonable definition and standard of identity, a reasonable standard of quality, and/or reasonable standards of fill of container. . . .

Standards of identity or quality cannot be established, however, for fresh or dried fruits, fresh or dried vegetables, or butter [butter is controlled under a separate act specific to it, 21 U.S.C. Sect. 321(a), which is administered by FDA], except that standards of identity are permissible for avocadoes, cantaloupes, citrus fruits, and melons.

The concept of a standard of identity is really quite simple. A standard of identity sets out a formula for a particular food so that, within relatively narrow limits, all foods sold under that name may be relied upon to meet the requirements of the applicable standard. As a consequence, a standardized food containing only mandatory ingredients may be sold under the established name without the need for a listing of ingredients. This is not the case with optional ingredients; as to these, Sect. 401 provides:

> In prescribing a definition and standard of identity for any food or class of food in which optional ingredients are permitted, the Secretary shall, for the purpose of promoting honest and fair dealing in the interest of consumers, designate the optional ingredients which shall be named on the label.

Further, as to labeling standardized foods and their ingredients, Sect. 403 (g) [21 U.S.C. Sect. 343(g)] of the *FD& C Act* provides:

> A food shall be deemed to be misbranded —

* * * * *

(g) If it purports to be or is represented as a food for which a definition and standard of identity has been prescribed by regulations. . . ., unless (1) it conforms to such definition and standard, and (2) its label bears the name of the food specified in the definition and standard, and, insofar as may be required by such regulations, the common names of optional ingredients (other than spices, flavoring and coloring) present in such food.

Therefore, optional ingredients included in standardized foods may be required to be specifically declared on the label, with the exception of spices, flavors and colors, which for the most part, may be stated generically. In general, FDA favors full ingredient labeling pursuant to the "consumer-right-to-know" idea, although with standardized foods this cannot be required, except for optional ingredients.

For many years, the standard of identity approach was central to FDA's control over foods. While standards are still important, they have diminished somewhat because they are difficult to establish or amend and build in a high degree of inflexibility. FDA has recognized this, and in more recent years has tended to be less specific in terms of optional additives. For example, instead of providing for a specific list of optional sweeteners such as sucrose, dextrose, lactose or fructose, the tendency now is merely to state "safe and suitable carbohydrate sweeteners."

In controlling the composition of a large number of important food products, standards of identity perforce control nutrient additions to those foods as well. Therefore, they are an important part of the regulations controlling food fortification. In allowing the addition of key micronutrients to basic food products, standards of identity played an instrumental part in overcoming overt nutritional deficiency diseases such as pellagra and rickets, which were serious public health problems earlier in this century. Standards of identity are still playing an important role in helping people achieve recommended levels of micronutrients, although changes in eating habits away from such dietary constituents as bread and fat-containing products have perhaps diminished their contribution somewhat.

In any event, with relation to standards of identity and food fortification, no nutrient may be added to a standardized food unless it is specifically allowed by the standard. If addition of a nutrient is mandatory, it must be added to achieve the level specified. If addition is optional, and it is decided to add a nutrient, again it must be at the level provided and, further, it may be required to be shown on the label. Table 20.3 summarizes the mandatory and optional micronutrient additions provided in the standards as of the time this chapter was written.

While the scope of this review is on regulation at the federal level, readers should be advised that there are regulations at the state level which should be reviewed in certain circumstances. Without diverting our attention to issues of federal preemption and individual state rights, as a general rule state regulatory activities in this area are directed to products manufactured and distributed at the intrastate level. For example, many states have adopted standards for flour and bread and others for cornmeal, corn grits, rice, macaroni, noodles, farina and other products. My home state of New Jersey has a number of standards of identity under the jurisdic-

TABLE 20.3
NUTRIENT FORTIFICATION UNDER STANDARDS OF IDENTITY

Food	Regulation	Mandatory
Milk	131.110(b)(1) 131.110(b)(2)	
Acidified Milk	131.111(b)(1) 131.111(b)(2)	
Cultured Milk	131.112(b)(1) 131.112(b)(2)	
Concentrated Milk	131.115(b)	
Lowfat Dry Milk	131.123(b)(1) 131.123(b)(2)	Vitamin A
Nonfat Dry Milk Fortified with Vitamins A & D	131.127(b)(1) 131.127(b)(2)	Vitamin A Vitamin D
Evaporated Milk	131.130(b)(1) 131.130(b)(2)	Vitamin D
Evaporated Skim Milk	131.132(b)(1) 131.132(b)(2)	Vitamin D Vitamin A
Lowfat Milk	131.135(b)(1) 131.135(b)(2)	Vitamin A
Acidified Lowfat Milk	131.136(b)(1) 131.136(b)(2)	
Cultured Lowfat Milk	131.138(b)(1) 131.138(b)(2)	
Skim Milk	131.143(b)(1) 131.143(b)(2)	Vitamin A

Optional	Amount	Labeling
Vitamin A	2,000 I.U./qt	131.110(e)(1)(i)
Vitamin D	400 I.U./qt	131.110(e)(1)(i)
Vitamin A	2,000 I.U./qt	131.111(g)(1)(i)
Vitamin D	400 I.U./qt	131.111(g)(1)(i)
Vitamin A	2,000 I.U./qt	131.112(f)(1)(i)
Vitamin D	400 I.U./qt	131.112(f)(1)(i)
Vitamin D	25 I.U./fl oz	131.115(e)
	2,000 I.U./qt (As Reconstituted)	131.123(e)(2)
Vitamin D	400 I.U./qt (As Reconstituted)	131.123(e)(2)
	2,000 I.U./qt (As Reconstituted)	131.127(e)
	400 I.U./qt (As Reconstituted)	131.127(e)
Vitamin A	25 I.U./fl oz	131.130(e)
	125 I.U./fl oz	131.130(e)
	25 I.U./fl oz	131.132(e)
	125 I.U./fl oz	131.132(e)
Vitamin D	2,000 I.U./qt	131.135(e)(1)(ii)
	400 I.U./qt	131.135(e)(1)(ii)
Vitamin A	2,000 I.U./qt	131.136(g)(1)(iii)
Vitamin D	400 I.U./qt	131.136(g)(1)(iii)
Vitamin A	2,000 I.U./qt	131.138(f)(1)(i)
Vitamin D	400 I.U./qt	131.138(f)(1)(i)
Vitamin D	2,000 I.U./qt	131.143(e)(1)(i)
	400 I.U./qt	131.143(e)(1)(i) 131.143(e)(1)(iii) (As to Protein) (Based on stay order)

TABLE 20.3 (*Continued*)

Food	Regulation	Mandatory
Acidified Skim Milk	131.144(b)(1) 131.144(b)(2)	
Cultured Skim Milk	131.146(b)(1) 131.146(b)(2)	
Dry Whole Milk	131.147(b)(1) 131.147(b)(2)	
Yogurt	131.200(b)(1) 131.200(b)(2)	
Lowfat Yogurt	131.203(b)(1) 131.203(b)(2)	
Nonfat Yogurt	131.206(b)(1) 131.206(b)(2)	
Asiago Cheese (Fresh & Soft) Medium Old	133.102(c)(2) 133.103 133.104	Vitamin A (If Milk Bleached)
Blue Cheese	133.106(b)(3)(v)	Vitamin A (If Milk Bleached)
Caciocavallo Siciliano Cheese	133.111(c)(2)	Vitamin A (If Milk Bleached)
Gorgonzola Cheese	133.141(c)(2)	Vitamin A (If Milk Bleached)
Parmesan and Reggiano Cheese	133.165(c)(2)	Vitamin A (If Milk Bleached)
Provolone Cheese	133.181(b)(3)(v)	Vitamin A (If Milk Bleached)
Provolone and Pasta Filata Cheese	133.181(c)(3)	Vitamin A (If Milk Bleached)

Optional	Amount	Labeling
Vitamin A	2,000 I.U./qt	131.144(g)(1)(i)
Vitamin D	400 I.U./qt	131.144(g)(1)(i)
Vitamin A	2,000 I.U./qt	131.146(f)(1)(i)
Vitamin D	400 I.U./qt	131.146(f)(1)(i)
Vitamin A	2,000 I.U./qt (As Reconstituted)	131.147(e)(1)(ii)
Vitamin D	400 I.U./qt (As Reconstituted)	131.147(e)(1)(ii)
Vitamin A	2,000 I.U./qt	131.200(f)(1)(iii)
Vitamin D	400 I.U./qt	131.200(f)(1)(iii)
Vitamin A	2,000 I.U./qt	131.203(f)(1)(iv)
Vitamin D	400 I.U./qt	131.203(f)(1)(iv)
Vitamin A	2,000 I.U./qt	131.206(f)(1)(iii)
Vitamin D	400 I.U./qt	131.206(f)(1)(iii)
	Compensate for Loss	
	Compensate for Loss	
	Compensate for Loss	
	Compensate for Loss	
	Compensate for Loss	
	Compensate for Loss	
	Compensate for Loss	

TABLE 20.3 (*Continued*)

Food	Regulation	Mandatory
Romano Cheese	133.183(c)(2)	Vitamin A (If Milk Bleached)
Swiss & Emmentaler Cheese	133.195(b)(3)(v)	Vitamin A (If Milk Bleached)
Mellorine	135.130(b)	Vitamin A
Enriched Bread, Rolls and Buns; Enriched Egg Bread, Egg Rolls & Egg Buns; Enriched Milk Bread, Milk Rolls & Milk Buns	136.115(a)(1)	(Thiamin (Riboflavin (Niacin (Iron
Enriched Flour Enriched Bromated Flour (See 137.160) Instantized Flours (See 137.170)	137.165(a)	(Thiamin (Riboflavin (Niacin (Iron
Enriched Self-Rising Flour	137.185(a) 137.185(a) 137.185(a) 137.185(a) 137.185(b)	Thiamin Riboflavin Niacin Iron
Enriched Corn Grits Quick & Quick Cooking Grits (See 137.240) Yellow Grits (See 137.245)	137.235(a)(1) 137.235(a)(1) 137.235(a)(1) 137.235(a)(1) 137.235(a)(2) 137.235(a)(3)	Thiamin Riboflavin Niacin Iron
Enriched Corn Meal, White Corn Meal, Bolted White Corn Meal, Degerminated White Corn Meal Self-Rising White Corn Meal, Yellow Corn Meal, Bolted Yellow Corn Meal and Self-Rising Yellow Corn Meal	137.260(a)(1) 137.235(a)(2) 137.235(a)(3)	(Thiamin (Riboflavin (Niacin (Iron

Optional	Amount	Labeling
	Compensate for Loss	
	Compensate for Loss	
	40 I.U./gm of Fat	
	1.8 mg/lb)	136.115(b)
	1.1 mg/lb)	
	15 mg/lb)	
	12.5 mg/lb)	
Calcium	Up to 600 mg Total	136.115(a)(2)
	2.9 mg/lb)	See 137.160
	1.8 mg/lb)	(Enriched Bromated)
	24 mg/lb)	and 137.170(c)
	20 mg/lb	(Instantized Flours)
Calcium	Up to 960 mg Total	137.165(b)
	2.9 mg/lb	
	1.8 mg/lb	
	24 mg/lb	
	20 mg/lb	
Calcium	Up to 960 mg Total	137.185(b)
	2.0 to 3.0 mg/lb)	
	1.2 to 1.8 mg/lb)	
	16 to 24 mg/lb)	137.135(b)
	13 to 26 mg/lb)	
Vitamin D	250 to 1,000 USP Units/lb)	
Calcium	500 to 750 mg/lb)	
	2.0 to 3.0 mg/lb)	137.260(b)
	1.2 to 1.8 mg/lb)	
	16 to 24 mg/lb)	
	13 to 26 mg/lb)	
Vitamin D	250 to 1,000 USP Units/lb.	
Calcium	500 to 750 mg/lb (Not more than 1,750 mg/lb for enriched self-rising corn meals)	

TABLE 20.3 (*Continued*)

Food	Regulation	Mandatory
Enriched Farina	137.305(a)(1)	Thiamin Riboflavin Niacin Iron
	137.305(a)(2)	
	137.305(a)(3)	
Enriched Rice	137.350(a)(1)	Thiamin Riboflavin Niacin Iron
	137.350(a)(2)	
	137.350(a)(3)	
Enriched Macaroni Products	139.115(a)(1)	Thiamin Riboflavin Niacin or Niacinamide Iron
	139.115(a)(2)	
	139.115(a)(3)	
Enriched Macaroni Products with Fortified Protein	139.117 (a)(1) & (a)(2)(i)	Protein
	139.117(b)(1)	Thiamin Riboflavin Niacin or Niacinamide
	139.117(b)(2)	Iron
Enriched Nonfat Milk Macaroni Products	139.122(a)(3)	Thiamin Riboflavin Niacin or Niacinamide Iron
Enriched Vegetable Macaroni Products	139.135(a)	Thiamin Riboflavin Niacin or Niacinamide Iron

Optional	Amount	Labeling
	2.0 to 2.5 mg/lb	
	1.2 to 1.5 mg/lb	
	16 to 20 mg/lb	
	Not Less Than 13 mg/lb	
Vitamin D	Not Less Than 250 USP Units/lb	
Calcium	Not Less Than 500 mg/lb	
	2.0 to 4.0 mg/lb)	137.350(c) & (d)
	1.2 to 2.4 mg/lb)	(Riboflavin Re-
	16 to 32 mg/lb)	quirement Subject
	13 to 26 mg/lb)	to stay order)
Vitamin D	250 to 1,000 USP Units/lb	
Calcium	500 to 1,000 mg/lb	
	4 to 5 mg/lb	139.115(e)
	1.7 to 2.2 mg/lb	
	27 to 34 mg/lb	
	13 to 16.5 mg/lb	
Vitamin D	250 to 1,000 USP Units/lb	
Calcium	500 to 625 mg/lb	
	20% by Weight	139.117(d) & (e)
	5 mg/lb	
	2.2 mg/lb	
	34 mg/lb	
	16 mg/lb	
Calcium	625 mg/lb	
	4 to 5 mg/lb	139.122(b)
	1.7 to 2.2 mg/lb	
	27 to 34 mg/lb	
	13 to 16.5 mg/lb	
	4 to 5 mg/lb	139.135(b)
	1.7 to 2.2 mg/lb	
	27 to 34 mg/lb	
	13 to 16.5 mg/lb	
Vitamin D	250 to 1,000 USP Units/lb	
Calcium	500 to 625 mg/lb	

TABLE 20.3 (*Continued*)

Food	Regulation	Mandatory
Enriched Noodle Products	139.155(a)(1)	(Thiamin (Riboflavin (Niacin or Niacinamide
	139.155(a)(2)	(Iron
	139.155(a)(3)	
Enriched Vegetable Noodle Products	139.165(a)	Thiamin Riboflavin Niacin or Niacinamide Iron
Canned Applesauce	145.110(a)(2)(viii)(<u>b</u>)	
Cranberry Juice Cocktail & Artificially Sweetened Cranberry Juice Cocktail & Artificially Sweetened Cranberry Juice (See 146.111)	146.110(c)	
Canned Fruit Nectars	146.133(e)(3)	
Pineapple Juice	146.185(a)(1)	
Canned Prune Juice	146.187(a)&(b)(3)	
Canned Mushrooms	155.201(a)(3)(vii)	
Margarine	166.110(a)(3) 166.110(b)(1)	Vitamin A

Optional	Amount	Labeling
Vitamin D Calcium	4 to 5 mg/lb 1.7 to 2.2 mg/lb 27 to 34 mg/lb 13 to 16.5 mg/lb 250 to 1,000 USP Units/lb 500 to 625 mg/lb	139.155(f)
Vitamin D Calcium	4 to 5 mg/lb 1.7 to 2.2 mg/lb 27 to 34 mg/lb 13 to 16.5 mg/lb 250 to 1,000 USP Units/lb 500 to 625 mg/lb	139.165(b)
Ascorbic Acid (Vitamin C)	60 mg/113 g (4 oz)	145.110(a)(4)
Vitamin C	30 to 60 mg/6 fl oz	146.110(e)(i) (Revocation subject to stay order)
Ascorbic Acid	30 to 60 mg/4 fl oz	146.113(g)
Vitamin C	30 to 60 mg/4 fl oz	146.185(a)(3)
Vitamin C	30 to 50 mg/fl oz	146.187(c)(2)(iv)
Ascorbic Acid (Vitamin C)	Up to 132 mg/100 g (37.5 mg/oz) (Drained Weight)	155.201(a)(4)(ii)
Vitamin D	Not less than 15,000 I.U./lb Not less than 1,500 I.U./lb	166.110(d)

tion of the state Department of Health, which are found in Title 8 of the *New Jersey Administrative Code*. A number of these standards either require fortification or permit it on an optional basis. The types of products covered are mellorine [N.J.A.C. 8:21-7.6], dietary or lowfat frozen deserts [N.J.A.C. 8:21-7.15], imitation milk [N.J.A.C. 8:21-8.1] and milk, cultured milk, lowfat milk, and skim milk [N.J.A.C. 8:21-10.1]. For the most part these involve vitamins A and D, although, in the case of the frozen deserts, fortification with GRAS vitamins generally is allowed at levels of 8-20% of the USRDA per 4-ounce serving. The specifics will vary from jurisdiction to jurisdiction, but the key point is that those considering operation within a particular jurisdiction should review the local regulations.

COMMON OR USUAL NAME REGULATIONS

Reference has previously been made to the food misbranding section of the *FD& C Act*. Section 403(c) [21 U.S.C. Sect. 343(c)] provides:

A food shall be deemed to be misbranded —

* * * * *

(c) If it is an imitation of another food, unless its label bears, in type of uniform size and prominence, the word "imitation" and, immediately thereafter, the name of the food imitated.

This provision is very clear, especially where a food product is similar to a standardized food, but deviates in some way from the requirements of the regulation setting the standard. In such case, the noncomplying food would have to be marked clearly as "Imitation," a word that is generally considered pejorative by marketers.

Recognizing that the strict formulas of the standards of identity coupled with the imitation labeling requirement presented a severe deterrent to new products that consumers might well find desirable, FDA adopted common or usual name procedures for nonstandardized foods [21 CFR Sect. 101.3(e)]. Under this concept, a food is deemed to be an "imitation," "if it is a substitute for and resembles another food, but is nutritionally inferior to that food. However, such a food shall not be deemed to be an "imitation," if "(1) it is not nutritionally inferior . . ., and (2) its label bears a common or usual name in compliance with the regulations." [21 CFR Sect. 101.3(e)(3)]. Nutritional inferiority includes "any reduction in the content of an essential nutrient that is present in a measurable amount," other than fat and calories [21 CFR Sect. 101.3(e)(3)(i)]. For this purpose a measurable amount of an essential nutrient is 2% of the USRDA for protein or any vitamin or mineral listed under Sect. 101.9(c)(7)(iv) of the Nutrition Labeling regulations [21 CFR Sect. 101.3(e)(3)(ii)]. Specific regulations may be adopted to cover other types of inferiority [21 CFR Sect. 101.3(e)(3)(iii)], and labels "may be required to bear the percentage(s) of a characterizing ingredient(s) or information concerning the presence or absence of an ingredient(s) or the need to add an ingredient(s) . . ." [21 CFR Sect. 101.3(f)].

A number of common or usual name regulations have been adopted covering a variety of foods. (21 CFR Part 102). While these are subject to the general provisions on nutritional inferiority discussed above, only the one for peanut spreads (21 CFR Sect. 102.23) has specific nutrient requirements. In addition to setting out minimum protein levels, the levels of micronutrients are specified per 100 g of a peanut-spread product in Table 20.4. Interestingly, at the time this regulation was proposed (40 Fed. Reg. 51052, Nov. 3, 1975), FDA specifically requested information on the vitamin E content of peanut butter. Such information was determined and submitted, but FDA, nevertheless, chose to ignore it and not include a vitamin E requirement (42 Fed. Reg. 36452, Jul. 15, 1977).

Peanut spread deviates from the standard of identity for peanut butter (21 CFR Sect. 164.150) in that its peanut content is less than 90% by weight of the finished product.

NUTRITIONAL QUALITY GUIDELINES

As the FDA's food regulations are organized, the Guidelines for Addition of Nutrients to Foods discussed above are included under Part 104, "Nutritional Quality Guidelines for Foods," under the subheading, "Fortification Policy" (21 CFR Sect. 104.20). In addition to the policy or guidelines, which have already been discussed, there are some general provisions applicable to specific nutritional quality guidelines (21 CFR Sect. 104.5).

The purpose of a specific nutritional quality guideline is to prescribe "the minimum level or range of nutrient composition (nutritional quality) appropriate for a given class of food" [21 CFR Sect. 104.5(a)]. If there is compliance, the food label may state: "This product provides nutrients in amounts appropriate for this class of food as determined by the U.S. Government" [21 CFR Sect. 104.5(b)]. A product bearing that label statement must bear the common or usual name of the food and utilize nutrition labeling (to be discussed later), both in compliance with applicable regulations [21 CFR Sect. 104.5(c)(i) and (ii)]. Except for inclusion of added nutrients in the list of ingredients, "no claim or statement may be made on the label or in the labeling representing, suggesting, or implying any nutritional or other differences between a product to which nutrient addition has or has not been made in order to meet the guideline . . ." [21 CFR Sect. 104.5(d)]. The procedures set forth that the nutrition labeling regulations [21 CFR Sect. 101.9(e)] must be used to determine compliance with a specified nutrient level [21 CFR Sect. 104.5(e)]. Lastly, under various conditions, a product deviation from the requirements of a specific nutritional quality guideline may be required, in order not to be deemed misbranded, to carry a negative label statement, i.e., "The addition of _____ to (or "The addition of _____ at the level contained in) this product has been

TABLE 20.4
MICRONUTRIENTS SPECIFIED PER 100G
OF A PEANUT SPREAD

Nutrient	Amount (mg)
Niacin	15.3
Vitamin B_6	0.33
Folic acid	0.08
Iron	2.0
Zinc	2.9
Magnesium	173.0
Copper	0.6

determined by the U.S. Government to be unnecessary and inappropriate and does not increase the dietary value of the food" [21 CFR Sect. 104.5(f)].

After all of that, we find that there is only one specific nutritional quality guideline presently included in the regulations, namely, frozen "heat and serve" dinners (21 CFR Sect. 104.47). In addition to specifying appropriate components of such dinners, including a protein requirement, the regulation provides the minimum nutrient levels set forth in Table 20.5 [21 CFR Sect. 104.47(d)]. If it is necessary to add a nutrient to meet a prescribed level, the addition cannot bring that level to more than 150% of the minimum and the added nutrient must be biologically available in the final product [21 CFR Sect. 104.47(c)]. Use of the components specified in the guideline would also result in the presence of folic acid, magnesium, iodine, calcium, and zinc, but these are not subject to minimum levels [21 CFR Sect. 104.47(d)(1)]. The minimum levels specified for pantothenic acid, vitamin B_6 and vitamin B_{12} are tentative and "until final levels are established, a product containing less than the tentative levels will not be deemed to be misbranded . . ." [21 CFR Sect. 104.47(d)(2)]. Where practical, "iodized salt shall be used or iodine shall be present at a level equivalent to that which would be present if iodized salt were used . . ." [21 CFR Sect. 104.47(d)(3)]. When practical, "components and ingredients shall be selected to obtain the desirable calcium to phosphorus ratio of 1:1" [21 CFR Sect. 104.47(d)(4)].

It is fortunate that there is the one specific nutritional quality guideline to illustrate the style and detail of such a regulation. Why aren't there more? This is difficult to say. There were a number of others proposed in 1974: Breakfast Beverage Products; Fortified Hot Breakfast Cereals; Fortified Ready-to-Eat Breakfast Cereals; Formulated Meal Replacements, Formulated Meal Bases; and Main Dish Products [39 Fed. Reg. 20895, 20896, 20898, 20905, 20906; Jun. 14, 1974]. These proposals were all withdrawn in 1986. (See *Food Chem. News,* Nov. 3, 1986, p. 39; Feb. 9, 1987, p. 13.)

However, the procedures are still in place, and proposals for issuance, revision,

TABLE 20.5
MINIMUM LEVELS FOR FROZEN "HEAT AND SERVE" DINNER

Nutrient	For each 100 Calories (kcal) of the Total Components Specified in Par. (a)	For the Total Components Specified in Par. (a)
Protein, g	4.60	16.0
Vitamin A, IU	150.00	520.0
Thiamin, mg	0.05	0.2
Riboflavin, mg	0.06	0.2
Niacin, mg	0.99	3.4
Pantothenic acid, mg	0.32	1.1
Vitamin B_6, mg	0.15	0.5
Vitamin B_{12}, mcg	0.33	1.1
Iron, mg	0.62	2.2

or revocation of specific nutritional quality guidelines may be made by the "Commissioner of Food and Drugs on his own initiative, on the advice of the National Academy of Sciences or other experts, or on behalf of any interested person who has submitted a petition . . ." [21 CFR Sect. 104.19].

NUTRITION LABELING OF FOOD

With certain specified exceptions, "inclusion of any added vitamin, mineral, or protein in a product or of any nutrition claim or information, other than sodium content, on a label or in advertising for a food . . .," subjects that food to the requirements of nutrition labeling [21 CFR Sect. 101.9(a)]. However, assuming there is no added nutrient and no other nutritional claim is made, nutritional labeling is not required, if a statement, "For Nutrition Information Write To _____," is employed or there is a reply to solicited or unsolicited requests, provided "the reply to the request conforms to the requirements" of the nutrition labeling section [21 CFR Sect. 101.9(a)(1)]. The specifics as to nutrition labeling are set forth in 21 CFR Sect. 101.9 and should be studied carefully by anyone who is or may be subject to these requirements. There are, however, some key features which should be discussed.

As a starting point it may be helpful to review those foods which are either exempt from nutrition labeling or are subject to special labeling requirements.

(1) Infant, baby and junior-type food promoted for infants and children under four years of age "shall include nutrition information on the label and

in labeling in accordance with this section," except where expressly covered by 21 CFR Sect. 105.65 (hypoallergenic foods) [21 CFR Sect. 101.9(h)(1)(i)]. Dual declaration may be made (with equal prominence required) of the USRDA for both infants and children under four years of age for foods represented or intended for use by either [21 CFR Sect. 101.9(h)(1)(ii)]. Provisions are also included for declaring protein in terms of USRDA depending on the protein efficiency ratio (PER) compared to casein. For example, the USRDA for protein for infants is 18 g, if the PER is equal to or greater than casein, and 25 g, if it is between 40–100% of casein [21 CFR Sect. 101.9(h)(1)(iii) and (iv)].

(2) Dietary supplements are exempted from the nutritional labeling requirements, unless they are in food form, such as breakfast cereals which are fortified at levels of 50% or more of the USRDA for micronutrients [21 CFR Sect. 101.9(h)(2). See also 21 CFR Sect. 101.9(a)(2)]. (Labeling of dietary supplements is an issue in and of itself. Suffice it to say that the usual format for the traditional capsule and tablet forms is in accordance with the long-since revoked regulations published by the FDA on Oct. 19, 1976, Fed. Reg. *41* (203), 46170 et seq. These regulations continue to be used as guidelines.)

(3) Foods "represented for use as the sole item of the diet" are special dietary foods (21 CFR Part 105) and are subject to additional labeling requirements [21 CFR Sect. 101.9(h)(3)].

(4) The same applies to those special dietary foods "represented for use solely under medical supervision to meet medical requirements in specific medical conditions" [21 CFR Sect. 101.9(h)(4)].

(5) If iodized salt is added to a food, the food itself is exempt from the nutrition labeling requirements, provided the iodized salt is merely listed as such in the ingredient listing "and neither iodine nor iodized salt is otherwise referred to on the label or in labeling or advertising" [21 CFR Sect. 101.9(h)(5)].

Labeling of salt and iodized salt themselves are covered by specific regulatory provisions [21 CFR Sect. 100.155]. "Iodized salt" or "iodized table salt" is salt (sodium chloride) "for human food use to which iodide has been added in the form of cuprous iodide or potassium iodide. . . ." Immediately following the product name this statement must appear: "This salt supplies iodide, a necessary nutrient." There are also specific type-size and positioning requirements [21 CFR Sect. 100.155(a)]. Iodine, of course, is essential in preventing goiter, and using salt as a vehicle for distributing this substance to eliminate what was once a commonly encountered condition is one of the major success stories in the history of adding nutrients to foods. As a corollary to the required statement on iodized salt, it is also required that, when distributed for human use, salt which does not have added iodide must bear the statement: "This salt does not supply iodide, a necessary nutrient" [21 CFR Sect. 100.155(b)].

On the topic of salt, it should be mentioned that there are specific provisions requiring, in the case of frozen vegetables, that the presence of salt must be declared on the label, even though it may be there indirectly through the use of a brine solution in processing, rather than through direct addition as seasoning (21 CFR Sect. 100.140).

(6) Nutrition labeling is not required where nutrients are added for technological purposes and the same are listed only in the ingredient statement and are not "otherwise referred to on the label or in labeling or in advertising" [21 CFR Sect. 101.9(h)(6)]. As indicated earlier, the subject of addition of nutrients to foods for technological purposes is beyond the scope of this chapter. However, as mentioned earlier, examples are ascorbic acid (vitamin C) (21 CFR Sect. 182.3013) and tocopherols (vitamin E) (21 CFR Sect. 182.3890) as generally recognized as safe (GRAS) preservatives (antioxidants), and beta carotene (21 CFR Sect. 73.95) and riboflavin (21 CFR Sect. 73.450) as color additives. (For further information on technical uses of nutrients in foods, see Reference 10.)

(7) Standardized foods containing added nutrients (such as enriched flour) used as components of other foods may be listed in the ingredient statement by their standardized names without triggering nutrition labeling, provided neither the standardized foods nor their added nutrients are otherwise mentioned either "on the label or in labeling or in advertising" [21 CFR Sect. 101.9(h)(7)].

(8) An exemption is also provided for distribution of bulk food products to be used solely for manufacture of other foods and not for distribution to consumers in bulk form [21 CFR Sect. 101.9(h)(8)].

(9) Foods which would otherwise meet the criteria for nutrition labeling, i.e., they have added vitamin, mineral, or protein, or a nutritional claim on the label or in labeling or advertising, are, nevertheless, exempt, if they are supplied for institutional food service only. The proviso here, however, is that the manufacturer or distributor must provide the required nutrition information to the institution on a current basis [21 CFR Sect. 101.9(h)(9)].

(10) In the absence of specific regulations (there are none at present), fresh fruits and fresh vegetables are exempt. Here, of course, the issue to be addressed is not addition of nutrients, but representations as to nutrient content [21 CFR Sect. 101.9(h)(10)].

(11) The last exemption provides that the percentage declarations of fat (milkfat, butterfat) content "in the ingredient statement on the label of a food listed in Sect. 1.24(a)(7)(i) of this chapter" is not to be considered

a nutrition claim, if certain criteria (e.g., type size and label location) are met [21 CFR Sect. 101.9(h)(11)].

With these exceptions aside, as stated at the outset of the discussion of this topic, when a nutrient is added or a nutrition claim is made, it is required that certain nutrition information be provided on the label of the food product. The nutrient quantities (including vitamins, minerals, calories, protein, carbohydrate and fat) must be declared in relation to the "average or usual serving" (where the food is consumed directly) or the "average or usual portion" (where the food is customarily not consumed directly). Where there are reliable data that a food is customarily consumed more than once a day and as to the amount usually consumed, another column of figures may be added giving that additional information [21 CFR Sect. 101.9(b)].

The definition of serving is "that reasonable quantity of a food suited for or practicable of consumption as part of a meal." Depending on the intended consumer this could be stated for an infant, child under four years of age, or an adult. The criterion employed for an adult is "an adult male engaged in light physical activity." The latter standard is employed because it is the one used by FDA in establishing the USRDA, although the word "young" should be added before "adult." The definition of "portion" is "the amount of a food customarily used only as an ingredient in the preparation of a meal component (e.g., ½ cup flour, ½ tablespoon cooking oil or ¼ cup tomato paste)." Whatever, it must be expressed in a convenient measuring unit that can be easily identified as an average or usual serving and readily understood by purchasers [21 CFR Sect. 101.9(b)(1)]. Definitions are also provided for teaspoonful, tablespoon and cupful, with provision that statements of weight "may also be expressed in grams" [21 CFR Sect. 101.9(b)(2)].

Nutrient quantities must be declared on the basis of the food as packaged. However, another column of figures may be added to show the nutrient quantities of the food as cooked or otherwise prepared. In the latter case, there must be a prominent disclosure of the method of cooking or preparation [21 CFR Sect. 101.9(b)(3)].

Nutrition information is included in the form of a table which, not surprisingly, must be headed exactly that: "Nutrition Information." The producer has an option to add either following as part of or directly below the headline the words "Per Serving" or "Per Portion," as may be applicable [21 CFR Sect. 107.9(c)]. The first item under the headline is a statement of the number of servings or portions in the container [21 CFR Sect. 101.9(c)(2)].

Caloric content is the next item to be included expressed, of course, per serving or portion. The actual calories are rounded to the nearest 2 calories up to 20, to the nearest 5 calories up to 50, and to the nearest 10 calories above 50. The standard employed in determining calories is the Atwater method (described in Merrill and Watt,[11] which is incorporated in the regulations). Caloric value for protein, carbohydrate and fat may be calculated on the basis of 4, 4, and 9 calories per gram, respectively, "unless the use of these values gives a caloric value more than 20%

greater than the caloric value obtained when using . . . the Atwater Method . . ." [21 CFR Sect. 101.9(c)(3)].

The next item in the table is the number of grams of protein per serving or portion. This is to be determined on the basis of "the factor of 6.25 the nitrogen content of the food, as determined by the appropriate method of analysis[12] . . . except when the official procedure for a specific food requires another factor." If a serving or portion contains less than one gram of protein, a statement to that effect, e.g., "Contains less than one gram" may be used as an alternative [21 CFR Sect. 101.9(c)(4)].

Following protein is a statement of the number of grams of carbohydrate per serving or portion, with the same alternative as protein, if there is less than one gram [21 CFR Sect. 101.9(c)(5)]. This is followed by the number of grams of fat, with the same alternative where there is less than one gram. As an option at this point, a statement of fatty acid composition and cholesterol content may be included [21 CFR Sect. 101.9(c)(6)].

When fatty acid composition is declared it must follow immediately the declaration of the fat content. [21 CFR Sect. 101.9(c)(6)(i)], and when cholesterol content is declared it must follow immediately after the fat content or the fatty acid composition, if the latter is declared [21 CFR Sect. 101.9(c)(6)(ii)]. Both may also be combined [21 CFR Sect. 101.9(c)(iii)]. The above applies to inclusion in nutrition labeling, but labeling requirements regarding fatty acid composition and cholesterol are covered in detail by separate regulations [21 CFR Sect. 101.25(d)]. However, this is a matter which strays from the topic of fortification and interested readers are referred to the specific regulatory sections on fatty acid composition and cholesterol.

The number of milligrams of sodium in the specified serving of the food "shall be placed on the nutrition label immediately following the statement on fat content (and fatty acid and/or cholesterol, if stated)." However, in the case of sodium, even in the absence of nutrition labeling, a statement "Contains _____ milligrams sodium per _____ serving (portion)" is permissible on the principal display panel or information panel. This, of course, is a concession to encourage declaration of sodium, since many persons, such as hypertensives, are interested in this information. Declaration should be zero when a serving or portion contains less than 5 mg, to the nearest 5 mg increment when 5–140 mg is present and to the nearest 10 mg when there is more than 140 mg. Determination of the amount present is by the appropriate method[12] as specified in the regulation [21 CFR Sect. 101.9(c)(8)(i)].

Potassium may be declared voluntarily on the label immediately following the declaration of sodium content. The manner of declaring potassium levels in terms of milligrams is the same as for sodium and the method of analysis is also specified[12] [21 CFR Sect. 101.9(c)(8)(ii)].

The heart of nutrition labeling from the standpoint of protein and micronutrient content is the regulatory section which sets forth how they are to be declared in the nutrition labeling format. This begins with a requirement that they be stated in terms of the amount per serving or portion as a percentage of the USRDA [21 CFR Sect. 101.9(c)(7)]. How this is done, however, is not quite so simple because of certain rounding and other factors which are to be employed. Up to and including the 10% level the declaration is in 2% increments, it is in 5% increments above 10% up to and including 50% and in 10% increments thereafter. Below 2% there are some options, including declaring the level as zero; use of an asterisk(s) with a corresponding asterisked statement at the bottom "contains less than 2% of the USRDA of this (these) nutrient (nutrients)." Where no more than 3 of the 8 micronutrients required to be declared have 2% or more of the USRDA, this statement may be used: "contains less than 2% of the USRDA of _____." (filling in the blank with the applicable nutrients in the same type size as those listed in the table) [21 CFR Sect. 101.9(c)(7)(i)]. It appears that there is a misleading element below the 2% level, if the level is actually zero. While not a regulatory requirement, from a consumer information perspective an argument can be made that a nutrient not present at a measurable level should be declared as zero, rather than "less than 2%."

In the table of those nutrients required to be listed in terms of the USRDA, protein is first [21 CFR Sect. 101.9(c)(7)(iii)]. The USRDA for protein in a food is 45 g, if the protein efficiency ratio (PER) of the total protein in the product is equal to or greater than that of casein, and 65 g, if the PER is less than that of casein. The protein USRDA declaration is subject to the rounding factors discussed above [21 CFR Sect. 101.9(c)(7)(ii)(*a*)]. Where the total protein PER compared to casein is less than 20%, protein must not be stated on the label in terms of the USRDA, but rather the statement of protein in grams must be modified to say "not a significant source of protein" immediately adjacent to the protein content statement regardless of the number of grams [21 CFR Sect. 101.9(c)(7)(ii)(*b*)].

Immediately following the protein declaration in terms of the USRDA (except when not allowed based on the PER), is the listing of vitamins and minerals in terms of the percentage of the USRDA. Listing of the following seven nutrients is required in the order stated: vitamin A, vitamin C, thiamin, riboflavin, niacin, calcium, and iron. Other added micronutrients must be listed and other naturally occurring ones may be listed, if they are included in the list shown in Table 20.6 below and, if listed, must be in the order shown [21 CFR Sect. 101.9(c)(7)(iii)]. Table 20.6 is derived from the regulations [21 CFR Sect. 101.9(c)(7)(iv)] and is obviously key to this discussion. The listing shows the established USRDA and nomenclature for the designated vitamins and minerals, which are found to be essential for human nutrition. Some further explanation is in order. Where an alternative name (synonym) is shown in parentheses, this is optional and may or may not be included on the label. The reference to IU, of course, means International Units. These are the same as USP (*United States Pharmacopeia*) units, found on vitamins in drug products, and occasionally referred to in this manner with relation to foods, such as in the standard of identity for enriched farina [21 CFR Sect. 137.305(a)(2) and (3)]. IU, however, are not the same as retinol equivalents (RE for vitamin A) or tocopherol

TABLE 20.6
USRDA ESTABLISHED FOR NUTRITION LABELING

Nutrient	USRDA
Vitamin A	5,000 IU
Vitamin C (Ascorbic Acid)	60 mg
Thiamin (Vitamin B_1)	1.5 mg
Riboflavin (Vitamin B_2)	1.7 mg
Niacin	20 mg
Calcium	1.0 g
Iron	18 mg
Vitamin D	400 IU
Vitamin E	30 IU
Vitamin B_6	2.0 mg
Folic Acid (Folacin)	0.4 mg
Vitamin B_{12}	6 mcg
Phosphorus	1.0 g
Iodine	150 mcg
Magnesium	400 mg
Zinc	15 mg
Copper	2.0 mg
Biotin	0.3 mg
Pantothenic Acid	10 mg

equivalents (TE for vitamin E), confusing elements introduced into later editions of *Recommended Dietary Allowances*, in 1974 as to vitamin A [7] and in 1980 as to vitamin E.[8] For example, 10 TE are equivalent to 14.9 (rounded to 15) IU of vitamin E. This merely moves the reference compound from 1 mg of dl-alpha tocopheryl acetate, the longstanding, traditional measuring standard for vitamin E to 1 mg, of d-alpha tocopherol, which is equivalent to 1.49 mg of dl-alpha tocopheryl acetate based on long-accepted biological equivalence measures. At the time the change from IU to TE was introduced into the RDA table, some commentators were clearly confused in reporting that the vitamin E RDA had been lowered, which it had not. Also, virtually all studies have been reported based on IU and a change to TE would require calculation to report results on a comparable basis, a needless exercise.

Further regarding Table 20.6, the list obviously does not encompass all of the micronutrients known to be essential, but includes only those for which an RDA or at least an estimated daily intake had been established at the time when the nutrition labeling regulations were first enacted. It is provided in the regulation that the nutrients and their levels "are subject to amendment from time to time as more information on human nutrition becomes available" [21 CFR Sect. 101.9(c)(7)(iv)]. Still further, regarding Table 20.6, the levels given, with minor deviations, track the USRDA as they were established for adults and children four or more years of age.

The nutrition labeling regulations contain a number of miscellaneous provisions. These include labeling of products which have separately packaged ingredients or as to which other ingredients are added by the user [21 CFR Sect. 101.9(d)], and the sampling method to determine compliance [21 CFR Sect. 101.9(e)]. Regarding the latter, two classes of nutrients are defined, namely, Class I for added nutrients and Class II for naturally occurring (indigenous) ingredients. When an ingredient containing a naturally occurring nutrient is added to a food, the total amount in the final food is subject to Class II requirements, unless the same nutrient is also added separately [21 CFR Sect. 101.9(e)(3)].

Regarding claims, the regulations provide that no claim can be made that a food containing less than 10% of a nutrient per serving is a significant source of that nutrient. The same principle applies in making a comparative claim, that is, a food cannot be claimed to be nutritionally superior to another food, unless it contains at least 10% more per serving of the nutrient giving rise to the claim [21 CFR Sect. 101.9(c)(7)(v)].

When a food has a label declaration as to a vitamin, mineral, or protein it shall be deemed misbranded under Sect. 403(a) of the *FD& C Act* [21 USC Sect. 343(a)] unless it meets the following requirements:

(1) For Class I (added nutrient) the nutrient content is at least equal to the amount declared on the label [21 CFR Sect. 101.9(e)(4)(i)], and for Class II (naturally occurring) the nutrient content of the composite is equal to at least 80% of the stated label value [21 CFR Sect. 101.9(e)(4)(ii)]. The above determinations are subject to an allowance for the generally recognized variability in the analytical method employed.

(2) In the case of calories, carbohydrates, fat, or sodium, the misbranding occurs, if the content of the composite exceeds the stated label value by more than 20% [21 CFR Sect. 101.9(e)(5)].

(3) Excesses of vitamins, minerals or protein and deficiencies of calories, fat or sodium are acceptable, if they are reasonable within good manufacturing practices [21 CFR Sect. 101.9(e)(6)].

An example of what is involved in the third requirement would be addition of a reasonable overage of a vitamin to assure label claim during the anticipated shelf-life. Since a number of nutrients are inherently unstable, the limitations of food technology require some flexibility here, since a substantial number of variables apply and it would not be feasible to cover every possibility in the regulations.

The regulations provide that nutrition information provided directly to professionals such as physicians, dietitians and educators may vary from the regulatory requirements, as long as the nutrition information is provided at the same time exactly as required [21 CFR Sect. 101.9(f)]. The location of the nutrition information must comply with Sect. 101.2 (21 CFR Sect. 101.2). The latter section contains much technical detail which preparers of food packages should review carefully in any case. Therefore, a review of these provisions and others which are not specific to fortification of foods is not included here.

There is one more important aspect of the nutrition labeling regulations, namely, the misbranding provisions [21 CFR Sect. 101.9(i)]. This section is premised on labeling representations, suggestions, or implications in six separate areas:

(1) That a food is "effective in the prevention, cure, mitigation, or treatment of any disease or symptom" [21 CFR Sect. 101.9(i)(1)].
(2) That adequate amounts of nutrients cannot be adequately supplied by a balanced diet of ordinary foods [21 CFR Sect. 101.9(i)(2)].
(3) That inadequacies in the daily diet based on lack of optimum nutritive quality of foods results from the soil in which it is grown [21 CFR Sect. 101.9(i)(3)].
(4) That dietary inadequacy results from "the storage, transportation, processing or cooking" of food [21 CFR Sect. 101.9(i)(4)].
(5) "That the food has dietary properties when such properties are of no significant value or need in human nutrition" [21 CFR Sect. 101.9(i)(5)]. This subsection goes into additional detail and contains specific limitations regarding "rutin, other bioflavinoids, para-amino-benzoic acid, inositol, and similar substances." Anyone intending to use any such substance should review this subsection carefully.
(6) "That a natural vitamin in a food is superior to an added or synthetic vitamin, or to differentiate between vitamins naturally present from those added" [21 CFR Sect. 101.9(i)(6)]. This last subsection could be the subject of an extensive treatise in and of itself. It is an amazingly persistent misconception that "natural" is better than "synthetic" as a general rule. While this is best left to the scientists, the simple facts are that a molecule is a molecule from whatever source, and, where vitamin forms differ, such as with vitamin E, weight adjustments are made to maintain the biological equivalence.

Regarding these misbranding subprovisions, the one which has developed as the most controversial is the first, relating to nutrition and disease. In recent years, much of the thinking of medical science has turned to prevention rather than cure. As the data have developed on the relationship between diet and disease, e.g., cholesterol and heart disease, salt and hypertension, beta carotene and cancer, it is clear that the demarcation between the definition of "drug" under Sect. 201(g) of the *FD& C Act* [21 USC Sect. 321(g)] and "food" under Sect. 201(f) [21 USC Sect. 321(f)] is becoming a barrier to communication of sound health information. This issue was joined with the label association made by Kellogg on its All-Bran cereal between fiber and cancer protection. [This was based on National Cancer Institute (NCI) publication.[13]] The Kellogg action had the support of both the NCI and the Federal Trade Commission (FTC), although clearly the product label and labeling is within the jurisdiction of the FDA. Product advertising of food products and over-the-counter (OTC) drug products, of course, comes under the jurisdiction of the FTC.

In any event, it was clear that the FDA would now have to develop some way to handle the so-called "health claim" or "health message" issue. In fact, these are both misnomers. Obviously, many claims can be made for foods and food constituents which are related to health: the calcium in milk is important for strong bones, vitamin A is necessary for good vision, the calories in food are required to assure proper growth and energy. Even drug claims may be permitted, it being universally accepted, for example, that a vitamin C deficiency can cause scurvy and vitamin B_{12} prevents pernicious anemia.

The true issue is whether "new drug" claims can be allowed for food. For instance, a large and growing body of evidence indicates that a diet high in beta carotene rich foods is associated with a reduced risk of certain forms of cancer. Based on this the NCI alone is sponsoring some 14 studies on beta carotene individually or in combination with other vitamins and minerals. To determine this in a controlled way is not only expensive, but can take many years, especially since dietary factors can have a cumulative impact over the course of a lifetime. In the meantime, what to do? The FDA is the nation's most prestigious health agency, but it also has the responsibility to regulate under the provisions of the *FD& C Act*. If someone includes information on beta carotene in connection with the sale of carrots, broccoli or spinach — all good sources — should these common vegetables be declared new drugs? If the "claim" made is accurate and well balanced, should it be prohibited because it is not based on double-blind, controlled studies on carrots conducted by scientists qualified to determine safety and efficacy?

These questions seem to be ridiculous on their face, and, in common sense terms it appears to be absolutely ludicrous to consider a carrot to be a new drug. Yet, despite all the inherent difficulties in such a concept, in legal contemplation, as part of the statutory scheme enacted by Congress under the *FD& C Act*, these questions are very real ones with which the FDA must contend. In finding ways around these strictures, however, the FDA must also find a way to allow fair and well-balanced information without at the same time opening a floodgate of highly speculative and exaggerated claims. Essential to this is a determination of what standard to use. The more conservative argue for a "consensus" standard (almost impossible to achieve with most nutrition issues), specifically approved claims developed by or under the supervision of FDA, or claim preclearance. They argue, in essence, that to do otherwise would be to open a floodgate which would inundate a gullible public with waves of misleading information.

The more liberal forces argue for a substantiation standard akin to that used by the FTC for advertising, scientific evidence short of consensus, and the right to include accurate, fairly balanced information. They argue, in essence, that under our democratic system the public has a right to be informed and make individual health decisions based on rational benefit/risk evaluations rather than having to wait years for conclusive scientific proof.

The FDA's original position was to prepare a set of guidelines to outline what was allowable and what was not. Even in draft form this unleashed a debate and generated citizens' petitions from interested groups. Among those significantly involved were the dietary supplement proponents who felt that their products were unfairly being given discriminatory treatment in favor of more traditional foods. In any case, after a long period of review by the Office of Management and Budget, what eventually emerged was a proposed regulation amending the misbranding provisions of nutritional labeling [21 CFR Sect. 101.9(i)] to allow "health messages" under a standard similar to that employed by FTC in advertising.

Some hundreds of comments ensued with sharp distinctions between the conservative and liberal forces. In addition, FDA's already difficult task was complicated further by Congressional inquiry and hearings. This is all related to the main theme of food fortification because it generates the potential for increased addition of ingredients such as vitamins and minerals. The FDA is apparently also concerned about this, since key personnel have made a number of negative public statements including warnings of possible toxicity from excessive fortification. (See Food Chem. News, Dec. 22, 1986, p. 12; Jun. 22, 1987, p. 27; Oct. 19, 1987, p. 3; Feb. 2, 1987, p. 52; Feb. 15, 1988, p. 19). Conspicuously absent from these statements is any evidence that food fortification has ever caused a problem in the United States.

As of this writing, the FDA has reviewed the comments on its proposal (52 Fed. Reg. 28843, Aug. 4, 1987) and redrafted it in a way that is more directed to a specific monograph approach. Since the matter is in flux, there is nothing to be gained by speculating further on the outcome or to detail the provisions of the latest unpublished draft. It is, however, a very important development, much less from the standpoint of allowable claims, than as a reflection of a fundamental change in the medico-scientific approach, i.e., a much greater research emphasis on prevention, as opposed to treatment. (For an excellent review of the legal/regulatory background of the health messages issue, see Taylor.[14])

FDA requested public comment on food labeling requirements, including "Health Messages" (54 Fed. Reg., 32610, Aug. 8, 1989), thus indicating that its 1987 "Health Message" initiative was not viable; and consumerist groups became more active. (See, for example, "Food Labeling Chaos"[15]). Anticipated congressional action based on the introduction of a number of bills (see, for example, Food Chem. News, Jul. 17, 1989, p. 51), ultimately materialized in the form of new legislation as this book was in press, and will directly impact FDA's final regulations on "Health Messages." (See Addendum.)

NUTRITION LABELING OF RESTAURANT FOOD

There is a special section of the regulations relating to nutrition labeling of restaurant foods (21 CFR Sect. 101.10) which is worth mentioning briefly. This provides that nutrition information or claims may be made in advertising or labeling (other than an actual label) without triggering a requirement for a nutrition label on the articles of foods served. However, it would be necessary to display nutrition labeling in the established format at the time the food is ordered or consumed on the specific combination of foods served (rather than each individual article).

One or two of the "fast-food" chains have been exploring the benefits of nutrition information. While it is unlikely to become a standard practice, with the continuing emphasis on good dietary habits, often in the form of what not to eat, and with increasing scientific information, the major chains especially may begin movements in this direction to support their marketing efforts. Such a trend could well impact on fortification practices.

TEMPORARY EXEMPTIONS FOR FOOD LABELING EXPERIMENTS

One last item on nutrition labeling is a special regulatory provision (21 CFR Sect. 101.108) under which the FDA may authorize exemptions from various food labeling requirements for the purpose of food labeling experiments on "graphics and other formats for presenting nutrition and other related food labeling information. . . ." The FDA has been concerned about the meaningfulness of nutrition information and its ready comprehensibility to consumers. There has been little, if any, activity in this regard in recent years. In a way this is unfortunate, since industry has not taken the opportunity through this means of cooperating in a proactive way with FDA in developing suitable formats. As indicated earlier, it is likely that in the reasonably near future either Congress or FDA will undertake significant changes regarding nutrition labeling, which will put industry in a reactive position.

FOODS FOR SPECIAL DIETARY USE

As defined in the regulations (21 CFR Sect. 105.3), "special dietary uses" as applied to human food means "particular (as opposed to general) use. . . ." In general, these fall into four categories:

(1) Those which address special dietary needs in physical, physiological, pathological, or other conditions such as disease, convalescence, pregnancy, lactation, allergic hypersensitivity, underweight, and overweight [21 CFR Sect. 105.3(a)(1)(i)].

(2) Those which address special dietary needs related to age such as infancy [21 CFR Sect. 105.3(a)(1)(ii)].

(3) Those used for supplementing or fortifying the usual diet with "any vitamin, mineral, or other dietary property." A food in this category is a special dietary food, if it has a particular use, even though it is also represented for general use [21 CFR Sect. 105.3(a)(1)(iii)].

(4) Those foods which use artificial sweeteners are considered special dietary foods for caloric regulation or diabetic use, unless the artificial sweetener is used to achieve a physical characteristic in the food, which could not be achieved with a nutritive sweetener [21 CFR Sect. 105.3(a)(2)].

This regulatory section also defines "infant" (up to 12 months), "child" (between 12 months and 12 years), and "adult" (12 years or more) [21 CFR Sect. 105.3(e)].

The third category above includes dietary supplements, which are generally beyond the scope of the present discussion. However, dietary supplements are not always in the form of tablets, capsules and the like. During the regulatory process described at the beginning of this chapter, the FDA established a premise that unless fortified based on some other regulation that would exclude the application of the special dietary food definitions, even a food for general use would be considered a dietary supplement, if fortified with a vitamin or mineral at a level of 50% or more of the USRDA. The outstanding examples of foods falling into this category are the breakfast cereals fortified up to 100% of the USRDA with vitamins and minerals.

Even though the so-called vitamin-mineral regulations were revoked in 1979 (44 Fed. Reg. 16005, Mar. 16, 1979) this dividing line, i.e., the 50% level for dietary supplement status continues to apply [21 CFR Sect. 101.9(a)(2)]. Other than for this passing explanation, an excursion into the intricacies of dietary supplements would be extraneous to the subject of food fortification. Special dietary foods other than dietary supplements may obviously involve fortification, but will not be discussed herein other than the following brief discussion of infant formula.

INFANT FORMULA

This topic is covered in a separate chapter devoted to special foods. By definition in the *FD& C Act* "the term 'infant formula' means a food which purports to be or is represented for special dietary use solely as a food for infants by reason of its simulation of human milk or its suitability as a complete or partial substitute for human milk" [*FD& C Act* Sect. 201(aa), 21 USC Sect. 321 (aa)].

The specific requirements for this class of food were set forth in the *Infant Formula Act* [P.L. 96-359, Sept. 26, 1980; *FD& C Act* Sect. 412; 21 USC Sect. 350a] in reaction to some unfortunate incidents involving the nutrient content of such products. Since these products are presently used as the sole sustenance of non-breast-fed infants for significant periods, the failure to include adequate levels or addition of excessive levels of essential nutrients can have truly tragic consequences. This is an area involving great sensitivity and special quality considerations apply (21 CFR Sect. 106.1 et seq.). The FDA does have the authority to revise the nutrient requirements set forth in this statute, both for general use and where special conditions exist such as inborn errors of metabolism, low birth weight, or other unusual medical or dietary problems. Since revisions may occur, it is always wise to review the current regulations (21 CFR Sect. 107.3 et seq.).

As is often the case, however, not everything is found in the regulations. Obviously, it is reasonable to include in infant formula beneficial or potentially beneficial constituents found in mothers' milk. On this basis manufacturers are adding such ingredients as the amino acids L-carnitine and taurine on the basis of independent determinations that they are GRAS at levels not greater than those normally found in mothers' milk; it being noted, however, that the formulations for these products are reported to the FDA.

ALLOWABLE NUTRIENT INGREDIENTS

Two statutory definitions form the starting point for this discussion. The first is the definition of "food," [*FD& C Act* Sect. 201(f); 21 U.S.C. Sect. 321 (f)] which reads as follows:

> The term "food" means (1) articles used for food or drink for man or other animals, (2) chewing gum and (3) articles used for components of any such articles.

This seems simple enough, but can be deceptive. Thus, we turn to the second definition, that of a "food additive," [*FD& C Act* Sect. 201(b), 21 U.S.C. Sect. 321 (s)] which is quoted here only in part:

> The term "food additive" means any substance the intended use of which results or may reasonably be expected to result, directly or indirectly, in its becoming a component or otherwise affecting the characteristics of any food. . . ., if such substance is not generally recognized, among experts qualified by scientific training and experience to evaluate its safety, as having been adequately shown through scientific procedures (or, in the case of a substance used in food prior to January 1, 1958, through either scientific procedures or experience based on common use in food) to be safe under the conditions of its intended use; except that such term does not include —
>
> * * * * * *
>
> (4) any substance used in accordance with a sanction or approval granted prior to the enactment of this paragraph pursuant to this Act, the Poultry Products Inspection Act (21 U.S.C. 451 and the following) or the Meat Inspection Act of March 4, 1907 (34 Stat. 1260), as amended and extended (21 U.S.C. 71 and the following). . . .

Thus, there are four regulatory bases for adding a substance to food: (1) through another food ingredient, (2) as allowed by a food additive regulation, (3) on the basis that it is generally recognized as safe (GRAS), or (4) under a prior sanction.

1. Food Ingredients

The addition of food ingredients, especially traditional ones, e.g., nuts, lemon juice, chocolate and the like, does not require much discussion. Adding flour, especially enriched flour, to a cake would enhance the nutritional content of the cake, but does not require any special regulatory consideration, provided the standardized food is merely listed in the ingredient statement and is, thus, within the exception from nutrition labeling set forth in the regulations [21 CFR Sect. 101.9(h)(7)]. Questions can and do arise, however, when we begin to "engineer" traditional ingredients and proceed to condense them or extract from them, perform simple hydrogenations of fats and oils or effect other molecular manipulations. Without leaving our main subject, the point where the food "engineering" changes the essential character of something such that it becomes a food additive (or possibly a GRAS substance requiring affirmation from FDA), rather than merely a food ingredient, can give rise to a very difficult decision with significant regulatory overtones, since the preparation and approval process for a food additive or GRAS affirmation petition can be lengthy and expensive.

2. Food Additives

The food additive regulations (21 CFR Part 172) contain a separate section — subpart D — covering direct additions of "Special Dietary and Nutritional Additives." These substances may be added in accordance with the conditions specified in the regulations. Anyone wishing to use a substance listed in this category should check the regulatory requirements carefully to assure compliance. Food additives included in these regulations which are of interest from the nutritional standpoint are the following:

(a) Aluminum nicotinate (21 CFR 172.310). May be used as a source of niacin in foods for special dietary use and is expressed on the label in terms of niacin activity.

(b) Nicotinamide-ascorbic acid complex (21 CFR Sect. 172.315). May be used as a source of both ascorbic acid and niacin in multivitamin preparations.

(c) Amino acids (21 CFR Sect. 172.320). Those specified in the regulations may be used "to significantly improve the biological quality of the total protein in a food containing naturally occurring primarily intact protein that is considered a significant dietary protein source . . ." [21 CFR Sect. 172.320 (c)]. Specific requirements for determining "significant" are set forth in the regulations [21 CFR Sect. 172.320 (c)(1)(2) and (3)], as are upper limits [21 CFR Sect. 172.320(c)(4)], the method for determining the protein efficiency ratio (PER) and record keeping [21 CFR Sect. 172.320(d)], and labeling requirements [21 CFR Sect. 172.320(e)]. Exemption from certain of the requirements is provided for "special dietary foods that are intended for use solely under medical supervision to meet nutritional requirements in specific medical conditions . . .," as long as they comply with the special dietary food regulations (21 CFR Part 105).

The following amino acids, which may be "in the free, hydrated or anhydrous form or as the hydrochloride, sodium or potassium salts" and may be used in combination, are listed in the regulations [21 CFR Sect. 172.320(a)]:

L-Alanine	L-Leucine
L-Arginine	L-Lysine
L-Asparagine	DL-Methionine (not for infant foods)
L-Aspartic acid	L-Methionine
L-Cysteine	L-Phenylalanine
L-Cystine	L-Proline
L-Glutamic acid	L-Serine
L-Glutamine	L-Threonine
Aminoacetic acid (glycine)	L-Tryptophan
L-Histidine	L-Tyrosine
L-Isoleucine	L-Valine

For most of these the applicable specifications [21 CFR Sect. 172.320(b)(i)] are found in *Food Chemicals Codex (FCC)*,[16] but for a few (L-Asparagine, L-Aspartic acid, L-Glutamine, and L-Histidine) they are set forth in "Specifications and Criteria for Biochemical Compounds." [NAS/NRC Publication 3rd Ed. (1972)].

(d) Bakers yeast protein (21 CFR Sect. 172.325). Meeting the specifications in the regulation may be used as a nutrient supplement.

(e) Calcium pantothenate, calcium chloride double salt (21 CFR Sect. 172.330). Is allowed in foods for special dietary uses. Either the *d* (dextrorotatory) or the *dl* (racemic) form of calcium pantothenate is allowed. The reference form for label declaration is pantothenic acid.

(f) D-Pantothenamide (21 CFR Sect. 172.335). Is allowed as a source of pantothenic acid in foods for special dietary use.

(g) Fish protein isolate (21 CFR Sect. 172.340). May be used as a food supplement when it is derived from the edible portions of bony fish, which are safe for human consumption, is properly handled, and when it is extracted according to the method and meets the specifications prescribed by the regulations.

(h) Folic acid (folacin) (21 CFR Sect. 172.345). A very safe, water-soluble vitamin in and of itself, but, since it has the potential to mask pernicious anemia, it created a level of concern sufficient to place it in the food additive, rather than the GRAS category. It may be used in food or dietary supplements for its dietary function based on maximum levels determined by one-day's intake, as follows:

Food Labeled	Maximum
Without reference to age or physiological state	0.4 mg
Infants (under 1 year of age)	0.1 mg
Children under 4 years of age	0.3 mg
Adults and children 4 or more years of age	0.4 mg
Pregnant or lactating women	0.8 mg

(i) Fumaric acid and salts of fumaric acid (21 CFR Sect. 172.350). May be used as a source of iron in foods for special dietary use in accordance with the specifications and requirements of the regulation. The allowable salts are calcium, ferrous, magnesium, potassium and sodium.

(j) Kelp (21 CFR Sect. 172.365). Dehydrated and ground, from *Macrocystis pyrifera, Laminaria digitata, Laminaria saccharina*, and *Laminaria cloustoni* may be added to a food or dietary supplement as a source of the essential mineral iodine. As in the case of folic acid, this is subject to maximum levels based on daily intake, as follows:

Food Labeled	Maximum
Without reference to age or physiological state	225 mcg
Infants (under 1 year of age)	45 mcg
Children under 4 years of age	105 mcg
Adults and children 4 or more years of age	225 mcg
Pregnant or lactating women	300 mcg

(k) Iron-choline citrate complex (21 CFR Sect. 172.370). Made from reacting equimolar quantities of ferric hydroxide, choline and citric acid may be used in foods for special dietary use as a source of iron.

(l) N-Acetyl-L-methionine (21 CFR Sect. 172.372). May be "added to food (except infant foods and food containing added nitrites/nitrates) as a source of L-methionine (amino acid) to improve significantly the biological quality of the total protein" in the food. As in the case of the amino acids discussed above, this is subject to specifications and requirements detailed at some length in the regulation.

(m) Potassium iodide (21 CFR Sect. 172.375). May be used in foods or dietary supplements as a source of iodine. It is subject to exactly the same maximums in iodine levels as are set forth above for kelp.

(n) Whole fish concentrate (21 CFR Sect. 172.385). May be used as a protein supplement added to food in the household or as a protein supplement in manufactured foods. It is subject to the same types of requirements and specifications as indicated for fish protein isolate discussed above. Anyone involved with this food additive should review the requirements carefully, including the limitations on fluoride content (100 ppm in the additive itself or 8 ppm based on dry weight of the finished food product) and on consumption by children (not over 20 g/day up to 8 years of age).

(o) Xylitol (21 CFR Sect. 172.395). Does not properly fit in a discussion on food fortification. Xylitol is a sugar alcohol calorically equivalent to sucrose, and other carbohydrate sweeteners, but having a cool, refreshing taste quality and non-cariogenic, if not anticariogenic, properties. It is these latter properties which make it of interest in foods for special dietary use and not any nutrient benefit. (As an aside, this author was involved with regulatory issues surrounding Xylitol for many years and remains convinced that it may be used safely and beneficially in a variety of ways, especially in chewing gums, confections, and chewable dietary supplement products.)

(p) Zinc methionine sulfate (21 CFR Sect. 172.399). Is limited to use as a source of zinc in tablets. It is derived from a reaction of equimolar amounts of zinc sulfate and DL-methionine in purified water and is subject to the regulatory specifications.

3. GRAS Substances

As indicated above regarding distinctions between "engineered" food ingredients and food additives, so too it is also difficult at times to distinguish whether a substance should be considered as a food additive or a GRAS substance. With new substances this has become less important where FDA approval is deemed to be required, if FDA accepts a GRAS affirmation petition procedure rather than a food additive petition approach.

When using a GRAS substance in strict accordance with an FDA regulation, there is no problem. However, the GRAS regulations specifically state:

> It is impracticable to list all substances that are generally recognized as safe for their intended use. However, by way of illustration, the Commissioner regards such common food ingredients as salt, pepper, sugar, vinegar, baking powder, and monosodium glutamate as safe for their intended use" [21 CFR Sect. 182.1(a)].

In any case, for many years FDA listed GRAS substances under simple regulations. The category of interest to us was a combined one of dietary supplements and nutrients. While industry sat back passively unaware of the consequences, FDA broke these into two separate categories, each containing the identical substances with identical conditions of use, i.e., "This substance is generally recognized safe when used in accordance with good manufacturing practice" (45 Fed. Reg. 58837, Sept. 5, 1980). This separation was innocent on its face until FDA began the process of substituting new GRAS affirmation regulations for nutrients in place of the older GRAS regulations. This process is not yet complete, and has so far not been extended to dietary supplements. The GRAS affirmation regulations are much more detailed and, in fact, are akin to food additive regulations, although the regulations allow that deviations may be allowable, if the manufacturer "shall independently establish that the use is GRAS or shall use the ingredient in accordance with a food additive regulation" [21 CFR Sect. 184.1(b)(1)].

The above is far from clear; if there were an appropriate food additive regulation, why should a manufacturer need to make an independent GRAS decision? As to independent GRAS determinations, they are fine as long as FDA agrees, but if FDA does not, they will simply state that, since they are experts and do not accept that the substance is safe, the "generally" part of generally recognized as safe is missing, hence, it is not GRAS.

FDA, on incomplete information; without evidence of unsafe use in foods; with incomplete data, including outworn surveys on use (not safety); and side-stepping GRAS recognition evidenced by its own longstanding regulations; has added limitations to traditional nutrients with regard to manufacturing methods and allowable food categories in which they may be used. [FDA has established 43 general food categories under 21 CFR Sect. 170.3(n) and 32 physical or technical functional effects for which direct human food ingredients may be added to food under 21 CFR Sect. 170.3(o).]

One suspects that, to some extent, the motivation for GRAS affirmation decisions on nutrients was not really safety, but an indirect means of controlling food fortification. Food processors should be able to act based on a clear regulatory scheme in keeping with statutory requirements. They should not have to rely on individual interpretations of individual members of FDA, or, in the alternative, make risk decisions or engage in protracted proceedings to satisfy regulatory requirements having limited scientific basis. This climate can have a stultifying effect on development of new food products.

For the convenience of the reader, Table 20.7 lists all of the remaining GRAS regulations on nutrients with the warning that the current regulations should always be checked, since these will eventually all be replaced by GRAS affirmation regulations. Substances for which GRAS affirmation regulations have already been adopted are listed in Table 20.8.

PRIOR SANCTIONS

" 'Prior Sanction' means an explicit approval granted with respect to use of a substance in food prior to Sept. 6, 1958, by the Food and Drug Administration or the United States Department of Agriculture pursuant to the *Federal Food, Drug, and Cosmetic Act*, the *Poultry Products Inspection Act*, or the *Meat Inspection Act*" [21 CFR Sect. 170.3(1), see also 21 CFR Sect. 181.5(a)]. While there are a number of prior-sanctioned substances listed in the regulations, (21 CFR Part 181) there are no nutrients presently listed.

As part of the GRAS affirmation procedures being conducted by FDA, the *Federal Register* proposals call for information on prior sanctions, providing that, if not produced in response to the notice, the same will be waived. However, more than 30 years have already gone by since the critical date of Sept. 6, 1958, and fewer and fewer of the old files continue to exist. It would certainly be a good idea to check all corporate sources where old GRAS letters may still exist. These may be valuable and should be placed in a centralized, permanent file. It would also be advisable to furnish copies to the appropriate trade associations for their information.

UNITED STATES DEPARTMENT OF AGRICULTURE (USDA)

The USDA, through its Food Safety and Inspection Service (FSIS), exercises jurisdiction over meat and meat food products under the *Federal Meat Inspection Act* [34 Stat. 1260, as amended 81 Stat. 584, 84 Stat. 438, 92 Stat. 1069, 21 USC Sect. 601 et seq.] and the *Poultry Products Inspection Act* [71 Stat. 441, as amended by the *Wholesome Poultry Products Act*, 82 Stat. 791; 21 U.S.C. 451 et seq.]. By

TABLE 20.7
SUBSTANCES GENERALLY RECOGNIZED AS SAFE AS NUTRIENTS[1]

21 CFR Part 182 Sect. No.	Substance
8013	Ascorbic acid
8159	Biotin
8195	Calcium citrate
8201	Calcium glycerophosphate
8217	Calcium phosphate
8223	Calcium pyrophosphate
8250	Choline bitartrate
8252	Choline chloride
8455	Manganese glycerophosphate
8458	Manganese hypophosphite
8628	Potassium glycerophosphate
8778	Sodium phosphate
8890	Tocopherols
8892	a-Tocopherol acetate
8985	Zinc chloride
8988	Zinc gluconate
8991	Zinc oxide
8994	Zinc stearate
8997	Zinc sulfate

[1] In each of these cases the regulation merely names the product as indicated above and states under "(b) *Conditions of Use*": "This substance is generally recognized as safe when used in accordance with good manufacturing practice."

regulation, FSIS has established lists of allowable substances for such products. [See 9 CFR Sect. 318.7(c)(4) as to meat and 9 CFR Sect. 381.147(f) as to poultry.]

While these lists include some readily recognizable nutrients, e.g., ascorbic acid, sodium ascorbate, and tocopherols, the uses specified in these lists are for technological purposes such as antioxidants, color accelerators, and curing accelerators, and not as nutrients. With regard to these lists of approved substances, it should be noted that FSIS will not approve any new substances, new uses, or new levels which have not been approved previously by FDA for use in meat or meat food products [9 CFR Sect. 318.7(2)(i)] or in poultry or poultry products [9 CFR Sect. 381.147(f)(2)(i)] "as a food additive, color additive or as a substance generally recognized as safe. . . ."

The overlying role of FDA is also indicated by the fact that the FDA regulations take precedence in the case of labeling of meat food products and poultry products intended or represented for special dietary use. [See 9 CFR Sect. 317.2(j)(2) and Sect. 381.124 respectively.]

TABLE 20.8
DIRECT FOOD SUBSTANCES AFFIRMED AS GENERALLY RECOGNIZED AS SAFE AS NUTRIENT SUPPLEMENTS

21 CFR Part 184 Sect. No.	Substance*	Footnotes
1065	Linoleic acid	(1)(4)
1193	Calcium chloride	(1)(3)
1207	Calcium lactate	(1)(5)
1212	Calcium pantothenate	(4)
1230	Calcium sulfate	(1)(3)
1245	Beta carotene	(2)(4)
1260	Copper gluconate	(1)(4)
1261	Copper sulfate	(1)(4)
1265	Cuprous iodate	(2)(3)(6)
1296	Ferric ammonium citrate	(4)
1298	Ferric citrate	(4)
1301	Ferric phosphate	(4)
1304	Ferric pyrophosphate	(4)
1307(a)	Ferrous ascorbate	(4)
1307(b)	Ferrous carbonate	(4)
1307(c)	Ferrous citrate	(4)
1307(d)	ferrous fumarate	(4)
1308	Ferrous gluconate	(4)
1311	Ferrous lactate	(4)
1315	Ferrous sulfate	(1)(4)
1321	Corn gluten	(1)
1322	Wheat gluten	(1)
1370	Inositol	(2)(4)(7)
1375	Iron, elemental	
1425	Magnesium carbonate	(1)
1426	Magnesium chloride	(1)(4)
1428	Magnesium hydroxide	(1)
1431	Magnesium oxide	(1)(4)
1434	Magnesium phosphate	(1)(4)
1440	Magnesium stearate	(1)
1443	Magnesium sulfate	(1)
1446	Manganese chloride	(4)
1449	Manganese citrate	(2)(4)
1452	Manganese gluconate	(2)(4)
1461	Manganese sulfate	(2)(4)
1530	Niacin	(4)
1535	Niacinamide	(4)
1553	Peptones	(1)
1613	Potassium bicarbonate	(1)
1619	Potassium carbonate	(1)

TABLE 20.8 (*Continued*)

21 CFR Part 184 Sect. No.	Substance*	Footnotes
1662	Potassium chloride	(1)(4)
1634	Potassium iodide	(2)(3)(6)
1676	Pyridoxine hydrochloride	(2)(4)
1695	Riboflavin	(4)
1697	Riboflavin-5'-phosphate (Sodium)	(2)(4)
1875	Thiamin hydrochloride	(1)(4)
1878	Thiamin mononitrate	(4)
1890	a-Tocopherols	(8)
1930	Vitamin A	(4)(9)
1945	Vitamin B_{12}	(4)
1950	Vitamin D	(2)(4)(10)

*In addition to the substances listed in this table, there are others of possible interest which have been affirmed as GRAS in foods generally without any specified functional use. These are as follows, with the 21 CFR Part 184 Sect. in parentheses: calcium carbonate (1191), calcium hydroxide (1205), calcium oxide (1210), lecithin (1400), ground limestone (1409), maltodextrin (1444), whey (1979), reduced lactose whey (1979a), reduced minerals whey (1979b), and whey protein concentrate (1979c).

[1]Regulation includes use(s) other than as a nutrient.
[2]Regulation limits use(s) to specific food category or categories.
[3]Regulation specifies maximum level(s).
[4]Regulation specifically allows use in infant formula.
[5]Regulation specifically disallows use in infant foods or formula.
[6]May be used in table salt at a maximum of 0.01% as a source of dietary iodine.
[7]May be used only in special dietary foods.
[8]Alpha-tocopherols are affirmed as GRAS to inhibit nitrosamine formation in pump-cured bacon. The comparable USDA approval is found in 9 CFR Sect. 318.7(c)(4). This is in addition to the general GRAS regulation covering tocopherols as nutrients, 21 CFR Sect. 182.8890. Inclusion in this table is for purposes of clarity only, since the use in bacon is for a technical purpose and not to provide vitamin E activity.
[9]Includes retinol and the acetate and palmitate (retinyl) esters. A careful reading of the virtually identical monographs in *USP* and *FCC* indicates that other fatty acid esters, such as propionate, should also be considered GRAS.
[10]Includes crystalline and resin forms of Vitamins D_2 and D_3.

Both in the case of meat food products and poultry products, FSIS has its own standards of identity. (See 9 CFR Part 319 and Part 381, Subpart P, respectively.) While there are a number of these, the only one which specifically provides for fortification is the standard for margarine or oleomargarine. (9 CFR Sect. 319.700). In this case the required fortification to provide 15,000 IU/lb (33,000 IU/kg) of vitamin A and, optionally, 1,500 IU/lb (3,300 IU/kg) of vitamin D is equivalent to the FDA standard. The reason for having two standards is that FDA has jurisdiction over margarines made from vegetable sources and USDA has jurisdiction over those made with meat products, i.e., rendered animal fats from cattle, sheep, swine or goats.

SUMMARY

While the elements that form the regulatory pattern regarding food fortification have a certain theoretical logic, they do not work so well in practice. Too often in the workaday world of food processing, what is allowable is not clear from reference to the regulations; too often the practical realities of securing regulatory approvals for minor changes, where safety is not at issue, can cause considerable expense and delays running into years; and too often we find that what is allowable is influenced by the personal views and opinions of regulators, rather than being dependent upon clear regulatory provisions.

The fundamental nature of the system elevates the issue of control to a dominant position over the underlying advances in science and food technology. Obviously, the interested agencies must fulfill their roles in assuring a safe food supply and this leads to a basic conservatism, especially as the trend continues away from a farm-fresh food supply toward more highly processed and engineered foods. For whatever reasons and despite whatever denials there appears to be a regulatory bias toward "natural" as opposed to "synthetic" foods and especially with regard to nutrients such as the essential vitamins and minerals.

For years this has manifested itself in a negative regulatory attitude toward dietary supplement products, but more recently it has been displayed in warnings about the dangers of overfortification. This despite the fact that there is no evidence that food fortification has presented a safety problem in the United States. The possibility exists that regulatory attention to the dangers of food fortification is a reaction to increasing scientific evidence that intakes of certain substances above normal dietary levels may have advantageous health effects that are distinct from the deficiency prevention levels, and a concern that this might set off a "horsepower" race. Of course, there are some within FDA who, while recognizing the need to keep fortification rational, do not have significant concerns about overfortification and see opportunities through this means to provide better nutritional balance to target populations. Nevertheless, despite changes in the availability of fresh farm produce and its increasingly high cost; social changes which have impacted on how, where and what we eat; nutritional survey evidence that many people fall short of recommended amounts of essential nutrients; increasing scientific evidence that higher amounts of certain nutrient substances may be beneficial to health; rampant institutional malnutrition; an aging population whose special nutritional needs are not well defined; significant advances in food technology; and a third world whose increasing population growth and concern about future decreasing food supplies threaten a human tragedy of immense proportions; regulatory emphasis on control and resistance to change in areas such as food fortification continues.

Although long-term nutrient impacts are difficult to study, in the long term science will ultimately prevail over opinion. In the meantime, while the struggle for nutritional enlightenment continues and scientific knowledge accumulates, we must continue to abide by the applicable statutory and regulatory provisions. It is hoped that this review will be of assistance in understanding these mechanisms.

REFERENCES

1. HUTT, P. B. 1980. FDA food fortification policy. Cereal World 25(7), 397–400.
2. VETTER, J. L. 1982. Adding Nutrients to Foods: Where do we go from here? Am. Assoc. Cereal Chem., St. Paul, Minn.
3. FRATTALI, V. P., VANDERVEEN, J. E. and FORBES, A. L. 1987. The role of the United States government in regulating the nutritional value of the food supply. In Nutritional Evaluation of Food Processing, 3rd Ed., E. Ramas and R. S. Harris (eds.). Van Nostrand Reinhold. New York.
4. United States v. 119 cases . . . "New Dextra Brand Fortified Cane Sugar," 231 F. Supp. 551 (S.D. FLA. 1963), aff'd 334 F. 2d 238 (5th Cir. 1964).
5. Committee Print No. 11, Vitamin, Mineral and Diet Supplements, Oct. 1973, prepared by the staff for the use of the Committee on Interstate and Foreign Commerce, U.S. House of Representatives and its Subcommittee on Public Health and Environment, U.S. Gov. Printing Office, Washington, DC.
6. As set forth in Recommended Dietary Allowances, Publication 1694 of the National Academy of Sciences, 7th Rev. Ed., 1968, A Report of the Food and Nutrition Board, National Research Council.
7. NAS/NRC. 1974. Recommended Dietary Allowances, 8th Ed., National Academy of Sciences/National Research Council, Washington, DC.
8. NAS/NRC. 1980. Recommended Dietary Allowances, 9th Ed., National Academy of Sciences/National Research Council, Washington, DC.
9. NAS/NRC. 1989. Recommended Dietary Allowances, 10th Ed., National Academy of Sciences/National Research Council, Washington, DC.
10. NEWSOME, DR. R. L. 1987. Use of vitamins as additives in processed foods. Food Technol., Sept., 163–168.
11. MERRILL, A. L. and WATT, B. K. 1955. Energy Value of Foods — Basis and Derivation. USDA Handbook 74.
12. AOAC. 1980. Official Methods of Analysis of the Association of Official Analytical Chemists, 13th Ed.
13. National Cancer Institute's (NCI) 1981 publication Diet, Nutrition and Cancer.
14. TAYLOR, S. E. 1988. Health Claims for Foods: Present Law, Future Policy. 43 Food Cosmetic Law J. May, 603–635.
15. "Food Labeling Chaos: The Case for Reform," a Report by the Center for Science in the Public Interest; July, 1989.
16. NAS/NRC. 1981. Food Chemicals Codex, 3rd Ed. National Academy of Sciences/National Research Council, Washington, DC

ADDENDUM

Introduction and Background

As indicated in the main text, at the time of its completion in manuscript form major issues regarding labeling were in a state of flux. This continues to be the case as the manuscript goes to press. While at this point nothing has been finalized, there have been some major developments that should be briefly noted so the reader will be adequately forewarned of impending changes.

On March 7, 1989, Dr. Louis W. Sullivan, Secretary of Health and Human Services, announced a comprehensive food labeling initiative to be undertaken by FDA. This was at least partly a reaction to congressional interest in matters relating to food labeling, largely arising from the emergence of the "health messages" controversy and the increasing scientific evidence on and public interest in relationships between diet and disease. In essence, a race had begun to implement a difficult regulatory process quickly with the hope that congressional legislation might thereby be forestalled. As we shall see the regulatory and legislative process eventually overlapped.

As mentioned in the main text, on August 8, 1989, FDA published an advance notice of proposed rulemaking (ANPRM) in the *Federal Register* [54 *Fed Reg* 32610]. The ANPRM sought public response and comment on food labeling issues in five major areas: requirements for nutrition labeling, nutrition labeling format, requirements for ingredient labeling, definition of food descriptors and use of food standards, and "health messages." FDA also held four national public meetings throughout the country on various labeling subjects: Chicago, Illinois, October 16, 1989, focusing on nutrition labeling content; San Antonio, Texas, November 1, 1989, on ingredient labeling, food standards and descriptors; Seattle, Washington, December 7, 1989, "health messages"; and Atlanta, Georgia, December 13, 1989, on nutrition labeling format. Thousands of responses to the ANPRM were received (approximately 2,000 letters and comments and 5,000 survey forms distributed by a consumer organization and printed in local newspapers), and approximately 200 people offered oral testimony at the public meetings. [The above is detailed in the Jul. 19, 1990 *Fed. Reg.* 55 (139), 29476, 29487-88.] This all created the impression of swift action, while furnishing FDA with whatever support it chose to select to support its ultimate proposals.

FDA began unveiling its new labeling proposals in the July 19, 1990 *Federal Register* cited above. The first four proposed rules, each prefaced with the general heading "Food Labeling" are (1) "Definitions of the Terms Cholesterol Free, Low Cholesterol, and Reduced Cholesterol; Tentative Final Rule" (p. 29456), (2) "Reference Daily Intakes and Daily Reference Values" (p. 29476), (3) "Mandatory Status of Nutrition Labeling and Nutrient Content Revision Sizes" (p. 29487) and (4) "Serving Sizes" (p. 29517). The proposal on cholesterol labeling is not relevant to the discussion of food fortification and the proposal on serving sizes is only indirectly relevant in that the size may affect nutrient density, i.e., a half-ounce serving fortified to a specific level would provide greater nutrient density than a one-ounce serving fortified to the same level.

FDA Proposal on "Daily Values"

The proposal on reference daily intakes (RDI) and daily reference values (DRV) is very significant both in terms of nutrition labeling and public health. In short, partly on the basis of consumer confusion, FDA proposed, not merely to adjust the easily explainable USRDA, but to replace them entirely with a far more complex combination of RDI and DRV, to be known collectively as "Daily Values." To give some idea of the complexity, the RDI for zinc for a "person 4 or more years of age" would be determined by taking every RDA age category for both males and females (12 categories), multiplying the RDA for each category by the number of people in the population in that category (based on the 1980 census, already 10 years old), totaling the number of milligrams in the 12 categories (3,042,401,000) and dividing it by the total population (232,373,000) to yield an RDI of 13 mg. The comparable USRDA (15 mg), based on the 7th Edition of *Recommended Dietary Allowances* published in 1968,[6] was simply the highest RDA for the adult category (excluding pregnant and lactating women). I will leave the readers to judge which method is more confusing, particularly since the RDI apply only to micronutrients and one still must contend with both the DRV, applicable to macronutrients, and the combined term "Daily Values."

It is not the purpose here to go through the proposed RDI and DRV for each of the micro- and macronutrients. However, specific to the micronutrients, the proposed RDI are based on the 10th edition of *Recommended Dietary Allowances* published in 1989.[9] The 1989 RDA already lowered the recommendations for several important micronutrients significantly below those of earlier committees in 1968, 1974 and 1980,[6,7,8] and the averaging technique proposed by FDA results in RDI which are lower still. For example, the USRDA and RDA for folate (folic acid, folacin), uniformly 400 mcg, since 1968 in the adult category, has been lowered to 200 mcg by the 1989 committee and the proposed RDI is 180 mcg. This is a matter of serious concern in that nutritional surveys will now show a phantom improvement in the American diet. Suddenly, problem nutrients will no longer be problems. At the very time when an outflow of scientific evidence is showing that people need more micronutrient intake from a health standpoint, FDA, supported by nutritional conservatives, is indicating the need for less. For example, in the face of several excellent studies showing that women in the periconceptional period need adequate folic acid to reduce the incidence of neural tube defects, the proposed RDI for folate is less than half the former level. FDA will counter that the "Daily Values" are only reference standards for labels and not recommendations for individuals, but there seems little question that they will be interpreted as the latter, not the former. An even larger concern is that government feeding programs will ultimately be impacted by these lowered standards to the nutritional detriment of the elderly, the poor and certain minorities.

FDA is proposing to split the present Pregnant and Lactating Women category into two separate categories; to change the reference standard for calories from 2,000 Kcal to 2,350 Kcal (impacting negatively on nutrient density); to adopt the NAS/NRC's use of retinol equivalents (RE) for vitamin A in place of International Units (IU), even though Ph.D. nutritional scientists have trouble calculating RE; and to change from IU for vitamin E to tocopherol equivalents (TE), which, while easy to calculate, causes its own confusion. On the other hand, FDA has not addressed the issue of nutrient recommendations for the elderly (the RDA stop at 51+), or the matter of separate label listing or reference values for beta carotene, despite dozens of studies showing associations between diets high in this important micronutrient and lowered incidence of certain types of cancer and other diseases.

Instead of using independent judgment, FDA has chosen to rely almost entirely on a few expert reports, which in turn rely on each other. The problem is that each of these reports is the product of a closed process, so the net result is that national nutrition policy, with all its far-reaching implications, is being set by a nutritional inner sanctum despite the notice and review procedure FDA is bound to follow by law. This leads to a traditional stance, which has never been successful in practice, as exemplified by this quotation from the proposal on "Daily Values," referring to the expert reports on which FDA is relying:

> The recommendations and guidelines place their emphasis on the total diet, not on individual foods. There is a general consensus among them that nutritional and health goals should be achieved through changes in food consumption patterns rather than through fortification and supplementation practices. In consideration of this emphasis, the agency has decided that as part of its efforts to respond to the changing nutrition information needs of consumers, a revision of nutrition labeling, including updating of the USRDAs, is needed.

The irony is that at the same time FDA is promoting government recommended diets that are high in vegetables and fruits and lower in fats, it is proposing RDI for micronutrients which are significantly lower in a number of instances than the levels consumers would attain through eating the very diets being recommended. In any case, the apparent negative attitude of FDA toward fortification and supplementation, combined with the lowering of the reference standards have obvious implications.

FDA's Proposal on Nutrition Labeling

FDA's July 19, 1990 proposal on nutrition labeling is premised on expanding required information on nutrient content to many more foods, including fresh fruits and vegetables. The overall approach is to make nutrition labeling mandatory unless the food product falls within one of 13 defined exemptions. The proposal, of course, is impacted by the federal legislation discussed below.

Regarding macronutrients, for the most part the nutrition labeling proposal is not directly relevant to fortification. As to this, however, FDA proposed that the following be included in a formatted way: serving size; servings per container; calories per serving (in designated increments); calories from fat (in designated increments) and on a voluntary basis calories from saturated fatty acids, unsaturated fatty acids, carbohydrate and protein; fat and saturated fatty acids in grams per serving, and on a voluntary basis unsaturated fatty acids, which may be further broken down into poly- and monounsaturated; cholesterol per serving in milligrams; carbohydrate in grams (of total digestible) per serving, and on a voluntary basis complex carbohydrate, sugars and sugar alcohols; fiber in grams per serving, and on a voluntary basis soluble and insoluble fiber; protein, sodium; and potassium on a voluntary basis.

Regarding micronutrients, FDA is proposing substantial changes. Thiamin, riboflavin and niacin would no longer be included in the nutrition labeling table on a mandatory basis. Only vitamin A, vitamin C, calcium, and iron would be required to be shown in the nutrition labeling table. Other micronutrients for which FDA has established an intake standard [under 21 CFR Sect. 101.9(c)(10)(iv)] would be required to be included, if added or the subject of a claim, and otherwise would be includible on a voluntary basis. These would be stated in specified increments (2% as the lowest) of the proposed RDI, but the label would refer to "Daily Value," supposedly to avoid consumer confusion.

Allowable synonyms would be ascorbic acid for vitamin C (but not its salts), folacin for the preferred folate (no longer to be called folic acid), and energy for calories. Inconceivably, vitamin B_1 and vitamin B_2 (in use longer than many readers have been alive) would not be allowable synonyms for thiamin (no longer to end with an "e") and riboflavin, respectively. The reason: according to the FDA proposal, the 10th edition of *Recommended Dietary Allowances* did not refer to them, therefore they "can be considered outdated." So much for the rest of the nutritional world, which had no previous opportunity to input on the issue whether through FDA's ANPRM of August 8, 1989, or otherwise. Also, FDA continues to include beta carotene under the vitamin A designation despite very persuasive scientific evidence that it has nutritional significance beyond its provitamin A function and despite growing public interest in this important nutrient.

Congressional Legislation

While the comment period on the FDA proposals discussed above was still open, Congress passed H.R. 3562, the "Nutrition Labeling and Education Act of 1990" (the "Act"). This was signed into law by the President on November 8, 1990. The Act will necessitate some revisions to the FDA proposals, mainly in the area of nutrition labeling.

The Act provides that covered products will be misbranded, if they do not contain required information. The basic information called for by the Act includes serving size, number of servings, and, on a per serving basis, calories derived from any source and from total fat, saturated fat, cholesterol, sodium, total carbohydrates, complex carbohydrates, sugars, dietary fiber and total protein. FDA is given fairly wide discretion regarding inclusion and exclusion, especially regarding vitamins, minerals and other nutrients in addition to those mentioned.

There are also provisions regarding nutrition information for raw fish and raw agricultural commodities (fruits and vegetables). Various exemptions are included, such as for restaurant foods, infant formula, medical foods, small packages and small businesses. There are limitations on claims regarding cholesterol, and dietary fiber, as well as regarding implied claims contained in the brand names of foods.

The Act addresses the "Health Messages" issue directly. The Secretary of Health and Human Services is specifically required to "determine whether claims respecting the following nutrients and diseases" should be allowed for food products: calcium and osteoporosis, dietary fiber and cancer, lipids and cardiovascular disease, lipids and cancer, sodium and hypertension, and dietary fiber and cardiovascular disease.

Interestingly, late amendments in the Senate provide for the establishment of a separate "procedure and standard respecting the validity of claims made with respect to a dietary supplement of vitamins, minerals, herbs, or other similar substances . . . ." In this respect a specific requirement is included requiring determination of the validity of claims for "folic acid and neural tube defects, antioxidant vitamins and cancer, zinc and immune function in the elderly, and omega-3 fatty acids and heart disease." (See *Congressional Record*, S16607-S16612, Oct. 24, 1990.) Other important aspects of the Act include limited preemption provisions and strict time limits for the completion of regulations to implement these amendments to the *FD& C Act*.

Since most of this does not impact directly on food fortification, more detailed analysis is not warranted. It is hoped, however, that this Addendum has served its purpose of alerting the reader to the impending new and amended regulations involving cholesterol labeling, changes regarding the USRDA, nutrition labeling, "Health Messages," and others, e.g., product descriptors. Food fortification will continue to be an important modality in assuring adequate nutrition in a changing world. Advances in food technology and rational fortification practices based on rapidly emerging nutritional science can be important weapons in the fight for good health and the dietary war against chronic diseases, if they are not impeded by overly restrictive regulatory policies. Working with the government, academia, consumer groups, trade and professional associations and all the others interested in good nutrition to assure sound fortification regulations and policies will be a continuing challenge for the food industry.

CHAPTER 21

REGULATION OF FOOD FORTIFICATION: OTHER COUNTRIES[1]

IRINA DU BOIS

Food enrichment generally designates the addition of nutrients to foods in order to improve their nutritional value; this addition is meant to help prevent, treat or eliminate nutrient deficiencies. According to the Codex Alimentarius,[2] a *nutrient* means any substance normally consumed as a constituent of food, (1) which provides energy, or (2) which is needed for growth, development and maintenance of life or (3) a deficit of which will cause characteristic biochemical or physiological changes.

Nutrients together with food components and technological additives form the ingredients of an industrial food product. They have to comply with certain legal prescriptions as far as their *addition* to food and their *declaration* on the label are concerned. This paper deals specifically with the addition of vitamins and minerals.

When discussing the general topic of enrichment, various terms are usually utilized: fortification, restoration, standardization and supplementation. Without going into details of definitions, it should be pointed out that, generally, *fortification* or *enrichment* means specifically the addition of nutrients to a food above the level normally found in that food. *Restoration* means the addition of nutrients to a food to compensate for losses during processing or storage. *Standardization* means the addition of nutrients to a food to compensate for natural variations. A more general term of *supplementation* which is sometimes used means the addition to a food of nutrients which are not contained naturally in that food or only in minute quantities.

In this paper, the following aspects of legislation on food *enrichment* will be considered: (1) the compulsory addition of vitamins and minerals; (2) the optional addition of vitamins and minerals, also in relation to permitted claims on the label; (3) example of restrictive regulations on addition of vitamins and minerals, and (4) the declaration of vitamins and minerals on the label trying to show the problems encountered by food manufacturers.

---

[1]Reprinted with permission of S. Karger AG, Basel.
[2]FAO/WHO Food Standards Programme.

COMPULSORY ADDITION OF VITAMINS AND MINERALS

One can distinguish four categories of foodstuffs where addition of vitamins and minerals is compulsory in some countries: (1) foods for special dietary uses; (2) staple foods representing an ideal vehicle for nutrients; (3) foods resembling a common food (replacement products), and (4) foods having lost nutrients during manufacturing.

Foods for Special Dietary Uses

According to the EC (European Community) definition, foods for special dietary uses or foods for particular nutritional uses are foodstuffs which, owing to their special composition or manufacturing process, are clearly distinguishable from foodstuffs for normal consumption, which are suitable for their claimed nutritional purposes and which are marketed in such a way as to indicate such suitability. A particular nutritional use must fulfil the particular nutritional requirements: (1) of certain categories of persons whose digestive processes or metabolism are disturbed: or (2) of certain categories of person who are in a special physiological condition and who are therefore able to obtain a special benefit from a controlled consumption of certain substances in foodstuffs, or (3) of infants or young children in good health.

The addition of vitamins and minerals is compulsory practically all over the world for one category of foods for special dietary uses, viz., for *infant formulae*. Infant formulae are special products, *complete* foods intended for use where necessary as a substitute for human milk in meeting the normal nutritional requirements of infants up to 4–6 months of age. The term "infant" in the terminology of Codex Alimentarius designates a person of not more than 12 months. As an example, we may mention the requirements of the Codex standard for infant formulae regarding the composition of such products Table 21.1.

There are other subcategories of foods for special dietary uses where the addition of vitamins and minerals is compulsory. E.g., Germany, the addition of vitamins A, B_1, B_2, B_6, C, D, E, calcium and iron to meal replacements for weight control or weight reduction is compulsory with minima per meal and per daily portion. However, the discussion on foods for special dietary uses goes beyond the scope of our presentation on general food enrichment. We shall come back to these when discussing the French legislation.

Staple Foods

Many countries advocate the enrichment of staple foods with nutrients in order to reach the majority of the population. Of course, staple foods vary from one geographical area to another and from one population to another.

The father or grandfather of such a fortification was certainly the French chemist

TABLE 21.1
CODEX STANDARD FOR INFANT FORMULAE (STAN 72—1981)

	Per 100 kcal	
	Minimum	Maximum
Protein, g	1.8	4
Fat, g	3.3	6
Carbohydrates, g	—	—
Linoleic acid, mg	300	—
Vitamin A, IU	250	500
as retinol, μg	75	150
Vitamin D, IU	40	80
Vitamin E, IU	0.7	—
Vitamin C, mg	8	—
Thiamin (B_1), μg	40	—
Riboflavin (B_2), μg	60	—
Nicotinamide, μg	250	—
Vitamin B_6, μg	35	—
Folic acid, μg	4	—
Panotothenic acid, μg	300	—
Vitamin B_{12}, μg	0.15	—
Vitamin K_1, μg	4	—
Biotin, μg	1.5	—
Choline, mg	7	—
Sodium, mg	20	60
Potassium, mg	80	200
Chloride, mg	55	150
Calcium, mg	50	—
Phosphorus, mg	25	—
Magnesium, mg	6	—
Iron, mg	0.15 1[1]	—
Iodine, μg	5	—
Copper, μg	60	—
Zinc, mg	0.5	—
Manganese, μg	5	—
Ca/P ratio	1.2	2.0

—Not specified.
[1] To be labelled "Infant formula with iron".

Boussingault who started in 1833 to recommend the addition of iodine to *salt* in order to prevent goiter. Little by little, the addition of iodine to salt spread worldwide and became one of the most effective public health measures. The situation today in Europe is shown in Table 21.2: countries like Austria, Switzerland, the Netherlands and Poland require a compulsory supplementation of salt with iodine, whereas it

TABLE 21.2
ADDITION OF IODINE AND FLUORINE TO TABLE SALT (NACL)

Country	I^-, F^-	Limits, mg/kg Minimum	Limits, mg/kg Maximum	Salts	Remarks
Austria	I^-	7.5 (= 10KI)	10.7 (= 14 KI)	KI	Compulsory for "complete salt"[1]
France	I^-	10	15	NaI	Permitted with declaration
	F^-		250	KF	Permitted with declaration
Germany	I^-	15	25	KIO_3 $NaIO_3$	Compulsory in *dietetic* "iodized salt"
Greece	I^-	31 ± 3.1 (= 40 KI)	46 ± 4.6 (= 60 KI)	KI	Permitted with declaration
Italy	I^-		15 (= 20 KI)	KI	
The Netherlands	I^-	18 (= 23 KI)	22 (= 29 KI)	KI, KIO_3	Compulsory for salt used in bread
Norway	I^-		25		Permitted with declaration[2]
Spain	I^-		60 ± 9	KI, KIO_3	Permitted with declaration[3]
	F^-	90	225	NaF	Permitted with declaration[4]
Sweden	I^-	40	70	NaI, KI	Permitted with declaration[5]
Switzerland	I^-	15		KI	Compulsory[5]
	F^-	250		KF	Compulsory[5]
UK	I^-	25	30		Recommended, not regulated

[1]Salt without the addition of KI must be labelled "not iodized."
[2]Not regarded as necessary, since high sea food consumption.
[3]It is permitted to have salt with both I^- and F^- added.
[4]Level to be declared: 50 mg/kg.
[5]Salt without addition of KI and KF is available.

is optional everywhere else. In Germany, iodized salt is considered as a food for special dietary use.

Other examples of public health measures by fortification of staple foods are the addition of vitamin D to *milk*, in order to prevent rickets (compulsory for instance in Canada and in evaporated milk in the United States), the addition of fluorine to *potable water* or *salt* to prevent caries (compulsory for instance in Switzerland).

Vitamin A deficiency and xerophthalmia are among the most widespread nutritional disorders that affect man, particularly in tropical and subtropical countries. To fight against these disorders, vitamin A is customarily added to various foodstuffs for the purpose of restoration and enrichment; e.g., its addition to *skim milk powder* is compulsory in Canada, in the United States and for distribution through supplementary feeding projects in countries where xerophthalmia is a public health problem. In Europe, the restoration or enrichment of skim milk powder with vitamin A is permitted in Germany, Switzerland, the United Kingdom, Sweden, Greece and France. Other vehicles have been used for enrichment with vitamin A: *rice, white sugar* (Guatemala, 1969), *tea* (India) and *monosodium glutamate* (Philippines).

Food Resembling a Common Food (Replacement Products)

In many countries, the addition of vitamins and minerals is compulsory to foodstuffs resembling common foodstuffs and intended for consumption in place of the latter. The best example of course is the addition of vitamins A and D to *margarine*. Table 21.3 shows the current situation in Europe: compulsory addition in Belgium, Denmark, the Netherlands, Norway, Sweden, the United Kingdom and, as far as we know, Poland and Hungary.

Another example is *texturized vegetable protein foods*, which simulate meat. In the UK and Italy they shall contain minima of vitamins per 100 g: B_1, 2 mg; vitamin B_2, 0.8 mg; vitamin B_{12}, 5 μg; and iron 10 mg.

Foods Having Lost Nutrients during Manufacturing

It is a quite common practice to restore foodstuffs with vitamins and minerals lost during manufacturing. The best known example is the restoration of vitamin B_1, B_2, niacin and iron to *flour*. This restoration, prescribed by law for instance in Canada, is compulsory in Europe to the best of our knowledge only in the United Kingdom and Denmark. In the United Kingdom, all types of flour other than wholemeal shall contain minima of vitamins per 100 g: B_1, 0.24 mg; niacin, 1.60 mg; and iron, 1.65 mg. In Denmark, flour shall contain per kg: vitamin B_1, 5 mg; vitamin B_2, 5 mg; calcium, 2 g; and iron 30 mg. Furthermore, in Denmark, rye flour shall contain calcium (4 g/kg) and iron (30 mg/kg), and rolled oats shall contain calcium (2.3 g/kg) and phosphorus (1.8 g/kg). The addition of vitamins A and D to *skim milk powder*, which we have considered already, is of course also a form of vitamin restoration.

OPTIONAL ADDITION OF VITAMINS AND MINERALS

In many countries, the addition of vitamins and minerals to food is optional, provided the resulting product is properly labeled. One of the oldest existing legislations which represents a "modèle du genre," is the Swiss legislation. In Switzerland, vitamins may be added to any foodstuff, except to alcoholic drinks (and tobacco).

Priority should be given to restoration, but addition of vitamins above the natural

TABLE 21.3
ADDITION OF VITAMINS A AND D TO MARGARINE

Country	Vitamin A IU/100 g		Vitamin D IU/100 g		Remarks
	Minimum	Maximum	Minimum	Maximum	
Austria	1,000	2,000	100		Optional
Belgium	2,500	3,000	250	300	Compulsory, also for minarine
Denmark		2,400		50	Compulsory, also for minarine
Finland		1,800		280	
Germany		3,333		100	Optional, also for minarine
Greece		2,500		150	Optional
The Netherlands	2,000[1]	300[2]			
Norway		2,000		250	Compulsory
Sweden	3,000	5,000	300	400	Compulsory, also for minarine
Switzerland		~2,800[3] ~8,400[4]		~250[3] ~750[4]	Optional
UK	2,680	3,315	283	352	Compulsory

[1] Compulsory.
[2] Optional.
[3] If reference to vitamin content.
[4] If claim "rich in. . .".

level is permitted in Switzerland, provided it does not exceed three times the recommended daily allowance (RDA) in a daily food portion (this is specified in an official table). However, vitamin D RDA cannot be exceeded. A reference on the label to a given vitamin may only be made if at least one-third of the RDA is contained in the daily food portion, and a specific claim; e.g., "rich in," is permitted only if 100% of the RDA is contained in the daily portion.

In Germany, the optional addition of all watersoluble vitamins, vitamin K and E is permitted to all foodstuffs for the purpose of restoration, enrichment and supplementation. The relation between claims on the label and minimum vitamin content is exactly the same as in Switzerland. The maxima permitted are three times the RDA. RDAs are defined. However, vitamins A and D may be added only to margarine and minarine (half-fat margarine) and to half-fat milk products. No specific regulations exist on the addition of minerals.

In the United Kingdom, the addition of vitamins and minerals is permitted to all foodstuffs except alcoholic drinks. Claims may be made in respect to the following vitamins: A, B_1, B_2, niacin, folic acid, B_{12}, C and D, and in respect to calcium, iodine and iron. If a claim is made on the label that a food is a *rich* or *excellent* source of vitamins or minerals, then the daily food portion must contain at least one-half of the RDA for that nutrient. For any other claim, the daily portion must contain at least one-sixth of the RDA. A list of RDAs is established and the daily food portion is defined as "the quantity of the food that can reasonably be expected to be consumed in one day."

In Sweden, general permissions exist to add vitamins A and D to low-fat milk and edible oils, and vitamins B_1, B_2, B_6 and iron to wheat flour, mixtures of rye and wheat flour, macaroni, spaghetti and other pasta products. Authorizations for special enrichments may be given.

In Belgium, the optional addition of vitamins and minerals to foodstuffs is, in principle, permitted. Special regulations govern the addition of vitamins A and D to margarine, the addition of vitamins B_1, B_2 and niacin to breakfast cereals and other specified additions. Italy, Portugal and Spain have no regulations on vitamins and minerals. Special permissions may be given for their use.

RESTRICTIVE REGULATIONS ON THE ADDITION OF VITAMINS AND MINERALS

There are several countries in Europe where a rather reluctant attitude towards the addition of vitamins and minerals to foods prevails. France belongs to this category of countries.

According to French legislation, enrichment, standardization and supplementation with vitamins are permitted only for foods for special dietary used, e.g., infant foods or low-calorie foods. There are only two situations when normal foods for healthy adults may bear the label claim "with a guaranteed vitamin content": (1) in the case of special processing which maintains the natural amount of vitamins unaltered, and (2) in the case of restoration with vitamins to compensate losses during manufacturing (the aim of restoration is 80–200% of the naturally occurring vitamin content in the raw materials). However, normal foods labeled "with a guaranteed vitamin content" are regulated like the foods for special dietary uses.

In the framework of a general anti-additive policy, the Netherlands also have a very restrictive legislation where no optional addition of vitamins and minerals to food is permitted. Exceptions are made only for infant formulae, special low-calorie foods and margarine. Vitamins lost by processing may not be restored.

In Norway and Finland, general addition of vitamins and minerals to foodstuffs is forbidden. Special permissions for particular types of products may be issued.

DECLARATION OF VITAMINS AND MINERALS ON THE LABEL

We have seen how regulations on the addition of vitamins and minerals vary from one country to another; labelling regulations are also quite divergent, when they exist at all, and cannot be discussed in detail in this presentation.

Generally, vitamins and minerals must appear in the list of ingredients, either in descending order of proportion or as a separate group. In addition, the numerical declaration per 100 g or 100 ml of food must be given. The manufacturer must ensure that the declared values are still present in the product until the end of the minimum durability, respectively expiry period, according to national legislations.

In this context, a very important document on nutrition labeling exists and should become the basis for further regulation: the Codex Alimentarius Guidelines on Nutrition Labelling, which were adopted by the Codex in 1985 and will be sent to governments for acceptance very soon.

CONCLUSION

To conclude, we have tried to show how regulations concerning food enrichment vary from one country to another, depending on a rather liberal or rather restrictive philosophy on this matter. Many problems arise for food manufacturers due to the lack of harmonization in this field.

Addition to foods of vitamins and minerals implies in some countries that these foods are perishable (France and Italy), are foods for special dietary uses (France), or even drugs (foods containing vitamin D in France).

The authorizations to make claims are quite divergent from one country to another.

The definitions themselves of the vitamins may differ: are substances like choline, biotin, pantothenic acid and vitamin K considered to be vitamins everywhere?

The lists of RDAs often vary from one country to another.

Methods of analysis sometimes differ.

In some countries, the reference for addition of nutrients is 100 g or 100 kcal, whereas in some others this is the food serving (or edible portion or daily portion). However, serving sizes or daily portions of a given food substance are totally different from one population to another according to eating habits.

If existing at all, regulations on tolerances for nutrient declaration differ from one country to another Table 21.4.

Last but not least, the only food category where the addition of vitamins and minerals may be of concern because of the "megavitamin" doses, the so-called "health foods," is not regulated at all.

With science progressing continuously, regulations have to be adjusted accordingly. Therefore, we stress the need for cooperation between scientists, legislators and food manufacturers. A significant example of cooperation is the Food Standards Programme sponsored by FAO/WHO within the Codex Alimentarius scheme.

TABLE 21.4
TOLERANCES ON DECLARATION OF VITAMINS AND MINERALS

Country	Tolerances	Remarks
USA	− 0% TO + GMP	For added vitamins and/or minerals
	−20% TO + GMP	For naturally occurring vitamins and/or minerals
Denmark	−10%	For normal foods
	− 0%	For infant foods
Italy	−20 TO + 30%	For vitamins B group, A, K, D
	−20 TO + 50%	For vitamins C, E
	−75 TO + 75%	If amount < 0.5 mg/100 g or 250 IU/100 g
Greece	± 5%	For infant formulae (agreement)
Germany	±15%	Not regulated, general agreement
The Netherlands	−20 TO + 100%	For infant formulae
Norway	±15%	
UK	±10%	Not regulated, general agreement

GMP = Good manufacturing practice.

APPENDIX

Regulatory Prescriptions

Austria
Lebensmittelkennzeichnungsverordnung   07.12.1973
Österreichisches Lebensmittelbuch, chapter A7: Diätetische Lebensmittel

Belgium
Arrêté Royal fixant la liste des additifs autorisés dans les denrées alimentaires
   (avec les modifications)   27.07.1978
Arrêté Royal sur la fabrication et à la mise dans le commerce   02.10.1980
   de la margarine et des graisses comestibles (avec les modifications)

Codex Alimentarius
Codex Standard for Infant Formula
(Codex STAN 72-1981 in Codex Alimentarius, vol. 9; 1st ed. Rome 1982)
Alinorm 85/26
   Annex 2 to appendix V: Proposed Draft Guidelines for the Use of Codex Committees on the Inclusion of Provisions on Nutritional Quality in Food Standards and other Codex Texts (at Step 5)
   Appendix VII: General Principles for the Addition of Nutrients to Foods
Codex Alimentarius Guidelines on Nutrition Labelling
(Alinorm 85/22 A Appendix III)

Denmark
Executive Order on Foods for Special Dietary Uses,   06.06.1973
Bekendtgorelse om levnedsmidler bestemt til en saerling ernaering (with modification)
Food Additives, "Godkendte tilsaetningsstoffer til levnedsmidler-positivlisten"   1983
See also "Produktliste Vurdering og regulering av Helsekostproduker; NORDEN"   1985
PNUN, Rapport 1985:1

EC
Directive du Conseil relative au rapprochement des législations des Etats   21.12.1976
membres concernant les denrées alimentaires destinées à une alimentation particulière
(No. 77/94/CEE).J.O.C.E. No. L 26 du 31.01.1977

Finland
Decree No. 281 on the addition of vitamins and   14.04.1972
certain other substances to foodstuffs, "Förordning om tillsättning av vitaminer och vissa andra ämnen i livsmedel" (with modifications)
See also: "Produktliste Vurdering og regulering av Helsekostprodukter i NORDEN"1985
PNUN, Rapport 1985:1

France
Produits diététiques et de régime
J.O.R.F., 1ère ed., 1983, No. 1545 (et amendements)

Germany
Verordnung über vitaminisierte Lebensmittel   01.09.1942
(last modification of 06.11.1984)
"Empfehlungen für die Vitaminisierung von Lebensmitteln"
Lebensmittelchem. Gerichtl. Chemie 36: 150–154 (1982)
Empfehlungen der GDCH-Arbeitsgruppe "Fragen der Ernährung"
(Protokoll vom 20.06.1985)
Diätverordnung   21.01.1982
Entwurf einer Verordnung zur Änderung der
Nährwert-Kennzeichnungsverordnung und der Diätverordnung. Stand: 15.08.1985
Zusatzstoff-Zulassungs-Verordnung   22.12.1981
(with modifications)
Zusatzstoff-Verkehrs-Verordnung   10.07.1984
Empfehlungen für die Nährstoffzufuhr.
Viete erweiterte Überarbeitung, 1985
Umschau Verlag, Frankfurt am Main

Greece
Greek Food Codex   1971
(Art 38.6)

Italy
Decreto Ministeriale.   18.07.1979
Autorizzazione alla produzione, importazione e commercio di farina
di soja sgrassata ristrutturata e di proteine di soja concentrate ristrutturate nonchè
di prodotti a base di tali sostanze. Gazzetta Uffic. Rep. Italiana di 4.8.1979

Circolare No. 27 di Ministero della Sanità nel quale sono stati   22.03.1984
fissati limiti di accettabilità dei titoli riscontrati in sede di analisi preventiva
sugli alimenti per la prima infanzia ed i prodotti dietetici

Norway
General regulations No. 1252 concerning the production and marketing   08.07.1983
of foodstuffs (III. Additives, minerals, vitamins)
See also: "Produktliste Vurdering og regulering av Helsekostprodukter i NORDEN"
PNUN, Rapport 1985:1

Spain
Real Decreto 2685   16.10.1976

Reglamentacion para preparados alimenticios
para regimenes dietéticos y/o especiales
(with modifications)
Real Decreto 1424 27.04.1983
Reglamentacion de la Sal
Codigo Sanitario Espanol 1967
Seccion 5 a: Alimentos Enriquecidos y sustancias enriquecedoras

Sweden
Enrichment Substances in Food 04.02.1983
(SLV FS 1983:2)
See also: "Produktliste Vurdering og regulering av Helsekostprodukter i NORDEN"
PNUN, Rapport 1985:1

Switzerland
Verfügung des Eidgenössischen Departements des Innern 07.03.1957
über Zusatz und Anpreisung von Vitaminen bei Lebensmitteln

UK
Food Labelling Regulations 1984 S.I. 1984 No. 1305; 15.08.1984
Bread and Flour Regulations 1984 S.I. 1984 No. 1304; 15.08.1984
Margarine Regulations 1967 (S.I. 1967 No. 1867 as amended) 14.12.1967
Butterworths Law of Food & Drugs
Report on Novel Protein Foods MAFF, 1974
Food Standards Committee
FSC/REP/62

Others
"Produktliste Vurdering og regulering av Helsekostprodukter I NORDEN"
PNUN, Rapport 1985:1

Addition of Vitamins to Foodstuffs— October 1980
Analysis and Comparison of the Regulations of some Developed Countries.
J.P. Matthieu, J.P. Mareschi,
Hoffmann-La Roche & Co. Ltd., Basel, Switzerland

DIRECTORY

JOINT FAO/WHO CODEX ALIMENTARIUS COMMISSION 1990 LIST OF CODEX CONTACT POINTS[1]

ALGERIA
Ministère du Commerce
Direction générale du commerce intérieur
Service du contrôle de la qualité et de la répression des fraudes
Rue Mohamed Belouizdad 44
Alger

ANGOLA
Ministère des relations extérieures de la République populaire d'Angola
Départment des affaires politiques
Secteur des organisations internationales
Luanda

ANTIGUA & BARBUDA
Mr. Roland A. Thomas
Director, Bureau of Antigua and Barbuda Standards
c/o Ministry of Agriculture, Fisheries, Lands and Housing
High Street
St. Johns
Antigua

ARGENTINA
Dr. A. M. Sanchez
Coordinador del Codex Alimentarius
Secretaría de Estado de Comercio y Negociaciones Económicas Internacionales
Avenida Julio A. Rocca 651, 5° Piso
Sector 13
100 Buenos Aires

AUSTRALIA
Director
Food Inspection and Support Services
Australian Quarantine and Insp. Service
Department of Primary Industries and Energy
Edmund Barton Building
Broughton Street
Canberra, A.C.T. 2600

AUSTRIA
Bundesministerium für Land und Forstwirtschaft (Division III/A/3)
Stubenring 1
A-1010 Vienna

BAHRAIN
Dr. Rifa'at Abdul Hameed
Director of Public Health
P.O. Box 42
Manama

BANGLADESH
The Director-General
Bangladesh Standards and Testing Institution (BSTI)
116/A, Tejgaon Industrial Area
Dhaka 8

BARBADOS
Director
Barbados National Standards Institution
"Flodden," Culloden Road
St. Michael

---

[1]Inquiries regarding current regulations on nutrient additives to foods or acceptance of specific nutrified foods in countries outside the United States might be directed to these listed sources with the request that the inquiry be directed to the proper governmental agency and personnel dealing with such matters.

BELGIUM
Comité Belge du Codex Alimentarius
Service du commerce international des
  matières premières et produits
  agricoles (B14)
Ministère des relations extérieures rue
  Quatre-Bras, 2
B-1000 Bruxelles

BENIN
Secrétariat de la Commission nationale
  du Codex ALimentarius
Direction de l'Alimentation et de la
  Nutrition appliquée (DANA)
Boîte Postale N° 295
Porto Novo

BOLIVIA
Director, Departmento de Nutrición
Ministerio de Salud Pública
Mariscal Sta. Cruz, Ed. de la Loteria, P.
La Paz

BOTSWANA
The Director of Veterinary Services
Private Bag 0032
Gaborone

BRAZIL
DIE—Divisao de Organismos Internacionales Especializados
Ministerio das Relacoes Exteriores
Espl. dos Ministerios, Pal. do
  Itamaraty
70.170 Brasilia

BULGARIA
Monsieur le Chef de la Section de la
  Commission du Codex Alimentarius
Union nationale agro-industrielle
55, boul. Botev
Sofia

BURKINA FASO
Ministre du développement rural
Ministère du développement rural
Ouagadougou

BURUNDI
M. le Directeur général de
  l'agriculture
Ministère de l'agriculture et de
  l'élevage
B.P. 1850
Bujumbura

CAMEROON
Ministre d'Etat chargé du plan et de
  l'amenagement du territoir
Ministère du plan et de l'amenagement
  du territoire
B.P. 1004
Yaoundé

CANADA
Mr. B. L. Smith
Vice-Chairman,
Canadian Interdepartmental Committee
  on Codex Alimentarius
Health and Welfare Canada
Room 200, H.P.B. Building
Tunney's Pasture
Ottawa, Ontario K1A 0L2

CAPE VERDE
Gabinete de Estudos e Planeamento
Ministerio do Desenvolvimento Rural e
  Pescas
Caixa Postal 115
Cidade de Praia

CENTRAL AFRICAN REP.
Ministère d'Etat chargé du développement rural
Ministère du développement rural
Bangui

CHAD
Direction du génie sanitaire et de
  l'assainissement—Sous-direction de
  l'assainissement
B.P. 440
N'Djamena

CHILE
Ministerio de Salud Pública
Monjitas 689, 5° Piso
Santiago

CHINA
Mr. Xu Guanghua
Department of Science & Technology
Ministry of Agriculture, Animal Husbandry and Fisheries
Beijing

COLOMBIA
Dr. Guillermo Benitez Bejarano Jefe
Sección Control de Alimentos
Dirección General de Saneamiento
Calle 55, N° 10-32, Oficina 308
Bogotà, D.E.

CONGO
Représentant de la FAO au Congo et à Sao Tomé-et-Principe
B.P. 972
Brazzaville

COSTA RICA
Comité Nacional del Codex Alimentarius
Oficina Nacional de Normas y Unidades de Medida
Ministerio de Economia, Industria y Comercio
Apartado 10216
1000 San José

COTE D'IVOIRE
M. le Secrétaire général
Comité national pour l'alimentation et le développement
B.P. V 190
Abidjan

CUBA
Sr. Director
Relaciones Internacionales
Comité Estatal de Normalización
Egido 610 e/ Gloria y Apodaca
Zona Postal 2
La Habana

CYPRUS
Dr. Ioannis G. Karis
Director,
Cyprus Organization for Standards and Control of Quality
Ministry of Commerce and Industry
Nicosia

CZCHOSLOVAKIA
Czechoslovak National FAO Committee
International Department
Federal Ministry of Agriculture and Food
Tesnov 17
110 06 Praha 1

DENMARK
Veterinaerdirektoratet
Rolighedsvej 25
1958 Frederiksberg C

DOMINICAN REP.
Secretaría de Estado de Salud Pública y Asistencia Social
(Sección de Control de Alimentos)
Ensanche La Fe
Santo Domingo

ECUADOR
Sr. Director General
Instituto Ecuatoriano de Normalización
Calle Baquerizo Moreno 454 y Avenida 6 de Diciembre
P.O. Box 3999
Quito

EGYPT
The President
Egyptian Organization for Standardization (EOS)
2 Latin America Street
Garden City
Cairo

EL SALVADOR
Dirección General
Centro de Tecnología Agrícola
Santa Tecla

EQUATORIAL GUINEA
Mr. Alejandro Ndjoli Mediko
Jefe Nacional de Estadísticas Agropecuarias
Ministerio de Agricultura, Ganadería y Desarrollo Rural
Malabo (Bioko Norte)

ETHIOPIA
Ethiopian Standards Institution
P.O. Box 2310
Addis Ababa

FIJI
The Permanent Secretary
Ministry of Agriculture and Fisheries
P.O. Box 358
Suva

FINLAND
Ministry of Trade and Industry
Advisory Committee on Foodstuffs
General Secretary
Box 230
00171 Helsinki

FRANCE
Mme J. Vergnettes
Secrétaire Général, Comité national du
 Codex Alimentarius
Direction Générale de la Concurrence,
 de la Consommation et de la
 Répression des fraudes
13, rue St. Georges
75436 Paris Cedex 09

GABON
Commission nationale de la FAO
Ministère de l'agriculture, de l'élevage
 et de l'économie rurale
B.P. 551
Libreville

GAMBIA
The Director of Agriculture
Department of Agriculture
Ministry of Agriculture
Central Bank Bldg.
Buckle Street
Banjul

GERMANY
International Relations Department
Ministry of Public Health
Rathausstrasse 3
1020 Berlin

Prof. Dr. D. Eckert
Ministerialdirektor
Bundesministerium für Jugend,
 Familie, Frauen und Gesundheit
Deutschherrenstrasse 87
Postfach 20 02 20
D-5300 Bonn 2

GHANA
The Director
Ghana Standards Board
P.O. Box M-245
Accra

GREECE
Division of Processing & Marketing of
 Agricultural Products
Dept. of Standardization & Quality
 Control of Processed Agricultural
 Products
Ministry of Agriculture
2 rue Acharnon
104 32 Athens

GRENADA
Dr. Peter Radix
Director, Grenada Bureau of Standards
c/o Produce Chemist Laboratory
Tanteen
St. George's

GUATEMALA
Dr. L. H. Díaz López,
Director-Técnico
Inspección Sanitaria y Control de
 Alimentos de Origen Animal
Ministerio de Agric., Gan., y
 Alimentación
Avenida Reforma 8-60, Zona 9
Ciudad Guatemala

GUINEA
M. le Directeur
Institut de Normalisation et de
 Métrologie
c/o Ministère de l'Industrie, du Com-
 merce et de l'Artisanat
B.P. 468
Conakry

GUINEA-BISSAU
Ministère du développement rural
B.P. 71
BISSAU

GUYANA
Cde. Lorna Lawrence,
Director (Designate)
Guyana National Bureau of Standards
Ministry of Works Compound
P.O. Box 10926—Fort Street
Kingston, Georgetown

HAITI
Direction normalisation et contrôle de qualité
Ministère du commerce
8, rue Légitime, Champ de Mars
Port-au-Prince

HONDURAS
Ing. Manuel Antonio Cáceres Pineda
Director General de Alimentación y Nutrición
Ministerio de Salud Pública
Tegucigalpa, D.C.

HUNGARY
The Vice President
Hungarian Office for Standardization
Hungarian National Committee for the Food and Agriculture Organization of the UN
P.O. Box 24
1450 Budapest

ICELAND
Mr. J. Gislason
Chief of Division
National Center for Hygiene, Food Control and Environmental Protection
P.O. Box 8953
IS-128 Reykjavik

INDIA
The Secretary
Central Committee for Food Standards and Liaison Officer NCC
Directorate General of Health Services
Kotla Road
New Delhi 110 002

INDONESIA
Attn. M. Bambang H. Hadiwiardjo
Dewan Standardisasi Nasional—DSN
(Standardization Council of Indonesia)
Gedung PDIN—LIPI
Jl. Jen. Gatot Subroto
P.O. Box 3123
Jakarta 12190

ISLAMIC REP. OF IRAN
Institute of Standards and Industrial Research of Iran
Ministry of Industries
P.O. Box 11365-7594
Tehran

IRAQ
Planning Board
Central Organization for Standardization and Quality Control
P.O. Box N⁰ 13032
Aljadiria, Baghdad

IRELAND
The Secretary
Irish National FAO Committee
Dept. of Agriculture and Fisheries
Agriculture House
Dublin 2

ISRAEL
Mr. L. Volman
Israel Codex Alimentarius Committee
Ministry of Industry and Trade
P.O. Box 299
91002 Jerusalem

ITALY
Sig. Presidente, Comitato Nazionale Italiano per il Codex Alimentarius
Direzione Generale della Tutela Economica dei Prodotti Agricoli
Via Sallustiana, 10
00187 Roma

JAMAICA
The Director
Bureau of Standards
6 Winchester Road
Kingstown 10

JAPAN
Director, Resource Division
Planning Bureau
Science and Technology Agency
2-2-1 Kasumigaseki, Chiyoda-ku
Tokyo 100

JORDAN
National Committee for Codex Alimentarius Directorate of Standards
Ministry of Industry and Trade
P.O. Box 2019
Amman

KAMPUCHEA
Relations ext., Direction générale de la Santé
Ministère de la santé publique
c/o Mission per. du Kampuchea dem. auprès de la CESAP
Radjadamnern Ave. UN Bldg.
Bangkok, Thailand

KENYA
The Director
Kenya Bureau of Standards
P.O. Box 54974
NHC House, Harambee Avenue
Nairobi

KOREA, DEM. PEOPLE'S REP. OF
Director
Foodstuffs Institute
P.O. Box 901
Pyongyang

KOREA, REP. OF
International Affairs Officer
Office of Planning & Coordination
Ministry of Health and Social Affairs
1, Choong Ang Dong, Kwa Chon Myon
Shi Heung Kun (Kyung Ki Prov.)

KUWAIT
Dr. Adnan Shalfan
Director, Standards and Metrology Dept.
Ministry of Oil and Industry
c/o UNDP Resident Representative
P.O. Box 2993
Safat

LEBANON
LIBNOR Institut libanais des normes et spécifications
B.P. 2806
Beyrouth

LESOTHO
Mr. C. S. Chobokoane
Acting Director
Food and Nutrition Coordination Office
Private Bag A78
Maseru 100

LIBERIA
Mr. Joseph M. Coleman
Director of Standards
Ministry of Commerce, Industry
P.O. Box 10-9041
1000 Monrovia

LIBYA
The Chief
Nutrition and Food Control Section
Secretariat of the General People's Committee for Health
P.O. Box 1583
Tripoli

LUXEMBOURG
M. François Arendt
Ingénieur-chef de Division
Laboratoire national de santé
1 A rue Auguste Lumière
Luxembourg

MADAGASCAR
Ministère des affaires étrangères
Antananarivo

MALAWI
The Director
Malawi Bureau of Standards
P.O. Box 946
Blantyre

MALAYSIA
The Director
Standards Division
SIRIM—Standards and Industrial Research Institute of Malaysia
P.O. Box 35
Shah Alam, Selangor

MALTA
Mr. V. Gatt
Chief Laboratory Officer
Standards Laboratory, Dept. of Industry
Evans Building, Merchants Street
Valletta

MAURITIUS
The Chief Agricultural Officer
Agricultural Services
Ministry of Agriculture, Fisheries and Natural Resources
Government House
Port Louis

MEXICO
Dirección General de Normas
Secretaría de comercio y Fomento Industrial
Puente de Tecamachalco N^O 6
Lomas de Tecamachalco, Sección Fuentes
Naucalpan de Juarez, Edo, de Mexico
53950 Mexico DF

MOROCCO
Division de la Répression des Fraudes
Ministère de l'Agriculture et de la réforme agraire
25, Avenue des Alaouiyines
Rabat

MOZAMBIQUE
Mr. Rufino Manuel de Melo
Ministerio da Saúde
Secção de Higiene de Aguas e Alimentos
P.O. Box 264
Maputo

MYANMAR
The Director
National Health Laboratory
35, Stewart Road
Yangon

NEPAL
The Chief Food Research Officer
Food Research Section, Marketing Service
Ministry of Agriculture and Land Reforms

NETHERLANDS
Mr. P. Ritsema
Deputy Director-General for Rural Areas and Quality Management
Director, Nutrition and Quality Affairs
Ministry of Agriculture & Fisheries
Room 9327
P.O. Box 20401
2500 EK The Hague

NEW ZEALAND
The Codex Officer
MAFQual, Ministry of Agriculture and Fisheries
P.O. Box 2526
Wellington

NICARAGUA
Progrma Normalización, Metrología y Control de Calidad (NMCC)
Dirección de Tecnología Industrial
Del Sandy's Carretera Masaya
1c arriba
apartado postal N^O 8
Managua

NIGERIA
The Secretary
Nigerian National Codex Committee
c/o Nigerian Standards Organization
Federal Ministry of Industries
P.M.B. 12614
11 Kofo Abayomi Street
Victoria Island, Lagos

NORWAY
Mr. John Race
Norwegian Food Control Authority
Postboks 8187
0034 Oslo 1

OMAN, SULTANATE OF
The Director of Public Health
Ministry of Health
Muskat

PAKISTAN
The Director General for Health
Ministry of Health, Social Welfare and Population Planning
Government of Pakistan
Secretariat Block C
Islamabad

PANAMA
Ing. Ramón Garcia
Director de COPANIT
Ministerio de comercio e Industrias
Departamento de Comisión de Normas
Panamá

PAPUA NEW GUINEA
Dr. M. J. Nunn
Director (Agricultural Protection)
Department of Agriculture and
  Livestock
P.O. Box 2141
Boroko

PARAGUAY
Dr. José Martino
Director, Instituto Nacional de
  Tecnología y Normalización
CC 967
Asunción

PERU
Dirección de Normalización y Control
  de Calidad—ITINTEC
Apartado 145 (Lima 100)
Av. Guardia Civil 400
Lima 41

PHILIPPINES
UNIO—Office of the United Nations
  International Organizations
Ministry of Foreign Affairs
Padre Faure
Manila

POLAND
Ministry of Foreign Economic Relations Quality Inspection Office
P.O. Box 25
00-950 Warszawa

PORTUGAL
Sub-Commissao do Codex
  Alimentarius
Commissao Nacional da FAO
Ministerio dos Negocios Estrangeiros
Pal. das Necessidades,
Largo do Rilvas
1354 Lisboa

QATAR
H.E. The Minister for Public Health
Ministry of Public Health
P.O. Box 42
Doha

ROMANIA
Institutul Roman de Standardizare
Str. Edgar Quinet 6
Casuta Postala 10
Bucaresti 1

RWANDA
Direction de l'Hygiène publique
Ministère de la Santé
P.B. 84
Kigali

SAMOA
Chief, Public Health Division
Health Department
P.O. Box 192
Apia

SAUDI ARABIA
Director-General
Saudi Arabian Standards Organization
  (SASO)
P.O. Box 3437
Riyadh 11471

SENEGAL
Comité national du Codex
Service de l'alimentation et de la nutrition appliquée au Sénégal (SANAS)
Ministère de la Santé Publique
Dakar

SEYCHELLES
Mr. R. Weber
Director, Seychelles Bureau of Standards
Ministry of National Development
P.O. Box 199
Victoria (Mahe)

SIERRA LEONE
Mr. A. B. Turay
Chief of Standards Central Contact
Codex Alimentarius Com.
National Bureau of Standards
Ministry of Trade and Industry
George Street
Freetown

SINGAPORE
Chia Hong Kuan
Head, Food Control Department
Ministry of the Environment
Environment Building
40 Scotts Road
Singapore 0922

SPAIN
Ilmo. Sr. D. F. Tovar Hernández
Secretario General, CIOA
Ministerio de Sanidad y Consumo
Subsecretaría para el Consumo
Paseo del Prado, 18-20, 4ª planta
Madrid 28014

SRI LANKA
The Permanent Secretary
Ministry of Health
P.O. Box 500
Colombo

ST. LUCIA
Produce Chemist
Ministry of Agriculture, Lands, Fisheries and Cooperatives
Government Buildings
Castries

SUDAN
The Secretary, National Codex Committee Chemical Laboratories
Ministry of Health
P.O. Box 287
Khartoum

SURINAME
Ir. G. Hindorie
Head—Division of Foreign Relations
Ministry of Agriculture, Animal Husbandry, Fisheries and Forestry
P.O. Box 1807
Paramaribo

SWAZILAND
The Permanent Secretary
Att: Chief Medical Officer
Ministry of Health
Mbabane

SWEDEN
National Swedish Food Administration
Codex Alimentarius Contact Point
Box 622
S-751 26 Uppsala

SWITZERLAND
Secrétariat, Comité national suisse du Codex Alimentarius
Office fédéral de la santé publique
Haslerstrasse 16
3008 Berne

SYRIA
Syrian Arab Oreganization for Standardization and Metrology
P.O. Box 11836
Damascus

TANZANIA
The Tanzania Bureau of Standards
P.O. Box 9524
Dar-es-Salaam

THAILAND
The Secretary
National Codex Alimentarius Committee of Thailand, TISI
Ministry of Industry
Rama VI Street
Bangkok 10400

TOGO
M. le Chargé de liaison du Codex Alimentarius
Division de la nutrition et de la technologie alimentaire
B.P. 1242
Lomé

TRINIDAD AND TOBAGO
The Chief Chemist and Director of
 Food and Drugs Chemistry
Food and Drugs Division
Ministry of Health and Environment
35-37 Sackville Street
Port-of-Spain

TUNISIA
Dr. Amor Jilani
Directeur général adjoint
Institut national de la normalisation et
 de la propriété industrielle
 (INNORPI)
B.P. 23
1012 Tunis-Belvedere

TURKEY
General Directorate of Protection &
 Control
Min. of Agric., Forestry & Rural
 Affairs
(Tarim Orman ve Köyisleri Bakanligi,
 Koruma ve Kontrol Genen
 Müdürlügü)
Akay Cad. N° 3 Bakanliklar
Ankara

UGANDA
Principal Medical Officer
Ministry of Health
P.O. Box 8
Entebbe

U.S.S.R.
Dr. V. E. Kovshilo
Chief, Main Sanitary-Epidemiological
 Board
Ministry of Health of the U.S.S.R.
T. Rakhmanovski Pereulok 3
101431 GSP Moskva K-51

UNITED ARAB EMIRATES
Federal Director
Department of Preventive Medicine
Ministry of Health
P.O. Box 848
Abu Dhabi

UNITED KINGDOM
The Principal
Food Standards Divisions—Branch B
Ministry of Agriculture, Fisheries and
 Food, Room 310
Ergon House, c/o Nobel House
17 Smith Square
London SW1P 2HX

URUGUAY
Ing. Ind. Enrique D. Bia
Presidente
Laboratorio Tecnológico del Uruguay
 (LATU)
Ministerio de Industria y Energía
Galicia 1133
Montevideo

VENEZUELA
Sr. Jefe, Sección de Registro de
 Alimentos
Ministerio de Sanidad y Asistencia
 Social
Centro Simón Bolivar, Edif. Sur 2
Caracas

VIETNAM
Hoang Manh Tuan
Deputy Director-General
General Department for Standardization
Metrology and Quality Control S.R.
70 Tran Hung Dao Str.
Hanoi

YEMEN ARAB REP.
General Director for Measurements
Ministry of Economy, Supply & Trade
Sana'a

YEMEN, PEOPLE'S DEM. REP.
The Permanent Secretary
Ministry of Agriculture and Agrarian
 Reform
Khor Maksar (105) — P.O. Box 4200
Aden

YUGOSLAVIA
Federal Institution for Standardization
Slobodana Penezica Krcuna br. 35
Postanski pregradak 933
Beograd

ZAIRE
  1ère Direction des études et de la
    politique agricoles
  Département de l'agriculture et du
    développement rural
  B.P. 8722
  Kinshasa 1

ZAMBIA
  Secretary, Food and Drugs Control
  Ministry of Health
  P.O. Box 30205
  Lusaka

ZIMBABWE
  The Government Analyst
  The Government Analyst's Laboratory
  P.O. Box 8042
  Causeway
  Harare

INDEX

Amino acids, added to foods, 21, 77, 138, 199, 214, 220, 226, 232, 325, 401, 406, 409
  as additives, 135–139
  deficiency, 136
  functions, 138
  limitations, 135, 217, 231
  losses, 231, 246
  profile, 213–215, 217
  requirements, 138–139, 214
  safety/toxicity, 138, 403
  stability, 136, 337
  structure, 137
Analogs. (*See* Food analogs)
Antioxidants, as additives, 72, 440–442
  ascorbates, added to food, 435–436
    properties, 434, 437
    structure, 435
  oxidation scheme, 441
  regulatory aspects, United States, 447–451
    other countries, 448–455
  tocopherols, properties, 441
    structure, 439
  uses in foods, bread, 445
    dairy products, 387, 445
    fats, 276, 447
    fish, 446
    flour, 445
    fruits, 443–444
    juices and beverages, 292, 299, 308, 310, 444–445
    meat, 446
    oils, 276, 447
    vegetables, 443–444
Apocarotenal, added, to fats and oils, 269
  to juices and beverages, 303–305
  as additive, 72, 295
  structure, 113
Ascorbates. (*See* Antioxidants)

Beta-carotene, added to beverages, 300, 303–305, 309
  application forms, 295–296
  as additive, 131, 295
  as antioxidant, 268, 447
    baked food, 174
    potato foods, 246
  bioavailability, 273, 275, 295
  nutrition and health, 496, 503–505
  structure, 113
Beverages. (*See* Juices and beverages)
Bioavailability, carotenoids, 273, 275, 295
  concerns, 466
  effect of disease, 467, 469
  effect of drugs, 9, 11, 460
  effect of processing, 97, 102–103, 325, 335
  effect of solubility, 98
  effect of toxicants, 11, 21–23
  electronic configuration, 97
  enhancers, 70, 99–101, 466–467
  functionality, compared to, 92, 95, 97
  inhibitors, 23, 99–101, 466–467
  measuring, 461–462
  mineral sensitivities, 92, 96, 102, 362
  minerals, trace elements, 463, 468
  nutrient interactions, 97, 99–101, 117
  vitamins, 116–117, 257, 274, 464–466
Blended food mixtures, added nutrients, 214, 216–220
  approaches to mixtures, 214, 216
  blend designs, 219–220
  costs, economics, 221, 224–225, 227
  donations of surplus, 213–214
  equipment, 224–225
  formulation, U.S. blends, 223
  history, use, 211–213
  mixture types, guidelines, INCAP, 218, 220–222
  PAG, 217–218

UNICEF, 213, 217
USDA/AID/NIH, 217, 219
nutrified blends, Ceplapro, 221
CSM, WSB, 166, 222–223
Incaparina, 77, 221
protein-based (soybean), 220–229
soy infant formulas, 401
weaning food needs, 64, 212
Bread (*See also* Cereal grain products)
enrichment, 72, 74, 77, 94, 156–158, 165–172, 179
nutrition studies, 74–77, 197
vitamin stability, 187–189

Carbohydrates, added to snacks, 326
to special purpose foods, 399, 410–411, 415
Carotenoids, 243, 283, 287, 300, 305, 308, 370
Cassava, 247–249
Cereal grain products (*See also* Nutrification)
annual production, 144–145
calorie, protein source, 145–146
cereal grain history, 143–145
enrichment practices, history, 156–164
present status, 165–171
extraction rate, 29, 30, 146–150, 153
kernel structure, 148–151
milling practices, 146–150, 154–155
nutrient losses, 151–156
U.S. consumption, 147
Condiments (*See also* Nutrification)
monosodium glutamate, history, 347
mineral carrier, 352
palatability, 348
safety/toxicity, 348
vitamin carrier, 348–353
other condiments, 363
salt (sodium chloride), history, 354
mineral carrier, 356–363
palatability, 354
vitamin carrier, 354–355
Confections. (*See* Snacks)
Consumer nutrient labeling issues (*See also* Regulations)
background, 519–520, 535–537
international interest, 522–524, 596
labeling costs, 520–521

NAS/IOM report, 521
revised nutrition labeling, consumer choice, 529–530
effect on nutrification, 531, 533, 585
NAS/IOM comments, 531
survey of consumers,
FMI study, 525
FDA/CRK, 521
findings, attention, nutrition, 527
health claims, 528
important factors, 526
label reading, 527, 529
useful sources, 526
IFIC/ADA, 521
NFPA study, 526
Corn (maize) products, 143, 150, 154, 158, 166, 169, 182, 187, 194–195, 198 (*See also* Cereal grains)
Costs, 65, 67, 95–96, 184, 194, 202, 221, 224–225, 227–228, 259, 335, 359, 363, 489, 491–492

Dairy products (*See also* Nutrification)
dairy product consumption, 370–371
loss of nutrients, 370
milk base infant formulas, 401
milk consumption, 284
nutrient content, 368–371
nutrification, 371–388
processing aspects, 377–380
standards of identity, 373
storage aspects, 380–386
variety of products, 367
Dietary allowances, amino acids, 139, 214
military, 59–60
minerals, 90–91, 114–115, 339, 512
vitamins, 114–116, 339, 512
Dietary guidelines, basic food groups, 35–39
food labeling, 37, 41, 339, 518, 559, 585
international, 44
NAS/NAP, 44–45
Surgeon General, 44
USDA/DHHS, 43
menu planning, 35
Diets, balanced diet, 34, 37, 40, 58
chemically defined, 21
federal monitoring, 42, 45–58

infant formulas, 397–405
meal replacers, 68, 406–408
military rations, 59–62
nutrients reported, 50–51
reducing diets, 45, 405
U.S. surveys, NFCS, 3, 5–6, 31, 36, 39, 42–43, 50–51, 57, 145, 283, 321–322, 333–334, 338, 342, 372
NHANES, 5, 38, 42, 50–51, 57

Eating habits, 31–35, 45, 321, 324
Engineering aspects (*See also* Technology)
 guideline additions to food, 477
 methods of nutrient addition
  feeders, 477–479
   roll-type, 478
   screw-type, 479
  mixers, 477, 479–481
   ribbon type, 480
   vertical-conical, 481
  sprayers, 481
 nutrification case studies, cereal enrichment, 484
  flour flow chart, 485
  rice premix process, 484, 486–487
  salt, iodination, 490
   iodine process, 490
   plant operations, 491–492
  tea nutrification, 487, 489
   costs, 489
   flow sheet, 488
Enrichment, 72–79, 156–171, 539, 591 (*See also* Nutrification)
Enteral nutritional foods. (*See* Formulated special purpose foods)
Extruded food blends (*See also* Blended food mixtures)
 added nutrients, 226
 blends, low cost, 224–225, 227
 extrusion equipment, 225
 thermal treatment, 222, 224–226
 use, indigenous crops, 225
 vegetable food mixes, 227

Fats and oils (*See also* Nutrification)
 added to, blended foods, 222
  snacks, 325
  special foods, 399, 401, 410

composition, fatty acids, 327
consumption pattern, 265–268, 271
fat substitutes, 24, 278, 329
functions, 266
loss of vitamin E, 275–276
metabolic aspects, 277–278
processing procedures, 265, 272–273
use in edible products, 270–271
Fiber, 25, 327–328, 411
Flour (*See also* Cereal grain products)
 added iron, 93
 blended foods, 221–223, 234, 249
 enrichment, 156–157, 161–179, 184–187, 194, 199, 201
 flour types, 146–148
 loss of nutrients, 28–30, 151–153
Food, away-from-home, 24, 31–34
 description, 20
 distribution equalities, 19
 fat substitutes, 24, 278
 Food for Peace, 160, 213–214, 223
 industry trends, 24–25
 new sources, 21, 24
 noncaloric sweeteners, 25, 329
 nutrient delivery vs food delivery, 34
 processed foods, 24–25
 shoppers concerns, 35, 40, 526–529
 snack foods, 31, 34, 319–323
 types of foods, 395–396
 USDA/WIC foods, 59
Food analogs, consumer acceptance, 226, 235
 description, history, 226
 economics, 227
 flavored, colored pieces, 230
 governmental regulations, 232–234
 guidelines, nomenclature, 234
 marketing strategy, 226, 235
 meat vs plant protein, 226–228, 232–233
 nutrient losses, 232
 nutrification, 231–232
 nutrified product, 233, 237
 pioneer processors, 226
 production, utility, 234–235
 protein quality, 231
 school lunch use, 233
 texturization, 228–232
 US analog producers, 236

Food processing, effect on bioavailability, 97–101
  effect of processing, 101–103
    canning, 28
    dehydrating, 244
    extrusion, 102, 226, 232
    fat extraction, 375
    freezing, 26–27
    milling, 28–30, 151
    refining, 275
  loss of nutrients, amino acids, 25
    minerals, 25, 30, 151–155
    vitamins, 25–31, 151–155, 245, 275, 375
Formulated special purpose foods, complex nature, 395–396
  enteral nutritional foods, disease management, 406, 408
    evaluation, use, 405
    nutritional support, 406, 408
    weight reduction, 408
  infant formulas, clinical testing, 404
    design, 398–401
    evaluation, use, 395–399
    ingredients involved, 395, 402–403, 417, 423
    nutrient losses, 401
    nutrient systems, 417
    routine formulas, 401–402
    specialty formulas, 402–403
  manufacturing, systems, 413–416
  process development, macronutrients, 409, 411, 417
    micronutrients, 411, 417
    nutrient flow, 415
    premix control, 416
    vitamin premixes, 413, 415
  quality control systems, 416–420
  regulatory considerations, 421–426
  required specifications, 423
Fortification (*See also* Nutrification)
  mineral fortification, 87–89, 103, 175, 260, 356, 359
  policy, 55, 57–59, 539, 589
  pro and con, 49–53
  vitamin fortification, 109–113, 253, 273, 298, 348, 371

Infant formulas (*See* Formulated special purpose foods)

Iodine (*See* Minerals)
Iron (*See* Minerals)

Juices and beverages (*See also* Nutrification)
  beverage consumption, 287, 384–385
  effect of container, 311–312
  effect of light and air, 308–309
  effects of metals, 309–310
  fruit product consumption, 283
  kinetic studies, 307–308
  nutrient content, juices and beverages, 286–292
  raw fruit, 283–284
  nutrification, 292–307
  product use patterns, 282–287
  soft drink usage, 42, 52, 287, 321–322, 342
  variety of drinks, 281–283

Labeling. (*See* Consumer nutrient labeling issues)
Legislation (*See also* Regulations)
  condiments, 363
  food analogs, 232–234
  sugar, 259
Living/marketing patterns, 31–34
Loss of nutrients, 25–31, 151–155, 245, 275, 375

Marginal nutrient deficiency, concept, 9
  corrective measures, education, 12
    nutrification, 12
    supplements, 13
  criteria for adequacy, 3
  effect, behavior, 9–10
    drugs, chemicals, 11
    immune response, 11
    performance, 10–12
  evaluation methods, 1–4
  five stage pattern, 10
  in alcoholics, 6, 42
  in children, 5
  in elderly, 6, 11, 12
  in other countries, 7–8, 63
  in sport participants, 6
  in US surveys, 3–7, 41–45, 333–335
  in women, 6, 43
  MMPI scoring, 9–11
  Military rations, 59–62

Milk. (*See* Dairy products)
Minerals, added to, beverages, 343
　　cereal grains, 59, 89, 175-176, 178, 179
　　condiments, 352, 356-361
　　dairy products, 77, 371, 377
　　rice, 75
　　snacks, 328
　　special foods, 401-402, 411, 415
　as additives, 87-104
　criteria, fortified foods, 103
　decrease of anemia, 63, 89, 359, 361
　dietary allowances, 90-91, 114-115, 339
　effect on milling, 30, 152-153
　effect of mineral activity, bioavailability, 97, 102
　　color, 91-92, 362
　　flavor, 92-94
　　protein, 94
　　texture, 92, 96
　　viscosity, 94
　effect of processing, 101-102
　enhancers, inhibitors, 63, 70, 99-100, 102
　forms, added minerals, 88, 96
　function versus availability, 92, 95, 97, 362-363
　iodine, 356-360, 489-492
　iron, 352, 359-363
　mineral complexes, 89, 93, 98-99
　mineral deficiencies, 6, 42, 63, 71
　policy of addition, 87, 89
　safety/toxicity, 95, 97
　toxicants, availability, 22-23
Mixtures. (*See* Blended food mixtures)
Monosodium glutamate. (*See* Condiments)

Nutrification, alternatives, 55-56, 64-65
　barriers, economics, 138, 202
　　legislation, 58, 71, 203, 539, 595
　　technological, 89-94, 201
　benefits (potential), allaying disease, 71
　　bioavailability, improved, 70
　　cereal improvement, 69
　　changing economics, 71
　　environmental deficiency, 71
　　food standardization, 68
　　GI tract problems, 70
　　nutrient/calorie balance, 69

　　nutrient restoration, 68
　　protective foods, 70
　　special purpose foods, 69
　　technological use, 72
　concept, 49
　costs, economics, 65, 67, 95-96, 184
　developing countries, interventions, 63-65
　　malnutrition, 62-63
　　refugee foods, 77
　military, 59-62
　of cereal grains, consumer acceptance, 170-171, 179, 183-184, 195-199, 202
　　enriched products, corn (maize), 158, 182-183
　　exported foods, 160
　　rice, 179-182
　　RTE cereals, 159, 483
　　wheat foods, 156-161, 178
　　enrichment, costs, 184, 194
　　current status, 165, 171
　　equipment, 177, 477-482
　　feasibility, 164, 166-167
　　methods, 177-183, 484-487
　　nutrient forms, 174
　　nutrient labeling, 170-171
　　nutritional effects, 72-77, 195-199
　　process, 171-184
　　rationale, 152-162
　　stability, nutrients, 184-193
　　standards, 168-169, 173
　　type 4, other countries, 161-162
　　United States, 156-160
　　vs type 10, 156, 163, 172
　　type 10, 162-163, 172-173
　of condiments, calcium to salt, 356
　costs, 359, 363
　iodine, salt, 356-360
　iron, curry powder, 363
　　fish sauce, 363
　　MSG, 352
　　salt, 359-362
　nutritional benefits, 350-351
　rationale, 66, 347
　vitamin A, MSG, 348-359
　　salt, 354-355
　vitamin C, salt, 355
　of dairy products, calcium, fluid milk, 379

618 NUTRIENT ADDITIONS TO FOOD

carotenoids, butter, 269
  cheese, 383
  influence of carrier, 379, 387
  iron, fluid milk, 378
  multinutrients, fluid milk, 380
    infant foods, 386
    yogurt, 380, 548
  nutrient forms, 376-377
  packaging, 387-388
  processing, 377-380
  rationale, 373, 375-376
  stability, nutrients, 381, 384-386
  storage, 380-387
  vitamin A and D, condensed milk, 378, 382
    dry milk, 379, 383
    fluid milk, 377, 380, 382
    mellorine, 380, 550
    reconstituted, 385-386
  vitamin C, cultured milk, 380
    evaporated milk, 378, 382
    fluid milk, 378, 382
of fats and oils, carotene, 266, 273
  heat stability, E acetate, 276
  omega-3 fatty acids, 276-278
  vitamin A, 273, 275
  vitamin E, 274-276
    dual role, 275, 442
of juices and beverages, carotenoids, 295-297, 300, 303-305
  minerals, 294-295
  multinutrients, 305-308, 343
  nutrient application forms, 294-297
  nutrification, rationale, 292, 294
  soft drinks, 299, 308-309
  packaging, 311-312
  processing, 295-300, 307-311
  stability, added nutrients, 301-302, 304, 306, 308
  vitamin C, dual role, 292, 442, 445
  vitamins, 294, 298-304
of snacks and confections, criteria of addition, 333
  nutrient costs, 335
  nutrient safety index, 336
  nutrient stability, 334-335, 337
  nutrients to add, 323-328
  nutrifying confections, 336-338
  nutrifying snacks, 331-335

physiological availability, 335
rationale, 328, 333
of sugar, calcium, 261
  iron, 260-261
  multinutrients, 261
  vitamin A, bioavailability, 257
    consumer acceptance, 257
    costs, economics, 259
    nutrification process, 256-257
    premix formulation, 253, 255, 257
    quality control, 257-258
    stability, 253-254
policy aspects, FDA, 57-58, 87, 539-544
  NAS/AMA, 55, 57, 87
  USDA, 59, 577
trends in future, 78-79, 587
Nutrified foods, analogs, 68, 231-232, 234-237
baked goods, 274
beverage powder, 62, 101
beverages, 286-307
blended foods, 77, 160, 217-223
bread, 48, 62, 72, 76-77, 94, 156-179, 188-189
brownies, 62
bun, 77
butter, 269
candy, 62, 72
cassava products, 249
cereal mixes, 167
cereal products, 69, 156-171
cheese, 62, 383, 548
cocoa, 62
coffee, 52, 62
combat foods, 60-61
condiments, 66, 76, 348-363
confections, 336-338
corn (maize) products, 74, 76, 158, 164, 166, 182-183, 192-193, 198
crackers, 62, 167
curry powder, 363
dairy products, 371-376, 546-550
dietary products, 91-92
doughnuts, 187
enteral foods, 405
exported foods, 160, 213-214
extruded blends, 226
farina, 159, 166, 190, 197, 552

INDEX

fats, 267–269, 363
fish sauce, 363
flour, 49, 72–73, 75, 77, 94, 156–179, 186–187, 484, 550
frozen desserts, 383
infant formulas, 72, 89, 92, 409–417
instant breakfast, 68
juices, 68, 293–305, 554
margarine, 49, 57, 73, 267–269, 274, 276, 554
meal, ready-to-go, 60
meal replacer, 68
military rations, 59–62
milk products, 49, 57, 72–73, 76–77, 92, 160, 371–386, 546–548
monosodium glutamate, 76, 348–353
pasta, 59, 77, 93, 158, 179, 189, 197, 552
peanut butter, 62, 68, 274
potato products, 52, 59, 68, 244, 247
ready-to-eat cereal, 93, 159, 183, 189–190, 483
rice, 75, 158, 166, 179–182, 191, 198, 484, 486, 552
salad oil, 267–269, 273–277
salt, 49, 57, 63, 66, 73, 354–363, 489–492
snacks, 51, 57, 69, 328, 331–335
soft drinks, 299, 307, 308–309
special purpose foods, 69, 395
sugar, 52, 66, 76, 253–261
tea, 52, 66, 76, 487–489
weaning foods, 77, 212, 214
Nutrition, balanced diet, 34, 37, 40
  basic food guide, 35–39
  benefits, nutrification, 72–77, 87, 89, 194–199
  caloric intake, 13, 31, 45
  calorie/nutrient ratio, 58, 61
  consumer concerns, 31, 34–35, 40, 342, 526–529
  developed countries, 5–9
  developing countries, 62–64
  dietary allowances, 90–91, 114–116, 139, 214, 339, 512
  eating habits, 31–34, 45, 324, 507
  empty calories, 319
  enteral foods, 405–408
  fat substitutes, 24, 278, 329

  implication of deficiency, 11–12
  infant formulas, 397–404
  influence of drugs, 460
  influence on immunity, 11
  influence on performance, 10–12
  influence of toxicants, 22–23
  labeling (*See also* Regulations)
    evaluation, 40
    history, 37–41, 339, 519–520, 559, 569, 585–586
    international interest, 521–523, 596
    labeling food analogs, 232–234
    labeling projections, 40–41, 530, 585
    labeling special purpose foods, 421, 425
    snacks, sodium labeling, 331
  malnutrition, 36, 63, 211–213, 407
  marginal deficiencies, 1–14
  military rations, 59–62
  noncaloric sweeteners, 25, 281, 329
  nutrient deficiencies, iodine, 356–361
    iron, 63, 89, 352, 359–361
    protein calorie, 63, 212
    vitamin A, 352–353
  nutrient losses, 25–31, 102, 151–155, 231, 234
  nutrient monitoring, 46–48, 50–51
  nutrient vs food delivery, 34, 36
  nutrition education, 12, 37, 45, 49, 53–55, 331
  nutritional status, 5, 8, 11, 13
  risk factors, stress, 8, 11, 13, 42
  school lunch, 5–6, 37, 123, 214, 232–233, 246
  snacking practices, 34, 319–322
  test of adequacy, 3–4
  USDA/WIC foods, 59
Nutrition-health interrelationships, absorption of vitamins, 499–503
  deficiencies, secondary, 497
    subclinical, 5–9, 497
  nutrient interactions, 508–511
  nutrition-health influence, 44–45, 71, 76, 406, 408, 495, 497
  optimal eating patterns, 507
  pathogenetic basis, 500–503
  prevention with nutrients, 498–507
  recommended allowances, 512

role of selected nutrients, carotene, 503
  folate, 504
  minerals, 507
  vitamin A, 503
  vitamin B_6, 504
  vitamin C, 505
  vitamin E, 506

Oils. (*See* Fats and oils)

Pasta, 158, 167, 179, 189, 197 (*See also* Cereal grains)
Population growth, 19–21
Potatoes, 68, 243–247 (*See also* Roots and tubers)
Processing. (*See* Food processing)
Protein, added to beverages, 343
  flour, 160, 403, 409, 415
  snacks, 324
  special purpose foods, 400
  amino acids, composition, 215
    limiting, 135
  blends, 217–218
  types, 216
  cereal grain source, 145
  deficiency, 138, 212–213
    protein-calorie, 212–213
  new protein foods, 21
  quality standards, 213
  requirements, 138, 213

Ready-to-eat cereals, 59, 93, 159–160, 183, 190–191, 197 (*See also* Cereal grain products)
Regulations, international, ascorbate and tocopherol, 451–455
  ascorbic acid addition to flour, 451
  ascorbic acid/tocopherol, JECFA, 452
  ascorbic esters/tocopherol, Codex, 453
  ascorbates/tocopherol to foods, Codex, 454–455
  compulsory addition of nutrients, foods, special dietary use, 590
    iodine, fluorine to salt, 592
    nutrient losses during manufacture, 593
    replacement food products, 593
    staple foods, 590

label declaration of nutrients, 596
  tolerances on declaration, 597
optional addition of nutrients, 593–595
  added nutrients to margarine, 594
  restrictive regulations on addition, 595
United States, allowable nutrient ingredients, food additives, 572–575
  food ingredients, 572–573
  GRAS basis, 572, 576–577
  prior sanction, 572, 577
  ascorbate and tocopherol, ascorbic acid to alcoholic items, 449
    ascorbic acid/tocopherol to meat, 449
    ascorbic acid additions to foods, 450–451
  common or usual name regulations, standard food, 556–557
    imitation food, 556
    peanut spread, 557
  Congressional legislation, Labeling and Education Act, 586
    labeling requirements, 586
    health message issues, 587
    USRDA proposed changes, 587
  definition of fortification, addition, technical, 538–539
    additions to add, 538
    additions to increase, 538
    additions to restore, 538–539
    enrichment vs fortification, 539
  FDA proposal of Daily Values, new RDI and DRV, 583–584
    replacements for USRDA, 584
  FDA proposal on nutrition labeling, new labeling format, 585–586
    substantial changes, 586
  foods for special dietary use, dietary supplements, 570–571
    dietetic or lo-cal foods, 571
    higher fortified RTE cereals, 571
    infancy or age needs, 570
    physiological, pathological needs, 570
  formulated special purpose foods, good manufacturing practices, 424
    Infant Formula Act, 420, 422, 571
    infant formula regulations, 422

label and records requirements, 425
nutrients required, 422, 591
quality factors and control, 423
guidelines, addition of nutrients, bases for nutrient addition, 540
correction for insufficiency, 540–541
1980 Federal Regulation policy, 540
fortification to caloric content, 542–543
restoration of lost nutrients, 542
specific applicable regulation, 543–544
nutrition labeling of food, Class I vs Class II nutrients, 566
foods exempt from labeling, 559–562
health message issues, 568–569
mineral vitamin requirements, 563–566
misbranding provisions, 567
required labeling format, 562–563
synthetic vs natural vitamins, 567
nutrition labeling of restaurant foods, advertised nutrition claims, 569
display nutrition labeling, 570
nutritional quality guidelines, appropriate nutrient provision, 557
example, heat-serve dinners, 558–559
specific quality guides, 557
prior sanctions, approval granted prior 9/6/58, 577
prior-sanctioned substances, 577
Standards of Identity (SI), federal and state laws, 545
fixed food formulas, 544
nutrient fortification under SI, 546–556
possible optional ingredients, 545
SI control, fortification, 545
Restoration, 57, 68, 156, 244, 275, 539, 589 (*See also* Nutrification)
Rice, 143, 151, 154, 158, 166, 169, 179, 181, 191, 198 (*See also* Cereal grain products)
  premix, 180, 182, 484
Roots and tubers, cassava, composition, 248

history, 247
nutrification, 249
processed products, 248–249
potato products, composition, 243
history, 243
nutrient losses, 244–245
nutrification, 245–247
processed products, 243–244
production, 245–246
school lunch, WIC use, 59, 246
stability, added nutrients, 245, 247

Salt. (*See* Condiments)
Snacks and confections (*See also* Nutrification)
adding nutrients, 51, 324–333
caffeine content, 332
caloric contribution, 319, 322
foods consumed as snacks, 321
frequency of snacking, 31, 321, 323
nutritional contribution, 51, 325, 340–342
nutritional labeling, 339–340
nutritional profile, 338
role of snacking, 31, 34, 319
snack market, 320–323
sodium content, 328–329
soft drink consumption, 42, 287, 321–322, 342
type of snack food, 321
Sugars (*See also* Nutrification)
as nutrient carrier, 251–253
consumption pattern, 252
countries involved, 252, 259
legislation, regulation, 259

Technology, addition method, feeders, 477, 480
infusion, 482
mixers, 477–481
sprayers, 481
addition site, nutrients, 473–476
analog food, nutrification, 232, 234
processing, 228–232
blended food, mixtures, 214–222
cereal grain, corn, 182
enrichment, 171–184, 484, 487
equipment, 177, 472, 477
feasibility, 163–164, 166–167

flour, 178, 484
milling, 146–151
rice, 179–182, 484–487
RTE cereals, 159, 183
condiment, MSG/vitamin A, 348–350, 352
salt/iodine, 358–359, 489–492
salt/iron, 359–363
container influence, 311–312, 387, 388
dairy product, nutrification, 377–380
packaging, 387–388
extruded food blend, equipment, 225
processing, 224–225
fats and oil, nutrification, 269, 273–274, 276
packaging, 311
processing, 265, 272–273
juices and beverage nutrification, 299–300
precautions, 297–298, 309–310
root and tuber, cassava, 248–249
potato, 244–247
special purpose food, 409–418
sugar, nutrification, 253–259, 260, 261
tea product, nutrification, 228–231, 487–489
Tocopherols. (*See* Antioxidants)
Toxicity/safety, minerals, 95–97, 334, 336
vitamins, 117–138, 334, 336
Tubers. (*See* Roots and tubers)

Vitamins, adding to foods, cereal grains, 156–171
condiments, 348–355
dairy products, 377–386
fats and oils, 266–276
food analogs, 231–232
food blends, 214, 216–220
juices and beverages, 294, 298–304
roots and tubers, 245–247, 249
snacks, 331–338
special foods, 409–417
sugars, 253–257
application forms, 112–113, 174, 177, 294, 376
as additives, biotin, 128
carotene, 131
multirole nature, 131, 268, 293, 503
folate, 117
niacin, 124
pantothenate, 127
vitamin A, 129, 348, 350–351
vitamin B_1, 122
vitamin B_2, 123
vitamin B_6, 125
vitamin B_{12}, 119
vitamin C, 121
multirole nature, 121, 292, 433, 440, 445, 505
vitamin D, 131
vitamin E, 133
multirole nature, 133, 276, 438, 440, 447, 506
vitamin K, 134
as antioxidants, 276, 292, 299, 308, 310, 387, 443–447
bioavailability, 116–117, 257, 274
chemical properties, 118–135
deficiencies, 5–13, 42–43, 352–353
dietary allowances, 114–116, 339, 512
effect of milling, 29–30, 151–155
effect of processing, 26–28, 275–276, 370
history, dates, 109, 111
interactions, 11, 116, 508–511
safety/toxicity, 117–135